Chronic Pancreatitis

Novel Concepts in Biology and Therapy

Chronic Pancreatitis

Novel Concepts in Biology and Therapy

Edited by

Prof. Dr. M. W. BÜCHLER, PD Dr. H. FRIESS, PD Dr. W. UHL
Department of General Surgery
University of Heidelberg
Heidelberg, Germany

Prof. Dr. P. MALFERTHEINER
Department of Gastroenterology,
Hepatology and Infectious Diseases
Otto-von-Guericke University
Magdeburg, Germany

Blackwell
Science

Editorial Offices:

Blackwell Science Ltd
A Blackwell Publishing Company
Osney Mead, Oxford OX2 0EL, UK

Blackwell Science, Inc.
350 Main Street, Malden,
MA 02148-5018, USA

Blackwell Science Asia Pty,
54 University Street, Carlton
Victoria 3053, Australia

Blackwell Wissenschafts-Verlag GmbH
Kurfürstendamm 57, 10707 Berlin, Germany
Firmiangasse 7, 1130 Wien, Austria

Editors' addresses:

Prof. Dr. M. W. Büchler
PD Dr. H. Friess
PD Dr. W. Uhl
Universität Heidelberg
Abteilung für Allgemeine, Viszerale,
Unfallchirurgie und Poliklinik
Im Neuenheimer Feld 110
69120 Heidelberg, Germany

Prof. Dr. P. Malfertheiner
Otto-von-Guericke-Universität
Zentrum für Innere Medizin
Klinik für Gastroenterologie, Hepatologie
und Infektiologie
Leipziger Straße 4
39120 Magdeburg, Germany

A catalogue record for this title
is available from the British Library

ISBN 0-632-06399-8

Library of Congress Cataloging-in-Publication Data

Set by: Type-Design, Berlin
Printed and bound by: Druckhaus Köthen GmbH

For further information on Blackwell Science, visit our website: www.blacksci.co.uk

Preface

Chronic pancreatitis is on the rise in the Western world, and this incidence is attributed mainly to higher alcohol consumption. Chronic pancreatitis was described in 1946 by Comfort and co-workers as an ongoing inflammatory disorder associated with loss of exocrine and endocrine pancreatic parenchyma and replacement by fibrotic tissue, resulting in maldigestion and diabetes mellitus. But even today the exact mechanisms initiating and perpetuating the disease are not fully understood. However, the knowledge has increased during the last few years and molecular and cellular events contributing to the chronic inflammatory destructive process are better defined. In the last few years we have learnt that there is another factor in chronic pancreatitis besides alcohol, gene mutations regulating the pancreatic enzyme activating cascades, and their inhibitors which are associated with a hereditary form of the disease. In addition, new pathophysiological concepts of pain based on molecular alterations and interactions between pancreatic nerves and the exocrine parenchyma and/or inflammatory cells have been presented.

Advances in the understanding of pathophysiological aspects have positively influenced our diagnostic approach and assessment of chronic pancreatitis. Imaging techniques such as contrast-enhanced computed tomography (CT) and endoscopic ultrasound (EUS) have been further refined and the introduction and development of new imaging procedures such as magnetic resonance imaging (MRI) and magnetic resonance cholangiopancreatography (MRCP) have further enhanced our ability to diagnose chronic pancreatitis in the various stages of disease evolution.

There is a general agreement that the initial treatment of choice in chronic pancreatitis is medical. However, the frequent appearance of complications requires interdisciplinary management with a careful selection of conservative, endoscopic or surgical intervention. All of the available options for their integrative use are presented and discussed here. A special topic is devoted to different surgical procedures. The use of various procedures for a range of indications points to uncertainties we still have in this field and the undisputed need for good clinical results.

The present book summarizes the contributions made by leading pancreatologists around the world during a conference held at the University of Bern from August 31 till September 2, 2000. New aspects of the etiology, pathophysiology, diagnostics and conservative, interventional and surgical treatment of chronic pancreatitis are presented.

The book summarizes the latest developments in the field of chronic pancreatitis with an update on all aspects of this disease.

We take this opportunity to thank all contributors and hope that his book rekindles interest in our colleagues working on the pancreas and related chronic inflammatory pathologies. We further hope that this book serves as a platform for further basic and clinical research into pancreatic diseases.

Heidelberg, Magdeburg, Winter 2001

Markus W. Büchler
Helmut Friess
Waldemar Uhl
Peter Malfertheiner

Contents

Contributors

Adler, Guido, M.D.
Department of Internal Medicine I
University of Ulm
89081 Ulm
Germany

Ammann, Rudolf W., M.D.
Division of Gastroenterology
Department of Internal Medicine
University Hospital of Zürich
8091 Zürich
Switzerland

Apte, Minoti V., M.D., PhD
Pancreatic Research Group
Level 4, Liverpool Hospital
The University of New South Wales
Liverpool, NSW 2170
Australia

Arendt, Thomas, M.D.
Clinic of Internal Medicine
University of Rostock
18057 Rostock
Germany

Astudillo, Emiliano, M.D.
Department of Surgery
Hospital Clinic
University of Barcelona
08034 Barcelona
Spain

Bachem, Max G., M.D.
Department of Clinical Chemistry
and Pathobiochemistry
University Hospital of Ulm
89070 Ulm
Germany

Bauer, Annette, M.D.
Department of Anaesthesiology
University of Heidelberg
69120 Heidelberg
Germany

Bauerfeind, Peter, M.D.
Department of Internal Medicine
Division of Gastroenterology
University Hospital of Zürich
8091 Zürich
Switzerland

Beger, Hans Günther, M.D.
Department of General Surgery
University of Ulm
89075 Ulm
Germany

Bloechle, C., M.D.
Department of General Surgery
University Hospital of Hamburg/
Eppendorf
20246 Hamburg
Germany

Bockman, Dale E., Ph.D.
The Medical College of Georgia
Department of Cellular Biology
and Anatomy
Augusta, GA 30912-2000
USA

Boerma, Djamila, M.D.
Department of Surgery
Academic Medical Center
University of Amsterdam
1105 AZ Amsterdam
The Netherlands

Büchler, Markus W., M.D.
Department of General Surgery
University of Heidelberg
69120 Heidelberg
Germany

Busch, C., M.D.
Department of General Surgery
University Hospital of Hamburg/
Eppendorf
20246 Hamburg
Germany

Clain, Jonathan, M.D.
Mayo Clinic
Division of Gastroenterology
and Hepatology
Rochester, Minnesota 55905
USA

Diem, Peter, M.D.
Division of Endocrinology and Diabetes
Inselspital, University of Bern
3010 Bern
Switzerland

DiMagno, Eugene P., M.D.
Division of Gastroenterology
and Hepatology
Gastroenterology Research Unit
Mayo Clinic
Rochester, Minnesota 55905
USA

Di Mola, Fabio F., M.D.
Department of Surgery
University of Chieti
66100 Chieti
Italy

Ding, J., M.D.
Roche Genomic and Information Sciences
Hoffmann-La Roche, Inc.
Nutley, New Jersey
USA

Di Sebastiano, Pierluigi, M.D.
Department of General Surgery
Bolzano General Hospital
39100 Bolzano
Italy

Domínguez-Muñoz, J. Enrique, M.D.
Department of Gastroenterology
University Hospital of Santiago
de Compostela
15706 Santiago de Compostela
Spain

Ebert, Matthias P. A., M.D.
Department of Gastroenterology,
Hepatology and Infectious Diseases
Otto-von-Guericke University
39120 Magdeburg
Germany

Eickhoff, Axel, M.D.
Department of Internal Medicine C
Municipal Clinic of Ludwigshafen/Rhein
Academic Teaching Hospital
of the University of Mainz
67063 Ludwigshafen a. Rhein
Germany

Fassmann, Carsten, Dr. med. vet.
Department of Animal Nutrition
School of Veterinary Medicine
30173 Hannover
Germany

Fernandez-Cruz, Laureano, M.D.
Department of Surgery
Hospital Clinic
University of Barcelona
08034 Barcelona
Spain

Fernandez-del Castillo, Carlos, M.D.
Massachusetts General Hospital
Harvard Medical School
Boston, Massachusetts 02114
USA

Fitzsimmons, Deborah, PhD
School of Nursing
University of Southampton
Southampton SO17 1 BF
UK

Flautner, Lajos E., M.D., D.Sc.
1st Department of Surgery
Faculty of Medicine
Semmelweis University of Medicine
11-1082 Budapest
Hungary

Fölsch, Ulrich R., M.D.
1st Department of Medicine
Christian-Albrechts University
24105 Kiel
Germany

Freeny, Patrick C., M.D.
Department of Radiology
University of Washington School
of Medicine
Seattle, WA 98195
USA

Friess, Helmut, M.D.
Department of General Surgery
University of Heidelberg
69120 Heidelberg
Germany

Gansauge, Frank, M.D.
Division of Molecular Oncology
Department of General Surgery
University of Ulm
89075 Ulm
Germany

Gansauge, Susanne, M.D.
Division of Molecular Oncology
Department of General Surgery
University of Ulm
89075 Ulm
Germany

Garvey, Conall J., MB, BS, FRCR
Department of Radiology
Royal Liverpool University Hospital
Liverpool L69 3GA
UK

Ghaneh, Paula, MB, BS, FRCS
Department of Surgery
Royal Liverpool University Hospital
Liverpool L69 3GA
UK

Giger, Urs, M.D.
Department of Visceral and Transplantation Surgery
University of Zürich
8091 Zürich
Switzerland

Gilmore, Ian, MA, MB, BChir, M.D., FRCP
Department of Gastroenterology
Royal Liverpool University Hospital
Liverpool L69 3GA
UK

Glasbrenner, Bernhard, M.D.
Department of Internal Medicine II
St. Franziskus Hospital
48145 Münster
Germany

Göke, Burkhard, M.D.
Medical Clinic II
Ludwig-Maximilians University
of Munich
81377 Munich
Germany

Göke, Rüdiger, M.D.
Clinical Research Unit
Philipps University of Marburg
35033 Marburg
Germany

Gorelick, Fred S., M.D.
GI Research Laboratory
The Department of Medicine
Yale University
Connecticut VA Healthcare
West Haven, Connecticut 06516
USA

Gouma, Dirk J., M.D.
Department of Surgery
Academic Medical Center
University of Amsterdam
1105 AZ Amsterdam
The Netherlands

Gregory, Peter C., BSc, PhD
Department of Pharmacology Research
Solvay Pharmaceuticals
30173 Hannover
Germany

Gress, Thomas M., M.D.
Department of Internal Medicine I
University of Ulm
89081 Ulm
Germany

Greten, Florian R., M.D.
Department of Internal Medicine I
University of Ulm
89081 Ulm
Germany

Gross, Hans-Jürgen, M.D.
Department of Clinical Chemistry
and Pathobiochemistry
University Hospital of Ulm
89070 Ulm
Germany

Grünert, Adolf, M.D.
Department of Clinical Chemistry
and Pathobiochemistry
University Hospital of Ulm
89070 Ulm
Germany

Gullo, Lucio, M.D.
Department of Internal Medicine and
Gastroenterology
St. Orsola Hospital
40138 Bologna
Italy

Hammer, Jürgen, M.D.
Roche Genomic and Information Sciences
Hoffmann-La Roche, Inc.
Nutley, New Jersey
USA

Hartley, Mark, MB, BS, FRCS
Department of Surgery
Royal Liverpool University Hospital
Liverpool L69 3GA
UK

Hinoue, Toshi, BS
Department of Surgery
Yale University School of Medicine
New Haven CT 06520-8062
USA

Hughes, Mark, MB, BS, FRCR
Department of Radiology
Royal Liverpool University Hospital
Liverpool L69 3GA
UK

Hults, Christopher, M.D.
Department of Surgery
Yale University School of Medicine
New Haven CT 06520-8062
USA

Izbicki, Jakob R., M.D.
Department of General Surgery
University Hospital of Hamburg/
Eppendorf
20246 Hamburg
Germany

Johnson, Colin D., M.Chir., FRCS
University Surgical Unit
Southhampton General Hospital
Southhampton SO16 6YD
UK

Kahl, Stefan, M.D.
Department of Gastroenterology,
Hepatology and Infectious Diseases
Otto-von-Guericke University
of Magdeburg
39120 Magdeburg
Germany

Kamphues, Josef, Prof. Dr. med. vet.
Department of Animal Nutrition
School of Veterinary Medicine
30173 Hannover
Germany

Keller, Jutta, M.D.
Department of Medicine
Israelitic Hospital
22297 Hamburg
Germany

Kidd, Mark, PhD
Department of Surgery
Yale University School of Medicine
New Haven CT 06520-8062
USA

Kleeff, Jörg, M.D.
Department of Visceral
and Transplantation Surgery
Inselspital, University of Bern
3010 Bern
Switzerland

Knoefel, W. T., M.D.
Department of General Surgery
University Hospital of Hamburg/
Eppendorf
20246 Hamburg
Germany

Korc, Murray, M.D.
Division of Endocrinology, Diabetes and
Metabolism
Departments of Medicine, Biological
Chemistry and Pharmacology
University of California
Irvine, CA 92697
USA

Kozarek, Richard A., M.D.
Department of Gastroenterology
Virginia Mason Medical Center
Seattle WA 98111-0900
USA

Krähenbühl, Lukas, M.D.
Department of Visceral
and Transplantation Surgery
University of Zürich
8091 Zürich
Switzerland

Lankisch, Paul Georg, M.D.
Department of Internal Medicine
Municipal Clinic of Lüneburg
21339 Lüneburg
Germany

Laugier, René, M.D.
Department of Gastroenterology
University of Marseille
Hospital La Timone
13385 Marseille
France

Layer, Peter, M.D.
Department of Medicine
Israelitic Hospital
22297 Hamburg
Germany

Leodolter, Andreas, M.D.
Department of Gastroenterology,
Hepatology and Infectious Diseases
Otto-von-Guericke University
of Magdeburg
39120 Magdeburg
Germany

Lerch, Markus M., M.D.
Department of Medicine B
Wilhelms-University of Westphalia
48129 Münster
Germany

Löhr, J.-Matthias, M.D.
Department of Medicine IV
Faculty of Clinical Medicine, Mannheim
Ruprecht-Karls University of Heidelberg
68167 Mannheim
Germany

Lombard, Martin, MD, FRCB(I), FRCP
Department of Gastroenterology
Royal Liverpool University Hospital
Liverpool L69 3GA
UK

Lowenfels, Albert B., M.D.
Department of Surgery
New York Medical College
Valhalla, New York 10595
USA

Lügering, Andreas, M.D.
Department of Medicine B
Wilhelms-University of Westphalia
48129 Münster
Germany

Magyar, Ambrus, M.D., PhD
1st. Department of Surgery
Faculty of Medicine
Semmelweis University of Medicine
11-1082 Budapest
Hungary

Maisonneuve, Patrick, Ing.
Unit of Clinical Epidemiology
European Institute of Oncology
20141 Milan
Italy

Malfertheiner, Peter, M.D.
Department of Gastroenterology,
Hepatology and Infectious Diseases
Otto-von-Guericke University
of Magdeburg
39120 Magdeburg
Germany

Meier, Rémy, M.D.
Department of Gastroenterology
University Hospital
4410 Liestal
Switzerland

Menke, Andre, M.D.
Department of Internal Medicine I
University Hospital of Ulm
89070 Ulm
Germany

Modlin Irvin M., M.D., PhD
Department of Surgery
Yale University School of Medicine
New Haven, Connecticut 06520-8062
USA

Mössner, Joachim, M.D.
Department of Internal Medicine II
University of Leipzig
04103 Leipzig
Germany

Mueller, Christoph, M.D.
Division of Immunopathology
Institute of Pathology
University of Bern
3010 Bern
Switzerland

Navarro, Salvador, M.D.
Department of Surgery
Hospital Clinic
University of Barcelona
08034 Barcelona
Spain

Nealon, William H., M.D.
UTMB Department of Surgery
6.112 John Sealy Hospital
Galveston, TX 77555-0544
USA

Neoptolemos, John P., MA, MB, BChir, M.D., FRCS
Department of Surgery
Royal Liverpool University Hospital
Liverpool L69 3GA
UK

Obertop, Huug, M.D.
Department of Surgery
Academic Medical Center
University of Amsterdam
1105 AZ Amsterdam
The Netherlands

Pantoja, Juan Pablo, M.D.
Department of Surgery
Hospital Clinic
University of Barcelona
08034 Barcelona
Spain

Prinz, Richard A., M.D.
Department of General Surgery
St. Luke's Medical Center
Rush University
Chicago, Illinois 60612-3833
USA

Pulay, Istvan, M.D., PhD
1st. Department of Surgery
Faculty of Medicine
Semmelweis University of Medicine
11-1082 Budapest
Hungary

Ramesh, Hariharan, M.D.
PVS Memorial Hospital
Cochin
India

Rattner, David W., M.D.
Massachusetts General Hospital
Harvard Medical School
Boston, Massachusetts 02114
U.S.A.

Reber, Howard A., M.D.
Gastrointestinal Surgery
Division of General Surgery
UCLA School of Medicine
Los Angeles, CA 90024-6904
USA

Reichen, Jürg, M.D.
Department of Clinical Pharmacology
Inselspital, University of Bern
3010 Bern
Switzerland

Riemann, Jürgen F., M.D.
Department of Internal Medicine C
Municipal Clinic of Ludwigshafen/Rhein
Academic Teaching Hospital
of the University
of Mainz
67063 Ludwigshafen a. Rhein
Germany

Robles-Diaz, Guillermo, M.D.
Department of Gastroenterology
National Institute of Nutrition
Tlalpan, Mexico D.F. 14000
Mexico

Roggo, Antoine, M.D.
Department of Visceral
and Transplantation Surgery
Inselspital, University of Bern
3010 Bern
Switzerland

Rudmann, Martin A., M.D.
Global Scientific Communication
Solvay Pharmaceuticals GmbH
30173 Hannover
Germany

Sáenz, Alejandro, M.D.
Department of Surgery
Hospital Clinic
University of Barcelona
08034 Barcelona
Spain

Saurer, Leslie, Ph.D.
Division of Immunopathology
Institute of Pathology
University of Bern
3010 Bern
Switzerland

Schäfer, Markus, M.D.
Department of Visceral
and Transplantation Surgery
University of Zürich
8091 Zürich
Switzerland

Schlosser, Wolfgang, M.D.
Department of General Surgery
University of Ulm
89075 Ulm
Germany

Schmid, Roland M., M.D.
Department of Internal Medicine I
University of Ulm
89081 Ulm
Germany

Schmid-Kotsas, Alexandra, M.D.
Department of Clinical Chemistry
and Pathobiochemistry
University Hospital of Ulm
89070 Ulm
Germany

Schmied, Bruno M., M.D.
Department of General Surgery
University of Heidelberg
69120 Heidelberg
Germany

Schneider, Eric, M.D.
Department of Internal Medicine I
University Hospital of Ulm
89070 Ulm
Germany

Schulz, Hans-Ulrich, M.D.
Department of Surgery
Otto-von-Guericke University
of Magedeburg
39120 Magdeburg
Germany

Seiler, Christian A., M.D.
Department of Visceral
and Transplantation Surgery
Inselspital, University of Bern
3010 Bern
Switzerland

Shedd Keith, Helen, M.D.
Department of General Surgery
St. Luke's Medical Center
Rush University
Chicago, Illinois 60612-3833
USA

Shrikhande, Shailesh, MBBS, MS
Shrikhande Clinic
Hindu Colony, Dadar
Mumbai (Bombay) – 400014
India

Siech, Marco, M.D.
Department of General Surgery
University Hospital of Ulm
89070 Ulm
Germany

Smart, Howard, MB, BS, FRCP
Department of Gastroenterology
Royal Liverpool University Hospital
Liverpool L69 3GA
UK

Strate, T., M.D.
Department of General Surgery
University Hospital of Hamburg/
Eppendorf
20246 Hamburg
Germany

Sutton, Robert, MB, BS, DPhil, FRCS
Department of Surgery
Royal Liverpool University Hospital
Liverpool L69 3GA
UK

Tabeling, Robert, Dr. med. vet.
Department of Animal Nutrition
School of Veterinary Medicine
30173 Hannover
Germany

Takada, Koichi, M.D.
Department of Radiology
Teikyo University School of Medicine
Tokyo 173-8605
Japan

Takada, Tadahiro, M.D., F.A.C.S.
First Department of Surgery
Teikyo University School of Medicine
Tokyo 173-8605
Japan

Takada, Yukiko, M.D.
Department of Medicine
Teikyo University School of Medicine
Tokyo 173-8605
Japan

Tcholakov, Oleg, M.D.
First Surgical Clinic
"Pirogov" Emergency Medical Institute
1606 Sofia
Bulgaria

Tihanyi, Tibor F., M.D., PhD
1st. Department of Surgery
Faculty of Medicine
Semmelweis University of Medicine
11-1082 Budapest
Hungary

Toskes, Phillip P., M.D.
Divison of Gastroenterology, Hepatology
and Nutrition
College of Medicine
University of Florida
32610-Gainesville
USA

Traverso, L. William, M.D.
Department of General Surgery
Virginia Mason Medical Center
P.O. Box 900 C6-N
Seattle WA 98111-0900
USA

Tsiotos, Gregory G., M.D.
Hepatobiliary and Pancreatic Surgery
Athens Medical Center
Athens 11521
Greece

Uhl, Waldemar, M.D.
Department of General Surgery
University of Heidelberg
69120 Heidelberg
Germany

Wagner, Andreas C. C., M.D.
Department of Gastroenterology
Inselspital, University of Bern
3010 Bern
Switzerland

Wagner, Markus, M.D.
Department of Visceral
and Transplantation Surgery
Inselspital, University of Bern
3010 Bern
Switzerland

Wagner, Martin, M.D.
Department of Internal Medicine I
University of Ulm
89081 Ulm
Germany

Warshaw, Andrew L., M.D.
Massachusetts General Hospital
Harvard Medical School
Boston, Massachusetts 02114
USA

Weber, Christoph K., M.D.
Department of Internal Medicine I
University of Ulm
89081 Ulm
Germany

Weidenbach, Hans, M.D.
Department of Internal Medicine I
University Hospital of Ulm
89070 Ulm
Germany

Weihe, Eberhard, M.D.
Institute of Anatomy and Cell Biology
Philipps-University of Marburg
35033 Marburg
Germany

Whitcomb, David C., M.D., PhD
Division of Gastroenterology, Hepatology
and Nutrition
Departments of Medicine, Cell Biology
& Physiology and Human Genetics
Center for Genomic Sciences
University of Pittsburgh
Pittsburgh, PA 15213
USA

Wilson, Jeremy S., M.D., PhD, FRACP
Pancreatic Research Group
Level 4, Bankstown-Lidcombe Hospital
The University of New South Wales
Bankstown, NSW 2200
Australia

Z'graggen, Kaspar, M.D.
Department of General Surgery
University of Heidelberg
69120 Heidelberg
Germany

Zimmermann, Arthur, M.D.
Institute of Pathology
Inselspital, University of Bern
3010 Bern
Switzerland

1 The history of chronic pancreatitis

1.1 A historical and critical appraisal of chronic pancreatitis

I. M. Modlin, Ch. Hults, M. Kidd, T. Hinoue

Early concepts of the pancreas

Although the Greeks were thought to be the first to recognize the pancreas as a distinct organ, rabbis in the earlier Babylonian Talmud refer to a structure designated by them as the *"finger of the liver"*[1]. While Galen provided a modest description of the organ, neither he, Hippocrates, Erasistratus nor Herophilus were able to identify a relationship to disease. These ancient anatomists regarded the pancreas as unusual, given that it had no cartilage or bone present, and Rufus of Ephesus (c. 100 AD) named the organ pancreas (Greek *pan:* all and *kreas:* flesh or meat) [2]. Andreas Vesalius referred to the pancreas in the fifth book of his opus as a *"glandulous organ or kannelly body of substance growing in the neather pannicle of the caule (omentum)"* and presumed the pancreas to exert a protective effect on the stomach by serving as a cushion *(Schutzorgan)* upon which it rested (Fig. 1.1-1).

Even though the main duct of the human pancreas was described in 1642, it was utterly misunderstood since contemporary views considered that *"chyme"* from the duode-

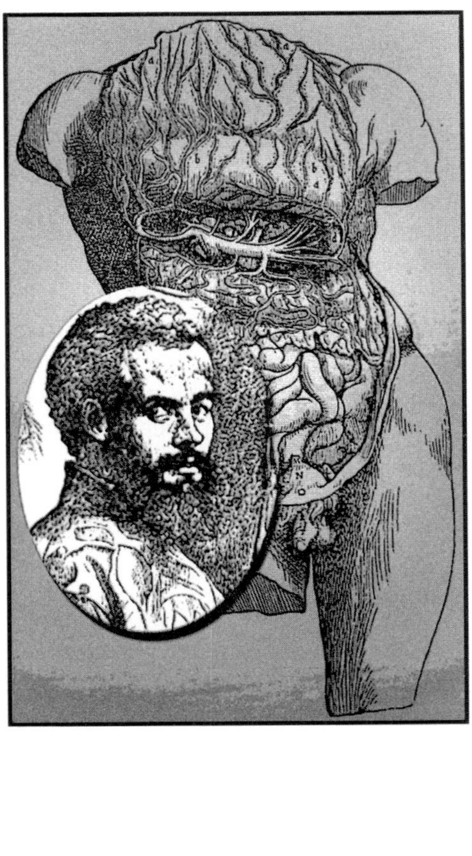

Figure 1.1-1. Andreas Vesalius (inset) (1514 to 1564) was one of the first anatomists to depict the pancreas. Despite a relatively accurate assessment of its structure there was little appreciation of its function. Vesalius referred to it as a "kannelly body" and considered it to act as a "cushion" for the stomach. Subsequent concepts of its function embraced the prescient notion that it was an abdominal salivary gland.

num ascended into the pancreas to provoke secretion of a *"sharp juice not unlike to the gall."* Sylvius and his brilliant pupil, Regnier de Graaf of Delft, ingeniously developed a method for the direct investigation of the nature of pancreatic juice utilizing canine pancreatic fistula through which he inserted feather quills into the pancreatic duct orifice to obtain *succus pancreaticus.* They believed that pancreatic juice *effervesced* with bile, and that this combination of acids and alkalis was a critical component of digestion. They also postulated that pancreatic juice exhibited a dual function by both *"attenuating the mucous lining of the gut as well as initiating segregation of the useful food elements."* The use of the acid secreting complex gastric pyloric ceca from fish complicated this work and it was not until the end of the 17th century that Johann Bohn successfully demonstrated that the pancreatic juice was not acid.

By 1682, Brunner noted that his pancreatectomized dogs survived for up to a year despite polyuria, polydypsia, and bulimia, but failed to identify the presence of sugar in the urine. The clinical correlation of pancreatic disease and diabetes was only recognized in 1788 when Thomas Cawley broadly alluded to such a disease entity [3]. The subject of the duct and the structure of the gland led Sommering (1755–1830) to first employ the vernacular term *Bauchspeicheldrüse* (abdominal salivary gland) in the medical and scientific literature and as a result, the pancreas was until the late 19th century considered to be an abdominal salivary gland. During the 18th century, Albrecht von Haller (1708–1777) noted the close relationship of the pancreatic duct to the bile duct and proposed that pancreatic juice and bile interacted in the process of digestion. Further contributions included Santorini's identification of the accessory duct (1742) while a detailed description of the embryology of the pancreas was provided by Meckel (1806). Trypsin was identified by Willy Kuhne (1837–1900) and in 1815, Alexander Marcet (1770–1822) identified lipase. Between 1849 and 1856 Claude Bernard (1813–1878) of Paris unified the concepts of pancreatic digestion by demonstrating that gastric digestion *"is only a preparation act"* and that pancreatic juice emulsified fatty foods, splitting them into glycerin and fatty acids. In addition, he demonstrated the power of the pancreas to convert starch into sugar and its solvent action upon the *"proteides that have not been cleaved in the stomach."* Further work by Eberle in 1843 demonstrated that pancreatic juice emulsified fat, and a year later Valentin demonstrated its activity on starch. Differences in the exocrine and endocrine pancreas were elucidated by Paul Langhans (1869) while in 1882, Kuhne and Lea noted the complex capillary network which embraced the collection of islets. The regulation of pancreatic secretion led IP Pavlov (1849–1936) and his pupils to use novel pancreatic fistula preparations to demonstrate the role of the vagus nerve in the neural regulation of pancreatic secretion. Thereafter Dolinski noted that acid introduced into the duodenum stimulated pancreatic secretion and interpreted this as indicative of a local neural reflex, while Chepovalnikov demonstrated that pancreatic juice acquired and exerted a powerful solvent action on *proteids* only after contact with either the duodenal membrane or extracts thereof. This led to the discovery of enterokinase. It was left to Bayliss and Starling to introduce the concept of hormonal regulation of the organ [4].

Pancreatitis

Since the anatomic location of the organ was not well known and its physiological functions ill defined, pathological conditions of the pancreas were difficult to delineate. Descriptions of pancreatic abnormalities from antiquity refer mostly to *"scirrhous"* disease,

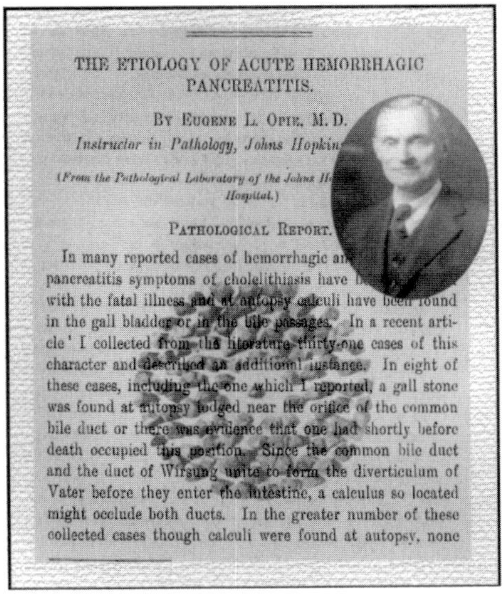
THE ETIOLOGY OF ACUTE HEMORRHAGIC PANCREATITIS.

BY EUGENE L. OPIE, M.D.

Instructor in Pathology, Johns Hopkin

(From the Pathological Laboratory of the Johns H
Hospital.)

PATHOLOGICAL REPORT.

In many reported cases of hemorrhagic a
pancreatitis symptoms of cholelithiasis have
with the fatal illness and at autopsy calculi have been found in the gall bladder or in the bile passages. In a recent article [1] I collected from the literature thirty-one cases of this character and described an additional instance. In eight of these cases, including the one which I reported, a gall stone was found at autopsy lodged near the orifice of the common bile duct or there was evidence that one had shortly before death occupied this position. Since the common bile duct and the duct of Wirsung unite to form the diverticulum of Vater before they enter the intestine, a calculus so located might occlude both ducts. In the greater number of these collected cases though calculi were found at autopsy, none

Figure 1.1-2. Eugene Opie in 1901 proposed the "common channel theory" of pancreatitis and correctly implicated gallstones in the pathogenesis of the disease.

without any specific identification of pathology. In Germany Friedreich and Claasen were prominent in establishing the role of alcohol in pancreatitis and defined its clinical and pathological sequel in the 1880s. Subsequently, Reginald Fitz of Boston, who had studied with Claasen, defined the signs and symptoms of pancreatitis and categorized the disease in terms of its gangrenous, hemorrhagic and suppurative forms. His reflections on the nature and causes of the disease were published in the Boston Medical and Surgical Journal of 1889, and have remained little changed in the centuries since their initial proposal [5]. Opie in 1901 further elucidated the pathogenesis of pancreatitis and proposed a *"common channel"* hypothesis whereby acute pancreatitis was the aftermath of the flow of infected bile into the pancreatic duct from the common bile duct (Fig. 1.1-2). He proposed that this clinical circumstance occurred when a gallstone became impacted in the ampulla of Vater and caused obstruction [6]. Further credence for this theory was provided by E. Archibald (1919) who experimentally demonstrated that spasm of the sphincter of Oddi increased biliary pressure and culminated in the development of acute pancreatitis [7]. Although alcohol and gallstones remain among the common denominators of the etiology of acute pancreatitis to this day, Rich and Duff in 1936 proposed that a combination of pathological vascular changes and local pancreatic enzyme damage were implicated in the pathogenesis. The diagnosis of acute pancreatitis, which had initially been purely clinical, was subsequently supported by the work of R. Elman of St. Louis who in 1929 described the quantitative determination of blood amylase using a viscometer. Subsequent investigations have proposed that the cytokine cascade of acute pancreatitis may be a consequence of disorganized intracellular trafficking or activation of acinar zymogen granules [8]. Unfortunately the etiology of both acute and especially chronic pancreatitis remains shrouded in dogma and conjecture.

Early observations on chronic pancreatitis

The identification of the etiology of chronic pancreatitis has frustrated physicians since the very earliest observations of the entity. Initially the pathological examination of the pancreas was the most defining focus in the diagnosis with clinical assessment of the patient as the only available diagnostic tool for the physician. As early as 1788, Cawley became the first to suggest a link between lifestyle and pancreatic disease. His patient, "a 34yr old man accustomed to free living and strong corporeal exertions in the pursuit of country living," was noted to have extensive pancreatic disease at autopsy [3].

One of the earliest reports of pancreatitis was by Edwin Klebs who reported a case of hemorrhagic pancreatitis in 1870. This was followed by many scattered reports throughout the medical literature without much focus toward a diagnosis before the patients' demise. At the turn of the 19th century Mayo Robson presumed the etiology to be due to bacterial infection; however, the distinction between acute, sub-acute and chronic pancreatitis was still controversial [9]. Other physicians, including Reginald Fitz, felt that the underlying insult was the hemorrhage of the pancreas which resulted in necrosis of the gland as evidenced at autopsy [5]. This assessment resulted in some prejudicial views, since cases described by pathologists represented advanced and fatal forms of pancreati-

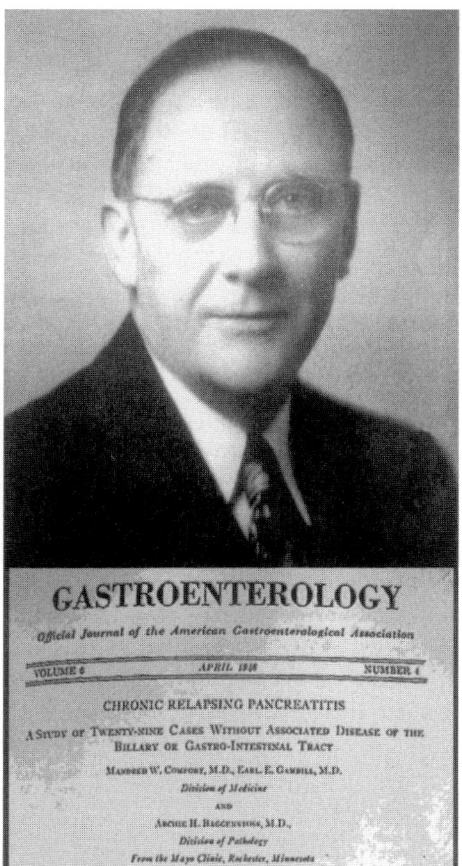

Figure 1.1-3. In 1946, Comfort published a clinical paper that provided the first coherent assessment of the nebulous entity of chronic pancreatitis.

tis. Thus many early attempts at classification resulted in contradictions as physicians and pathologists differed on the nature of the process and in addition lacked scientific data to address the question of etiology.

In 1946 Comfort provided a significant analysis of the clinical entity of chronic pancreatitis and in so doing produced the seminal manuscript on the subject that has for 50 years remained the critical commentary on the disease (Fig. 1.1-3) [10]. Although there had been references to the relationship between alcohol and chronic pancreatitis, there were no clinical studies and proof remained anecdotal until Comfort described in detail the connection between alcohol abuse and chronic pancreatitis. His study added considerable credibility to the much earlier description of the "drunkard's pancreas" by Friedrich in the 19th century [11]. The criteria utilized by Comfort to characterize the diagnosis included recurrent attacks of abdominal pain, disturbances of acinar function and alterations in endocrine function. During the last fifty years, despite the fact that much has been learned from studies of alcoholic pancreatitis the definitive mechanisms are for the most part obscure. The relative increase in the diagnosis of pancreatitis probably reflects a wide variety of factors including increased awareness, greater diagnostic skill and more sophisticated technology as well as an increase in alcohol consumption. Considerable debate has centered around the question of whether pancreatic lithogenesis is a diagnostic criterion of chronic pancreatitis or whether it merely represents a correlatible epiphenomenon. Prior to the twentieth century, pancreatic stones were thought of as exceedingly rare. Calcium carbonate was known to be the main chemical in the composition and, as might therefore be predicted, diagnosis of the condition increased substantially as the new technique of roentgenography facilitated visualization [12]. The similar increase in surgical recognition further dispelled the notion of rarity. While exhaustive analysis confirmed the composition of the calculi the mechanism of the initiation of the pancreatic precipitates eluded identification. A wide variety of agents including lactoferrin, alcohol, and the pancreatic stone protein lithostatine have been associated with pancreatic calculi [13]. The question however of whether the calculi are caused by an increase in calcium production, precipitation of proteins or a yet to be defined mechanism remains as yet unclear. Indeed the correlation between the mere presence of pancreatic calculi and the diagnosis of chronic pancreatitis itself remains debated. Thus in the condition of "senile pancreatitis", described by Amman, the presence of idiopathic asymptomatic pancreatic calculi in the elderly suggests that chronicity and calculi may not necessarily occur *pari passu* [14].

There is however little disagreement that pancreatic stones may obstruct the ducts and play a part in the development of pancreatic pain. This observation has resulted in efforts to remove stones by either medical dissolution (including HCl) or mechanical intervention. Thus lithotripsy, endoscopic sphincterotomy with or without stent placement and a wide variety of ductal and pancreatic surgical techniques have been proposed to eliminate calculous disease of the pancreas.

In 1959, Zuideman labeled dietary factors as an additional etiologic agent and proposed that the entity known as "tropical pancreatitis" in underdeveloped countries was associated with the standard low protein, fat-deficient diet prevalent in such areas [15]. Subsequent reports have suggested that the Cassava root (manioc) might be the agent implicated in tropical pancreatitis, but rigorous confirmation of this theory is still required. [16]. Despite considerable attention to the identification of the basis of chronic pancreatitis approximately 30% of patients diagnosed with the disease still are regarded as idiopathic with no known evidence of any associated disease or inciting event.

In the absence of minimal evidence for etiology the identification of a mechanistic explanation of the disease process has been similarly frustrating. Various theories have been propounded to explain the pathology, including the necrosis-fibrosis concept of Kloppel, the obstruction theory of Sarles, the toxic metabolic hypothesis of Bordalo and the oxidative stress hypothesis of Braganza [17–20]. No rigorous data in support of any of these hypotheses exists though each in its own right has attractive elements.

As a result of the absence of a defined etiology and the lack of a mechanism of disease, clinical attention to chronic pancreatitis has for the most part focused on establishing a diagnosis and thereafter management of the sequelae, including pain, ductal obstruction and the exocrine and endocrine deficits based upon acinar and islet cell destruction.

The evolution of management

The definition of chronic pancreatitis and its classification has changed with the advance of biochemical and scientific technology over the last 50 years. Thus the enhancement of radiographic methods for visualization of the pancreas, the development of ERCP and the assessment of pancreatic exocrine and endocrine function have greatly abetted identification and characterization of the disease. A major problem however has been and remains the lack of tissue for pathological examination. Thus, clinical acumen remains the first and foremost criterion available with recurrent or persistent abdominal pain a hallmark of the disease. The natural history of chronic pancreatitis with the development of endocrine and exocrine insufficiency, leading to diabetes and steatorrhea, provide further supportive clinical evidence. There exist no pathognomonic criteria for the disease but rather a constellation of symptoms and signs corroborated with radiographic, ERCP and biochemical data.

Despite numerous attempts no particular classification system has proved entirely satisfactory and the field of chronic pancreatitis has been troubled in the area of categorization. Recent attempts include the Marseilles and Cambridge classifications but neither has adequately resolved the dilemma.

The Marseilles system addressed a series of morphologic criteria including focal necrosis and segmental or diffuse fibrosis with or without calculi, while the Cambridge system focused mainly on the utility of imagery of the ductal system and the nature of the gland to provide a descriptive assessment of the pathology [21]. Overall the definition and clinical pictures of both acute and chronic pancreatitis intertwine, and separation often remains obscure. Since no definitive treatment exists the evolution of therapy has perforce been directed at dealing with the symptomatic manifestations of the disease.

Medical treatment

Pain. The first and predominant treatment regime of pancreatitis was pain control although in the early part of the 20th century the lack of accurate diagnosis often resulted in treatment delay. For the most part measures employed included high dosage opiates, especially morphine. Other strategies included the use of calomel to lessen distention and as a potential intestinal antiseptic. Overall the extent of the medical treatment in the early part of the century included little more than observation, although in dire circumstances such as shock hot saline enemas were advocated [9]. The dominant therapy however relied upon pain management; thus the introduction of intravenous agents greatly enhanced the ability to ameliorate acute discomfort. Orr in 1950 established the efficacy of the epidural technique, and its application to the management of pancreatic pain proved quite efficacious [22].

Although pain relief was predominantly a pharmacotherapeutic strategy, in 1946 Fontaine achieved some moderate success by resection of splanchnic nerves to relieve the pain associated with chronic pancreatitis [23]. As a result of this strategy and the adverse effects of long-term narcotic usage numerous permutations of denervation, including left splanchnic only, right only, thoracolumbar, and thoracolumbar associated with vagotomy were introduced [24]. Unfortunately, the results of such procedures varied drastically and as a consequence the inconsistent therapeutic relief rendered this a suboptimal management strategy. Despite the many different manipulations of the pain pathway that were attempted in the management of chronic pancreatitis, the first and simplest, the use of opiates, has remained the most widespread. As a result of the debate in regard to the clinical relevance of the morphine-induced sphincter of Oddi spasm, a shift from morphine to Demerol as the narcotic of choice has occurred (Fig. 1.1-4).

Exocrine deficiency. Aside from pain, complaints of chronic diarrhea and fatty stools proved to be issues of considerable discomfort to individuals with chronic pancreatitis. Complaints varied from simple "unrest in the abdomen" to major and even uncontrollable attacks of diarrhea. Although exocrine function *per se* had not been studied in detail, Fles in 1868 reportedly used oral extracts of pancreas to relieve the steatorrhea associated with the disease [25]. In 1902, Salomon effectively used a more defined role of diet and "fresh pancreas" with moderate success. [26] This substitution of exocrine produc-

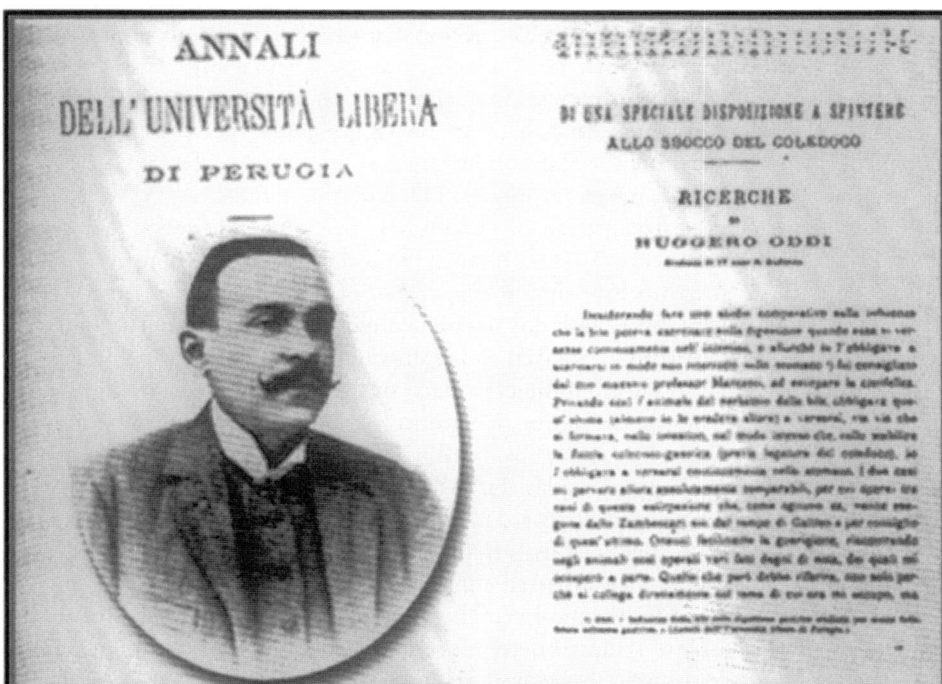

Figure 1.1-4. Ruggero Oddi, as a fourth year medical student in Perugia, Italy, described the choledochal sphincter and accurately defined its role in the regulation of bile flow.

tion, or *organotherapy*, was the precursor of later efforts to "cool" the pancreas to both alleviate pain and restore exocrine function. Although the oral supplementation of zymogens has proved to be highly beneficial in the symptomatic management of disordered digestion, rigorous data regarding the effects of "pancreatic cooling" has not been forthcoming. Similarly, the usage of subcutaneous Octreotide (an analog of somatostatin) that inhibited acinar secretory activity has been without significant benefit in decreasing the progress of the disease although some amelioration of pain has been claimed [27, 28].

Endocrine deficiency. The progressive pancreatic fibrosis associated with the inexorable progress of chronic pancreatitis culminates in diabetes in approximately 15% of patients. Although the overt manifestations of diabetes are not usually evident until the destruction of approximately 90% of the gland, subtle alterations in glucose homeostasis may predate such events by many years. The early institution of appropriate dietary and pharmacotherapeutic (insulin) measures thus became an important prophylactic strategy in stabilizing the adverse metabolic events noted during the evolution of chronic pancreatitis. Overall the goal of medical treatment thus remains directed at the control of pain and the reduction of the exocrine and endocrine consequences of pancreatic parenchyma destruction.

Surgical strategy

The development of a rationale for surgical intervention in chronic pancreatitis has been hindered by numerous difficulties. Firstly there was little appreciation of pancreatic disease itself. Secondly the inflammatory condition of acute pancreatitis was often so violent and rapidly terminal that little explicit surgical therapy other than simple exploration, incision and drainage was ever possible. The notion that various gradations of this disease process were related or even amenable to specific therapy was to a large extent obviated by the technical difficulties encountered in operating upon the pancreas itself. A further considerable problem has been the inability to exactly define the mechanism of the disease process and thus identify the appropriate target(s) for surgical intervention. Nevertheless, when faced with the relentless progress of the disease and the ravages inflicted by pain, narcotics and organ dysfunction, physicians have been driven to seek a therapeutic albeit symptomatic intervention. Thus despite the lack of any discernable cause for chronic pancreatitis surgeons have since the latter part of the 19th century applied themselves vigorously and in diverse fashions to the treatment of the disease. The solutions seemed initially obvious. Thus a damaged and dysfunctional gland causing pain might be best removed. Needless to say the technical aspects of this endeavor soon resulted in reconsideration of this concept. Biliary or pancreatic calculi capable of causing both pain and obstruction should be extracted, but this obvious remedy appeared to be relatively ineffective. The obvious target of a sphincter in "spasm" or fibrosed was attractive as a solution but its ablation once again appeared to effect little relief. The observation of a massively dilated duct system suggested that drainage would bring relief but neither disease amelioration nor pain abeyance appeared either to be predictable or occur with any acceptable regularity. Indeed for the most part the surgery of chronic pancreatitis has today come to rest in the hands of stalwarts determined to do what best they can fully aware of the absolute limitations of their procedures and those who confine their activities to the elimination of pain effected by means of nerve injection or ablation. The following sections address the evolution of surgical ideation in its attempts to deal with the relentless disease of chronic pancreatitis in the absence of any defined target demonstrably able on

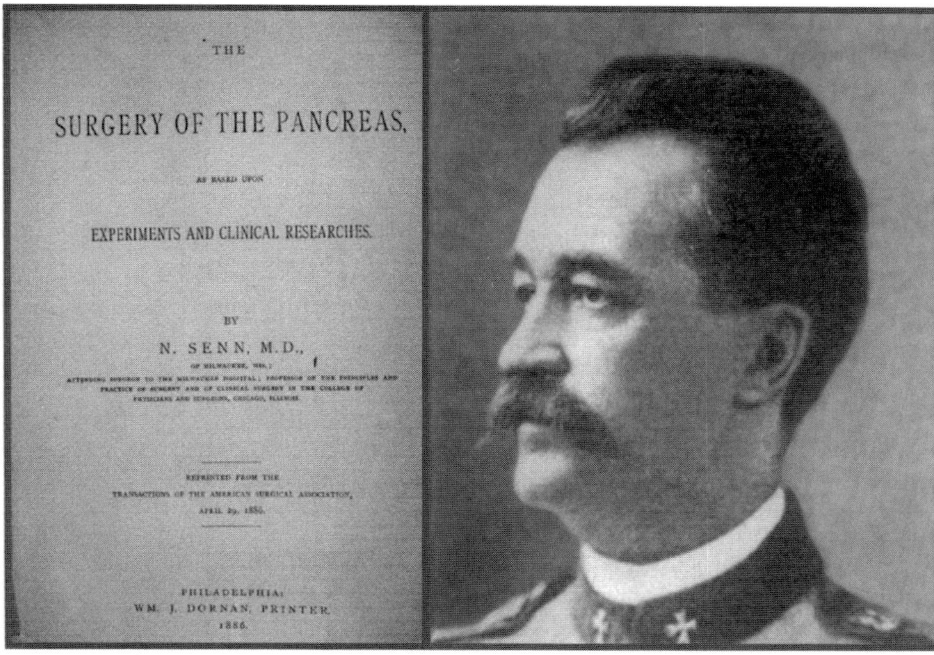

Figure 1.1-5. Nicholas Senn of Chicago was an early surgical pioneer of experimental pancreatic surgery. His evaluation of current work in the field led him to a pessimistic conclusion regarding the outcome of surgery on the pancreas. As a result he cautioned his colleagues regarding the utility of surgery for pancreatic disease.

a predictive basis to either counter the progress of the disease, effect its etiology or ameliorate its symptomatology.

Aware of the problems of pancreatic disease Nicholas Senn in 1886 commented in one of his earliest papers, "The surgery of the pancreas, as based upon experiments and clinical research," on what he recognized as a vexatious problem (Fig. 1.1-5). Senn demonstrated that experimental extirpation of the pancreas in animals was "invariably followed by death"[29]. Although prior separate experiments by both Brunner and Meiring had not drawn so absolute a conclusion [30], nevertheless it was evident to most surgeons of any experience that the vast majority of pancreatic surgery (whether major or minor) resulted in fatal consequences.

The general advances in surgery of the late 19th and early 20th century heralded the introduction and refinement of surgical treatment for pancreatic disease but as might have been predicted there were misadventures. Intervention in pancreatic disease was regarded as extremely dangerous and even the most experienced of the gastrointestinal surgeons such as Mayo Robson of Leeds advocated the surgical approach of "waiting until collapse of the patient with presumed pancreatitis" before surgery was undertaken. In fact Robson – an arbiter on such matters – maintained that "until collapse no surgery {was} justifiable" [31]. Out of therapeutic strategies of this type would grow the justifiably cynical medical comments of men such as Naunyn who described such surgery as little more than an autopsy *in vivo!* The lack of technical expertise and knowledge limited the ensuing surgery to a mere evacuation of the septic material and given the non-availability of antibiotics and the primitive state of knowledge of fluid and electrolyte balance the outcome was invariably fatal. In some circumstances surgeons performed an exploratory laparotomy under the belief of a hollow visceral source of the disease only to be confronted by a diagnosis of acute pancreatitis. In such instances, minimal intervention became the recognized order of the day, based upon a naive assumption that in the absence of "pus" exploratory surgery would do no harm. Such views were however soon discarded in the light of experience and the field of pancreatic surgery thus became a territory visited by few surgeons. Nevertheless such were the humble beginnings that led to the establishment of the field of pancreatic surgery. Indeed the early 20th century tenet of Kocher seemed most applicable when directed to the subject of pancreatic surgery: "A surgeon is a doctor who can operate and knows when not to."

The origins of pancreatic surgery

In order to understand the limitations of surgery for chronic pancreatitis and the difficulty in developing a rationale for such intervention a brief diversion into an assessment of the evolution of pancreatic surgery is helpful. The inaccessibility of the organ to both diagnosis and intervention coupled with an almost complete absence of its function and pathology rendered interfering with it worrisome.

Early experimental pancreatic surgery originated in 1673 when Regnier De Graaf constructed pancreatic fistulae on dogs to determine the nature of pancreatic secretion (Fig. 1.1-6). These experiments laid the foundation of pancreatic physiology and initiat-

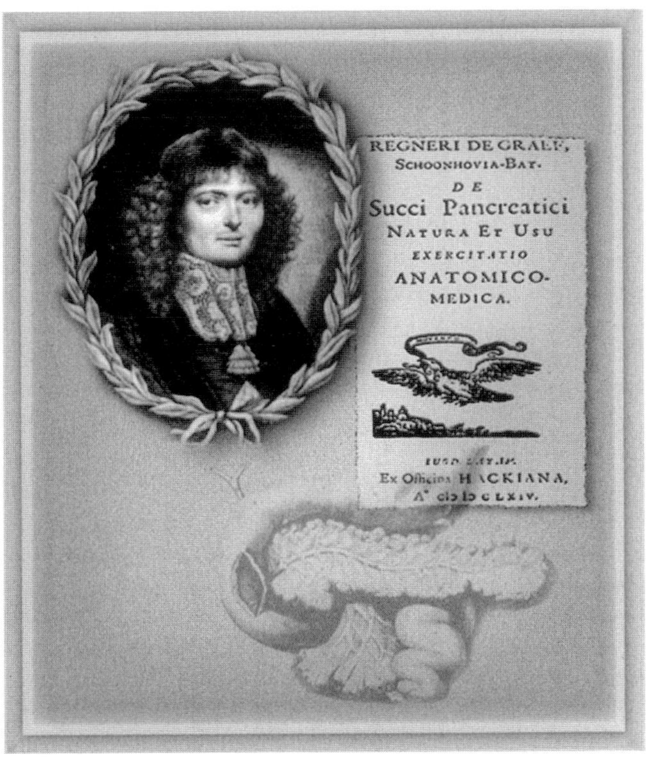

Figure 1.1-6. Regnier de Graaf developed an ingenious method for the creation of canine pancreatic fistulae and was able to elucidate the nature of *succus pancreaticus.*

ed further interest in the organ that had previously been inaccessible. His publication, *"De Succo Pancreatico"*, detailed the nature of pancreatic juice and described the technical requirements needed to create the fistula [32]. A decade later Johann Conrad Brunner (1683) expanded De Graaf's work by undertaking a series of partial resections of canine pancreas that were published as *"Experimenta Nova Circa Pancreas"*. Although this work determined that animals could survive without a pancreas, the interpretation of the significance of the concomitant observations of polydipsia and polyuria post-operatively sadly eluded Brunner, who might otherwise have been the first to identify the endocrine component of pancreatic function [33].

Resection

Other than the occasional acute dramatic incision and drainage of acute pancreatitis, the field of formal pancreatic surgery remained quiescent for over 200 years. Although the literature in the late nineteenth century periodically alluded to isolated cases of resection and extirpation no specific intervention for pancreatic disease was contemplated or described. At the turn of the 19th century more intrepid surgeons including Trendelburg, Halsted and Codvilla began to report pancreatic resections and suggest the possibility of formal intervention in "tumorous" disease processes that afflicted the organ. In 1898 William S. Halsted of Baltimore resected the first carcinoma of the "duodenal papilla and diverticulum Vateri" and in so doing demonstrated that pancreatic surgery was a feasible albeit risky proposition [34]. Although the patient survived the operation, a few months after discharge she succumbed to a recurrence in the head of the pancreas. Almost simultaneously Alessandro Codvilla of Bologna undertook an "en bloc" resection of the pancreas and duodenum, becoming in all likelihood the first to perform a pancreaticoduodenectomy [35]. An appreciation of the inherent risks associated with the presence of jaundice as well as the recognition of the appalling prognosis of pancreatic cancer led to the development of a two-stage operation to first relieve the "cholemia" and thereafter remove the tumor. In 1907 A. Desjardins described an experimental two-stage operation for resection of the pancreas based on his cadaveric resections [36]. In the following year, L. Sauve devised a one-staged operation and noted the loss of exocrine function as a necessary evil [35]. Neither Sauve nor Desjardins had the temerity to undertake these procedures in patients! Apart from the magnitude of the procedure itself a major surgical problem was presented by the anastomotic sites and even in the experimental setting limited results and certain mortality were associated with leakage. In 1909 Kausch, from Konigsberg, was able to document the successful re-implantation of the pancreas via pancreatico-enterostomy after ampullary resection for carcinoma [37]. Fearful surgeons, although unaware of the precise nature of the problem, proposed that the anastomotic failures were due in part to the inherent nature of the pancreatic juice, which caused leakage with resultant fatality [38]. As a result of the high mortality and morbidity of intervention the development of pancreatic surgery was slow and most surgeons refrained from undertaking such procedures, and isolated case studies dominated the literature and no definable approach could be discerned. Nevertheless isolated successful procedures led to a degree of progress.

Evarts A. Graham reported the first successful "as nearly a total resection of the pancreas as possible" in an infant suffering from hypoglycemia in 1934 and in so doing inspired the future efforts of Allen O. Whipple in undertaking radical pancreatic excisional surgery (Fig. 1.1-7) [39, 40].

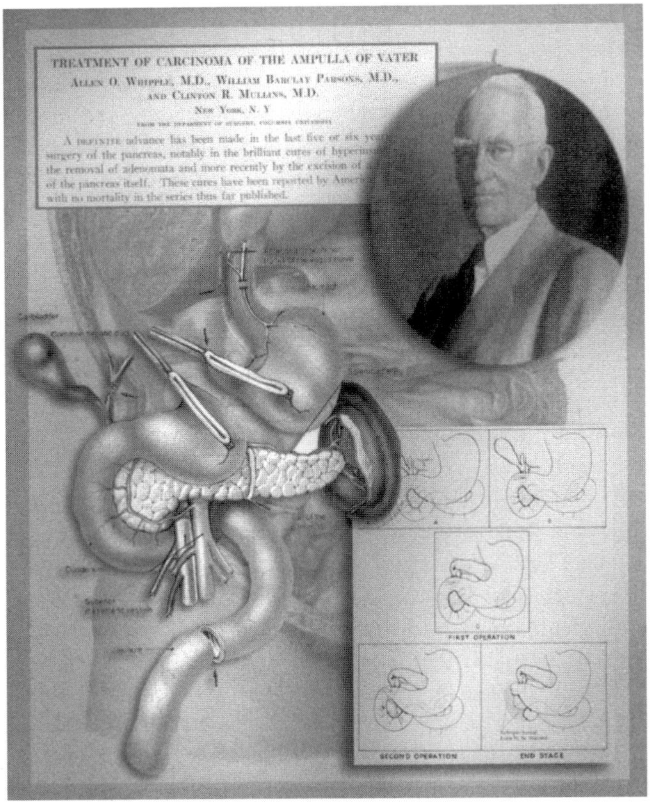

Figure 1.1-7. Allen Whipple successfully resected the pancreas and duodenum for adeno-carcinoma in 1934. This "radical" procedure was thereafter often applied to the management of the "benign" process of chronic pancreatitis.

Thus in 1935, Whipple published "Treatment of Carcinoma of the Ampulla of Vater," and in so doing laid the groundwork for modern pancreatic surgery. The operation was a two-staged procedure that initially involved a posterior gastroenterostomy and anterior cystogastrostomy. Three–four weeks later the second stage that included excision of the descending duodenum with V-shaped excision of the pancreatic head and over-sewing of the pancreatic ducts was undertaken. Whipple stated that the critical factors in the success of this operation included the determination of the extent of the disease process (thus a two-stage procedure), the avoidance of pancreatic anastamosis (pancreatic exclusion) and the use of silk suture [41]. Despite some initial failures Whipple was able to demonstrate successfully the feasibility of pancreatico-duodenal resection and confirm that a patient could not only survive the surgery but maintain an acceptable quality of life. Shortly thereafter, Alexander Brunschwig published his experience documenting the "Resection of the Head of the Pancreas and Duodenum for Carcinoma-Pancreatoduodenectomy." This description was the first radical resection of a carcinoma in the head of the pancreas and demonstrated that the complete removal of the duodenum could be undertaken without consequence [42]. In so doing, Brunschwig was the first to confirm Lester R. Dragstedt's proposal that the extirpation of the duodenum was compatible with life [43]. Despite the rigorous efforts of Brunschwig and Whipple the first total pancreatectomy is credited to Eugene W. Rockey who in 1942 undertook this atypical procedure under circumstances where the carcinoma had spread throughout the entire pancreas and no other method of treatment was possible [44]. Unfortunately, the patient died a couple of weeks after the operation, due to a presumed biliary anastamotic leak.

A further issue in the danger of pancreatic surgery was presented by the problems of excessive bleeding. As a result of prolonged biliary obstruction the resultant haemostatic diathesis rendered major surgery hazardous. The discovery of vitamin K, its biological effects and the profound relationship to hepatic function by Henrick Dam in 1938 initiated a major strategic evaluation of pancreatic surgery [45]. The entire concept of hemostasis in patients with jaundice was reviewed and as a result hemostasis in pancreatic surgery was addressed from the biliary obstructive perspective. Thus improvement of hepatic function consequent upon relief of biliary obstruction became a critical issue in defining a resolution of the bleeding. Armed with this knowledge, Whipple was able to successfully perform a one-stage procedure later that year modifying the two-stage procedure by re-anastamosis of the pancreatic duct into an enterostomy [38]. The rationale for this modification was the concern that fatty degeneration of the liver was a consequence of pancreatic exclusion. A short time previously, I. Ridgeway Trimble had independently published his own series of one-stage operations for carcinoma of the pancreas and ampulla [46]. The obvious benefit of one operation of removing anesthetic risk and avoiding adhesions soon transformed this into the accepted standard in resection of pancreatic carcinoma. By 1940 sufficient experience had been developed in pancreatic carcinoma and resection that other diseases and other areas of the pancreas could be considered amenable to intervention.

Sphincterotomy

Although the first reported depiction of the sphincter of the common bile duct was by Francis Glissen of Oxford in 1681, Ruggeri Oddi of Perugia (1887) actually is credited with the delineation of its structure and function (Fig. 1.1-4). Since that time, a considerable amount of intellectual energy has been expended towards the elucidation of its role in pancreatitis as well as biliary function. In the earlier part of the century innumerable experimental investigations were conducted regarding the diverse mechanisms thought to determine resistance to biliary and pancreatic flow. Indeed as early as 1884 Langenbuch of Berlin proposed that biliary disease was related to sphincter stenosis and actually proposed division of the muscle fibers as a method of treatment [47]. In 1901, Eugene L. Opie described the common channel theory as a mechanism of pancreatitis secondary to bile reflux and in so doing was the first to provide a rationale linking biliary disease to pancreatic pathology [6]. E. Archibald provided the critical experiments that established a definitive link between the resistance of the sphincter and pancreatitis in 1913 [48]. Proof of concept was demonstrated by application of the theory when sphincteric ablation by Archibald of a patient with recurrent pancreatitis was reported to have successfully relieved the symptoms [7]. An extrapolation of this concept led to the notion that long-standing sphincter dysfunction (stenosis) might be an etiological factor (reflux of bile into the pancreas) in the development of chronic pancreatitis and that the condition could be ameliorated by sphincterotomy. Support for this notion was provided by the work of Henry Doubilet and Ralph Colp who in 1935 undertook a series of studies which confirmed the theories of Archibald. In patients with common bile duct T-tubes the infusion of diverse substances was noted to result in pressure changes as recorded by a kymograph. In particular they noted the immediate, sustained high pressure resulting from the administration of morphine and laid the basis for the avoidance of its usage in pan-

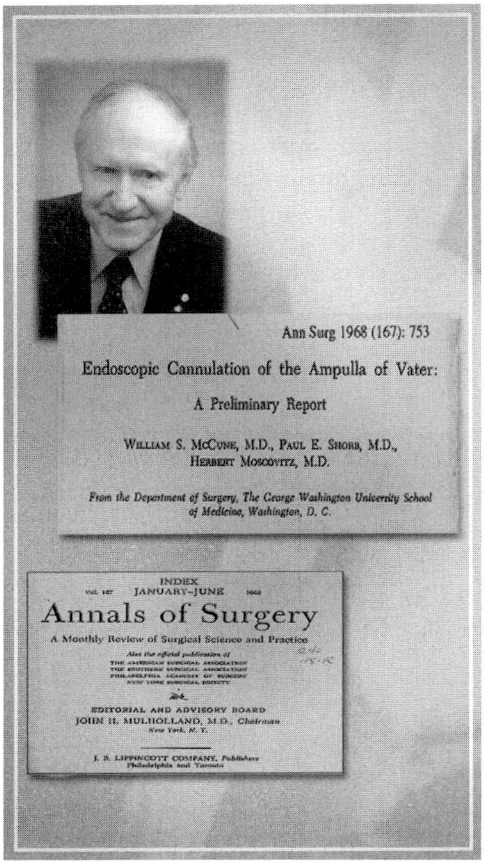

Figure 1.1-8. William S. McCune, a surgeon at George Washington University (Washington D.C.), was the first to describe the technique of endoscopic retrograde cannulation in 1968.

creatitis. Thus the demonstration of the nature of sphincteric resistance led to the conclusion that it must be of relevance to pancreatic (as well as biliary) disease in humans and laid the basis for the development of a variety of surgical interventions designed to decrease sphincteric tone and hence de facto pancreatico-biliary disease [49].

Although the classic initial sphincterotomy was credited to Archibald in 1919 the most active proponents of this concept were Henry Doubilet and John H. Mulholland, who pursued the subject over the course of many years. In 1956, they published the "Eight-Year Study of Pancreatitis and Sphincterotomy" [50].

In addition to performing a sphincterotomy, they mandated the surgical removal of the gallbladder due to alteration of dynamics of the biliary tree. In the summary of the paper, they claimed abolishment of pain, prevention of pancreatitis, and regeneration of the damaged pancreas [50]. Unfortunately, the efficacy of sphincterotomy did not live up to these miraculous claims. An amendment to the simple procedure of sphincter ablation was provided by Richard B. Cattell who utilized the technique of sphincterotomy in addition to adding a T-tube across the sphincter to stent-open the duct [51]. Although this procedure seemed ideal for patients whose disease consisted of fibrosis of the sphincter the technique was not deemed particularly effective (presumably since few had sphincter problems) and did not gain widespread acceptance.

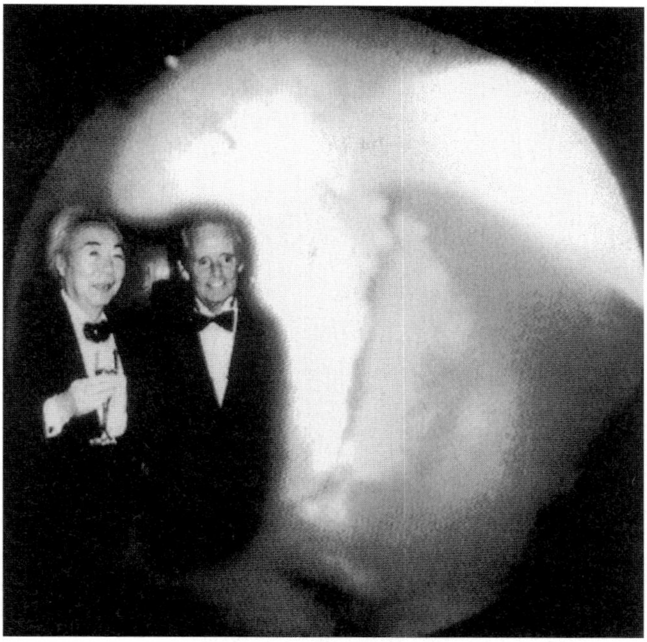

Figure 1.1-9. K. Kawai and M. Claasen (1973) independently developed the technique of endoscopic papillotomy and in so doing removed sphinterotomy from the armamentarium of the gastrointestinal surgeon.

A further diversion on the sphincterotomy odyssey was based upon a fanciful notion that sphincter spasm reflected the effects of acid from the stomach. Thus removal of acid by gastrectomy would decrease secretory function of the pancreas, diminish spasm and relieve pain. The rationale for this concept rested on the contemporary notion that chronic pancreatitis was the "summation of repeated attacks of acute pancreatitis," and that secretin generated by gastric secretion was involved in driving pancreatic ductal secretions. This theory accorded well with the then current ill-conceived understanding of the basis of chronic pancreatitis and Colp thus became a proponent of gastrectomy as a means of treating pancreatic disease of the "chronic pancreatitic type"[52]. Although seemingly based on physiological observations, this operation quickly fell into disrepute and was shortly abandoned as a pain relieving procedure.

The introduction of endoscopic retrograde cholangiopancreatography in 1968 by a surgeon McCune failed to excite initial interest in chronic pancreatic disease (Fig. 1.1-8) [53]. Subsequent advances in the development of sphincterotomy by Claasen and Kawai led to a further re-examination of the clinical efficacy of sphincterotomy (Fig. 1.1-9). P. Cotton was an early adept in the application of this novel modality to the treatment of pancreatitis culminating not only in the relief of putative obstruction by papillotomy but the introduction of stents and even the extraction of calculi which were deemed to play a role in obstruction and pain [54].

The extraction of pancreatic calculi

The first reports of pancreatic calculi as curious manifestations of the disease date as far back as the work of De Graaf in 1667 and Morgagni in 1765. However prior to1883 such case reports were for the most part confined to the realm of fascinating observations noted at postmortem study. The relationship of stones and chronic pancreatitis was however

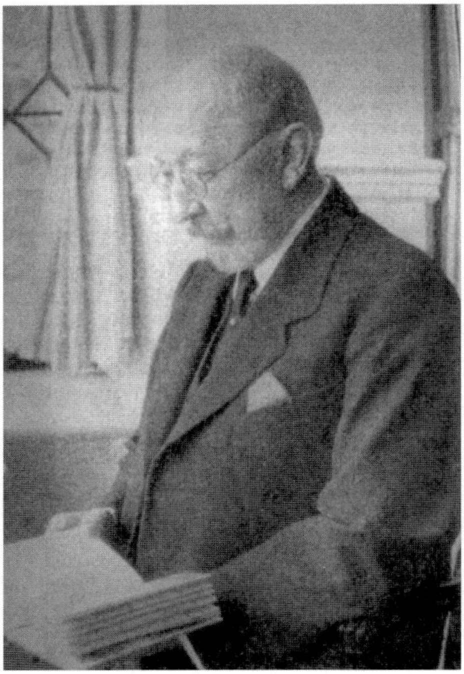

Figure 1.1-10. Sir Mayo Robson (Leeds, England) had initially proposed (in the latter part of the 19th century) that diseases of the pancreas should be non-operatively managed but thereafter became the first surgeon to perform a transpancreatic stone extraction early in the 20th century.

not specifically evident and a liberal interpretation of stones as abnormal matter and therefore likely to be the source of pain and disease (as found in kidney, salivary gland and gall bladder pathology) was therefore applied to surgical practice. In 1891, A. Pearce Gould was the first to remove pancreatic calculi from the duct of Wirsung [55], while in 1902, the first diagnosis and transduodenal surgical removal was undertaken by B. G. Moynihan of Leeds, England. Six years later, A. W. Mayo Robson, also of Leeds, performed the first transpancreatic stone extraction (Fig. 1.1-10). For the most part such surgical expeditions were random occurrences and not part of a recognizable management strategy. Indeed the entity of chronic pancreatitis was barely recognized at that time. A more interesting anecdote was provided by the interesting case of a baroness with an epigastric abscess, which after surgical drainage by Capparelli resulted in the development of a pancreatic fistula that produced hundreds of stones as observed over the subsequent six-year period [56].

Ductal drainage

Pancreatic. After the failure of sphincterotomy to adequately improve the condition of chronic pancreatitis it was proposed that the problem might lie with the inability of the former procedure to adequately decompress and allow drainage of a damaged and/or dilated distal ductal system. This inadequacy of sphincterotomy was accepted by many surgeons who thereupon embarked upon the development of strategies designed to adequately address the presumed distal component of the disease. Rather than rely upon a mere sphincter ablating procedure and its relatively local as well as possibly only transient effect, a novel direct surgical approach was proposed that would allow decompression of the pancreatic duct on a permanent basis. In 1909 Robert C. Coffey reported the effects of a variety of experimental techniques utilizing pancreatico-enterostomy and established the possibility of pancreatectomy and pancreatic anastamosis as a viable procedure. This seminal series of contributions would in fact define many of the further advances in pancreatic anastamosis and culminate in the development of the ductal drainage techniques that became ubiquitous in the management of chronic pancreatitis [57]. A report in 1921 by Walter Ellis Sistrunk was deemed important since it claimed that the successful achievement of a direct drainage procedure on the "pancreas proper" without complication had resulted in an improvement in the diabetic condition [58]. Despite such exciting initial reports the subject of direct pancreatic ductal drainage did not gain popularity until the early 1950s as most surgeons deemed direct address of the pancreas dangerous or considered pancreatic disease to be of biliary origin and therefore chose to preferentially address the subject of gall stones and bile duct drainage.

In 1954 Merlin K. Duval and Robert M. Zollinger separately and almost simultaneously published their innovative descriptions of experience using a caudal pancreaticojejunostomy [59, 60]. Duval stated that he did not accept Opie's common channel theory as *sine qua non* of pancreatitis and claimed that current information confirmed the presence of a bi-directional flow of pancreatic juice. This combined with Goethe Link's previous work on the subject of pancreatic fistula "cure" stimulated the concept of pancreatic duct obstruction as an etiology for the disease and further supported his proposal that ductal drainage would be beneficial [61]. Driven by this reasoning Duval proposed and implemented the procedure of caudal pancreaticojejunostomy drainage as an alternative treatment for chronic pancreatitis. This included mobilization of the tail of the pancreas and spleen, transection of the pancreatic duct at the junction of the body and tail with subsequent end to end anastamosis with a Roux-Y limb. In 1954 he published his positive experience, detailing a series of successful case studies although gracefully acknowledging that the final result would require the tincture of time before definitive conclusions could be drawn [59]. Zollinger claimed to be similarly encouraged by the initial results of this technique but commented on the need for further investigation as well as an "individualized surgical approach".

Despite the fact that a temporal tincture had not yet had the opportunity for review some surgeons were impressed with the logic of the Duval procedure and sought to amplify it. Thus in 1958 Puestow proposed an extension of the efficacy of drainage by opening the dilated duct of Wirsung lengthwise (filleting) and anastamosing the filleted duct to a loop of jejunum that had been similarly treated (Fig. 1.1-11) [62]. This mechanical arrangement was proposed as beneficial since each ductal branch was now able to drain directly into a new widely patent jejunal lumen rather than a single narrow distal anastamosis. Puestow termed the procedure a lateral pancreaticojejunostomy, and based upon early enthusiastic reports as to its efficacy it soon achieved a prominent role in the treatment of chronic pancreatitis associated with ductal disease. A criticism that had been leveled at the Puestow procedure was that it necessitated a splenectomy as well as mobilization of the pancreas itself to enable a distal pancreatectomy. In 1960 Robert E. Rochelle therefore proposed a judicious modification that retained the spleen and simply anastomosed the jejunum to the intact pancreas [63]. Other permutations and commutations of the ductal drainage scenario were entertained with modest success and have retained a defined, albeit limited, role in the surgical management of chronic pancreatitis.

Biliary. Despite the conclusion of the majority that a pancreatic drainage problem was the crux of the issue in chronic pancreatitis some surgeons clung steadfastly to the concept of biliary tract disease as the *modus operandi* in chronic pancreatitis. A body of liter-

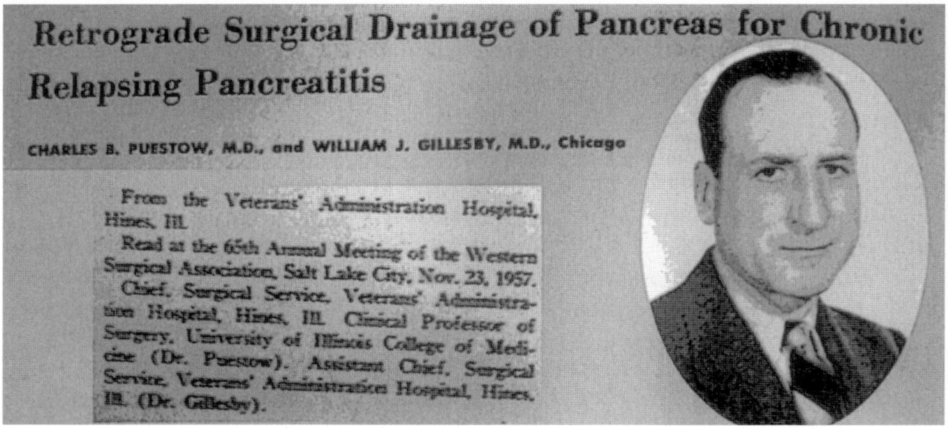
Retrograde Surgical Drainage of Pancreas for Chronic Relapsing Pancreatitis

CHARLES B. PUESTOW, M.D., and WILLIAM J. GILLESBY, M.D., Chicago

From the Veterans' Administration Hospital, Hines, Ill.

Read at the 65th Annual Meeting of the Western Surgical Association, Salt Lake City, Nov. 23, 1957.

Chief, Surgical Service, Veterans' Administration Hospital, Hines, Ill. Clinical Professor of Surgery, University of Illinois College of Medicine (Dr. Puestow). Assistant Chief, Surgical Service, Veterans' Administration Hospital, Hines, Ill. (Dr. Gillesby).

Figure 1.1-11. Charles Puestow (inset) devised the procedure of lateral pancreaticojejunostomy as a surgical treatment for "dilated duct chronic pancreatitis" in 1958.

ature therefore accumulated during the mid 20th century as attempts at relief were directed at the purported biliary component. Thus cholycystostomy, cholycystectomy, common bile duct exploration, bile duct drainage and sphincterotomy continued to be explored as avenues by which the disease could be dealt with [64–66]. Finally, as it became apparent that pancreatic drainage appeared to have some utility and biliary procedures seemed relatively unsatisfactory, attempts at transmogrifying the procedure to a biliary venue were undertaken. Thus in 1955, in an attempt to control the relapses noted with currently available biliary system intervention, Ralph F. Bowers in 1955 introduced choledochojejunostomy as a viable option [67]. This report, although not the first to propose this technique, presented criteria for the selection of patients and appeared to provide satisfactory long-term relief in most patients. This technique has however failed to withstand the Duval "acid test of time"!

Excisional surgery for chronic pancreatitis

Since the progress in the surgery of pancreatic carcinoma had resulted in a drastic reduction in morbidity and mortality it was soon accepted that an "excisional cure" for a malignant disease might have considerable merit if applied to a benign disease such as chronic pancreatitis (Table 1.1-1) (Fig. 1.1-12). Thus in 1946 O. T. Clagget performed a total pancreatectomy for chronic pancreatitis and in so doing became the first of a long line of surgeons who would undertake extensive and radical surgery for this "benign" condition [68]. Unfortunately the complications of the procedure and the severe metabolic consequences for the most part persuaded the majority that this course was less than effective and the procedure did not gain widespread acceptance. A further problem noted was that even in those who survived the operation and could come to terms with the disastrous metabolic sequelae, "phantom pain" still remained a major issue. Indeed the concept of a diabetic with no exocrine pancreatic function and dependent upon narcotics for pain relief proved to be a daunting specter for even the most hardened pancreatic surgeon.

In 1965, William J. Fry and Charles G. Child realized that the superfluity of surgical operations for the cure of pancreatitis was a result of the lack of an ideal treatment. Seek-

Table 1.1-1. Surgery for chronic pancreatitis – a timeline.

Date	Author	Procedure
1946	O.T. Clagget	*Total pancreatectomy*
	A.O. Whipple	*Pancreaticoduodenectomy*
1950	R. Colp	Gastrectomy
1954	M.K. Duva	*Caudal Pancreatojejunostomy*
1955	R.F. Bowers	*Choledochojejunostomy*
1956	H. Doubilet	*Sphincterotomy*
1958	C.B. Puestow	*Lateral Pancreatojejunostomy*
1965	W.J. Fry	*95% Distal Pancreatectomy*
1978	L.W. Traverso	*Pylorus-preserving "Whipple"*
1980	H.G. Beger	*Duodenum-preserving resection*

ing to ameliorate this state of affairs they proposed an alternative to complete resection and reported the results following a 95% distal pancreatectomy [69]. The rationale for their procedure was well conceived and addressed many of the concerns raised by the previous attempts to derive a solution for the surgical management of chronic pancreatitis. They noted that the results of sphincterotomy could not be reproduced, that resection by the technique of Whipple resulted in dissatisfaction (due to the post-operative complications entailed in the numerous anastomoses and jejunal ulceration) in addition to the fact that much residual diseased gland remained *in situ*. Lastly they were aware that there existed promising results with total pancreatectomy but that the magnitude of the resection left somewhat unacceptable metabolic consequences. They therefore proposed a procedure that would encompass the strong points of the previous excisional techniques yet obviate the disadvantages. The operation (95% distal pancreatectomy) entailed removal of the spleen, the uncinate process, and the body and the tail of the pancreas, i.e the majority of the diseased tissue, and was designed to be technically easier, reduce postoperative complications and have a higher success rate. Regrettably, this surgery also failed to absolutely attain its objectives and provided a further reminder that the surgical therapy for chronic pancreatitis remained an enigma.

Although Whipple's original two-stage pancreaticoduodenectomy spared the pylorus, he subsequently revised this and included removal of the distal stomach and entire duodenum in the one-stage procedure. A significant portion of these patients developed jejunal ulceration. Given the limited life expectancy of a patient with pancreatic carcinoma this was acceptable but in the more chronic condition of pancreatitis the issues of mucosal ulceration were significant in a population of this type. However Traverso and Longmire questioned the rationale of not preserving the pylorus for a benign condition and in 1978 applied this technique of preservation of the pylorus to patients with chronic pancreatitis with acceptable results [70].

Another refinement of the pancreaticoduodenectomy – the duodenum-preserving resection of the head of the pancreas (DPRHP) – was proposed by Hans G. Beger in 1980 [71]. Beger, having presciently noted the distinct nature of the discrete inflammatory mass in the head of the pancreas in some patients, devised a technique specifically designed to deal with this apparent subset of patients with chronic pancreatitis. It is of interest that this group of patients had been emphasized as early as 1925 by Mallet-Guy;

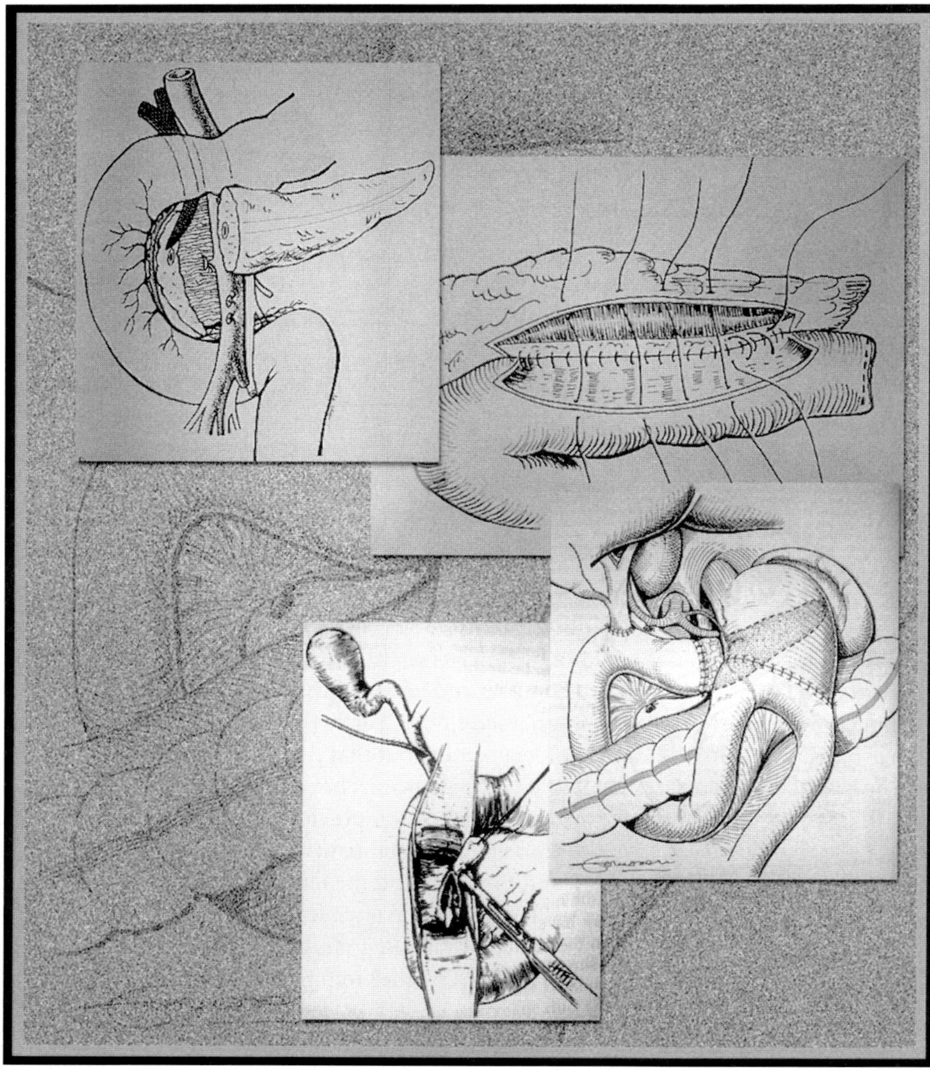

Figure 1.1-12. A variety of surgical techniques utilized in the palliation of the symptoms of chronic pancreatitis. Clockwise from top left: a) Resection of the head of the pancreas; b) lateral pancreaticojejunostomy; c) Whipple procedure and d) transduodenal sphincterotomy.

however, no surgical refinements resulted from his astute observations until the advent of Beger. The proposed surgical goal of this limited resection was relief of pain, decrease of the local complications due to the inflammation, and avoidance of the dramatic effects of exocrine and endocrine dysfunction that accompanied massive resection. Beger in fact suggested that this disease might well represent a separate phenomenon within the broad spectrum of chronic pancreatitis. Although initial reports were encouraging, it was apparent that the technique was significantly operator-dependent and that rigorous attention was required in terms of selection criteria to eliminate the majority of patients suffering from chronic pancreatitis and an emphasis on operative candidate selection was critical. Despite the fact that excision had become the favored methodology following the limited degree of success achieved with ductal drainage, W. Dean Warren in 1984 produced a brief report on the use of a denervated pancreatic flap to control pain in chronic pancreatitis [72]. The rationale of this intervention was based upon the observation that a minority of patients with chronic pancreatitis exhibited small ducts not ideally amenable to the Puestow procedure. The technique involved excision of most of the head of the pancreas while preserving the remaining pancreatic tissue but appeared to confer no special advantage and was relegated to the option section of surgical texts on the subject. Similarly dissatisfied with the results of available surgery, Frey proposed a further modification and introduced the combination of local head resection (LRH) of the pancreas with a lateral pancreaticojejunostomy [73]. This operation was designed for a specific subset of patients that had both discrete pancreatic head disease and multiple irregular segments of the pancreatic duct and initially appeared to have some advantage.

Coda

The evolution of surgery for pancreatitic disease has been arduous due both to the technical difficulties of addressing the organ and the lack of understanding of the mechanisms of the disease processes involving it. In particular the tardy advance of surgery in the management of chronic pancreatitis exemplifies these problems. Since no specific target has been identified mechanical intervention has for the most part reflected intuitive or creative attempts to address perceived pathological issues such as sphincter disease, calculi or fibrotic masses. Duct dilation and pain have often been viewed as synonymous, but neither drainage nor extirpation nor nerve section has ameliorated progress of the disease or provided predictable or effective symptomatic relief.

As regards chronic pancreatitis the past and present remain a confusion of etiology and diagnosis. Treatment remains for the most part a dramatically disappointing scenario and both patients and their physicians are frustrated. Although the remarkable technological progress exhibited by the odyssey of operative strategy from simple drainage to ductal drainage to the complex refinements of extensive resection is a testimonial to surgical skill and determination, it has been nullified to a large extent by the inability to either address the initiating factors of the disease or alter those that engender progress of the pathology. It is not unreasonable to recognize that we are facing an enigmatic disease process generically classified as "chronic pancreatitis" for want of any more specific terminology. In the light of our current knowledge and experience intervention should probably be modest in the extreme and limited to centers and individuals with expertise or involved in specific studies to determine the precise criteria and techniques necessary for optimum intervention. It is important that in charting such a course future surgeons involved in the management of chronic pancreatitis have an understanding of the historical evolution of the subject. As Theodor Billroth, the greatest of the surgical innovators, remarked: "An awareness of the past is necessary to comprehend the present and without it no consideration of the future is possible."

References

1. Metter CC. History of Medicine. Philadelphia: The Blakiston Co., 1947.
2. Daremberg C, Ruelle E. Oeuvres de Rufus d'Ephese. Paris, 1879.
3. Cawley T. A singular case of diabetes, consisting entirely in the quantity of urine with an inquiry into the different theories of that disease. Lond Med J 1788; 9: 286.
4. Modlin IM, Kidd M, Farhadi F. Bayliss and Starling and the nascence of endocrinology. Regul Pept 2000; 93(1–3): 109–23.
5. Fitz RH. Acute pancreatitis: a consideration of pancreatic hemorrhage, hemorrhagic, suppurative, and gangrenous pancreatitis, and of disseminated fat-necrosis. Medical monographs, no. 2. Boston: Cupples and Hurd, 1889: 91.
6. Opie EL. The Etiology of Acute Hemorrhagic Pancreatitis. Bull Johns Hopkins Hosp 1901; 12: 182–88.
7. Archibald E. Experimental Production of pancreatitis in animals as a result of common duct sphincter. Sugery, Gynecology and Obstetrics 1919; 28: 529.
8. Freedman S, Sakamoto K, Venu R. GP2, the homologue to the renal cast protein uromodulin, is a major component of intraductal plugs in chronic pancreatitis. J Clin Invest 1993; 92: 83.
9. Deaver JB. Chronic Pancreatitis: Its Symptomatology, Diagnosis and Treatment. Journal of American Medical Association 1911; 56: 1079.
10. Comfort M, Gambill E, Baggenstoss AH. Chronic relapsing pancreatitis: A study of 29 cases without associated disease of the biliary or gastrointestinal tract. Gastroenterology 1946; 6: 238–76.
11. Ziemssen H v. Cyclopaedia of the practice of Medicine. New York: William Wood & Co., 1878.
12. Pitchumoni CS, Viswanathan KV, GeeVarghese PJ. Ultrastructure and elemental composition of human pancreatic calculi. Pancreas 1987; 2: 152.
13. DeCaro A, Lohse J, Sarles H. Characterization of a protein isolated from pancreatic calculi of men suffering from chronic calcifying pancreatitis. Biochem Biophys Res Commun 1979; 87: 1176–82.
14. Ammann RW. Idiopathic "senile" chronic pancreatitis and pancreatic lithiasis in the aged. Gastroenterology 1984; 86: 253.
15. Zuideman P. Calcification and cirrhosis of the pancreas in patients with deficient nutrition. Doc Med Geograph Trop Amsterdam 1955; 5: 229–31.
16. Sarles H, Bernard JP, Johnson C. Pathogenesis and epidemiology of chronic pancreatitis. Annu Rev Med 1989; 40: 453–68.
17. Bordalo O et al. Newer concept for the pathogenesis of chronic alcoholic pancreatitis. Am J Gastroenterol 1977; 68(3): 278–85.
18. Braganza JM. The pathogenesis of chronic pancreatitis. Qjm 1996; 89(4): 243–50.
19. Kloeppel G. Pathology of chronic pancreatitis and pancreatic pain. Acta Chir Scand 1990; 156(4): 261–5.
20. Sahel J, Sarles H. Modifications of pure human pancreatic juice induced by chronic alcohol consumption. Dig Dis Sci 1979; 24(12): 897–905.
21. Singer M, Gyr K, Sarles H. Revised Classification of Pancreatitis. Gastroenterology 1985; 89: 683–90.
22. Orr RB, Warren KW. Continuous epidural analgesia in acute pancreatitis. Lahey Clin Bull 1950; 6: 204–10.
23. Fontaine R, Forster E, Stefanini C. Résultats éloignes de 63 splanchnicectomies pour diverse affections (en dehors de l'hypertension artérielle chronique permanente). Lyon chir 1946; 41: 279–300.
24. Leung JW, Bowen-Wright M, Aveling W. Celiac plexus block for pain control in pancreatic cancer and chronic pancreatitis. Br J Surg 1983; 70: 730.
25. Osler W. Comment on Medicine. American Journal of Medical Science 1902; 123: 904.
26. Salomon H. Organotherapie der Fettstühle bei Pankreaserkrankung. Klin Wochenschr 1902; 39: 45–8.

27. Malfertheiner P et al. Treatment of pain in chronic pancreatitis by inhibition of pancreatic secretion with octreotide. Gut 1995; 36(3): 450–4.
28. Toskes PP. Medical management of chronic pancreatitis. Scand J Gastroenterol Suppl 1995; 208: 74–80.
29. Senn N, American Surgical Association. The surgery of the pancreas, as based upon experiments and clinical researches. Trans Amer Surg Ass 1886; 4: 99–232.
30. Modlin IM. The History of Gastroenterology at the Millenium. Milano: Healthnext, 2000.
31. Robson M. Pancreatitis. American Journal of Medical Science 1902; 123: 168–9.
32. Graaf RD, Packe C. De succo pancreatico; or, A physical and anatomical treatise of the nature and office of the pancreatick juice. London: N. Brook, 1676: [24], 151, [17] plates.
33. Brunner JC v. Experimenta nova circa pancreas : accedit diatribe de lympha & genuino pancreatis usu. 1683, Amstelædami: apud Henr. Wetstenium [16], 168, [8], 4 leaves of plates (2 fold.).
34. Halsted WS. Contribution to the Surgery of the Bile Passages, especially of the Common Bile-Duct. Boston Medical and Surgical Journal 1899; 141(26): 645–54.
35. Sauve L. Des Pancréatectomies et Spécialement de la Pancréatectomie Céphalique. Rev Chir 1908; 37: 113–52, 335–85.
36. Desjardins A. Technique de la Pancreatectomie. Rev Chir 1907; 35: 945–73.
37. Kausch W. Das Carcinom der Papilla Duodeni und seine radikale Entfernung. Beitr klin Chir 1912; 78: 471–624.
38. Whipple AO. Present-Day Surgery of the Pancreas. The New England Journal of Medicine 1942; 226(13): 515–26.
39. Graham EA, Hartmann AF. Subtotal Resection of the Pancreas for Hypoglycaemia. Surgery, Gynecology and Obstetrics 1934; 59: 474–9.
40. Whipple AO. Observations on Radical Surgery for Lesions of the Pancreas. Surgery, Gynecology and Obstetrics 1946; 82(6): 623–31.
41. Whipple AO, Parsons WB, Mullins CR. Treatment of Carcinoma of the Ampulla of Vater. Annals of Surgery 1935; 102(4): 763–79.
42. Brunschwig A. Resection of the Head of Pancreas and Duodenum for Carcinoma-Pancreatoduodenectomy. Surg Gynecol Obstet 1937; 65: 681–4.
43. Dragstedt LR et al. Extirpation of Duodenum. Am J Physiol 1918; 46: 584.
44. Rockey EW. Total Pancreatectomy for Carcinoma. Annals of Surgery 1943; 118(4): 603–11.
45. Dam H, Glavind J. The Clotting Power of Human and Mammalian Blood in Relation to Vitamin K. Acta med Scandinav 1938; 96: 108–28.
46. Trimble IR, Parsons JW, Sherman CP. A One Stage Operation for the Cure of Carcinoma of the Ampulla of Vater and of the Head of the Pancreas. Sugery, Gynecology and Obstetrics 1941; 73: 711–22.
47. Grage TB et al. Stenosis of the Sphincter of Oddi. Surgery 1960; 48: 304.
48. Archibald E. Ideas Concerning the Causation of Some Cases of Pancreatitis. Canadian Journal of Medical Science 1913; 33: 263.
49. Doubilet H, Colp R. Resistance of the Sphincter of Oddi in the Human. Surgery, Gynecology and Obstetrics 1937; 64: 622–33.
50. Doubilet H, Mulholland JH. Eight-Year Study of Pancreatitis and Sphincterotomy. The Journal of the American Medical Association 1956; 160(7): 521–8.
51. Cattell RB, Warren KW. Surgery of the pancreas. Philadelphia: Saunders, 1953: 374.
52. Richman A, Colp R. Chronic Relapsing Pancreatitis Treatment by Subtotal Gastrectomy and Vagotomy. Annals of Surgery 1950; 131(2): 145–58.
53. McCune WS, Shorb PE, Moscovitz H. Endoscopic Cannulation of the ampulla of Vater: a preliminary report. Ann Surg 1968; 167: 752–6.
54. Cotton PB et al. Comparative clinical impact of endoscopic pancreatography, grey-scale ultrasonography, and computed tomography (EMI scanning) in pancreatic disease: preliminary report. Gut 1978; 19(8): 679–84.
55. Gould AP. A Case of acute intestinal obstruction relieved by operation: death from intestinal toxaemia on the ninth day after operation. Tr Clin Soc Lond 1897–98; xxxi: 47–55.

56. Haggard W, Kirtley JJA. Pancreatic Calculi. Annals of Surgery 1939; 109(5): 809–26.
57. Coffey RC. Pancreato-Enterostomy and Pancreatectomy. Annals of Surgery 1909; 50: 1238–64.
58. Sistrunk WE. The Surgical Removal of Pancreatic Stones. Annals of Surgery 1921; 74: 380–4.
59. DuVal MKJ. Caudal pancreatico-jejunostomy for chronic relapsing pancreatitis. Annals of Surgery 1954; 140(6): 775–85.
60. Zollinger RM, Luther J, Keith M, Ellison EH. Pancreatitis. The New England Journal of Medicine 1954; 251(13): 497–502.
61. Link G. The Treatment of Chronic Pancreatitis by Pancreatostomy. Annals of Surgery 1911; 138: 768–82.
62. Puestow CB, Gilleesby EJ. Retrograde surgical drainage of pancreas for chronic relapsing pancreatitis. Arch Surg 1958; 76: 898.
63. Partington PF, Rochelle RE. Modified Procedure for the Retrograde Drainage of the Pancreatic Duct. Annals of Surgery 1960; 6: 1037–43.
64. Rousselot LM, Sanchez-Ubeda R, Giannelli S. Choledochoenterostomy in Chronic Relapsing Pancreatitis: A Study of Five Cases with Prolonged Followup Observation. N Engl J Med 1954; 250: 268.
65. Barclay S. Operative Relief of Recurrent Pancreatitis. New Zealand M J 1950; 49: 419.
66. Bowers RF. Surgical Therapy for Chronic Pancreatitis. Surgery 1951; 30: 116.
67. Bowers RF. Choledochojejunostomy – Its Ability to Control Chronic Recurring Pancreatitis. Annals of Surgery 1955; 142(4): 682–9.
68. Clagget OT. Total Pancreatectomy; A Symposium Presenting Four Successful Cases with Metabolic Studies. Proc Staff Mayo Clinic 1946; 21: 25–46.
69. Fry WJ and C.G.D. Child. Ninety-five per cent distal pancreatectomy for chronic pancreatitis. Ann Surg 1965; 162(4): 543–9.
70. Traverso LW, Longmire WP Jr. Preservation of the pylorus in pancreaticoduodenectomy. Surg Gynecol Obstet 1978; 146(6): 959–62.
71. Beger HG, Witte C, Krautzberger W, Bittner R. [Experiences with duodenum-sparing pancreas head resection in chronic pancreatitis.] [Article in German] Chirurg 1980 May; 51(5): 303–7.
72. Warren WD et al. A denervated pancreatic flap for control of chronic pain in pancreatitis. Surg Gynecol Obstet 1984; 159(6): 581–3.
73. Frey CF, Smith GJ. Description and rationale of a new operation for chronic pancreatitis. Pancreas 1987; 2(6): 701–7.

2 Molecular pathogenesis and genetic alterations in chronic pancreatitis

2.1 Epidemiology of chronic pancreatitis and the risk of cancer

A. B. Lowenfels, P. Maisonneuve

Introduction

Chronic pancreatitis is a complex disease, afflicting heavy drinkers, but also associated with several other causes. Although much is known about the disease there is still a large group of patients, perhaps 20% of the total, where the exact cause is unknown. Even more confusing, the reasons why most heavy drinkers do not develop pancreatitis are unknown. In this section we will review the epidemiology of chronic pancreatitis and the relationship between chronic pancreatitis and cancer.

Descriptive characteristics

Frequency

Unlike pancreatic cancer or other forms of cancer, there are no registries that report the frequency of pancreatic disease in a systematic, organized, reliable manner. Information about chronic pancreatitis is particularly difficult to assess because of the confusion between acute pancreatitis, acute recurrent pancreatitis, and chronic pancreatitis. Furthermore, only recently have there been fairly uniform guidelines for the diagnosis of chronic pancreatitis.

The only available information regarding the occurrence of chronic pancreatitis comes from reports from centers with a large experience in treating this disorder. Such reports suffer from a bias in that patients with this difficult disease could be selectively referred to treatment centers specializing in the management of this pancreatitis.

Starting in about 1985 in northern Germany, Lankisch has maintained a population-based registry of patients with pancreatic disease who reside in the county of Luneburg, a region of approximately 150,000 persons. In this population, the estimated frequency is about 7/100,000 per year [1]. Nearly all of these patients had CAT scans, so the diagnosis of chronic pancreatitis seems especially secure.

In an earlier period in Copenhagen, the reported frequency of chronic pancreatitis was estimated to be about 7–10 per 100,000 – a figure that is similar to the estimate from the adjacent region of northern Germany [2].

In the United States, we can estimate the incidence of chronic pancreatitis from hospital discharge statistics. For white populations, the annual discharge rate in 1987, a period comparable to the two previously cited estimates, was 5.7 per 100,000 for males and 7.6 per 100,000 for females. These figures seem somewhat unreliable because chronic pancreatitis is known to be more frequent in males than females. Nevertheless, all three estimates – from Denmark, Germany, and the USA – are reasonably close. Chronic pancreatitis is clearly an uncommon disease – significantly less frequent than alcohol-induced liver cirrhosis.

Age

It is difficult to establish the exact date of onset of chronic pancreatitis, especially when it has been preceded by several attacks of acute pancreatitis. In a large collaborative report, the mean age of onset of chronic pancreatitis in all subjects was 44.6 ± 12.6 SD years [3]. The range of ages is wide, because certain types of pancreatitis, such as hereditary pancreatitis, begin in adolescence. The mean age at the onset of pancreatitis is usually several years earlier than the age at developing alcoholic cirrhosis.

Sex

Alcohol consumption is the strongest risk factor for chronic pancreatitis, so it is not surprising that males comprise about 75% of all patients in most centers. But when females do develop alcohol-induced chronic pancreatitis, the disease course resembles chronic alcoholic pancreatitis in males.

Race

There are significant racial differences in the frequency of chronic pancreatitis. Both male and female black populations in the USA have higher discharge rates for chronic pancreatitis than whites. Susceptibility to alcohol-related diseases differs by race: blacks are more likely to develop pancreatitis, whereas whites are more susceptible to cirrhosis [4]. The explanation for the uneven racial distribution is not immediately obvious. There is little evidence that black populations drink more than white populations. Smoking is another suggested risk factor for pancreatitis, but again, there is no strong evidence for excess smoking in black populations. The explanation might be that the ability to degrade and detoxify tobacco products differs in different racial groups.

In addition to the increased risk of chronic pancreatitis in blacks, there are several reports of tropical pancreatitis occurring in populations native to India and Africa. It is unknown whether this represents racial susceptibility based on genetic differences, or environmental factors, such as diet or climate.

Inherited forms of chronic pancreatitis

Hereditary pancreatitis

This rare form of pancreatitis, now known to be caused by mutations in the trypsinogen gene on chromosome 7q35 provides an excellent model to observe the progression from acute to chronic pancreatitis [5]. Attacks of pain, vomiting in the first decade or two of life are followed by progressive pancreatic dysfunction, characterized by calcification and diabetes. Eventually, about a third of patients will develop pancreas cancer.

Cystic fibrosis

Cystic fibrosis (CF) is the commonest autosomal recessive inherited disorder of Caucasian populations. In addition to the lungs, the pancreas is severely damaged *in utero* or soon after birth. Pancreatic dysfunction is of sufficient severity to require daily pancreatic enzyme replacement therapy in nearly all patients with CF. Only about 10% of CF patients are pancreatic sufficient; these patients can then develop pancreatitis.

Time trends

Since most cases of chronic pancreatitis are caused by alcohol, country or population-specific changes in alcohol consumption should be followed after a suitable lag period by similar changes in the frequency of chronic pancreatitis. Data from the United Kingdom confirms this hypothesis [6]. As seen in Figure 2.1-1, during the period from 1960–1984, alcohol consumption doubled and was followed after a lag period of six years, by a three-fold increase in the frequency of hospital discharges from chronic pancreatitis.

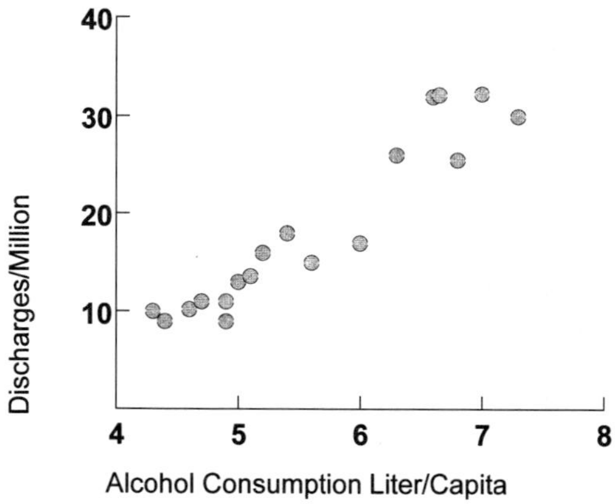

Figure 2.1-1. Relationship between alcohol consumption and hospital discharge rate for chronic pancreatitis in the UK during the years 1960–1984; (with permission from the BMJ Publishing Group, redrawn [6]).

Etiology

Alcohol

As pointed out in the introductory section, heavy consumption of alcohol is the major risk factor for pancreatitis. Although the type of alcohol consumed may be a risk factor, far more important is the quantity of alcohol consumed and the duration of heavy drinking. Figure 2.1-2 presents revised data from a case-control study in France comparing al-

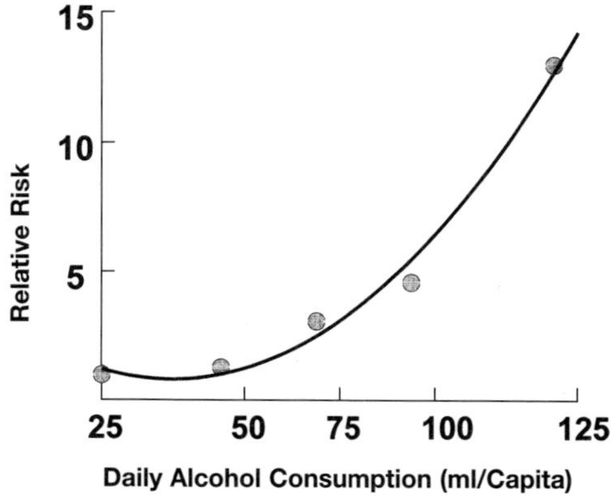

Figure 2.1-2. Alcohol consumption and the risk of chronic pancreatitis in male French patients from Marseille. Data based on 193 patients with chronic pancreatitis and 490 hospitalized patients without organic disease of the digestive tract. Relative risks are not corrected for smoking [7].

cohol consumption in 193 male patients with pancreatitis (with and without calcification) and alcohol consumption in 490 patients without pancreatic or hepatic disease [7]. As can be seen, the risk of chronic pancreatitis rises sharply with increased intake of alcohol. These findings are reminiscent of similar findings relating alcohol intake with liver cirrhosis.

Smoking

Heavy drinkers are usually heavy smokers, so it has been difficult to assess the importance of smoking as an independent risk factor for chronic pancreatitis. From several studies in different populations, it does appear that smoking is a separate cause for this disease. Nearly all case-control studies have found an association between smoking and chronic pancreatitis, independent of alcohol consumption [8–12].

Risk of cancer in chronic pancreatitis

Is there an increased risk of cancer in patients with chronic pancreatitis? Virchow, in the 19th century, believed that many cases of cancer could be explained by antecedent chronic inflammatory disease. Cancer following chronic pancreatitis would certainly fit this model. There are numerous anecdotal reports of individual patients with chronic pancreatitis who have subsequently developed pancreas cancer. Brat has reported several patients in whom premalignant changes were detected as long as ten years prior to tumor formation [13].

Most case-control studies of pancreatic cancer have shown that pancreatitis increases the risk of pancreas cancer, but because chronic pancreatitis is a relatively rare disease, few patients with pancreatic cancer will have had previous attacks of pancreatitis. Furthermore, a recent attack of pancreatitis unrelated to alcohol or gallstones may signify the onset of pancreatic cancer. Nevertheless, the majority of case-control studies show an association between pre-existing chronic pancreatitis and pancreatic cancer [14].

Record linkage studies also show an association between previous hospitalization for chronic pancreatitis and the eventual development of pancreatic cancer. Record linkage studies are dependent upon an accurate discharge diagnosis and upon the ability to obtain complete linkage of patients in two different data sets. Of the three record linkage studies which have been reported, all have shown a relationship between a hospital admission for pancreatitis and a later hospitalization for pancreas cancer [15–17].

Cohort studies are regarded as providing the strongest type of epidemiologic evidence. Three such studies have been published – all show a strong link between chronic pancreatitis and an eventual diagnosis of pancreatic cancer [3, 18, 19].

The available evidence confirms an association between chronic pancreatitis and pancreatic cancer. What is debatable is the strength of the relationship, which ranges from a two-fold increased risk in some studies to a 15-fold risk in other studies.

Special types of pancreatitis and pancreatic cancer

Recent studies on hereditary pancreatitis, a rare autosomal dominant disease, have demonstrated a remarkably high risk of cancer [20]. The disease resembles more common forms of pancreatitis with respect to symptoms and findings, but the onset is usually within the first two decades of life. Nearly always other family members in multiple generations have had attacks of pancreatitis. The risk of pancreas cancer is about 50 times greater than similarly aged patients and the life-type risk of pancreatic cancer is about 30%. Why do these patients have such a high risk of pancreas cancer? The long duration of pre-existing pancreatitis is the probable explanation. Although there are several different types of genetic defects in the trypsinogen gene that produces this disease, as yet there is insufficient evidence to determine if the risk of cancer is related to a particular genetic mutation.

Tropical pancreatitis is another unusual form of pancreatitis, occurring mainly in India and in sub-Saharan Africa – areas where pancreatic cancer is rare [21]. Similar to hereditary pancreatitis, the disease begins in early life, does not appear to be associated with alcohol, and has a high risk of pancreatic cancer. In one report six pancreatic cancers were observed compared to 0.06 expected, yielding a risk ratio of 100.

Chronic pancreatitis and pancreatic cancer: which patients are at risk?

The cumulative risk of pancreatic cancer in patients with common forms of pancreatitis over about a 20-year period is about 5%. Therefore, even though patients with chronic pancreatitis are at increased risk of developing this lethal cancer, most patients will not develop cancer of the pancreas. Are there any subgroups that are at specially high risk?

Age and sex

Age is a strong predictor of pancreas cancer and therefore it is not surprising that most patients with chronic pancreatitis who develop pancreatic cancer are in their 60s or older. What is somewhat surprising is that the age at developing pancreas cancer is only a few years younger than observed in patients without a background history of pancreatitis. Even though there is an excess of male patients with chronic pancreatitis, sex does not appear to predict the subsequent development of cancer.

Duration of pancreatitis

Patients who develop pancreatitis at an early age, as in the hereditary type, have a high risk of pancreatic cancer. It is unclear whether the high risk is caused by the prolonged duration of chronic pancreatitis or whether there are age-specific differences in the response of the pancreas to chronic pancreatitis. It is likely that in both hereditary pancreatitis and tropical pancreatitis, the excessive risk is associated with the early onset and prolonged duration of pancreatitis rather than with the specific type of pancreatitis.

Alcohol and smoking

In several case-control studies, alcohol has not been found to increase the risk of pancreatic cancer. This finding is somewhat surprising, given that heavy drinkers who develop pancreatitis are at increased risk of chronic pancreatitis. The explanation may be that in case-control studies, there are very few patients or controls who drink sufficient quantities of alcohol to produce chronic pancreatitis.

Smoking as an additional risk factor for developing pancreas cancer in patients with pre-existing pancreatitis has received little attention. However, in hereditary pancreatitis, smoking appears to be an independent risk factor. As in most case control studies of pancreas cancer, smoking doubles the already high risk of cancer in patients with this genetic abnormality.

Genetic factors, chronic pancreatitis, and pancreatic cancer

There are several genetic factors now known to increase the risk of pancreas cancer, but in only a few types does the mutation cause pancreatitis as part of the phenotype. Known current examples include hereditary pancreatitis, cystic fibrosis, and the unusual familial pancreatic cancer kindreds reported by Brentnall and co-workers [22].

K-ras

Oncogenes such as K-ras are found in a small percentage of patients with chronic pancreatitis and are known to be strongly associated with pancreatic cancer [23]. Additional long term follow-up of K-ras positive pancreatitis patients will be required before we can determine if K-ras positivity in patients with chronic pancreatitis predicts the future development of pancreatic cancer.

Table 2.1-1 lists some of the main factors that are currently believed to be predictors of pancreas cancer in patients with chronic pancreatitis.

Table 2.1-1. Risk factors for developing pancreas cancer in patients with chronic pancreatitis.

Factor	Association with pancreas cancer
Age	A risk for pancreas cancer in persons with and without a history of chronic pancreatitis
Smoking	Appears to be an independent risk factor in certain forms of pancreatitis
Type pancreatitis	High risk of pancreatic cancer in some types of pancreatitis may be explained by long duration of pancreatitis
Genetic factors	Probable interaction between smoking and genetic mutations associated with CP
Duration of pancreatitis	Risk increases with increased duration of pancreatitis
Pre-malignant changes	Anecdotal evidence links pre-malignant pathologic changes in patients with pancreatitis and subsequent development of pancreas cancer.
K-ras	Positive in about 5% of patients with chronic pancreatitis and about 80% of patients with pancreatic cancer. Additional prospective follow-up studies needed

Summary

In most westernized countries, heavy consumption of alcohol is the commonest cause of chronic pancreatitis. The few available population-based estimates of the frequency of chronic pancreatitis suggest that the incidence is about 5–10 per 100,000 per year. The frequency of chronic pancreatitis is much lower than the frequency of heavy drinking, and we do not know why so few heavy drinkers develop chronic pancreatitis. Several studies suggest that smoking is an additional important co-factor.

The combined evidence from several case-control, cohort, and record linkage studies confirms an association between chronic pancreatitis and the subsequent development of pancreatic cancer. Only about 5% of patients with common forms of pancreatitis will develop pancreatic cancer, but in patients with hereditary pancreatitis the risk is much higher. The risk of pancreatic cancer is strongly dependent upon the duration of the underlying pancreatitis.

Acknowledgments

Supported by grants from the C. D. Smithers Foundation, Inc. and Solvay Pharmaceuticals.

References

1. Lankisch PG, Assmus D, Pflichthofer D, Maisonneuve P, Lowenfels AB. The burden of pancreatic disease in a well-defined population. Gastroenterology 1998; 114[4]: A24. Ref Type: Abstract.
2. Copenhagen Pancreatitis Study Group. Copenhagen Pancreatitis Study. An interim report from a prospective epidemiological multicentre study. Scand J Gastroent 1981; 16: 305–12.
3. Lowenfels AB, Maisonneuve P, Cavallini G, Ammann RW, Lankisch PG, Andersen JR et al. Pancreatitis and the risk of pancreatic cancer. International Pancreatitis Study Group. N Engl J Med 1993; 328: 1433–7.
4. Lowenfels AB, Maisonneuve P, Grover H, Gerber E, Korsten MA, Antunes MT et al. Racial factors and the risk of chronic pancreatitis. Am J Gastroenterol 1999; 94(3): 790–4.
5. Whitcomb DC. Genetic predispositions to acute and chronic pancreatitis. Med Clin North Am 2000; 84(3): 531–47, vii.
6. Johnson CD, Hosking S. National statistics for diet, alcohol consumption, and chronic pancreatitis in England and Wales, 1960–88. Gut 1991; 32(11): 1401–5.
7. Durbec JP, Sarles H. Multicenter survey of the etiology of pancreatic diseases. Relationship between the relative risk of developing chronic pancreatitis and alcohol, protein and lipid consumption. Digestion 1978; 18(5–6): 337–50.
8. Bourliere M, Barthet M, Berthezene P, Durbec JP, Sarles H. Is tobacco a risk factor for chronic pancreatitis and alcoholic cirrhosis? Gut 1991; 32: 1392–5.
9. Lowenfels AB, Zwemer FL, Jhangiani S, Pitchumoni CS. Pancreatitis in a Native American Indian population. Pancreas 1987; 2: 694–7.
10. Talamini G, Bassi C, Falconi M, Frulloni L, Di Francesco V, Vaona B et al. Cigarette smoking: an independent risk factor in alcoholic pancreatitis. Pancreas 1996; 12: 131–7.
11. Yen S, Hsieh C, MacMahon B. Consumption of alcohol and tobacco and other risk factors for pancreatitis. Am J Epidemiol 1982; 116: 407–14.
12. Lin Y, Tamakoshi A, Matsuno S, Takeda K, Hayakawa T, Kitagawa M et al. Nationwide epidemiological survey of chronic pancreatitis in Japan [see comments]. J Gastroenterol 2000; 35(2): 136–41.
13. Brat DJ, Lillemoe KD, Yeo CJ, Warfield PB, Hruban RH. Progression of pancreatic intraductal neoplasias to infiltrating adenocarcinoma of the pancreas. Am J Surg Pathol 1998; 22(2): 163–9.
14. Lowenfels AB, Maisonneuve P, Lankisch PG. Chronic pancreatitis and other risk factors for pancreatic cancer. Gastroenterol Clin North Am 1999; 28(3): 673–85, x.
15. Bansal P, Sonnenberg A. Pancreatitis is a risk factor for pancreatic cancer. Gastronenterology 1995; 109: 247–51.
16. Ekbom A, McLaughlin JK, Karlsson BM, Nyren O, Gridley G, Adami HO et al. Pancreatitis and pancreatic cancer: a population-based study. J Natl Cancer Inst 1994; 86: 625–7.
17. Karlsson BM, Ekbom A, Josefsson S, McLaughlin JK, Fraumeni JF, Nyren O. The risk of pancreatic cancer following pancreatitis: an association due to confounding? Gastroenterology 1997; 113: 587–92.
18. Madeira J, Pessione D, Malka P et al. The risk of pancreatic adenocarcinoma (PA) in patients with chronic pancreatitis (CP): Myth or Reality? Gastroenterology 1998; 114: 481. Ref Type: Abstract.

19. Talamini G, Falconi M, Bassi C et al. Incidence of cancer in the course of chronic pancreatitis. Amer J Gastroenterol 1999; 94: 1253–60.
20. Lowenfels AB, Maisonneuve P, DiMagno EP, Elitsur Y, Gates LK Jr, Perrault J et al. Hereditary pancreatitis and the risk of pancreatic cancer. International Hereditary Pancreatitis Study Group. J Natl Cancer Inst 1997; 89(6): 442–6.
21. Chari ST, Mohan V, Pitchumoni CS, Viswanathan M, Madanagopalan N, Lowenfels AB. Risk of pancreatic carcinoma in tropical calcifying pancreatitis: an epidemiologic study. Pancreas 1994; 9: 62–6.
22. Brentnall TA, Bronner MP, Byrd DR, Haggitt RC, Kimmey MB. Early diagnosis and treatment of pancreatic dysplasia in patients with a family history of pancreatic cancer. Ann Intern Med 1999; 131(4): 247–55.
23. Lohr M, Maisonneuve P, Lowenfels AB. K-Ras mutations and benign pancreatic disease [In Process Citation]. Int J Pancreatol 2000; 27(2): 93–103.

2.2 Growth factors in repair and remodeling in chronic pancreatitis

M. Korc, H. Friess, J. Kleeff, M. W. Büchler

Introduction

The mammalian pancreas consists of acinar cells that synthesize and secrete digestive enzymes, duct cells that produce bicarbonate rich fluid, and islet cells that release insulin and other hormones into the circulation. The acinar cell of the exocrine pancreas constitutes the largest component of the pancreas by mass. Its function is regulated by gastrointestinal hormones and neurotransmitters, as well as by polypeptide growth factors. The locally produced growth factors can act through autocrine, paracrine, intracrine, and juxtacrine mechanisms to further regulate these functions. In addition, as a consequence of the presence of an intra-pancreatic portal circulation, acinar and ductal cells are exposed to high levels of islet cell hormones. These endocrine hormones act through a so-called proxicrine mechanism to further modulate pancreatic exocrine functions [1]. Partly as a result of the trophic actions of hormones and growth factors, the exocrine pancreas can synthesize large quantities of digestive enzymes throughout the life of an individual.

Chronic pancreatitis

Chronic pancreatitis (CP), an inflammatory disease of the pancreas, is characterized by dysplastic ducts, foci of proliferating ductal cells, acinar cell degeneration, and fibrosis [2]. Consequently, patients with CP can exhibit variable degrees of pancreatic exocrine and endocrine dysfunction [2]. Several underlying conditions can contribute to an increased incidence of CP. These include, but are not limited to, excessive ethanol intake, pancreatic stone formation, and recurrent episodes of acute pancreatitis [3]. In certain parts of the Indian subcontinent, a condition termed chronic calcific pancreatitis or tropical pancreatitis is relatively common [4]. It is often associated with insulin-resistant diabetes mellitus, which is sometimes described as fibrocalculous pancreatic diabetes [4]. In Western countries, subtle mutations in the CFTR gene have been implicated etiologically in the genesis of some cases of chronic pancreatitis [5, 6].

The molecular mechanisms that lead to the perturbations that occur in most patients with CP are not known. In general, however, genetic alterations such as K-*ras* mutations may be seen in lesions within the larger pancreatic ducts in CP, but not within the pancreatic parenchyma [7]. Furthermore, p53 mutations are rare in CP [8]. This review will focus on the role of tyrosine kinase receptors and their ligands, which have been implicated in the pathobiology of CP, and summarize the evidence that these growth factors may be involved in the repair and remodeling process that occurs in this condition.

Expression of tyrosine kinase receptors and their ligands in chronic pancreatitis

Multiple alterations in the expression of tyrosine kinase receptors and their ligands have been reported in CP (Table 2.2-1). Thus, the epidermal growth factor (EGF) receptor (EGFR) is overexpressed in the pancreatic acinar and ductal cells in CP to the same extent as in pancreatic cancer cells within the pancreas of pancreatic cancer patients [9]. However, by comparison with levels observed in pancreatic cancer, erbB-3 is only modestly overexpressed in CP [10], whereas erbB-2 expression is increased only in a rare condition in which CP is associated with enlargement of the head of the pancreas [11]. Some of the ligands that bind to EGFR, including EGF and transforming growth factor-alpha (TGF-α), are also expressed at high levels in CP [9], as is CRIPTO, an EGF-like growth factor that does not bind to EGFR [12].

Table 2.2-1. Examples of tyrosine kinase receptors and their ligands that are overexpressed in chronic pancreatitis.

Receptors	Ligands
EGF receptor	**EGF, TGF-α**
erbB2, rarely	
erbB3, mildly	
FGF receptors	FGF1, -2, -5, -7
PDGF receptor-β	PDGF B chain
TrkA	NGF
See text for details	

Several additional growth factors and their tyrosine kinase receptors are expressed at high levels in the pancreas in CP (Table 2.2-1). These include multiple fibroblast growth factors (FGF1, FGF2, FGF5, and FGF7) and their high affinity receptors, which are often found in the acinar and ductal cells in CP [13–16]. However, FGF-5 is also abundant in the inflammatory cells in CP [14]. By contrast, the β isoform of the platelet-derived growth factor (PDGF) receptor and its ligand (PDGF B chain) are present at relatively high levels in the acinar and ductal cells in CP, as well as in the endocrine islets, the adjoining fibroblasts, the endothelial cells and the inflammatory cells [17]. Furthermore, TrkA and its nerve growth factor (NGF) ligand are especially abundant in the perineurium and ganglia within the pancreas [18]. These findings indicate that in CP in humans there is overexpression of several important tyrosine kinase receptors and their ligands, which exhibit selective localization that implies specific regulatory functions. In addition, the fact that both IGF-II and insulin are abundant in the endocrine islets, in conjunction with the existence of an intra-pancreatic portal circulation, implies a potential for proxicrine-mediated activation of signaling pathways that may also contribute to regeneration and repair processes.

Pancreatic ductal adenocarcinomas (PDAC) also overexpress many of these receptors and their mitogenic growth factors, including EGFR and its ligands [19]. It could be argued, therefore, that this overexpression is an epi-phenomenon that is not biologically important. Numerous lines of evidence, however, mitigate against this possibility. Thus, the concomitant presence in PDAC of EGFR and either EGF or TGF-α is associated with disease progression and decreased patient survival [20]. Overexpression erbB-3 [10] or aberrant cytoplasmic localization of amphiregulin [21] is also associated with decreased survival. Inhibition of EGFR signaling, following transfection or retroviral infection with a construct encoding a truncated EGFR, markedly attenuates the growth of PANC-1 pancreatic cancer cells *in vitro*, and enhances their chemosensitivity to cisplatinum [22]. The overexpressed EGFR can serve as a portal of entry for pseudomonas-coupled TGF-α (TP-40), which then acts to inhibit the growth of pancreatic cancer cells [23]. An amphiregulin antisense oligonucleotide inhibits amphiregulin synthesis and release, and suppresses the growth of T3M4 human pancreatic cancer cells while causing an up-regulation of their cell-surface EGFR [24]. Furthermore, cyclin D1 overexpression in pancreatic cancer is associated with decreased patient survival [25], whereas stable expression of a cyclin D1 antisense construct in pancreatic cancer cells attenuates their growth *in vitro* and *in vivo* [26]. Transfected clones underexpress cyclin D1, are no longer growth stimulated by EGF in spite of the fact that EGF can still activate the mitogen activated protein kinases (MAPK) ERK1 and ERK2 in these cells [26]. These findings support the hypothesis that the tyrosine kinase may have an important role in enhancing the growth of pancreatic cancer cells, and, by extension, that they also have a role in the proliferation and regeneration that is observed in CP.

Evidence for regeneration in chronic pancreatitis

Regeneration is a process whereby cell proliferation occurs in conjunction with tissue remodeling and repair, either as a consequence of physiological mechanisms or following tissue damage. In rodents, regeneration of various components of the pancreas has been observed following partial pancreatectomy and following induction of pancreatitis, which is most commonly accomplished by injections of high levels of the pancreatic secretagogue caerulein [27–29]. Although the total mass of the pancreas is not restored following pancreatectomy, there is regeneration of both the endocrine and exocrine components [30].

Different types of studies suggest that the overexpression of EGF, TGF-α and EGFR may contribute to regeneration and repair of the exocrine components of the pancreas. Thus, EGF is necessary for the maintenance of acinar cells in serum-free culture, enhances acinar cell survival, potentiates cholecystokinin-mediated amylase secretion in cultured acini, and modulates adenylate cyclase and phospholipase C-gamma 1 (PLC-γ1) activities in acinar cell membranes [31–34]. When mouse pancreatic acini are plated on a collagen gel, the cells exhibit increased thymidine incorporation in the presence of 10 nM EGF [35]. EGF enhances thymidine incorporation in pancreatic acini and ductal cells in male Wistar rats [36], and causes pancreatic ductal cell proliferation in the pig pancreas [37]. EGF also reduces pancreatic damage and accelerates pancreatic healing in the cerulein-induced pancreatitis model [38]. Together, these studies suggest that EGFR may have a role in maintaining acinar cell integrity and differentiated functions, and in promoting duct cell proliferation, and that this pathway may thereby contribute to the regenerative process in the pancreas. However, it is likely that this regulation is complex, inasmuch as the pancreatic acinar cell exhibits a decreased capacity to bind EGF following a 90% partial pancreatectomy in the rat [39].

Insulin-like growth factor I (IGF-I) also enhances acinar cell survival [31]. Furthermore, IGF-I mRNA levels are increased 3 days following a 90% pancreatectomy in the rat

[40, 41], and this increased expression is most prominent in focal areas of regeneration, especially within proliferating ductules and connective tissue cells [40]. IGF-I mRNA levels are also increased following induction of acute pancreatitis with caerulein [41]. Taken together, these observations suggest that IGF-I may also have a role in the growth, regeneration and repair of the pancreas.

The evidence for the existence of pancreatic regeneration in humans is controversial, especially in the setting of partial surgical resections of the pancreas [42]. Nonetheless, already in 1919 it was reported that there is an increased mitotic index in pancreatic tissues from patients suffering from acute or chronic pancreatitis [43]. In addition, several recent studies have reported that there is histological evidence for regeneration of human pancreatic parenchyma following recovery from acute pancreatitis [44, 45]. In these studies, there were foci of pancreatic necrosis as well as foci of pancreatic regeneration. Within the foci of regeneration, there was increased EGFR erbB-3, FGFR-1, FGF-1 and FGF-2 immunoreactivity in the acinar and ductal cells, whereas erbB-2 immunoreactivity was only increased in the ductal cells [44, 45]. These findings suggest that members of the EGF and FGF families of growth factors may be involved in the process of pancreatic exocrine regeneration during recovery from acute pancreatitis.

Chronic pancreatitis and pancreatic cancer

Epidemiological studies have shown that the risk of developing pancreatic cancer is increased up-to 16-fold in patients with pre-existing CP in comparison to the risk in the general population [46]. The mechanisms that contribute to neoplastic transformation in CP are not known [47]. Furthermore, is not known why only a small percentage of patients with CP progress toward the development of PDAC. However, a number of alterations in oncogenes and tumor suppression genes occur in PDAC [48], but, with the exception of K-*ras* mutations, probably do not occur in CP.

Several additional mechanisms may protect the pancreas in CP from undergoing malignant transformation. First, in contrast to PDAC, which is resistant to apoptosis [49, 50], there is a considerable level of apoptosis in CP [51]. Activation of apoptotic pathways in CP may eliminate genetic alterations that could lead to neoplastic transformation. Second, while EGFR, erbB-2 and erbB-3 are often concomitantly overexpressed in PDAC [1], only EGFR is consistently expressed to high levels in CP [9]. EGFR-related receptors often heterodimerize with EGFR and thereby potentiate mitogenic signaling [52, 53]. Therefore, in pancreatic cancer cells there may be activation of signaling pathways through the EGFR family that are not normally activated in CP. Third, there is overexpression of glypican-1 in PDAC, but not in CP [54]. Glypican-1 is a membrane associated heparan sulfate proteoglycan (HSPG) that is attached to the plasma membrane via glycosylphophatidylinositol (GPI) anchor. It acts to facilitate the interaction between heparin-binding growth factors and their respective high-affinity cell surface receptors. Its abundance in PDAC suggests that glypican-1 may play a crucial role in the growth factor signaling pathways underlying an aggressive human cancer. Conversely, its relatively low expression in CP may prevent many heparin-binding growth factors from exerting their full mitogenic potential. Fourth, Id-1, -2, and -3 mRNA species are expressed at high levels in PDAC by comparison with CP samples [55, 56]. Inasmuch as Id proteins antagonize basic helix-loop-helix (bHLH) proteins, inhibit differentiation, and enhance cell proliferation (57, 58], their relative under-expression in CP may prevent excessive cellular proliferation. Interestingly, in dysplastic and atypical papillary ducts in CP, there is increased Id immunoreactivity [56]. These findings suggest that increased expression of Id-1, Id-2, and Id-3 may enhance the proliferative potential of dysplastic ductal cells in CP.

Summary

Multiple growth factors and their tyrosine kinase receptors are overexpressed in CP. Together, these growth factors may act as mitogens that induce duct cell and acinar cell proliferation during the process of tissue regeneration. It is evident, however, that during the process of injury and inflammation other polypeptides, including chemokines and cytokines, also contribute to the histological changes that occur in CP [59–61]. Together, these regulatory molecules dictate the balance between the deleterious and beneficial biological events that occur in the pancreas in CP. These processes include necrosis, apoptosis, and fibrosis on the one hand, and repair, regeneration, and cell survival on the other hand (Fig. 2.2-1). Together, these alterations result in a dual process that can lead to tissue repair and remodeling, but also to fibroblastic proliferation and pancreatic fibrosis. Occasionally, as a consequence of these changes, dysplastic cells may arise. These cells, upon acquiring K-*ras* mutations, have a greater potential to acquire additional genetic mutations and to ultimately undergo neoplastic transformation.

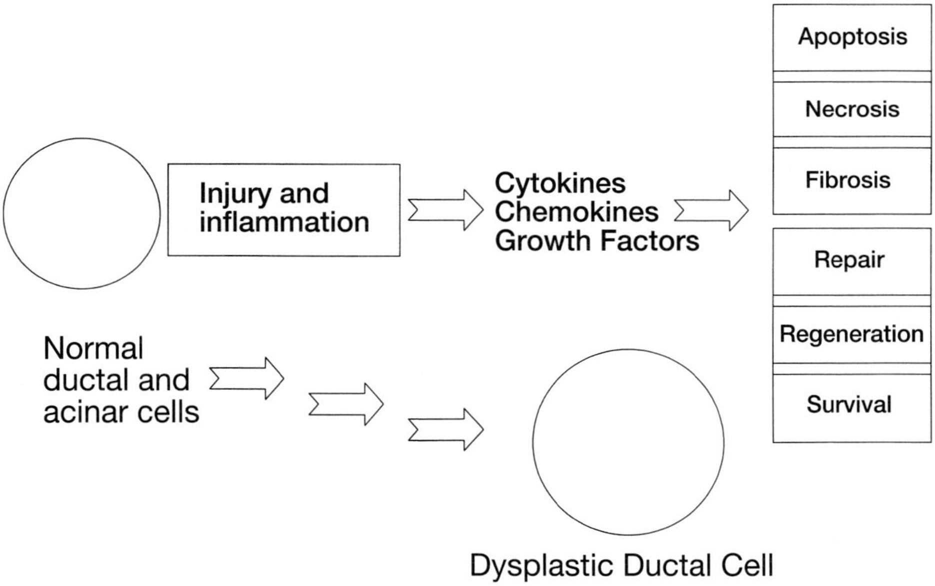

Figure 2.2-1. Potential epigenetic alterations in chronic pancreatitis. During the recovery from injury and inflammation, there is overexpression of certain growth factors and their tyrosine kinase receptors in the pancreatic exocrine cells, leading to activation of signaling pathways. There is concomitant production of various chemokines and cytokines in the pancreas. In addition to an ongoing process of apoptosis, necrosis, and fibrosis, these regulatory polypeptide molecules contribute to cell survival and regeneration, and, ultimately, to tissue repair. Repeated episodes of injury and repair can give rise to dysplastic cells, which have a greater propensity to undergo malignant transformation.

Acknowledgment

This work was supported by U.S. Public Health Service Grants CA-40162 and CA-75059 from the National Cancer Institute.

References

1. Korc M. Role of polypeptide growth factors and their receptors in human pancreatic cancer. In: Reber HA, ed. Pancreatic cancer: pathogenesis, diagnosis, and treatment. Totowa, New Jersey: Humana Press, 1998: 21–32.
2. Kloppel G. Progression from acute to chronic pancreatitis. A pathologist's view. Surg Clin North Am 1999; 79: 801–14.
3. Layer P, DiMagno EP. Early and late onset in idiopathic and alcoholic chronic pancreatitis. Different clinical courses. Surg Clin North Am 1999; 79: 847–60.
4. Mohan V, Premalatha G, Padma A, Chari ST, Pitchumoni CS. Fibrocalculous pancreatic diabetes. Long-term survival analysis. Diabetes Care 1996; 19: 1274–8.
5. Arduino C, Gallo M, Brusco A, Garnerone S, Piana MR, Di Maggio S, Gerbino Promis G, Ferrone M, Angeli A, Gaia E. Polyvariant mutant CFTR genes in patients with chronic pancreatitis. Clin Genet 1999; 56: 400–4.
6. Cohn JA, Bornstein JD, Jowell PS. Cystic fibrosis mutations and genetic predisposition to idiopathic chronic pancreatitis. Med Clin North Am 2000; 84: 621–31.
7. Hsiang D, Friess H, Büchler MW, Ebert M, Butler J, Korc M. Absence of K-ras mutations in the pancreatic parenchyma of patients with chronic pancreatitis. Am J Surg 1997; 174: 242–6.
8. Casey G, Yamanaka Y, Friess H, Kobrin MS, Lopez ME, Büchler MW, Beger HG, Korc M. p53 mutations are common in pancreatic cancer and are absent in chronic pancreatitis. Cancer Lett 1993; 69: 151–60.
9. Korc M, Friess H, Yamanaka Y, Kobrin MS, Büchler MW, Beger HG. Chronic pancreatitis is associated with increased concentrations of epidermal growth factor receptor, transforming growth factor alpha, and phospholipase C gamma. Gut 1994; 35: 1468–73.
10. Friess H, Yamanaka Y, Kobrin MS, Do D, Büchler MW, Korc M. Enhanced erbB-3 expression in human pancreatic cancer correlates with tumor progression. Clin Canc Res 1995; 1: 1413–20.
11. Friess H, Yamanaka Y, Büchler MW, Hammer K, Kobrin MS, Beger HG, Korc M. A subgroup of patients with chronic pancreatitis overexpress the c-erb B-2 protooncogene. Ann Surg 1994; 220: 183–92.
12. Friess H, Yamanaka Y, Büchler MW, Kobrin MS, Tahara E, Korc M. Cripto, a member of the epidermal growth factor family, is over-expressed inhuman pancreatic cancer and chronic pancreatitis. Int J Cancer 1994; 56: 668–74.
13. Yamanaka Y, Friess H, Büchler MW, Beger HG, Uchida E, Onda M, Kobrin MS, Korc M. Overexpression of acidic and basic fibroblast growth factors in human pancreatic cancer correlates with advanced tumor stage. Cancer Res 1993; 53: 5289–96.
14. Ishiwata T, Kornmann M, Beger HG, Korc M. Enhanced fibroblast growth factor 5 expression in stromal and exocrine elements of the pancreas in chronic pancreatitis. Gut 1998; 43: 134–9.
15. Kornmann M, Beger HG, Korc M. Role of fibroblast growth factors and their receptors in pancreatic cancer and chronic pancreatitis. Pancreas 1998; 17: 169–75.
16. Ishiwata T, Friess H, Büchler MW, Lopez ME, Korc M. Characterization of keratinocyte growth factor and receptor expression in human pancreatic cancer. Am J Pathol 1998; 153: 213–22.
17. Ebert M, Kasper HU, Hernberg S, Friess H, Büchler MW, Roessner A, Korc M, Malfertheiner P. Overexpression of platelet-derived growth factor (PDGF) B chain and type beta PDGF receptor in human chronic pancreatitis. Dig Dis Sci 1998; 43: 567–74.
18. Friess H, Zhu ZW, di Mola FF, Kulli C, Graber HU, Andren-Sandberg A, Zimmermann A, Korc M, Reinshagen M, Büchler MW. Nerve growth factor and its high-affinity receptor in chronic pancreatitis. Ann Surg 1999; 230: 615–24.

19. Korc M. Role of growth factors in pancreatic cancer. Surg Oncol Clin N Am 1998; 7: 25–41.
20. Yamanaka Y, Friess H, Kobrin MS, Büchler MW, Beger HG, Korc M. Coexpression of epidermal growth factor receptor and ligands in human pancreatic cancer is associated with enhanced tumor aggressiveness. Anticancer Res 1993; 13: 565–9.
21. Yokoyama M, Ebert M, Funatomi M, Friess H, Büchler MW, Johnson GR, Korc M. Amphiregulin is a potent mitogen in human pancreatic cancer cells: correlation with patient survival. Int J Oncol 1995; 6: 625–31.
22. Wagner M, Cao T, Lopez ME, Hope C, Van Nostrand K, Korbrin MS, Fan H, Büchler MW, Korc M. Expression of a truncated EGF receptor is associated with inhibition of pancreatic cancer cell growth and enhanced sensitivity to cisplatinum. Int J Canc 1996; 68: 782–7.
23. Baldwin RL, Kobrin MS, Tran T, Pastan I, Korc M. Cytotoxic effects of TGF-alpha-Pseudomonas exotoxin A fusion protein in human pancreatic carcinoma cells. Pancreas 1996; 13: 16–21.
24. Funatomi H, Itakura J, Ishiwata T, Pastan I, Thompson SA, Johnson GR, Korc M. Amphiregulin antisense oligonucleotide inhibits the growth of T3M4 human pancreatic cancer cells and sensitizes the cells to EGF receptor targeted therapy. Int J Cancer 1997; 72: 512–7.
25. Kornmann M, Ishiwata T, Itakura J, Tangvoranuntakul P, Beger HG, Korc M. Increased cyclin D1 in human pancreatic cancer is associated with decreased postoperative survival. Oncology 1998; 55: 363–569.
26. Kornmann M, Arber N, Korc M. Inhibition of basal and mitogen-stimulated pancreatic cancer cells growth by cyclin D1 antisense in associated with loss to tumorigenicity and protentiation of cytotoxicity to cisplatinum. J Clin Invest 1998; 101: 344–52.
27. Steinle AU, Weidenbach H, Wagner M, Adler G, Schmid RM. NF-kappaB/Rel activation in cerulein pancreatitis. Gastroenterology 1999; 116: 420–30.
28. Song M, Zaninovic V, Kim D, Gukovsky I, Gukovskaya A, Kang K, Pandol S. Amelioration of rat cerulein pancreatitis by guamerin-derived peptide, a novel elastase inhibitor. Pancreas 1999; 18: 231–9.
29. Saluja AK, Bhagat L, Lee HS, Bhatia M, Frossard JL, Steer ML. Secretagogue-induced digestive enzyme activation and cell injury in rat pancreatic acini. Am J Physiol 1999; 276: G835–42.
30. Brockenbrough JS, Weir GC, Bonner-Weir SE. Discordance of exocrine and endocrine growth after 90 % pancreatectomy in rats. Diabetes 1988; 37: 232–6.
31. Brannon PM, Hirschi K, Korc M. Effects of epidermal growth factor, insulin, and insulin-like growth factor on rat pancreatic acinar cells cultured in serum-free medium. Pancreas 1988; 3: 41–8.
32. Logsdon CD, Williams JA. Pancreatic acinar cell in monolayer culture: direct trophic effects of caerulein in vitro. Am J Physiol 1986; 250: G440–7.
33. Pipper A, Stryjek-Kaminska D, Zeuzem S. Epidermal growth factor activates phospholipase C-gamma 1 via G(i) 1-2 proteins in isolated pancreatic acinar membranes. Am J Physiol 1997; 272: 1276–84.
34. Stryjek-Kaminska D, Pipper A, Zeuzem S. Epidermal growth factor regulates adenylate cyclase activity via Gs and Gi 1-2 proteins in pancreatic acinar members. Biochem J 1996; 316: 87–91.
35. Logsdon CD. Stimulation of pancreatic acinar cell growth by CCK, EGF and insulin in vitro. Am J Physiol 1986; 251: G487–94.
36. Dembinski A, Gregory H, Konturek SJ, Polanski M. Trophic action of epidermal growth factor on the pancreas and gastroduodenal mucosa in rats. J Physiol 1982; 325: 35–40.
37. Vinter-Jensen L, Juhl CO, Teglbjaerg PS, Poulsen SS, Dajani EZ, Nexo E. Systemic treatment with EGF in pigs induces ductal proliferations in the pancreas. Gastroenterology 1997; 113: 1367–74.
38. Dembinski A, Warzecha Z, Konturek PC, Ceranowicz P, Stachura J, Tomaszewska R, Konturek SJ. Epidermal growth factor accelerates pancreatic recovery after caerulein-induced pancreatitis. Eur J Pharmacol 2000 Jun 9; 398(1): 159–68.
39. Brockenbrough JS, Weir GC, Korc M. Alterations in EGF binding to acini during pancreatic regeneration in the rat. Int J Pancreatol 1988; 3: 415–24.

40. Smith FE, Rosen KM, Villa-Komaroff L, Weir GC, Bonner-Weir. Enhanced insulin-like growth factor I gene expression in regenerating rat pancreas. Proc Natl Acad Sci USA 1991; 88: 6152–6.
41. Calvo EL, Bernatchez G, Pelletier G, Iovanna JL, Morisset J. Downregulation of IGF-I mRNA expression during postnatal pancreatic development and overexpression after subtotal pancreatectomy and acute pancreatitis in the rat pancreas. J Mol Endocrinol 1997; 18: 233–42.
42. Tsiotos GG, Barry MK, Johnson CD, Sarr MG. Pancreas regeneration after resection: does it occur in humans? Pancreas 1999; 19: 310–13.
43. Parker FJ. Toxic necrosis and regeneration of the acinar cells of the pancreas. J Med Res 1919; 40: 471–6.
44. Ebert M, Friess H, Büchler MW, Korc M. Differential distribution of human epidermal growth factor receptor family in acute pancreatitis. Dig Dis Sci 1995; 40: 2134–42.
45. Ebert M, Yokoyama M, Ishiwata T, Friess H, Büchler MW, Malfertheiner P, Korc M. Alteration of fibroblast growth factor and receptor expression after acute pancreatitis in humans. Pancreas 1999;18: 240–6.
46. Lowenfels AB, Maisonneuve P, Lankisch PG. Chronic pancreatitis and other risk factors for pancreatic cancer. Gastroenterol Clin North Am 1999; 28: 673–85.
47. Niederau C, Niederau MC, Heintges T, Lüthen R. Epidemiology: relation between chronic pancreatitis and pancreatic carcinoma. In: Beger HG, Büchler MW, Schoenberg MH, eds. Cancer of the pancreas. Ulm, Germany: Universitätsverlag Ulm GmbH, 1996: 6–9.
48. Moskaluk CA, Kern SE. Molecular genetics of pancreatic carcinoma. In: Reber HA, ed. Pancreatic cancer: pathogenesis, diagnosis, and treatment. Totowa, New Jersey: Humana Press, 1998: 3–20.
49. Ungefroren H, Voss M, Jansen M, Roeder C, Henne-Bruns D, Kremer B, Kalthoff H. Human Pancreatic Adenocarcinomas Express Fas and Fas-Ligand Yet Are Resistant to Fas-mediated Apoptosis. Cancer Res 1998; 58: 1741–9.
50. Kornmann M, Ishiwata T, Kleeff J, Beger HG, Korc M. Fas and Fas-ligand expression in human pancreatic cancer. Ann Surg 2000; 231: 368–79.
51. Kornmann M, Ishiwata T, Maruyama H, Beger HG, Korc M. Coexpression of FAS and FAS-ligand in chronic pancreatitis: correlation with apoptosis. Pancreas 2000; 20: 123–8.
52. Prigent SA, Lemoine NR. The type 1 (EGFR-related) family of growth factor receptors and their ligands. Prog Growth Factor Res 1992; 4: 1–24.
53. Carraway KL III, Cantley LC. A new acquaintance for erbB3 and erbB4. A role for receptor heterodimerization in growth signaling. Cell 1994; 78: 5–8.
54. Kleeff J, Ishiwata T, Kumbasar A, Friess H, Büchler MW, Lander AD, Korc M. The cell-surface heparan sulfate proteoglycan glypican-1 regulates growth factor action in pancreatic carcinoma cells and is overexpressed in human pancreatic cancer. J Clin Invest 1998; 102: 1662–73.
55. Kleeff J, Ishiwata T, Friess H, Büchler MW, Israel MA, Korc M. The helix-loop-helix protein Id2 is overexpressed in human pancreatic cancer. Cancer Res 1998; 58: 3769–3772.
56. Maruyama H, Kleeff J, Wildi S, Friess H, Büchler MW, Israel MA, Korc M. Id-1 and Id-2 are overexpressed in pancreatic cancer and in dysplastic lesions in chronic pancreatitis. Am J Pathol 1999; 155: 815–22.
57. Benezra R, Davis RL, Lockshon D, Turner DL, Weintraub H. The protein Id: a negative regulator of helix-loop-helix DNA binding proteins. Cell 1990; 61: 49–59.
58. Norton JD, Atherton GT. Coupling of cell growth control and apoptosis functions of Id proteins. Mol Cell Biol 1998; 18: 2371–81.
59. Berberat PO, Friess H, Büchler MW. Chronic pancreatitis – new pathophysiological concepts. Swiss Surg 2000; 6: 227–30.
60. Di Sebastiano P, Di Mola FF, Di Febbo C, Baccante G, Porreca E, Innocenti P, Friess H, Büchler MW. Expression of interleukin 8 (IL-8) and substance P in human chronic pancreatitis. Gut 2000; 47: 423–8.
61. Goecke H, Forssmann U, Uguccioni M, Friess H, Conejo-Garcia JR, Zimmermann A, Baggiolini M, Büchler MW. Macrophages infiltrating the tissue in chronic pancreatitis express the chemokine receptor CCR5. Surgery 2000; 128: 806–14.

2.3 Genetic alterations in chronic pancreatitis

D. C. Whitcomb

Introduction

Chronic pancreatitis is a terrible disease. Recognition of this condition by the clinician usually occurs rather late in the course of the disease when recurrent or unrelenting pain prompts a global evaluation of the abdomen. Only then are the characteristic morphologic or functional changes observed which reflect the widespread destruction of the normal gland. To make matters worse, the healing profession is incapable of altering the unrelenting progression of the chronic pancreatitis syndrome until the patient is left with total exocrine and endocrine failure [1].

Many investigators, motivated by the frustration of caring for these patients without offering a cure or legitimate hope, proposed various possible etiologies and disease mechanisms for chronic pancreatitis based on a number of interesting and tenable hypotheses. Despite many heroic efforts, the state-of-the-art in 1995 was accurately summarized in a statement by Steer et al. (Medical Progress Review in New England Journal of Medicine in 1995): "Chronic pancreatitis remains an enigmatic process of uncertain pathogenesis, unpredictable clinical course, and unclear treatment" [2]. Thus, new approaches were needed.

During the 1990s an incredibly powerful new resource became available to medical researchers: a draft sequence of the human genome. This resource provided the foundation for a number of new methods, including genetic linkage studies, positional cloning, and mutational analysis of candidate genes. It is the utilization of this resource that serves as a foundation and focus of this chapter.

Most people don't develop chronic pancreatitis

The human pancreas serves three primary functions: production of bicarbonate to neutralize gastric acid entering the duodenum, synthesis of digestive enzymes to hydrolyze organic macromolecules so they can be absorbed from the intestine, and release of hormones into the bloodstream to regulate utilization of circulating nutrients from a meal. As one considers the complexity, efficiency, and quantity of digestive enzymes that are synthesized by the pancreas, it is apparent that they contain sufficient enzymatic potential to transform an entire meal into a suspension of simple molecules. Indeed, the majority of pancreatic digestive enzymes are targeted for the dissolution of the exact types of proteins, lipids and nucleic acids of which humans are made. Thus, it is remarkable that in the vast majority of people, the pancreas synthesizes and delivers large quantities of these enzymes multiple times a day for up to 100 years or more without a problem.

From these observations, we must conclude that the pancreas contains a number of effective protective mechanisms that prevent the pancreas from self-destruction by these digestive enzymes. These processes have been summarized by Rinderknecht [3, 4]. The protective mechanisms that we currently recognize include: (a) synthesis of most digestive enzymes in an inactive or proenzyme form, (b) the segregation and compartmentalization of digestive enzymes within the acinar cell, (c) the maintenance of an environmental state of low intracellular calcium, (d) synthesis of protease inhibitors, (e) the appropriate release of zymogens from the pancreatic acinar cells, (f) the efficient delivery of the zymogens to the duodenum and (g) the remote site for enzymes activation mediated by the trypsin activation cascade. A number of theories have been advanced on how these protective mechanisms might be disrupted, but they have proven very difficult to prove, especially in humans. Progress in understanding the factors leading to acute and chronic pancreatitis remained slow, hindered in part by the lack of an adequate animal model and by the problems faced by investigators who are trying to reconstruct the trigger sequence at the end of a widely destructive process.

Genetic linkage studies in hereditary pancreatitis

The availability of large families with a clear genetic predisposition to acute and chronic pancreatitis, along with the construction of detailed marker maps of the human chromosomes, opened the door to new insights in pancreatic disease. These resources, along with large scale DNA sequencing efforts, provided the opportunity for detecting key molecules involved in protecting the pancreas from acute and chronic pancreatitis to be identified. At least three groups [5–7] with access to huge kindreds with hereditary pancreatitis converged on chromosome 7q in late 1995 and 1996. Within weeks of localization, the culprit gene was discovered.

In 1996, Whitcomb et al. [8] discovered the first mutation that was clearly associated with acute and chronic pancreatitis, the cationic trypsinogen codon 122 R122H mutation (Figure 2.3-1) (the same mutation is R117H using the chymotrypsinogen numbering system, or Chy#R117H) [9, 10]. The R122H mutation provided a series of critical insights into the mechanisms leading to acute and chronic pancreatitis. This mutation resulted in an amino acid substitution in a surprising location on the trypsin molecule. Arginine 122 (Chy#R117) is on the surface of the trypsinogen molecule opposite the catalytic site and the trypsinogen activation site [8]. Inspection of the three-dimensional structure of trypsinogen revealed that arginine 122 is located within a flexible connecting chain linking the two globular domains of the trypsinogen molecular. Biochemical studies [11, 12] had previously demonstrated that arginine 122 (Chy#R117) represents the initial site of attack of trypsin by a second trypsin molecule, thereby representing the initial site of trypsin autolysis. Taken together, we hypothesized that the R122H mutation eliminated a "fail-safe" self-destruction mechanism that prevented the rapid accumulation of large amounts of active trypsin within the pancreas [8, 13]. This self-destruct mechanism appears to function as a "last resort", since others had previously recognized that the pancreas synthesized the pancreatic secretory trypsin inhibitor PSTI (also known as serin

---

Figure 2.3-1. Cationic trypsinogen (CT) compared to anionic trypsinogen (AT), mesotrypsinogen (MT), the putative gene TRY6/trypsinogen C (TRY6) and chymotrypsinogen (Chy) from Whitcomb [10]. Cationic trypsinogen is divided according to the amino acids coded for in each of the 5 exons. The amino acids are numbered according to codon (top) and the numbering system is based on alignment with chymotrypsinogen at serine 195 (bottom). The sequences of cationic trypsino-

Tryspinogen Exons and Alignment with Other Proteases.

```
Exon 1    signal peptide
CODON  1          10  14
       |          |   |
CT     MNPLLILTFVAAAL
AT     MNLLLILTFVAAAV
MT     MNPFLILAFVGAAV
Chy    MAFLWLLSCWALLGTTF


Exon 2          TAP
CODON 15        16    23    29      40      50     60   67
      |         |     |     |       |       |      |    |
CT    A         APFDDDDK IVGGYNCEENSVPYQVSLN  SGYHFCGGSLINEQWVVSAGHCYKS
AT    A         APFDDDDK IVGGYICEENSVPYQVSLN  SGYHFCGGSLISEQWVVSAGHCYKS
MT    A         VPFDDDDK IVGGYTCEENSLPYQVSLN  SGSHFCGGSLISEQWVVSAAHCYKT
Chy   G CGVPAIHPVLSGLSR IVNGEDAVPGSWPWQVSLQDKTGFHFCGGSLISEDWVVTAAHCGVR
          |      |        ||     |       |      |    |
 Chy#            1               10      2021   30   40     50   57


Exon 3
CODON  68 70      80      90      100     110     120 122   130      140     150 152
       | |       |       |       |       |       | |     |        |       | |
CT     RIQVRL  GEHNIEVLEGNEQFINAAKIIRHPQYDRKTLNNDIMLIKLSSRAVINARVSTISLPT APPA TGTKCLISGWGNTASSGA
AT     RIQVRL  GEHNIEVLEGNEQFINAAKIIRHPKYNSRTLDNDILLIKLSSPAVINSRVSAISLPT APPA AGTESLISGWGNTLSSGA
MT     RIQVRL  GEHNIKVLEGNEQFINAAKIIRHPKYNRDTLDNDIMLIKLSSPAVINARVSTISLPT APPA AGTECLISGWGNTLSFGA
Chy    TSDVVVAGEFDQGSDEENIQVLKIAKVFKNPKFSILTVNNDITLLKLATPARFSQTVSAVCLPSADD DFPAGTLCATTGWGKTKYNAN
       |       |       |       |       | |     |    | |      * |       |
Chy#   62      70      80      90      100 102 110  117 120    130     140


Exon 4
CODON  153     160      170      180      190     197
       |       |        |        |        |       |
CT     DYPDELQCLDAPVLSQAKCEASYPGKITSNMFCVGFLEGGKDSCQ
AT     DYPDELQCLDAPVLSQAECEASYPGKITNNMFCVGFLEGGKDSCQ
MT     DYPDELKCLDAPVLTQAECKASYPGKITNSMFCVGFLEGGKDSCQ
Chy    KTPDKLQQAALPLLSNAECKKSWGRRITDVMICAG ASGV SSCM
       |       |        |        |     *    *s|
Chy#   150     160      170      180          190


Exon 5
CODON  198          210      220      230      240   247
       |            |        |        |        |     |
CT     GDSGGPVVCNGQ    LQGVVSWGD GCAQKNKPGVYTKVYNYVKWIKNTIAANS
AT     GDSGGPVVSNGE    LQGIVSWGY GCAQKNRPGVYTKVYNYVDWIKDTIAANS
MT     RDSGGPVVCNGQ    LQGVVSWGH GCAWKNRPGVYTKVYNYVDWIKDTIAANS
Chy    GDSGGPLVCQKDGAWTLVGIVSWGSDTCS TSSPGVYARVTKLIPWVQKILAAN
         |   |        |    |  | *   | |       |        *
Chy#    195  200      210  s  220  s 230      240
```

gen, anionic trypsinogen, and TRY6; mesotrypsinogen, and chymotrypsinogen from cDNA (introns unknown) are summarized by Whitcomb [10]. Signal peptides are in italics, activation peptides are underlined italics, the catalytic triad (H57, D102 and S195], N21 and R117 are bold. The amino acids determining specificity of the enzymes (D189, G216 and G226) are marked with "*s*". Amino acids in trypsinogen that occur between the chymotrypsinogen numbered residues are marked with an asterisk.

```
Exon 1
Codon #         1        10      18
 obs var        |        |    P  |
human           MKVTGIFLLSALALLSLS
porcine
rat             MKVAIIFLLSALALLNLA

Peptide #

Exon 2
Codon #              24   29
 obs var              |    |
human           GNTGADSLGRE
porcine              TSPQRE
rat             GNTTAKVIGKK
                     |    |
Peptide #            1    6

Exon 3
Codon #         30        40        50        60   65
 obs var        |   S     |*        E    S    |    |
human           AKCYNELNGCTKIYDPVCGTDGNTYPNECVLCFENR
porcine         ATCTSEVSGCPKIYNPVCGTDGITYSNECVLCSENK
rat             ANCPNTLIGCPRDYDPVCGTDGKTYANECILCFENR
                |   |        |         |         | |
Peptide #       7   11       20        30        40 42


Exon 4
Codon #         66  70       79
  obs var       |   |        |
human           KRQTSILIQKSGPC
porcine         KRQTPVLIQKSGPC
rat             KFGTSIRIQRRGLC
                |      |     |
Peptide #       43     50    56
```

Figure 2.3-2. Protein sequence alignments of SPINK1 (PSTI) from Pfützer et al. [27]. Comparison of human, porcine and rat. Obs var: observed variations in human protein sequence deduced from allele polymorphisms. Bold type: the position of N34S variant (changes human sequence to porcine sequence [28]). *: the "bait" lysine (K) in human and porcine, and arginine (R) in rat that projects into the specificity pocket of trypsin during trypsin inhibition.

protease inhibitor Kazal type I; SPINK1 (Fig. 2.3-2), with a capacity of inhibiting up to 20% of trypsinogen within the pancreas [3].

The cationic trypsinogen R122H mutation represents a "gain of function" mutation [13]. In this case, the gain of function develops because of the loss of a mechanism to inhibit trypsin once it is activated. Thus, the mutation becomes recognized only *after* trypsin has been activated through a different mechanism, and *after* other inhibitory mechanisms such as interaction with the SPINK1/PSTI are exhausted. Since a primary role of trypsin is to activate all of the other digestive proenzymes, it becomes clear that active trypsin is an important early step in the initiation of pancreatic autodigestion and pancreatitis driven by trypsin [14], elastase [15], and other digestive enzymes.

The trypsinogen mRNA is coded by alleles from the two copies of chromosome 7, yet the disease is present with only one allelic mutation. However, persistent activity of only ½ of the synthesized trypsin will result in a pancreatitis phenotype. This explains why hereditary pancreatitis presents as an autosomal dominant disorder [13]. To date, only a limited number of trypsin mutations have been identified in the families predisposed to acute and chronic pancreatitis, which is consistent with other diseases in which gain of function mutations are far less frequent than loss of function mutations [13]. Other trypsinogen mutations that have been identified and confirmed include the N29I mutation (Chy#N21I) [16], A16V mutation (Chy#A8V) [9, 17, 18], K23R [19], D22G [20], N29T, R122C and others. As expected, these gain-of-function mutations are rare in individuals with chronic pancreatitis but without a clear family history [21–23]. However, in endemic areas up to 19% of patients who were previously classified as having idiopathic chronic pancreatitis were found to have mutations in the cationic trypsinogen gene [24] and therefore represent cases of hereditary pancreatitis with an incomplete or inadequate family history.

In summary, the study of hereditary pancreatitis kindreds and the discovery of the cationic trypsinogen mutations have taught us that trypsinogen is central to the initiation of acute pancreatitis [8, 13, 14], that recurrent attacks of acute pancreatitis lead to classic chronic pancreatitis, and that certain genetic mutations clearly predispose some individuals to developing acute and chronic pancreatitis.

SPINK1/PSTI mutations

As a number of international groups studied their families with hereditary pancreatitis, it became clear that this disease was heterogeneous and that a number of kindreds with clustering of pancreatitis did not have mutations in the cationic trypsinogen gene. A genome wide scan to identify linkage between pancreatitis and a new pancreatitis gene was conducted in the J family with linkage clearly identified on chromosome 12 and excluded on chromosome 5 [25]. Both Chen et al. [26] and Pfützer et al. [27] performed segregation analyses on families with pancreatitis in whom the trypsinogen gene had been excluded to investigate a potential linkage on chromosome 5 in the region known to contain the SPINK1/PSTI gene. In both cases, an association with mutations in PSTI and autosomal dominant inheritance pattern of this gene was excluded. Furthermore, both Chen et al. and Pfützer et al. performed screening of representative control populations and identified the same mutations in the SPINK1/PSTI gene in the control population that were seen in several members of the hereditary pancreatitis families. These results led Chen et al. to conclude that these mutations were common polymorphisms [26]. However, Witt et al. [28] and later Pfützer et al. [27] also looked at patients with idiopathic chronic pancreatitis. Witt et al. sequenced the SPINK1 gene in 96 unrelated pediatric patients with idiopathic chronic pancreatitis [28]. They identified a SPINK1 mutation in 23% of these patients. Interestingly, both homozygous and heterozygous genotypes were observed (N34S/N34S = 6, N34S/WT = 12, plus several other polymorphisms not seen in 52 unrelated controls (MIT, L14P, P55S, –53C > T, IV53 + 2T > C). Witt et al. went on to speculate that this may represent an autosomal recessive disease [28]. The mutations appeared to have caused a loss of inhibitory function whereby the initial mechanism for inhibiting prematurely activated trypsinogen within the pancreas was lost. This was hypothesized to lead to an imbalance between serine proteases and inhibitors, thereby predisposing patients to pancreatitis.

Pfützer et al. [27] sequenced the entire SPINK1 gene plus intronic regions in 112 individuals with familial and/or idiopathic chronic pancreatitis in whom the major trypsinogen gene mutations had been excluded. In addition, Pfützer et al. sequenced 380 alleles from exon 2 and 190 alleles from all other exons of the SPINK1/PSTI gene from a control population. We identified several new mutations (D50 E, 1VS 3 + 125C > A, 1VS 3 + 184T > A) and confirmed the N34S and P55S mutations reported by Witt [28]. These mutations were present in 29 of 112 patients (25%). The results of this study closely matched the results of Witt et al. [26, 28] in which 23% of patients with idiopathic chronic pancreatitis had SPINK1 mutations. Furthermore, Pfützer et al. [27] identified three N34S (0.77%) and two P55S (0.53%) SPINK1/PSTI mutations in 380 control alleles, suggesting that SPINK1/PSTI mutations are present in ~2% of the population. This finding closely parallels the study of Chen et al. in the French control population [26]. Pfützer et al. went on to investigate the age of onset of symptoms in the heterozygous versus the homozygous mutation in individuals. There was no difference in age at onset, a potential marker of severity of the mutations blurring the distinction between the effect of the heterozygous and homozygous genotypes. This finding suggested that SPINK1 mutations were clearly associated with idiopathic pancreatitis, and that the disease was associated with both heterozygous and homozygous genotypes. However, it was estimated from the population studies that the penetrance of the heterozygous genotype mutation was less than 1%, whereas the penetrance of the homozygous genotype may be higher. Furthermore, ICP associated with SPINK1/PSTI mutations could not represent an autosomal recessive disease, but a disease modifier gene which probably lowers the threshold for unchecked trypsinogen activation.

Pfützer et al. also presented molecular modeling data based on composite x-ray crystallography data [27]. Inspection of the resulting model (comparing human SPINK1/PSTI to porcine SPINK1/PSTI, since the N34S mutation changes the human sequence to

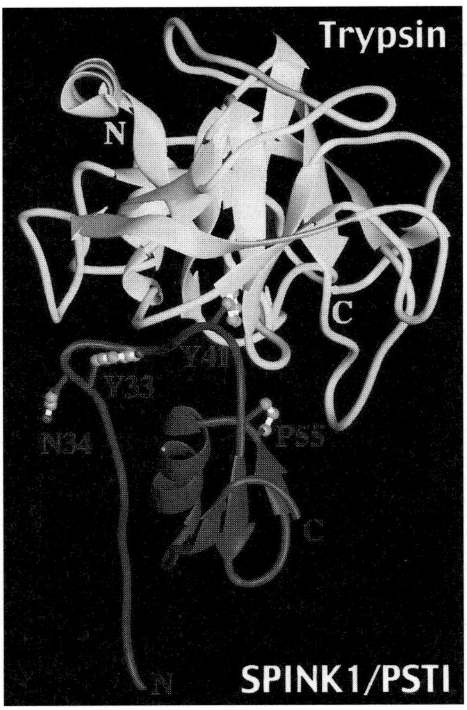

Figure 2.3-3. Structure of the free PSTI crystal structure and the PSTI-cationic trypsinogen complex.

porcine sequence) [27, 28] revealed that this mutation was within a flexible loop at the edge of the SPINK1/PSTI-cationic trypsinogen molecular interface. When the structure of the free PSTI crystal structure and the PSTI-cationic trypsinogen complex were compared, it appeared that this flexible loop rotates inward during PSTI binding, allowing Y33 to interact with the amino acids immediately associated with the trypsinogen specificity pocket "bait" at K41 (Fig. 2.3-3). It was also noted that there are several other amino acids that differ from the porcine and human SPINK1/PSTI molecules (Fig. 2.3-2).

Based on these observations, there are several possible explanations for the punitive loss of function mutations in human SPINK1/PSTI. The first is that the N34S substitution might interfere with the rotation of the side chain containing Y33 so that it would project into the aqueous phase rather than toward the interior of the SPINK1/PSTI molecular. This could interfere with the binding of SPINK1/PSTI to a trypsin molecule. It is also noted that the P55S mutation is located at the interface between SPINK1/PSTI and cationic trypsinogen and may act through a similar mechanism. Another possibility is that the N34S mutation could alter loop mobility and/or effect the interaction of Y33 with a key amino acid near K41, resulting in either easy hydrolysis of SPINK1/PSTI or marked reduction in the binding affinity to trypsinogen. However, these interpretations must be taken with caution, since the observed structural differences between the free and bound PSTI might be an artifact of crystallization.

Other chronic pancreatitis associated gene mutations

Mutations in the cystic fibrosis transmembrane conductance regulator (CFTR) are associated with chronic pancreatitis [29, 30]. The greatest relative risk appears to be associated with two mutations, CFTR R117H and the 5T allele [31]. Each of these mutations are normally considered mild CFTR mutations based on the observation that the combination of either of these mutations with a severe mutation (e.g. ΔF508) is associated with a form of cystic fibrosis with pancreatic sufficiency [32]. Of note, these two mutations are also associated with congenital bilateral aplasia of the vas deferens (CBAVD) which is a rare disorder associated with male infertility [33, 34]. Although these mutations are closely associated with idiopathic chronic pancreatitis, they are also frequent in the normal population (1:700) so that the penetrance of a 5T or R117H CFTR mutation is very low.

The question as to whether the CFTR or R117H or 5T allele represents a compound heterozygous CFTR associated disorder for our part of a polygenic disease [35] has not been determined. Answering this question remains difficult since over 900 CFTR polymorphisms have been identified. Thus, it becomes difficult to determine whether a compound heterozygous condition such as R117H plus another rare polymorphism represents a disease causing combination or whether the other mutation is completely silent. An important approach to understanding the genotype-phenotype correlation is reported by Cohn et al. [31]. Interestingly, only about half of the patients with idiopathic chronic pancreatitis and unusual CFTR mutations were found to have nasal impedance conductance measurements that were outside of the normal range [31]. This work is important because it suggests that many patients with the CFTR R117H or 5T allele mutations indeed have functional impairments of the CFTR, while the explanation for the others remains obscure. It should also be noted that the physiology of the pancreatic duct cells is likely different from nasal epithelium and it is the function of the pancreatic duct cells that is critical for preventing chronic pancreatitis.

The research into the association between CFTR mutations and idiopathic chronic pancreatitis is important but leaves many questions unanswered. First, why is there an apparent selection of several rare CFTR mutations such as the R117H and 5T allele? Second, what is the association between CFTR and chronic idiopathic pancreatitis? Does the pathophysiologic mechanism relate to an impairment of the delivery of digestive enzymes to the duodenum, a change in pH, or some other derangement of the duct cells? Third, are the identified CFTR mutations actually a part of a polygenic disorder [9]? These and other questions should be answered in the near future as a number of major groups investigate the molecular genetics of chronic pancreatitis.

Polygenic idiopathic chronic pancreatitis

Pfützer and Whitcomb [9] were the first to describe polygenic pancreatitis. This became evident in a family with the A16V mutation of cationic trypsin plus the CFTR R117H mutation. In this report, all individuals within the family that had both mutations had both acute and chronic pancreatitis. This is markedly different from the original A16V mutation identified by Witt et al. [17] in which a family with the A16V mutation was identified, but only one of 5 family members with the mutation had pancreatitis. Thus, the combination of a milder cationic trypsinogen gene mutation that apparently predisposed to premature activation of trypsin but was insufficient to cause pancreatitis by itself, became disease-causing in combination with a CFTR mutation.

Other mutations

There have been a variety of mutations that have been reported in preliminary reports to be associated with pancreatitis. These include the N-acetyltransferase 2 gene (NAT2) in patients with alcoholic pancreatitis [36]. In two recent preliminary reports from Scotland, Buter et al. [37] reported an association between the severity of acute pancreatitis and markers associated with patients that either overexpressed TNF, or underexpressed IL-10. The importance of these observations remains to be fully explored.

Several mutations in well characterized genes cause *secondary* acute and chronic pancreatitis. These include familial hyperparathryroidism with hypercalcemia and recurrent acute and chronic pancreatitis [38], families with mutations in the lipoprotein lipase gene [39], and/or apolipoprotein C-II mutations [40–42] resulting in severe hyperlipidema and pancreatitis. Both of these syndromes are confirmed by established clinical observations that hypercalcema and hyperlipidema are associated with pancreatic injury.

Genetic testing and gene therapy

With the identification of specific gene mutations that are associated with chronic pancreatitis, an immediate opportunity becomes available for developing specific tests that will identify the presence of any one of these mutations with 100% certainty in patients with idiopathic chronic pancreatitis. However, there are tremendous implications for this type of testing. Unlike other types of clinical laboratory testing which have immediate implications for the patient's management but have few other implications (e.g. hematocrit), genetic testing has lifelong implications for the patient, their ancestors, and their children. Furthermore, concern exists over possible discrimination associated with a positive test, such as insurance and/or job discrimination [43, 44]. A positive or negative test result may elicit unexpected psychological responses from other members of the patient's families, including mutation-free siblings with "survival guilt" or a parent feeling responsible for their child's disorder. The considerations that go into genetic testing have been addressed in detail elsewhere [43, 44]. However, several important principles must be considered. First, will the test change medical management? For trypsin and possibly SPINK1/PSTI mutations, genetic testing may be useful in confirming a suspected diagnosis in *symptomatic* patients, thereby eliminating expensive and intensive evaluation. Secondly, genetic testing may be useful in guiding specific therapy, which unfortunately does not exist yet for pancreatic diseases. Third, testing for gene mutations in autosomal dominant disorders such as the cationic trypsinogen gene associated hereditary pancreatitis syndrome may be useful in *presymptomatic* individuals in families with hereditary pancreatitis and with high risk of developing the disease. Presymptomatic testing may be useful if it is likely to assist the patient in making life style decisions (such as whether or not to drink alcohol or to smoke cigarettes) or for family planning. However, testing for SPINK1/PSTI and CFTR mutations in asymptomatic individuals is not warranted since the risk of pancreatic disease in a mutation positive person is low. Thus, at the present time, genetic testing for CFTR mutations or SPINK1/PSTI mutations should probably be limited to tertiary referral centers with an active research program.

Another important consideration with highly penetrant mutations such as the trypsinogen R122H or N29I mutations in hereditary pancreatitis is the genetic testing of asymptomatic minors. The problem centers on informed consent. Minors less than age 7 years generally do not understand enough about diseases to make an informed decision about testing. Around age 7 the child enters the concrete operational stage of psychological development, and could give assent to testing with parental consent [45] and [46]. Testing for the purposes of relieving anxiety, learning about their own personal health and life style decisions, may be legitimate reasons for testing, if appropriate counseling and parental involvement is available [45, 46]. By age 12, most children enter the formal operational stage of development (age of reason), and comprehend many concepts of disease and risk. Usually, the child's assent and parental consent are needed for testing until the age of majority is reached (e.g. 18 years of age).

Gene therapy

Gene therapy is another consideration when a specific gene mutation is associated with a severe disease. At the present time, however, effective gene therapy to prevent hereditary pancreatitis seems unlikely [47]. The major limitations are: (1) the cationic trypsinogen mutation causes a gain-of-function so that the mutated gene must be suppressed, rather than having its function replaced; (2) the disease (pancreatitis) is expressed only episodically (e.g. once every 4 to 12 months) so that most of the time the mutation is inconsequential; (3) the phenotypic expression is sudden and unpredictable, and the injury phase is probably completed rapidly; and (4) the pancreas is relatively inaccessible for targeted delivery of viral or nonviral vectors [47]. Therefore, although genetic analysis provides tremendous potential for identifying individuals at risk of pancreatic disease, and preventing development of this disease may be on the horizon, it remains in the future.

Future directions

The work that has been accomplished in the last five years on the role of specific genes and genetic mutations in the initiation and development of acute and chronic pancreatitis have been truly remarkable. These discoveries go far beyond the limited number of families with hereditary pancreatitis because they have given insight into initiating events, the critical role of trypsin, the role of protective mechanisms such as trypsin inhibitors and trypsin autolysis, conditions that enhance trypsin, possible synergistic interaction between the acinar cells and the duct cells in patients with a combination of trypsinogen and CFTR mutations, and hints that a number of other gene mutations are also important in predisposing individuals to pancreatic disease. These findings are also pertinent for chronic pancreatitis because they suggest that there may be genetic predispositions to chronic pancreatitis which are not manifest until there is a sentinel acute pancreatitis event [13] resulting in activation and infiltration of immune cells and pancreatic stellate cells. As we learn more about the complex interactions with the pancreas, routine investigation of a panel of key genes may be feasible, providing a profile of a patient's risk for pancreatic diseases, type of disease and progression of the disease. This information may also prove useful to guide preventative strategies and more specific treatments while the majority of the pancreatic glands' function remains intact. The author sees this scenario as the brightest light on the horizon: the chance to prevent the devastating consequences of a destructive disease that we presently cannot cure.

References

1. Ammann RW, Muellhaupt B, Group ZPS. The natural history of pain in alcoholic chronic pancreatitis. Gastroenterology 1999; 116: 1132–40.
2. Steer ML, Waxman I, Freedman S. Chronic pancreatitis. New England Journal of Medicine 1995; 332(22): 1482–90.
3. Rinderknecht H. Pancreatic Secretory Enzymes. In: Go VLW, DiMagno EP, Gardner JD, Lebenthal E, Reber HA, Scheele GA, eds. The Pancreas: Biology, Pathobiology, and Disease. Second ed. New York: Raven Press, 1993: 219–51.
4. Rinderknecht H. Activation of pancreatic zymogens. Normal activation, premature intrapancreatic activation, protective mechanims against inappropriate activation. Digestive Diseases and Sciences 1986; 31: 314–21.
5. Le Bodic L, Bignon JD, Raguenes O, Mercier B, Georgelin T, Schnee M et al. The hereditary pancreatitis gene maps to long arm of chromosome 7. Human Molecular Genetics 1996; 5(4): 549–54.
6. Whitcomb DC, Preston RA, Aston CE, Sossenheimer MJ, Barua PS, Zhang Y et al. A gene for hereditary pancreatitis maps to chromosome 7q35. Gastroenterology 1996; 110(6): 1975–80.
7. Pandya A, Blanton SH, Landa B, Javaheri R, Melvin E, Nance WE et al. Linkage studies in a large kindred with hereditary pancreatitis confirms mapping of the gene to a 16-cm region on 7q. Genomics 1996; 38(2): 227–30.
8. Whitcomb DC, Gorry MC, Preston RA, Furey W, Sossenheimer MJ, Ulrich CD et al. Hereditary pancreatitis is caused by a mutation in the cationic trypsinogen gene. Nature Genetics 1996; 14(2): 141–5.
9. Pfützer RH, Whitcomb DC. Trypsinogen mutations in chronic pancreatitis (letter). Gastroenterology 1999; 117: 1508–9.
10. Whitcomb DC. Genetic Predispositions to Acute and Chronic Pancreatitis. Medical Clinics of North America 2000; 84(2): 531–47.

11. Higaki JN, Light A. Independent refolding of domains in the pancreatic serine proteinases. Journal of Biological Chemistry 1986; 261(23): 10606–9.
12. Rovery M. Limited proteolysis in pancreatic chymotrypsinogens and trypsinogens. Biochimie 1988; 70(9): 1131–5.
13. Whitcomb DC. Hereditary Pancreatitis: New insights into acute and chronic pancreatitis. Gut 1999; 45: 317–22.
14. Whitcomb DC. Early Trypsinogen Activation in Acute Pancreatitis. Gastroenterology 1999; 116(3): 770–3.
15. Lerch MM, Gorlick FS. Early trypsinogen activation in acute pancreatitis. Medical Clinics of North America 2000; 84(3): 549–63.
16. Gorry MC, Gabbaizedeh D, Furey W, Gates LK Jr, Preston RA, Aston CE et al. Mutations in the cationic trypsinogen gene are associated with recurrent acute and chronic pancreatitis. Gastroenterology 1997; 113(4): 1063–8.
17. Witt H, Luck W, Becker M. A signal peptide cleavage site mutation in the cationic trypsinogen gene is strongly associated with chronic pancreatitis. Gastroenterology 1999; 117: 7–10.
18. Ford M, Whitcomb DC. Analysis of the hereditary pancreatitis-associated cationic trypsinogen gene mutations in exons 2 and 3 by enzymatic mutation detection from a single 2.2-kb polymerase chain reaction product. Molecular Diagnosis 1999; 4: 211–32.
19. Ferec C, Raguenes O, Salomon R, Roche C, Bernard JP, Guillot M et al. Mutations in the cationic trypsinogen gene and evidence for genetic heterogeneity in hereditary pancreatitis. Journal of Medical Genetics 1999; 36(3): 228–32.
20. Teich N, Ockenga J, Hoffmeister A, Manns M, Mössner J, Keim V. Chronic pancreatitis associated with an activation peptide mutation that facilitates trypsin activation. Gastroenterology 2000; 119: 461–5.
21. Teich N, Ockenga J, Manns MP, Mössner J, Keim V. Evidence for further mutations of the cationic trypsinogen in hereditary pancreatitis (abstract). Digestion 1999; 60: 401.
22. Böhm AK, Reinheckel T, Rosenstrauch D, Halangk W, Schulz HU. Screening for a point mutation of cationic trypsinogen in patients with pancreatic disease (abstract). Digestion 1999; 60: 369.
23. Cohn JA, Bornstein JD, Jowell PS, Noone PG, Zhou Z, Branch MS et al. Molecular pathogenesis of chronic pancreatitis associated with abnormal CFTR genotypes. Gastroenterology 2000; 118(4): A159.
24. Creighton J, Lyall R, Wilson DI, Curtis A, Charnley R. Mutations of the cationic trypsinogen gene in patients with chronic pancreatitis [letter]. Lancet 1999; 354(9172): 42–3.
25. Bartness MA, Duerr RH, Ford MA, Zhang L, Barmada MM, Aston CE et al. A new hereditary pancreatitis gene may map to chromosome 12. Pancreas 1998; 17(4): 426.
26. Chen JM, Mercier B, Audrezet MP, Ferec C. Mutational analysis of the human pancreatic secretory trypsin inhibitor (PSTI) gene in hereditary and sporadic chronic pancreatitis. Journal of Medical Genetics 2000; 37: 67–9.
27. Pfützer RH, Barmada MM, Brunskill APJ et al. SPINK1/PSTI polymorphisms act as disease modifiers in familial and idiopathic chronic pancreatitis. Gastroenterology 2000; 119: 615–23.
28. Witt H, Luck W, Hennies HC, Classen M, Kage A, Lass U et al. Mutations in the gene encoding the serine protease inhibitor, Kazal type 1 are associated with chronic pancreatitis. Nature Genetics 2000; 25(2): 213–6.
29. Sharer N, Schwarz M, Malone G, Howarth A, Painter J, Super M et al. Mutations of the cystic fibrosis gene in patients with chronic pancreatitis. New England Journal of Medicine 1998; 339(10): 645–52.
30. Cohn JA, Friedman KJ, Noone PG, Knowles MR, Silverman LM, Jowell PS. Relation between mutations of the cystic fibrosis gene and idiopathic pancreatitis. New England Journal of Medicine 1998; 339(10): 653–8.
31. Cohn JA, Bornstein JD, Jowell PS. Cystic Fibrosis Mutations and Genetic Predisposition to Idiopathic Chronic Pancreatitis. In: Whitcomb DC, Cohn JA, Ulrich II CD, eds. The Medical Clinics of North America. Philadelphia: W. B. Saunders, 2000: 621–32.

32. Durie PR. Pancreatitis and mutations of the cystic fibrosis gene [editorial; comment]. New England Journal of Medicine 1998; 339(10): 687–8.
33. Chillon M, Casals T, Mercier B, Bassas L, Lissens W, Silber S et al. Mutations in the cystic fibrosis gene in patients with congenital absence of the vas deferens. New England Journal of Medicine 1995; 332(22): 1475–80.
34. Kerem E, Rave-Harel N, Augarten A, Madgar I, Nissim-Rafinia M, Yahav Y et al. A cystic fibrosis transmembrane conductance regulator splice variant with partial penetrance associated with variable cystic fibrosis presentations. American Journal of Respiratory & Critical Care Medicine 1997; 155(6): 1914–20.
35. Pfutzer RL, Li HS, Thompson BS, Ford MA, Eagon PK, Whitcomb DC. Pancreatic cholesterol esterase mRNA expression is upregulated in vivo during chronic ethanol feeding in rats (abstract). Pancreas 1999; 19(4): 435.
36. Palmer KJ, Gough AC, Primrose JN, Johnson CD. Inherited susceptibility to alcohol-induced acute pancreatitis (abstract). Digestion 1998; 59: 250.
37. Buter A, Eskdale J, Gallagher G, Robertson SA, Evans S, Carter RR et al. Microsatellite polymorphism at the human TNF and IL-10 loci in acute pancreatitis. Gastroenterology 2000; 118(4): A195.
38. Carey MC, Fitzgerald O. Hyperparathyroidism associated with chronic pancreatitis in a family. Gut 1968; 9(6): 700–3.
39. Wilson DE, Hata A, Kwong LK, Lingam A, Shuhua J, Ridinger DN et al. Mutations in exon 3 of the lipoprotein lipase gene segregating in a family with hypertriglyceridemia, pancreatitis, and non-insulin-dependent diabetes. Journal of Clinical Investigation 1993; 92(1): 203–11.
40. Beil FU, Fojo SS, Brewer HJ, Greten H, Beisiegel U. Apolipoprotein C-II deficiency syndrome due to apo C-IIHamburg: clinical and biochemical features and HphI restriction enzyme polymorphism. European Journal of Clinical Investigation 1992; 22(2): 88–95.
41. Cox DW, Breckenridge WC, Little JA. Inheritance of apolipoprotein C-II deficiency with hypertriglyceridemia and pancreatitis. New England Journal of Medicine 1978; 299(26): 1421–4.
42. Fojo SS, Brewer HB. Hypertriglyceridaemia due to genetic defects in lipoprotein lipase and apolipoprotein C-II. Journal of Internal Medicine 1992; 231(6): 669–77.
43. Applebaum SE, Kant JA, Whitcomb DC, Ellis IH. Genetic testing: counseling, laboratory and regulatory issues and the EUROPAC protocol for ethical research in multi-center studies of inherited pancreatic diseases. Medical Clinics of North America 2000; 82(3): 575–88.
44. Applebaum SE, O'Connell JA, Aston CE, Whitcomb DC. Motivations and concerns of patients with access to genetic testing for hereditary pancreatitis. American Journal of Gastroenterology 2000; 96(5): 1610–7.
45. O'Connell JA. The process of childhood genetic testing and disclosure: Parental views and intentions [Masters Thesis]. Pittsburgh, PA: University of Pittsburgh, 2000.
46. Etemad B, Whitcomb DC. Chronic Pancreatitis: Diagnosis, Classification and New Genetic Developments. Gastroenterology 2001; 120: 682–707.
47. Whitcomb DC. The Spectrum in Complications of Hereditary Pancreatitis: Is this a model for future gene therapy? Gastroenterology Clinics of North America 1999; 28(3): 525–41.

2.4 Alterations of immunocompetent peripheral blood lymphocytes in chronic pancreatitis patients

F. Gansauge

Abstract

Chronic pancreatitis is a chronic inflammatory disease of the exocrine pancreas. In approximately 30% an inflammatory mass of the pancreatic head is found, representing an indication for surgery. In order to investigate whether the chronic inflammatory process in chronic pancreatitis patients affects the immune function in these patients we evaluated the distribution and the proliferation capacity of peripheral blood lymphocytes in 28 patients suffering from chronic pancreatitis. Sixteen patients were also re-evaluated 1 year following resection of the pancreatic head for chronic pancreatitis. In comparison with an age and gender matched control group, in chronic pancreatitis patients the number of CD3+ cells was significantly increased with an increase of both CD3+CD4+ and CD3+CD8+ cells. The number of natural killer cells or B-lymphocytes did not differ between chronic pancreatitis patients and the control group. Following stimulation with PHA or anti-CD3-antibodies the blastogenic response was significantly attenuated in chronic pancreatitis patients. One year following resection of the pancreatic head for chronic pancreatitis the distribution as well as the blastogenic response to PHA and anti-CD3-antibodies had normalized as compared to the preoperative values ($p < 0.01$ and $p < 0.005$ respectively). These data provide evidence that the chronic inflammatory process in chronic pancreatitis markedly affects the distribution and function of peripheral immunocompetent blood cells and that elimination of the chronic inflammatory focus by pancreatic head resection restores the suppressed immune function in these patients.

Introduction

Chronic pancreatitis is characterized by a painful progressive destruction of the pancreatic gland with increasing loss of exocrine and endocrine function. Approximately 30% of patients with chronic pancreatitis develop a pancreatic head enlargement. This enlargement of the pancreatic head can lead to various complications, like obstruction of the bile duct, the pancreatic duct and the duodenum or compression of the portal vein or the mesenteric artery. These complications represent an indication for surgical treatment [1–3]. Besides the removal of the local complication, the resection of the enlarged pancreatic head offers several other advantages, since the inflamed pancreatic head is suspected to be the locomotive element which supports chronic pancreatitis [4]. On the other hand recent studies provided evidence that chronic pancreatitis patients have an up to tenfold increased risk of developing pancreatic carcinoma [5].

In recent studies several groups investigated the infiltrating lymphocytes in tissue specimens of chronic pancreatitis [6–9]. All investigators found an increased number of infiltrating lymphocytes and most groups support the hypothesis of an involvement of cell-mediated cytotoxicity in the pathogenesis of chronic pancreatitis, as shown by elevated frequencies of perforin-expressing cells [10] or CD8+CD103+ T cells [6] in chronic pancreatitis. In contrast to this hypothesis of cell-mediated toxicity Emmrich and coworkers found a more common inflammatory type of infiltrating lymphocytes in chronic pancreatitis tissue specimens [8].

With regard to alterations of the systemic immune function only rare data are available. In previous studies we have investigated serum levels of immunological parameters like neopterin, sIL-2Rα, sCD44s and sCD44v6 in chronic pancreatitis. Interestingly, we found reduced serum levels of sCD44v6 whereas serum levels of sIL-2Rα and neopterin were not altered in chronic pancreatitis patients [11].

The aim of our study was to investigate the distribution and proliferation capacity to PHA, ConA, PWM and anti-CD3-antibodies of peripheral blood lymphocytes in comparison to a gender and age matched group of healthy volunteers. Furthermore, we compared these data in 16 chronic pancreatitis patients prior to and one year following resection of the pancreatic head in order to evaluate whether the resection of the inflamed pancreatic head leads to a normalization of the distribution and function of peripheral blood lymphocytes.

Patients and methods

Patients

Between March 1997 and December 1998 28 patients with the diagnosis of chronic pancreatitis were enrolled into the prospective study. In all patients included in this study the time between the last exacerbation of chronic pancreatitis and the immunological analyses was longer than 3 months in order to avoid an influence of the results by acute inflammatory processes. The main indication for pancreatic head resection was long lasting pain (20/21) and obstruction of the common bile duct (12/21). In all patients with compression of the common bile duct endoscopic stenting prior to operation had been performed. Twenty-one patients underwent resection of the pancreatic head due to chronic pancreatitis. In 19 patients a duodenum-preserving pancreatic head resection and in 2 patients a pylorus-preserving duodenopancreatectomy was performed. In one patient a resection of the pancreatic tail was performed. In 6 patients no resection was performed (1 cystojejunostomy, 1 Ligamentum arcuatum resection, 4 biopsies). In all patients the diagnosis was confirmed by histological examination. The mean age was 48 years ranging from 32 to 67 years. 25 patients were male, 3 patients were female. Twenty of the 28 patients had a history of chronic alcohol abuse (defined as alcohol consumption of more than 50 ml per day). In all patients 15 ml of heparinized blood and 4 ml of EDTA-blood was drawn prior to operation and immediately proceeded for the examinations concerning the immune status. In sixteen patients the immune status was again evaluated 1 year following pancreatic head resection. The control group of healthy volunteers comprised 20 patients (mean age 46.8 years ranging from 28 to 71 years), Four patients were female, 16 patients were male.

All patients gave informed consent to the study. The study was performed according to the local Ethic committee.

Determination of peripheral blood lymphocytes

For the identification of peripheral blood lymphocytes in whole blood we used a four-color immunofluorescence method as described previously [12]. Following directly labeled mouse-anti human antibodies were used: anti-CD3-FITC, anti-CD8-PE, anti-CD4-APC, anti-CD45-Percp, anti-CD56-PE, and anti-CD19-APC (all Dianova, Hamburg, Germany).

Determination of proliferation capacity of peripheral blood lymphocytes

The proliferation capacity of peripheral blood lymphocytes following stimulation with phytohemagglutinin (PHA), Concavalin A (ConA), Pokeweed mitogen (PWM) and anti-CD3-antibodies was determined by using a commercially available kit (Blastest, YLEM, Roma, Italy). Immediately following puncture 250 µl of heparinated whole blood were incubated in 3 ml of culture medium and incubated at 5% CO_2 atmosphere at 37°C in a glass vial. Every blood sample consisted of 5 probes, containing PHA-, ConA-, PWM-, anti-CD3-stimulation or control. After a 72 h incubation period nuclei were isolated and stained with propidium iodide according to the manufacturer's instructions. The nuclei were analyzed on a FACScan (Becton Dickinson, Germany) using the Cell Quest program. The corrected stimulation index (CSI) was calculated using the following formula: CSI = (S/G2-phase % stimulated culture) – (S/G2-phase % control culture).

Determination of TGF-β1 levels in peripheral blood

Levels of TGF-β1 were determined in EDTA plasma of the patients and the control group using a commercially available ELISA according to the manufacturer's instructions (R&D Systems Inc., Minneapolis, MN, USA).

Statistics

All statistics were calculated using the Medcalc Software Package. Significance was set at $p < 0.05$. Significances were calculated using the Student's t-test.

Results

Distribution and proliferation capacity following mitogenic stimulation of peripheral blood lymphocytes

No differences were observed between chronic pancreatitis patients and healthy blood donors concerning leukocyte count and red blood cell count. However, the number of lymphocytes per µl was significantly increased in chronic pancreatitis patients (Fig. 2.4-1, $p < 0.05$). This increased number of peripheral blood lymphocytes was mainly due to an increased number of CD3+ cells ($p < 0.005$). Further analyses showed that CD3+CD4+ and CD3+CD8+ lymphocytes were both elevated in peripheral blood of chronic pancreatitis patients ($p < 0.01$ and $p < 0.05$). The number of B-cells (CD19+) or NK-cells (CD16+) did not differ between chronic pancreatitis patients and healthy blood donors. When peripheral blood was stimulated with PWM or ConA, no differences were observed between chronic pancreatitis patients and healthy blood donors. However, when peripheral blood lymphocytes were stimulated by either PHA or anti-CD3, the CSIs differed significantly between chronic pancreatitis patients and healthy blood donors. Following stimulation with PHA, the CSI in CP was 19.9% (SEM 1.54) as compared to 25.3% (SEM

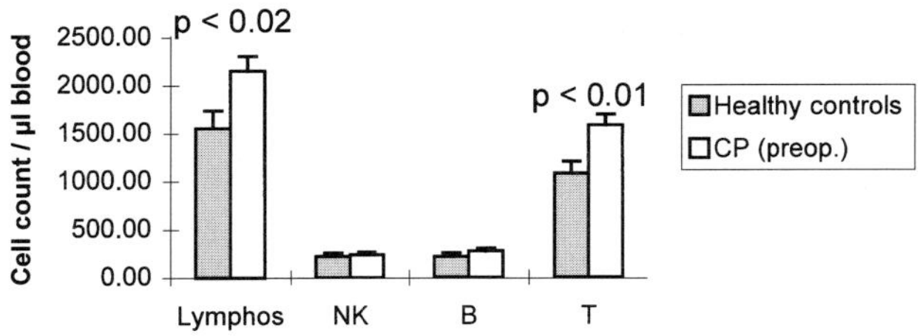

Figure 2.4-1. Cell count of lymphocytes and lymphocyte subsets in chronic pancreatitis patients and healthy controls. In chronic pancreatitis patients the total number of lymphocytes (lymph.) was significantly higher than in controls. This increase was mainly due to an increased number of CD3+ T cells (T). The number of natural killer cells (NK) or B-lymphocytes was not different between chronic pancreatitis patients and healthy controls.

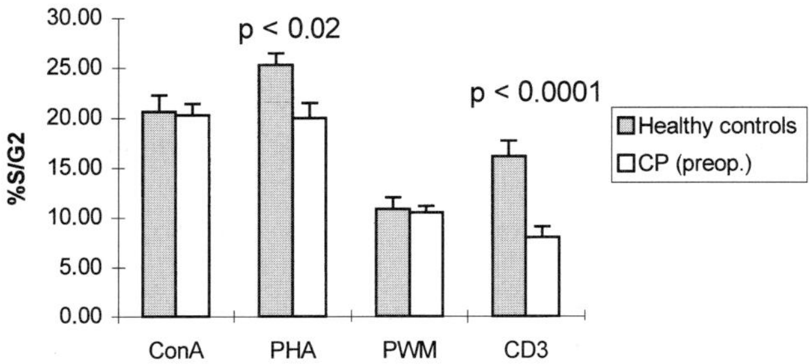

Figure 2.4-2. Blastogenic response of peripheral blood lymphocytes following stimulation with ConA, PHA, PWM or anti-CD3. In chronic pancreatitis patients the blastogenic response was significantly reduced following stimulation with PHA or anti-CD3 antibodies as compared to healthy controls.

1.2) in healthy blood donors ($p < 0.02$). Following stimulation with anti-CD3 these differences were even more visible, in CP the CSI was 7.99% (SEM 1.1) as compared to 16.1% (SEM 1.6) in HC ($p < 0.0001$), pointing to a possible immune dysfunction especially in CD3+ lymphocytes in chronic pancreatitis patients (Fig. 2.4-2).

Determination of TGF-β1 plasma levels revealed significantly increased TGF-β1 levels in chronic pancreatitis patients as compared to the group of healthy blood donors (CP: 5.9ng/mL, SEM 0.21; HC: 4.2ng/mL, SEM 0.3; $p < 0.005$).

Function of peripheral immunocytes

The function of peripheral immunocytes is not dependent on exocrine or endocrine pancreatic insufficiency in chronic pancreatitis patients. In order to test whether the distribution or function of peripheral immunocytes in chronic pancreatitis patients is dependent on risk factors or comorbidity (exocrine or endocrine insufficiency) the chronic pancreatitis patients were analyzed with regard to gender, age, duration of symptoms, diabetes, exocrine insufficiency, nutrition status (determined by body mass indices), and elevated levels of the acute phase parameter C-reactive protein. Neither gender, duration of symptoms, serum protein levels nor serum CRP levels had any influence on the distribution or function of peripheral blood lymphocytes. With regard to the nutritional status we found that patients with a BMI below 20 (6/28 patients) had an increased number of CD3+CD4+ peripheral blood lymphocytes (mean 1399.5/μl, SEM 127) as compared to patients with a BMI above 20 (22/28 patients, mean 947.5/μl, SEM 79; $p < 0.02$). The other measured parameters did not differ. With regard to the endocrine and exocrine function, patients with endocrine insufficiency (n = 15) had a significantly higher number of peripheral CD56+ cells (299/μl, SEM 56) than patients without endocrine insufficiency (n = 13, 192/μl, SEM 17, $p < 0.05$, Table 2.4-1). Furthermore, the T4/T8 ratio was significantly lower in diabetic patients with chronic pancreatitis than chronic pancreatitis patients without endocrine insufficiency (diabetes: 1.87, SEM 0.2, no diabetes: 2.58, SEM 0.2; $p < 0.05$, Table 2.4-1). This difference was mainly due to a higher number of CD3+CD8+ cells in diabetic patients, although this did not reach statistical significance (diabetes: 584/μl, SEM 69, no diabetes: 468/μl, SEM 56, p = 0.16). Patients with exocrine insufficiency as determined by pathologic Pancreato-Lauryl-Test (n = 20) had significantly higher amounts of peripheral blood CD19+ B-lymphocytes (337/μl, SEM 38) than chronic pancreatitis patients without exocrine insufficiency (n = 8, 179/μl, SEM 35, $p < 0.01$, Table 2.4-1). The other parameters were not dependent on endocrine or exocrine insufficiency. The proliferation capacity following mitogenic stimulation by ConA, PHA, PWM or anti-CD3 was not dependent on gender, age, duration of symptoms, diabetes, exocrine insufficiency, nutrition status, or C-reactive protein levels.

Patients with a history of chronic alcohol abuse had a tendency towards higher CSIs following stimulation with PHA, PWM or anti-CD-3 antibodies than patients without chronic alcohol abuse, although this did not reach statistical significance. The distribution of peripheral immunocytes was not significantly altered (Table 2.4-1). Nicotine abuse also had no influence on these parameters.

Table 2.4-1. Distribution and proliferation capacity of peripheral blood lymphocytes with regard to exocrine and endocrine function and alcohol consumption in chronic pancreatitis.

	Endocrine function		**Exocrine function**		**Alcohol abuse**	
	diabetes (n = 15)	no diabetes (n = 13)	PLT > 4 (n = 8)	PLT < 4 (n = 20)	no (n = 8)	yes (n = 20)
Lymphocytes/μl	2342 (247)	2009 (101)	1819 (208)	2286 (172)	1963 (202)	2215 (178)
CD56+/μl	**299 (56)***	**192 (17)***	173 (28)	263 (35)	241 (41)	
CD19+/μl	323 (45)	237 (21)	**179 (35)***	**337 (38)***	237 (54)	286 (31)
CD3+/μl	1664 (172)	1518 (90)	1446 (187)	1634 (125)	1442 (153)	1626 (131)
CD3+CD4+/μl	1055 (124)	1036 (66)	895 (125)	1104 (90)	821 (83)	1119 (93)
CD3+CD8+/μl	584 (69)	468 (56)	514 (92)	510 (50)	599 (81)	482 (51)
T4/T8	**1.87 (0.17)***	**2.58 (0.2)***	2.0 (0.3)	2.4 (0.2)	1.9 (0.3)	2.5 (0.2)
CSI						
ConA (%)	19.4 (1.5)	20.9 (1.1)	20.5 (2.6)	20.2 (1.1)	19.4 (2.2)	20.9 (1.1)
PHA (%)	20 (2.1)	20.1 (7.3)	17.6 (2.7)	20.9 (1.7)	18.4 (3.2)	21.1 (1.3)
PWM (%)	10.1 (1)	10.8 (0.5)	9.9 (0.9)	10.8 (0.8)	9.3 (1.3)	11.4 (0.6)
anti-CD3 (%)	6.9 (1.3)	8.9 (1.2)	7.3 (2.4)	8.3 (1.1)	6.2 (1.9)	9.5 (1.1)
TGF-β1 (ng/ml)	**6.4 (0.2)****	**5.4 (0.2)****	6.1 (0.4)	5.8 (0.2)	6.5 (0.3)	5.7 (0.2)

* $p < 0.05$
** $p < 0.01$

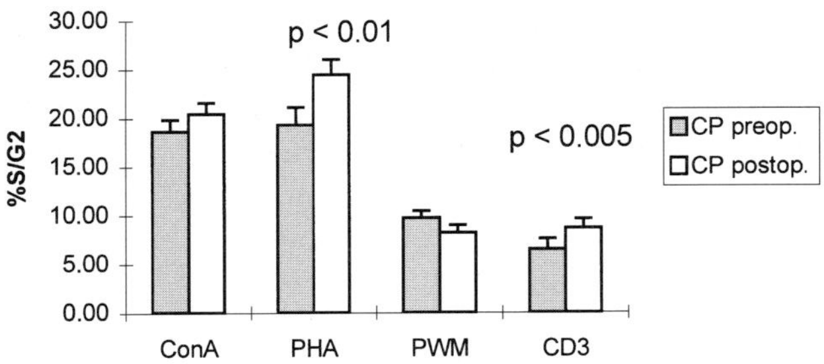

Figure 2.4-3. Blastogenic response of peripheral blood lymphocytes following stimulation with ConA, PHA, PWM or anti-CD3 in chronic pancreatitis patients before and one year after pancreatic head resection. Following pancreatic head resection the blastogenic response to PHA and anti-CD3 increased significantly.

We found a strong inverse correlation between the blastogenic response of peripheral blood following stimulation with anti-CD3 antibodies and plasma levels of TGF-β1 in chronic pancreatitis patients ($r = -0.68$, $p < 0.0001$), whereas the inverse correlation between blastogenic response following PHA stimulation and plasma TGF-β1 levels did not reach statistical significance ($r = -0.35$, $p = 0.08$) pointing to a direct relation between elevated levels of TGF-β1 and a reduced response to stimulation of peripheral T-lymphocytes in chronic pancreatitis.

Following resection of the pancreatic head in chronic pancreatitis the distribution and function of peripheral immunocytes normalize. Out of the 21 patients who underwent resection of the pancreatic head due to chronic pancreatitis sixteen patients were examined one year following resection of the pancreatic head. Interestingly, the number of peripheral blood lymphocytes, especially CD3+ cells, had normalized (Table 2.4-2). CD3+CD4+

Table 2.4-2. Distribution and proliferation capacity of peripheral blood lymphocytes before and one year after pancreatic head resection for chronic pancreatitis.

	Chronic pancreatitis patients (n=16)		
	preoperativ (SEM)	Postoperativ (SEM)	p-value
Lymphocytes/μl	2035 (199)	1652 (134)	0.07
CD56+/μl	248 (41)	205 (29)	0.34
CD19+/μl	261 (35)	239 (38)	0.54
CD3+/μl	1468 (143)	1181 (97)	***0.03***
CD3+CD4+/μl	939 (96)	739 (61)	***0.03***
CD3+CD8+/μl	512 (65)	420 (47)	0.08
T4/T8	2.08 (0.22)	2.06 (0.24)	0.65
CSI			
ConA (%)	18.6 (1.23)	20.4 (1.18)	0.08
PHA (%)	19.3 (1.79)	24.4 (1.59)	***0.01***
PWM (%)	9.71 (0.75)	8.18 (0.83)	0.11
Anti-CD3 (%)	6.5 (1.09)	8.67 (0.99)	***0.005***

CSI = corrected stimulation index, SEM = standard error of the mean and CD3+CD8+ cells had both decreased as compared to the preoperative values. Also in the blastogenic response to mitogens the preoperatively reduced values of CSIs following stimulation of peripheral blood with PHA or anti-CD3 increased significantly (PHA-stimulation CP pre vs. CP post. $p < 0.01$; anti-CD3-stimulation CP pre vs. CP post. $p < 0.005$, Fig. 2.4-3, Table 2.4-2).

Discussion

Chronic pancreatitis is a disease which primarily affects the exocrine pancreas. In the course of chronic pancreatitis continuous destruction of the pancreatic acinar and ductal cells occurs and these cells are replaced by fibrous tissue. An overproduction of extracellular matrix molecules may further compromise the remaining parenchyma leading to an ongoing process of tissue destruction which finally ends in exocrine and sometimes endocrine insufficiency. So far several hypotheses for the development of chronic pancreatitis have been postulated; however, the exact pathomechanisms of this disease still remain unclear. Recent studies provided evidence of an overproduction of several growth factors, like EGF or members of the TGF-β family [13–15]. Especially the overproduction of TGF-β in chronic pancreatitis seems to be an important factor in the excessive production of extracellular matrix molecules, inducing the connective tissue growth factor (CTGF) and subsequently leading to the production of collagen, fibronectin and proteoglycan [13, 16, 17]. However, TGF-β is also known to be a potent immunosuppressive agent *in vitro* and has been shown to effectively inhibit immune function in chronic inflammatory lesions *in vivo* [18]. Especially *in viral* or bacterial chronic inflammatory processes like hepatitis or streptococcal infections TGF-β is supposed to be one of the factors responsible for the immune dysfunction in the local inflammation site as well as the imbalance of the systemic immune cells [18, 19]. Corresponding to these results we found a direct inverse correlation between TGF-β1 plasma levels and a reduced blastogenic response of peripheral T-lymphocytes following stimulation with anti-CD3 antibodies.

In our study we found an increased number of peripheral CD3+ cells, with an increase of both CD3+CD4+ and CD3+CD8+ cells. However, stimulation of the peripheral blood lymphocytes with anti-CD3 antibodies resulted in decreased CSIs as compared to a gender and age matched control group, pointing to an immune dysbalance in the peripheral blood lymphocytes in chronic pancreatitis. Also, when peripheral blood was stimulated with PHA, the CSIs of chronic pancreatitis were markedly decreased as compared to the control group. These observations could offer new aspects for the discussion about whether chronic pancreatitis patients have an increased risk of developing pancreatic cancer. Recently, special entities of chronic pancreatitis like hereditary pancreatitis [20] or the tropical form of chronic pancreatitis [9] have been claimed to be associated with a highly increased risk for pancreatic cancer. Even in alcoholic pancreatitis the risk of pancreatic cancer seems to be elevated [5]. However, these patients also seem to have an overall increased cancer risk [21], which could be due to risk factors like alcohol and smoking. Anyhow, in our patients suffering from chronic pancreatitis neither alcohol consumption nor smoking had a negative influence on the distribution of peripheral blood cells. Interestingly, the CSIs following stimulation with PHA, PWM or anti-CD3 antibodies even had the tendency to be higher in chronic pancreatitis patients with a history of chronic alcohol abuse than in patients without, suggesting that the immune dysfunction and probably the reduced immunosurveillance in chronic pancreatitis patients is not related to alcohol consumption. Nicotine abuse had no influence on the distribution or function in chronic pancreatitis patients either.

In order to confirm our hypothesis that chronic inflammatory processes are the reason for the reduced proliferation capacity of peripheral blood lymphocytes we investigated the distribution and proliferation capacity of peripheral blood lymphocytes of 16 chronic pancreatitis patients one year following pancreatic head resection. We did indeed find a significant restoration of the CSIs as compared to the preoperative values and the distribution of peripheral blood lymphocytes had also normalized, which supports the idea that the local inflammatory process is the reason for the systemic immune dysfunction in chronic pancreatitis patients.

In conclusion, we demonstrated for the first time that the chronic inflammatory process in chronic pancreatitis markedly affects the distribution and function of peripheral immunocompetent blood cells and that elimination of the chronic inflammatory focus by pancreatic head resection restores the suppressed immune function in these patients.

References

1. Beger HG, Büchler MW, Bittner RR, Oettinger W, Roscher R. Duodenum-preserving resection of the head of the pancreas in severe chronic pancreatitis. Early and late results. Ann Surg 1989; 209: 273–8.
2. Beger HG, Krautzberger W, Bittner RR, Büchler MW, Limmer J. Duodenum-preserving resection of the head of the pancreas in patients with severe chronic pancreatitis. Surgery 1985; 97: 467–73.
3. Ammann RW, Akovbiantz A, Largiader F, Schueler G. Course and outcome of chronic pancreatitis. Longitudinal study of a mixed medical-surgical series of 245 patients. Gastroenterology 1984; 86: 820–8.
4. Frey CF, Bodai BI. Surgery in chronic pancreatitis. Clin Gastroenterol 1984; 13: 913–40.
5. Lowenfels AB, Maisonneuve P, Cavallini G, Ammann RW, Lankisch PG, Andersen JR, DiMagno EP, Andren-Sandberg A, Domellof L. Pancreatitis and the risk of pancreatic cancer. International Pancreatitis Study Group. N Engl J Med 1993; 328: 1433–7.
6. Ebert M, Ademmer K, Muller-Ostermeyer F, Friess H, Büchler MW, Schubert W, Malfertheiner P. CD8+CD103+ T cells analogous to intestinal intraepithelial lymphocytes infiltrate the pancreas in chronic pancreatitis. Am J Gastroenterol 1998; 93: 2141–7.
7. Muller-Ostermeyer F, Ebert M, Malfertheiner P, Schubert W. T-cell receptor alpha gene expression of infiltrating T cells in pancreatic cancer. Scand J Gastroenterol 1998; 33: 872–9.
8. Emmrich J, Weber I, Nausch M et al. Immunohistochemical characterization of the pancreatic cellular infiltrate in normal pancreas, chronic pancreatitis and pancreatic carcinoma. Digestion 1998; 59: 192–8.
9. Ramesh H. Tropical pancreatitis. Indian J Gastroenterol 1997; 16: 20–5.
10. Hunger RE, Mueller C, Zgraggen K, Friess H, Büchler MW. Cytotoxic cells are activated in cellular infiltrates of alcoholic chronic pancreatitis. Gastroenterology 1997; 112: 1656–63.
11. Birk D, Gansauge F, Gansauge S, Schwarz A, Beger HG. Levels of serum neopterin are increased in pancreatic cancer patients and correlate with prognosis. Eur J Med Res 1999; 4: 1–6.
12. von Laer D, Modrau B, Dietrich M, Kern P. Leukocyte differentiation antigens in the bone marrow of patients with HIV-related disease. Acta Haematol 1994; 92: 197–203.
13. Lee MS, Gu D, Feng L, Curriden S, Arnush M, Krahl T, Gurushanthaiah D, Wilson C, Loskutoff DL, Fox H, Sarvetnick N. Accumulation of extracellular matrix and developmental dysregulation in the pancreas by transgenic production of transforming growth factor β1. Am J Pathol 1995; 147: 42–52.

14. Van Laethem JL, Deviere J, Resibois A, Rickaert F, Vertongen P, Ohtani H, Cremer M, Miyazono K, Robberecht P. Localization of transforming growth factor β1 and its latent binding protein in human chronic pancreatitis. Gastroenterology 1995; 108: 1873–81.
15. Yamanaka Y, Friess H, Büchler MW, Beger HG, Gold LI, Korc M. Synthesis and expression of transforming growth factor beta-1, beta-2, and beta-3 in the endocrine and exocrine pancreas. Diabetes 1993; 42: 746–56.
16. Grotendorst GR, Okochi H, Hayashi N. A novel transforming growth factor beta response element controls the expression of the connective tissue growth factor gene. Cell Growth Differ 1996; 7: 469–80.
17. Wenger C, Ellenrieder V, Alber B et al. Expression and differential regulation of connective tissue growth factor in pancreatic cancer cells. Oncogene 1999; 18: 1073–80.
18. Wahl SM, Hunt DA, Bansal G, McCartney Francis N, Ellingsworth L, Allen JB. Bacterial cell wall-induced immunosuppression. Role of transforming growth factor beta. J Exp Med 1988; 168: 1403–17.
19. Banner BF, Allan C, Savas L, Baker S, Barnard G, Bonkovsky HL. Inflammatory markers in chronic hepatitis C. Virchows Arch 1997; 431: 181–7.
20. Lowenfels AB, Maisonneuve P, DiMagno EP et al. Hereditary pancreatitis and the risk of pancreatic cancer. International Hereditary Pancreatitis Study Group. J Natl Cancer Inst 1997; 89: 442–6.
21. Hansen TH, Laursen M, Christensen E, Worning H. Chronic pancreatitis and extrapancreatic cancer: a retrospective study among 181 patients with chronic pancreatitis. Int J Pancreatol 1995; 18: 235–9.

2.5 Comparison of alcoholic, tropical and idiopathic chronic pancreatitis on a molecular basis

S. Shrikhande, H. Friess, H. Ramesh, A. Zimmermann, M. W. Büchler

Introduction

Chronic pancreatitis (CP) is an inflammatory disease of the pancreas leading to progressive and irreversible morphological alterations along with functional derangement. The progression of the disease may be slow with long-term preservation of pancreatic function or rapidly progressive, and the extended fibrosis results in varying degrees of exocrine and in the later stages even endocrine pancreatic insufficiency [1, 2, 3]. While the clinical features in alcoholic, tropical and idiopathic CP are similar in many respects, tropical chronic pancreatitis has some unique clinical features; the patients are young without any history of alcoholism, the calculi are larger and invariably located intraductally and the disease appears to run an accelerated course in comparison to other forms of CP [4]. While alcoholic and idiopathic CP have been more intensively studied, they have not been compared with tropical CP on a molecular basis. Our group undertook such a study to evaluate whether irrespective of the underlying etiology, the disease approaches a "common stage" and progresses as a distinctive entity.

Etiology

In the Western world, the dominant etiological factor of CP is alcohol abuse, accounting for approximately 80% of the patients [5]. In a small percentage of patients (approximately 7%) with CP, alcohol abuse can be clearly ruled out as an etiological factor and in the absence of other known etiological factors (hypercalcemia, hyperlipoproteinemia, heredi-

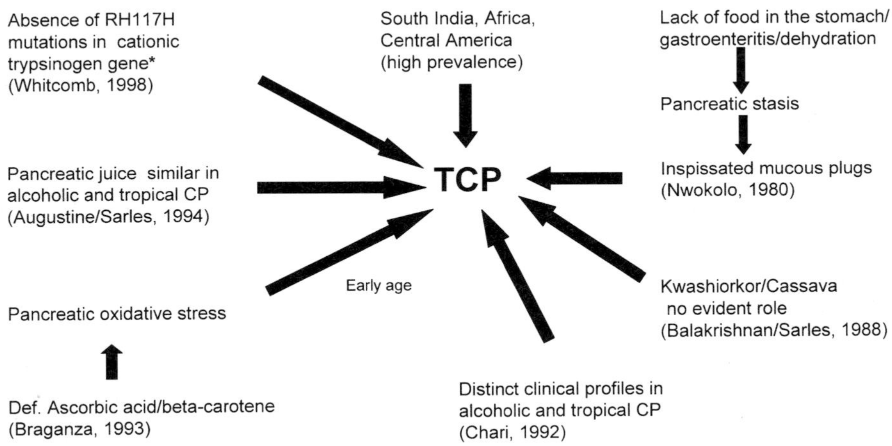

Figure 2.5-1. Pathogenetic facts and hypotheses on factors involved in the development of tropical chronic pancreatitis (TCP).

tary factors, tropical CP etc.), this group of patients are classed under idiopathic CP [2, 5–7]. In contrast to Western countries, in Southern India and other tropical belts of the world, an alcohol independent form of chronic pancreatitis – so called tropical pancreatitis – is common [4, 8–11]. Nutritional and environmental factors were propagated in the 70s and 80s as major causative factors in the pathogenesis of this form of chronic pancreatitis [12, 13]. However, etiological studies in 1988 [14] and 1994 [15] concluded that nutritional factors seem to have no evident role in the evolution of tropical CP. Thus, the etiology of tropical chronic pancreatitis remains largely unknown (Figure 2.5-1).

Genetic studies

In recent years a vast amount of research in chronic pancreatitis has focused on genetic analysis. A significant advance has been the discovery of mutations in the cystic fibrosis transmembrane conductance regulator gene in a sub-group of patients who were classified as idiopathic CP [16]. These mutations were noted in approximately 30% of patients with previously diagnosed idiopathic CP, suggesting that genetic alterations are of relevance in this group of patients with CP. The hypothesis of gene mutations in tropical CP has also been explored. However, RH 117H mutations of the cationic trypsinogen gene that are commonly observed in hereditary CP are absent in tropical CP patients, diminishing the etiological relevance of trypsinogen gene mutations in tropical CP [17].

Growth factors in chronic pancreatitis

Growth factors and growth factor receptors are known to play a role in the morphological changes that occur in chronic pancreatitis. The epidermal growth factor (EGF) receptor is a transmembrane protein that binds EGF and transforming growth factor alpha (TGF-alpha). Previous studies have shown that TGF-alpha may act through autocrine and paracrine mechanisms to excessively activate the overexpressed EGF receptor in the ductal and acinar cells of the exocrine pancreas, thereby contributing to the pathobiology of this disorder [18]; c-erb B-2 protooncogene regulates cell growth and differentiation. It has been demonstrated that c-erb B-2 is overexpressed in patients of chronic pancreatitis with an inflammatory mass in the head of the pancreas. Its overexpression has been suggested to contribute to processes leading to an inflammatory mass in the head of the pancreas [19]. Similarly, acidic fibroblast growth factor (aFGF) and basic fibroblast growth factor (bFGF) are mitogenic polypeptides that are involved in cellular proliferation and differentiation. Abundant overexpression of these growth factors in pancreatic acinar and ductal cells in chronic pancreatitis suggests their possible role in the fibrotic process that characterizes chronic pancreatitis [20]. Connective tissue growth factor (CTGF), which is regulated by transforming growth factor beta (TGF-beta), has recently been implicated in extracellular matrix synthesis and accumulation, resulting finally in the fibrogenesis observed in chronic pancreatitis [21]. Similarly, upregulation of phospholipase A2 isoforms (PLA2) such as PLA2 types II and IV in areas of chronic pancreatitis with increased histologic damage suggest that they might contribute to the morphologic changes that occur in chronic pancreatitis [22].

However, all these studies have been performed only in alcoholic chronic pancreatitis and it is not known whether these findings hold true even in other forms of chronic pancreatitis.

Neural changes and pain in chronic pancreatitis – The neuroimmune interaction

In alcoholic CP, neural changes involving neural proliferation with resultant increase in number of nerves and nerve diameter, damage of the perineurium, increase in sensory neurotransmitters and a neuroimmune interaction of inflammatory cells with altered nerves have been reported [23–26]. All these changes are implicated in the development of pain in alcoholic CP [26]. Upper abdominal pain in CP is the single most important link between the patient and the clinician and is also the most common indication for surgery. However, besides alcoholic CP, even other types of CP such as idiopathic [27] and tropical CP are associated with severe pain [28]. Therefore, if nerves are involved in the pathogenesis of pain in CP, similar neural alterations should be present in different etiological forms of CP such as idiopathic or tropical CP. To further test this hypothesis, neural changes in alcoholic, idiopathic and tropical CP were evaluated and compared.

Comparison of neural changes in alcoholic, tropical and idiopathic chronic pancreatitis

Neural changes were evaluated in three forms of CP, since similar neural changes in different forms of CP would provide further evidence as regards the significance of neural alterations in the pain pathogenesis of CP. The average area of nerves per tissue and the percentage of tissue occupied by nerves were calculated. Also, the innervation area per nerve and number of nerves per 10 mm^2 of tissue area were calculated. Since inflammatory cell infiltrates are regularly noted in alcoholic CP and a close interaction between inflammatory cells, pancreatic nerves and the presence of pain was recently reported, perineural inflammation was also evaluated. To quantify and to summarize the degree of perineural inflammation in CP tissues, a perineural inflammation number score and a perineural area score were calculated taking into account the total number of perineural inflammatory foci, the area of foci, the density of the cell infiltrates and the total area of the tissue sections evaluated.

Patients of different etiological groups included in the evaluation had a comparable pain syndrome with regard to pain intensity, frequency and duration and exhibited similar neural alterations (Figure 2.5-2A and B) with an increase in neuronal tissue, supporting the hypothesis that changes in innervation are of importance in the pain syndrome of CP. A point to note was that while the number of nerves per tissue section was more in alcoholic and idiopathic CP, the size of nerves, and not the number of nerves, was significantly more in tropical CP. We also found a similar pattern of perineural inflammatory cell infiltrates without any significant differences, irrespective of the etiological initiation of the disease (Figure 2.5-2B). These findings, considered together, indicate that comparable neural alterations occur in painful CP independent of the underlying etiology and possibly explain the similar course of pain observed in alcoholic and non-alcoholic chronic pancreatitis [27, 28].

Immune cells in chronic pancreatitis

It is well known that the morphological changes in alcoholic CP are associated with infiltration by inflammatory cells [6, 29]. The immune cell reaction in alcoholic CP appears

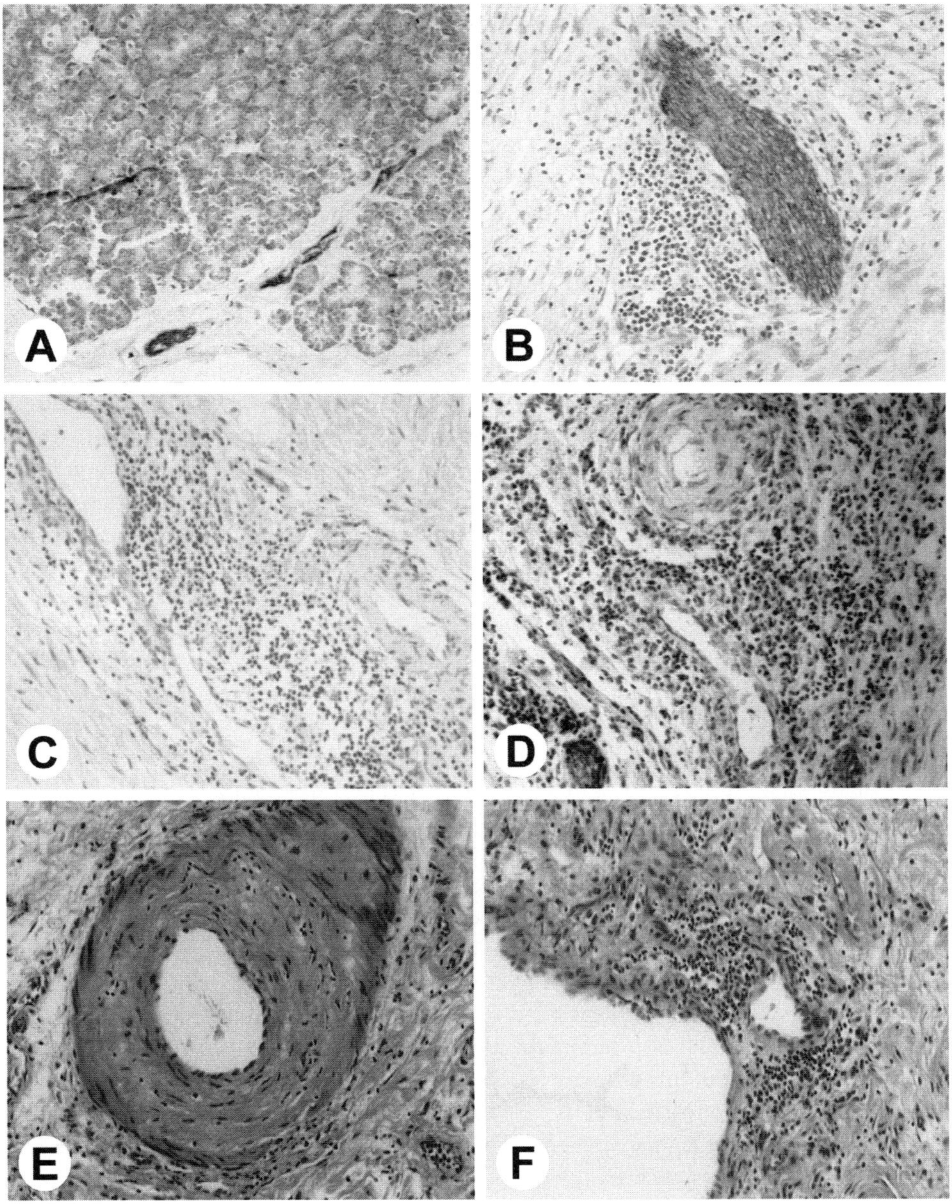

Figure 2.5-2A–F. Histological and immunohistochemical analysis of chronic pancreatitis. **A:** Visualization of pancreatic nerves by immunohistochemical staining with the panneuronal marker PGP 9.5 in the normal pancreas. **B:** Visualization of pancreatic nerves by immunohistochemical staining with the panneuronal marker PGP 9.5 in chronic pancreatitis. Nerve diameter in chronic pancreatitis is increased in comparison to the normal pancreas. **C:** Perivascular cellular infiltrate in non-tropical (alcoholic) CP. **D:** Typical intense perivascular cellular infiltrate in tropical CP. **E:** Arteriopathy as seen exclusively in tropical CP. **F:** Endophlebitis as seen exclusively in tropical CP.

to be varied. While one study reported that CD 4+ cells form the dominant subset of lymphocytes that infiltrate the pancreas in CP and CD 8+ and CD 103+ cells may play an important role in the first line of defense against deleterious epithelial events involved in chronic pancreatitis [30, 31, 32], others concluded that the inflammatory cell infiltrates in alcoholic CP are composed predominantly of CD 8+ lymphocytes [29]. Thus they are now considered to be important players in the pathogenesis of this disorder where the characteristic chronic inflammation is thought to be immune mediated [33, 34, 35, 36].

Comparison of immune cell infiltrates and histologic features in alcoholic, tropical and idiopathic chronic pancreatitis

In the second part of our study, we compared CD 4, CD 8, CD 45 and CD 68 cell populations and histological features and patterns of inflammatory cell infiltrates in the three etiologically different forms of chronic pancreatitis to evaluate whether the inflammatory reaction in CP is dependent upon and hence directed by the underlying etiology. In each tissue section, the number and location of the inflammatory cell infiltrates were recorded as in the fibrotic areas, within acini, around acini, periductally and perivascularly. For purposes of comparative evaluation between the different groups, the area of each inflammatory foci was measured with a computer-assisted video image system and the median area was calculated. To summarize the degree of inflammation in CP tissues, an inflammation number score and an area score were calculated taking into account the total number of inflammatory foci, area of foci, the density of the cell infiltrates and the area of the tissue sections evaluated.

The CD 4, CD 8, CD 45 and CD 68 cell populations in the three different forms of CP were essentially similar and no significant differences were observed.

On histologic examination, we observed a higher number of inflammatory infiltrates around blood vessels in tropical CP in comparison with non-tropical CP (Figure 2.5-2C and D). Arteriopathy and endophlebitis were significantly noted only in tropical CP; but were probably absent in the other two forms of CP (Figure 2.5-2 E and F). Thus it appears that vascular factors may be of significance in the evolution of tropical CP. Another interesting feature was the significantly greater number of plasma cells in tropical CP in comparison to alcoholic CP. This probably explains the greater fibrosis that typically characterizes tropical CP and also points to humoral mechanisms that could be associated with the development of this disorder. In all other parameters analyzed, no significant histological differences were noted in the three different forms of CP.

Therefore, though the initiating events in the various forms of CP are likely to be distinctively different, it appears that progression of the disease, at least as regards the various inflammatory cell infiltrates, is more or less unique.

Conclusion

While there were reasons to believe that different forms of CP follow different courses depending on the initiating etiological event, our findings suggest that the disease appears to approach a common stage where neural alterations, histological features and immune cell infiltrates are essentially similar irrespective of the underlying etiology and the activated pathobiological pathways follow a distinctive, etiology independent pattern in all forms of CP.

The observation that neural changes were almost uniform in all patients who experienced pain is a further pointer that pain mechanisms are due to "neuroimmune interactions" not only in alcoholic CP but also in non-alcoholic forms of CP. Furthermore, these findings could possibly influence the pathogenesis and progression of this disease.

However, it must be remembered that all pancreatic tissues were obtained during "advanced stage disease" of CP – the only stage when surgical intervention is normally considered necessary. Due to lack of early stage human CP tissue and the unavailability of relevant experimental models of CP that mimic the etiology and other features associated with human CP, the development of neural alterations and the relationship with perineural inflammatory cell infiltrates cannot be presently studied in a time dependent fashion.

On the background of our findings, potential areas for future research should concentrate on developing relevant experimental models of chronic pancreatitis and genetic studies in different forms of CP, especially in tropical CP.

References

1. Sarles H, Bernard JP, Johnson C, Chir M. Pathogenesis and epidemiology of chronic pancreatitis. Ann Rev Med 1989; 40: 453–68.
2. DiMagno EP, Layer P, Clain JE. Chronic pancreatitis. The exocrine pancreas: biology, pathobiology, and diseases. Edited by Go VLW, DiMagno EP, Gardner JD, Lebenthal E, Reber HA, Scheele GA. New York: Raven Press, 1993: 665–706.
3. DiMagno EP. A short, elective history of exocrine pancreatic insufficiency and chronic pancreatitis. Gastroenterology 1993; 104: 1255–62.
4. Pitchumoni CS. Special problems of tropical pancreatitis. Clin Gastroenterol 1984; 13: 941–59.
5. Pitchumoni CS. Chronic pancreatitis: a historical and clinical sketch of the pancreas and pancreatitis. Gastroenterologist 1998; 6: 24–33.
6. Ammann RW. Idiopathic "juvenile" chronic pancreatitis. Dtsch Med Wochenschr 1976; 101: 1789–94.
7. Ammann RW, Sulser H. "Senile" chronic pancreatitis; a new nosologic entity? Studies in 38 cases. Indications of a vascular origin and relationship to the primarily painless chronic pancreatitis. Schweiz Med Wochenschr 1976; 106: 429–37.
8. Zuidema PJ. Cirrhosis and disseminated calcification of the pancreas in patients with malnutrition. Trop Geog Med 1959; 11: 70–4.
9. Shaper AG. Chronic pancreatic disease and protein malnutrition. Lancet 1960; ii: 1223–4.
10. GeeVarghese PJ. Calcific Pancreatitis. Bombay: Varghese Publishing House, 1985.
11. GeeVarghese PJ, Pitchumoni CS. Pancreatic diabetes in Kerala. In: Patel JC, Talwalkar NG, eds. Diabetes in the tropics. Bombay: Diabetes Association of India, 1966: 233–9.
12. Nwokolo C, Oli J. Pathogenesis of juvenile tropical pancreatitis syndrome. Lancet 1980; 1: 456–9.
13. Braganza JM, Schofield D, Snehalatha C, Mohan V. Micronutrient antioxidant status in tropical compared with temperate-zone chronic pancreatitis. Scand J Gastroenterol 1993; 28: 1098–104.
14. Balakrishnan V, Sauniere JF, Hariharan M, Sarles H. Diet, pancreatic function, and chronic pancreatitis in south India and France. Pancreas 1988; 3: 30–5.
15. Narendranathan M, Cheriyan A. Lack of association between cassava consumption and tropical pancreatitis syndrome. J Gastroenterol Hepatol 1994; 9: 282–5.
16. Cohn JA, Friedman KJ, Noone PG, Knowles MR, Silverman LM, Jowell PS. Relation between mutations of the cystic fibrosis gene and idiopathic pancreatitis. N Engl J Med 1998; 339: 653–8.
17. Rossi L, Whitcomb DC, Ehrlich GD, Gorry MC, Parvin S, Sattar S, Ali L, Azad Khan AK, Gyr N. Lack of R117H mutation in the cationic trypsinogen gene in patients with tropical pancreatitis from Bangladesh. Pancreas 1998; 17: 278–80.

18. Korc M, Friess H, Yamanaka Y, Kobrin MS, Büchler MW, Beger HG. Chronic pancreatitis is associated with increased concentrations of epidermal growth factor receptor, transforming growth factor alpha, and phospholipase C gamma. Gut 1994; 35: 1468–73.
19. Friess H, Yamanaka Y, Büchler MW, Hammer K, Kobrin MS, Beger HG, Korc M. A subgroup of patients with chronic pancreatitis overexpress the c-erb B-2 protooncogene. Ann Surg 1994; 220: 183–92.
20. Friess H, Yamanaka Y, Büchler MW, Beger HG, Do DA, Kobrin MS, Korc M. Increased expression of acidic and basic fibroblast growth factors in chronic pancreatitis. Am J Pathol 1994; 144: 117–28.
21. Di Mola FF, Friess H, Martignoni ME, Di Sebastiano P, Zimmermann A, Innocenti P, Graber H, Gold LI, Korc M, Büchler MW. Connective tissue growth factor is a regulator for fibrosis in human chronic pancreatitis. Ann Surg 1999; 230: 63–71.
22. Kashiwagi M, Friess H, Uhl W, Graber H, Duarte R, Zimmermann A, Büchler MW. Phospholipase A2 isoforms are altered in chronic pancreatitis. Ann Surg 1998; 227: 220–8.
23. Keith RG, Keshavjee SH, Kerenyi NR. Neuropathology of chronic pancreatitis in humans. Can J Surg 1985; 28: 207–11.
24. Bockman DE, Büchler MW, Malfertheiner P, Beger HG. Analysis of nerves in chronic pancreatitis. Gastroenterology 1988; 94: 1459–69.
25. Büchler MW, Weihe E, Friess H, Malfertheiner P, Bockman E, Müller S, Nohr D, Beger HG. Changes in peptidergic innervation in chronic pancreatitis. Pancreas 1992; 7: 183–92.
26. Di Sebastiano P, Fink T, Weihe E, Friess H, Innocenti P, Beger HG, Büchler MW. Immune cell infiltration and growth-associated protein 43 expression correlate with pain in chronic pancreatitis. Gastroenterology 1997; 112: 1648–55.
27. Lankisch PG, Seidensticker F, Lohr-Happe A, Otto J, Cruetzfeldt W. The course of pain is the same in alcohol- and non-alcohol induced chronic pancreatitis. Pancreas 1995; 10: 338–41.
28. Chari ST, Mohan V, Jayanthi V, Snehalatha C, Malathi S, Viswanathan M, Madanagopalan N. Comparative study of the clinical profiles of alcoholic chronic pancreatitis and tropical chronic pancreatitis in Tamil Nadu, South India. Pancreas 1992; 7: 52–8.
29. Emmrich J, Weber I, Nausch M, Sparmann G, Koch K, Seyfarth M, Lohr M, Liebe S. Immunohistochemical characterization of the pancreatic cellular infiltrate in normal pancreas, chronic pancreatitis and pancreatic carcinoma. Digestion 1998; 59: 192–8.
30. Roberts AI, O'Connell SM, Ebert EC. Intestinal intraepithelial lymphocytes bind to colon cancer cells by HML-1 and CD11a. Cancer Res 1993; 53: 1608–11.
31. Taunk J, Roberts AI, Ebert EC. Spontaneous cytotoxicity of human intraepithelial lymphocytes against epithelial cell tumors. Gastroenterology 1992; 102: 69–75.
32. Ebert MP, Ademmer K, Muller-Ostermeyer F, Friess H, Büchler MW, Schubert W, Malfertheiner P. CD8+CD103+ T cells analogous to intestinal intraepithelial lymphocytes infiltrate the pancreas in chronic pancreatitis. Am J Gastroenterol 1998; 93: 2141–7.
33. Vallance BA, Hewlett BR, Snider DP, Collins SM. T cell-mediated exocrine pancreatic damage in major histocompatibility complex class II-deficient mice. Gastroenterology 1998; 115: 978–87.
34. Hunger R, Müller Ch, Zgraggen K, Friess H, Büchler MW. Cytotoxic cells are activated in cellular infiltrates of alcoholic chronic pancreatitis. Gastroenterology 1997; 112: 1656–63.
35. Saurer L, Reber P, Schaffner T, Büchler MW, Buri C, Kappeler A, Walz A, Friess H, Müller C. Differential expression of chemokines in normal pancreas and in chronic pancreatitis. Gastroenterology 2000; 118: 356–67.
36. Friess H, Büchler MW, Müller C, Malfertheiner P. Immunopathogenesis of chronic pancreatitis. Gastroenterology 1998; 115: 1018–22.

2.6 DNA microarrays in chronic pancreatitis

J. Kleeff, J. Ding, J. Hammer, H. Friess, M.W. Büchler

Introduction

Genome-wide gene expression analysis using DNA microarray technology will provide new insights into gene function and cause of disease. In this chapter we will give a short introduction of the technology behind DNA microarrays as well as a brief overview of the different applications and results obtained with DNA microarrays. We will then present some of our own data obtained with a DNA microarray representing 5,600 genes and analyzing the differential gene expression patterns in the normal pancreas, chronic pancreatitis, and pancreatic cancer. The potential use of the results and future research directions are discussed.

DNA microarrays

Understanding and evaluating biological systems with 30,000 genes, such as a human cell, requires new technologies; the traditional gene-by-gene or protein-by-protein approach is not sufficient to meet the magnitude of the task. DNA arrays represent a first step forward, providing a systematic way to survey concomitant RNA expression of a large number of genes. DNA microarrays are on the way to becoming standard tools for molecular research and clinical diagnostics, although they are presently still extremely expensive. Subsequently, future innovations will likely help to analyze protein expression, subcellular localization, and intermolecular interaction of protein products in a similar fashion (Fig. 2.6-1).

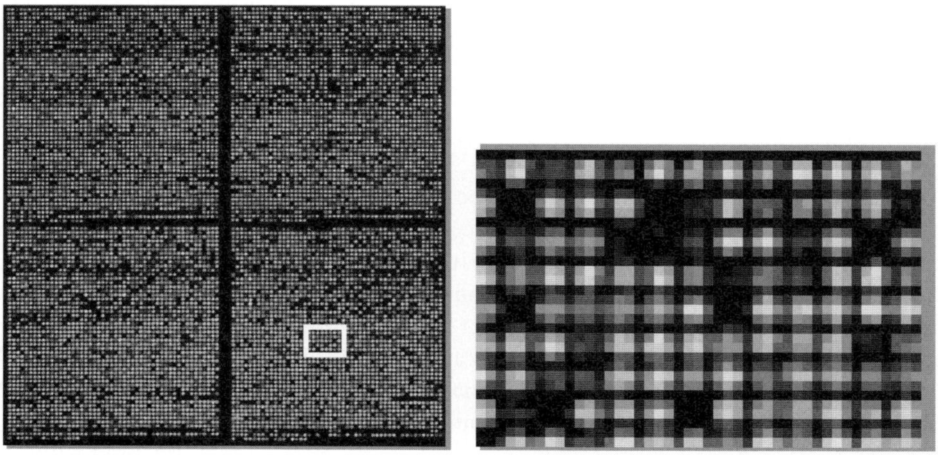

Figure 2.6-1. Example of a DNA microarray with different fluorescent color intensity. A magnification of the denoted area is shown on the right side.

History

The Southern blot was in a sense the first DNA array, involving hybridization between nucleic acids, one of which is immobilized on a matrix [1]. Subsequently, a number of different technologies have evolved to detect and quantify gene expression, such as Northern blotting [2], RNAse protection assays [3], differential display [4], and serial analysis of gene expression (SAGE) [5]. DNA microarrays are the latest innovation used to study expression of a large number of genes. This technology has been made possible through the use of non-porous solid supporters, such as glass, and the development of methods for high-density synthesis of oligonucleotides.

Chip design

Microarrays are made from a collection of purified cDNAs or oligonucleotides. A drop of each type of DNA in solution is placed onto a specially-prepared glass slide by an arraying machine. The advantages of glass compared to other materials are that DNA can be covalently attached to its surface, that it is a durable material that sustains high temperatures and washes, and that it is non-porous so the hybridization volume can be kept to a minimum. The arraying machine can quickly produce a regular grid of tens of thousands of spots. After DNA samples are arrayed onto a slide, they are air dried and immobilized by UV irradiation to form covalent bonds between the thymidine residues of the DNA and the positively charged amine groups on the silane slides (for review: [6]). The choice of DNA/oligonucleotides to be used in the spots on a microarray determines which genes can be detected in an assay. For organisms whose genomes have been completely sequenced, such as several bacteria and yeast, it is possible to array genomic DNA from every known gene of the organism. Each gene is amplified from total genomic DNA by PCR, or designed as a representative oligonucleotide. Since the human genome is almost completely sequenced, it will be possible in the near future to produce a comprehensive array for all human genes. However, currently the number of human genes has been estimated at somewhere around 30,000, so that several arrays will probably be required. Despite these current limitations, several strategies can be used today to design arrays for studying human genes. The location and sequence of the majority of human genes is known, so that it is possible to design human arrays with this information. There are even ways to produce arrayable DNA for unknown genes, such as amplifying clone inserts from human cDNA libraries, or synthesizing oligonucleotides directly from known expressed sequence information such as expressed sequence tags (EST's).

RNA/mRNA extraction

Genes which code for proteins are transcribed into messenger RNA (mRNA). The transcription level of a gene is taken to be the amount of its corresponding mRNA present in the cell. To prepare mRNA for use in a microarray assay, it must be purified from total cellular contents; mRNA accounts for only about 3% of all RNA in a cell. Common mRNA isolation methods take advantage of the fact that most mRNA species have a poly-adenine – poly(A) – tail. The poly(A) + mRNA can be purified by capturing it on oligo-(dT) molecules bound to a solid support. Alternatively, total RNA is used to maximize the amount of message that can be obtained from a given amount of tissue. In the next step, RNA/mRNA is reverse-transcribed into cDNA. One problem with cDNA production is that not all mRNA species are reverse-transcribed with the same efficiency. This fact leads to reverse transcription bias, which can change the relative amounts of different cDNA measured by the microarray assay, and which prohibits a quantitative comparison between different mRNA species on one microarray. Another problem is that some mRNA species are reverse-transcribed for only part of their lengths, making them less likely to bind and stay bound to their complement oligonucleotides on the array. In general, these problems do not interfere with the analysis of the same mRNA species from two samples (e.g., tissues, cells).

Fluorescent labeling

In order to detect cDNA bound to the microarray, the cDNA is most commonly labeled with a fluorescent dye, such as Cye3-dUTP or Cye5-dUTP. A different colored fluor is used for each sample to tell the two samples apart on the array. The number of fluor molecules needed in order to label each cDNA depends on its length and possibly its sequence composition, both of which are often unknown. This is one more reason why fluorescent intensities for different cDNAs cannot be quantitatively compared. However, identical cDNA from the two probes are still comparable as long as the same number of label molecules are added to the same DNA sequence in each probe. One of the disadvantages of the fluorescent labeling in this technology is the large amount of RNA required per target (approximately 50–200 µg total RNA, or 2–5 µg mRNA). With this amount of RNA/mRNA the detection limit is approximately 1 transcript per cell (around 1 transcript per 100,000 transcripts) [7]. A number of modifications are currently being tested to improve the sensitivity of this technology, including *in vitro* transcription [8] and post hybridization amplification [9].

Hybridization

Arrays hold typically more than 10,000 spots, each of which contains a different DNA sequence. If a probe contains a cDNA whose sequence is complementary to the DNA on a given spot, this cDNA will hybridize to this region. Thus, every spot on an array is an independent assay for the presence of a different cDNA. A number of factors influence hybridization of the cDNA with the target on the microarray, such as base composition, secondary structure, temperature, and buffer (for review see [10]).

Scanning

Once the cDNA probes have been hybridized to the array, the array is scanned to determine how much of each probe is bound to each spot. As mentioned, the probes are tagged with fluorescent reporter molecules which emit detectable light when stimulated by a laser. The emitted light is captured by a detector, for example a confocal microscope. The regular arrangement of elements that result from robotic printing and confocal imaging renders image data amenable to extraction by digital image processing procedures. Spots with more bound probe will fluoresce more intensely. Although the purpose of the scanner is to pick up light emitted by bound cDNA, it also records light from a few molecules that hybridized either to the wrong spot or nonspecifically to the glass slide. This extra light is the background of the scanned array image, and deciding the intensity threshold between spots and background can be difficult, especially when the spots fade gradually around their edges. Local sampling of background can be used to specify a threshold which true signals must exceed. Furthermore, there are a number of methods applied today to normalize the expression in a single set of experiments, either taking all genes on a certain array into account or designating a subset of constantly expressed genes. Validation of the experiments is furthermore achieved by subsequent re-analysis of the obtained data with current technologies, e.g., Northern blotting (for review see [7]).

Data analysis

The intensities provided by the array image can be quantified by measuring the average or integrated intensities of the spots. In comparative experiments (e.g., different cell populations, different tissues) the ratio of fluorescent intensities for a spot is interpreted as the ratio of concentrations for its corresponding mRNA in the two cell populations. Schena et al. [11] have demonstrated the ability to detect quantitative changes of as little as a factor of two, with reasonable agreement between expression ratios measured on the array and ratios measured by an alternate form of RNA blotting. The information on the expression of the genes represented on an array has to be managed in databases to examine and compare the outputs from single and multiple array experiments. A number of software programs are applied today to cope with the immense statistical and mathematical problems of this analysis.

Applications

Today, the main application of microarrays is expression analysis, such as comparative expression profiling of different tissues (e.g., diseased versus normal tissue) or cell lines (e.g., transformed versus normal cells). Currently, the vast number of available microarrays are designed for expression analysis. *Genotyping:* Variation in DNA sequence underlies most of the differences that are observed within species. Locating and identifying these genotypic differences is the first step in elucidating a link between genotypic and phenotypic changes in a disease state. There are currently microarrays designed to detect genetic changes through the identification of single-nucleotide polymorphisms (SNPs), which represent the most frequent type of variation in the human genome [12]. These arrays are currently being used in clinical settings [13; 14]. Furthermore, DNA microarrays can be designed to detect polymorphisms and mutations, for example in the p53 gene.

Results

Comparative expression profiling has been performed in a number of different settings. One of the main points of interest is the analysis of genes involved in carcinogenesis. Up to now, a number of different human tumors, such as ovarian cancer [15], lung cancer [16; 17], breast cancer [18–20], colon cancer [21], prostate cancer [22–24], rhabdomyosarcoma [25], melanoma [26], and head and neck cancers [27; 28], have been investigated by microarray analysis to identify cancer-specific genes, genes involved in metastasis formation [29], and genes that regulate the response towards chemotherapy [30]. With this information, new diagnostic and therapeutic strategies will be developed in the future.

Chronic pancreatitis

Chronic pancreatitis (CP) is an inflammatory disease of the pancreas characterized by irreversible and progressive destruction of the whole organ, resulting in severe exocrine and endocrine insufficiency [31; 32]. Heavy alcohol consumption is the main etiologic factor of chronic pancreatitis (CP) in Western industrialized countries [32–34]. Less common causes include nutritional factors, gene mutations (hereditary CP), metabolic disturbances, congenital anomalies of the ductal system *(pancreas divisum)* and acquired pancreatic duct obstructions [32; 33; 35; 36]. The origin of the disease is unknown in 15–20% of the cases (idiopathic pancreatitis) [34; 37].

The morphological changes of CP include acinar cell degeneration, dilatation of the duct system with intraductal protein plugs and stones, necrosis, and replacement of the lost parenchyma by dense fibrous tissue. The destruction of pancreatic parenchyma is accompanied by infiltrating leukocytes and followed by tissue remodeling, with ductal cell proliferation and ductular hyperplasia.

With the exception of hereditary CP, the pathogenetic mechanisms of CP remain enigmatic, and none of the recently proposed pathophysiological concepts [33; 35; 38] can fully explain the morphological, functional and clinical picture of the disease. Our knowledge about the mechanisms of tissue destruction and remodeling in CP is limited by the fact that the only tissue specimens available for detailed studies come from patients with advanced disease, for whom surgical treatment is indicated.

In recent years, modern molecular biology techniques have provided important clues to clarify morphological changes and pathophysiological aspects of CP. Genetic studies have been useful in expanding our knowledge of another intriguing and uncertain topic, the relationship between CP and pancreatic adenocarcinoma. A deeper understanding of the biological and molecular mechanisms underlying CP and of its relationship with pancreatic cancer could help to develop new diagnostic and therapeutic strategies.

Use of microarrays in chronic pancreatitis to identify disease-specific genes

The purpose of pairwise comparisons of tissue expression profiling is the identification of genes whose level of expression correlates with the disease phenotype. Although correlation with disease does not always imply causation, it provides a means to filter out candidate therapeutic and diagnostic targets.

Microarrays and designs

The custom arrays used in this study were fabricated by Affymetrix Inc. (Santa Clara, CA, USA). The array was designed from a database of high-quality sequences assembled from public and Incyte (Incyte Inc., Palo Alto, CA, USA) human expressed sequence tags (EST) sequences. The assemblies were built using very conservative overlap criteria to avoid creation of chimeric sequences. Quality criteria were length and average redundancy of the assemblies. The final design of the array represented 5,600 genes consisting of approximately 2,700 annotated and 3,300 non-annotated sequence assemblies.

Transcript profiling using microarrays

Total RNA was extracted from snap-frozen human tissues or cell lines. 5–20 μg total RNA was converted into double-stranded cDNA by reverse transcription. The double-strand cDNA product was cleaned up by Phenol/Chloroform/Isoamyl extraction and subsequently converted into cRNA by using the *in vitro* transcription T7 kit and biotinylated nucleotides, as described previously [39]. Hybridization to DNA microarrays was performed as suggested by the manufacturer (Affymetrix, Santa Clara, CA).

Computational analysis of data

Primary analysis of array data was performed using the Affymetrix GeneChip®, software. The program "DiseaseExpressionMap" was developed to evaluate expression data from profiling experiments over multiple matched pairs of diseased/normal samples. Differential expression was defined as ≥ 2-fold change versus respective controls. The detection specificity of the used chip was approximately 1 in 100,000 copies, the difference detection was two-fold changes, and the dynamic range approximately 500-fold.

Tissue samples

Eight normal human pancreatic tissues and all other normal tissues were obtained through an organ donor program. Eight CP tissues and 8 pancreatic cancer tissues were obtained from surgical specimens. All the CP patients had severe symptoms requiring surgery [40].

Analysis

We first analyzed normal pancreatic tissues in comparison with a panel of other normal tissues (e.g., bowel, liver). This analysis revealed 11 signature genes that were selectively expressed in the pancreas (triglyceride lipase, microsomal dipeptidase, pancreatic elastase IIA, pancreatic secretory trypsin inhibitor, pancreatic lipase-related protein 2, MAP kinase activated protein kinase, protein disulfide isomerase [PDIp], pancreatic zymogen granule membrane protein GP-2, Na,K-ATPase gamma subunit, carboxyl ester lipase [bile salt-stimulated lipase], and procarboxypeptidase A1) [40]. Comparison of the expression of 5,600 genes between the normal pancreas and CP as well as pancreatic cancer tissues demonstrated that the expression of 294 genes was increased in pancreatic cancer tissues in comparison with the normal pancreas (Fig. 2.6.-2). Of those, 152 genes were simultaneously increased in CP. In addition, the expression of 94 genes was decreased in pancreatic cancer tissues in comparison to normal pancreatic tissues, and the expression of 34 of these genes was simultaneously decreased in CP. Interestingly, only 5 of 5,600 genes were exclusively overexpressed in CP but not in pancreatic cancer (mucin-6, germline oligomeric matrix protein, tryptase-III, rearranged immunoglobulin lambda light chain, and cysteine-rich secretory protein-3) (Fig. 2.6.-3) [40].

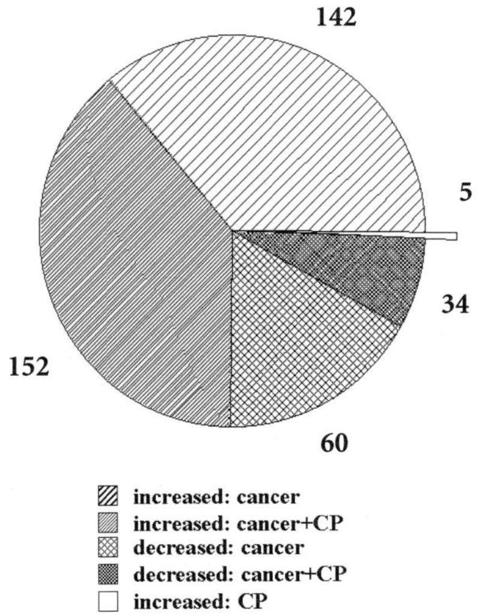

Figure 2.6-2. Summary of the 5,600 genes that were differentially regulated in pancreatic cancer and chronic pancreatitis as compared to normal pancreatic tissues. The number of the differentially expressed genes is denoted outside the pie chart.

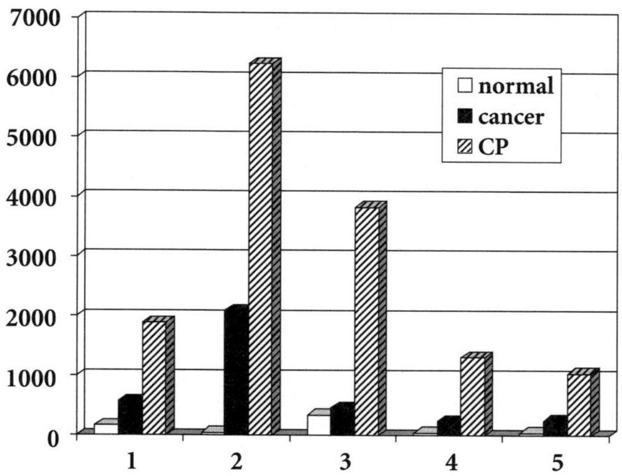

Figure 2.6-3. Summary of the 5 genes that were selectively overexpressed in chronic pancreatitis as compared to normal and cancerous pancreatic tissue samples. Relative expression units are denoted on the right axis.
1: mucin-6; 2: germline oligomeric matrix protein; 3: tryptase-III; 4: rearranged immunoglobulin lambda light chain; 5: cysteine-rich secretory protein-3.

In the future, it would be interesting to obtain microdissected tissue sections to compare expression profiles of different cellular subtypes in CP (e.g., normal ducts, proliferating ducts, hyperplastic ducts, etc.). However, at present, current protocols for fluorescent labeling of RNA/cDNA demand large quantities of RNA, which impedes the use of microdissected RNA on DNA microarrays. Future innovations will likely solve these problems.

Conclusion

DNA array expression analysis is a powerful technology that allows the simultaneous analysis of the expression of multiple genes. Our results indicate that the majority of epigenetic alterations observed in pancreatic cancer are already present in CP, and that the number of key genes whose expression is deregulated in CP is surprisingly small. These results provide new insight into the pathobiology of both CP and pancreatic cancer, and might also help to identify certain molecular alterations that could serve as targets for new therapies in pancreatic cancer and chronic pancreatitis.

References

1. Southern EM. Detection of specific sequences among DNA fragments separated by gel electrophoresis. J Mol Biol 1975; 98: 503–17.
2. Alwine JC, Kemp DJ, Stark GR. Method for detection of specific RNAs in agarose gels by transfer to diazobenzyloxymethyl paper and hybridization with DNA probes. Proc Natl Acad Sci USA 1977; 74: 5350–4.
3. Berk AJ, Sharp PA. Sizing and mapping of early adenovirus mRNAs by gel electrophoresis of S1 endonuclease-digested hybrids. Cell 1977; 12: 721–32.
4. Liang P, Pardee AB. Differential display of eukaryotic messenger RNA by means of the polymerase chain reaction. Science 1992; 257: 967–71.
5. Velculescu VE, Zhang L, Vogelstein B, Kinzler KW. Serial analysis of gene expression. Science 1995; 270: 484–7.
6. Cheung VG, Morley M, Aguilar F, Massimi A, Kucherlapati R, Childs G. Making and reading microarrays. Nat Genet 1999; 21: 15–9.
7. Duggan DJ, Bittner M, Chen Y, Meltzer P, Trent JM. Expression profiling using cDNA microarrays. Nat Genet 1999; 21: 10–4.

8. Lockhart DJ, Dong H, Byrne MC, Follettie MT, Gallo MV, Chee MS, Mittmann M, Wang C, Kobayashi M, Horton H, Brown EL. Expression monitoring by hybridization to high-density oligonucleotide arrays. Nat Biotechnol 1996; 14: 1675–80.
9. Chen JJ, Wu R, Yang PC, Huang JY, Sher YP, Han MH, Kao WC, Lee PJ, Chiu TF, Chang F, Chu YW, Wu CW, Peck K. Profiling expression patterns and isolating differentially expressed genes by cDNA microarray system with colorimetry detection. Genomics 1998; 51: 313–24.
10. Southern E, Mir K, Shchepinov M. Molecular interactions on microarrays. Nat Genet 1999; 21: 5–9.
11. Schena M, Shalon D, Heller R, Chai A, Brown PO, Davis RW. Parallel human genome analysis: microarray-based expression monitoring of 1000 genes. Proc Natl Acad Sci USA 1996; 93: 10614–9.
12. Wang DG, Fan JB, Siao CJ, Berno A, Young P, Sapolsky R, Ghandour G, Perkins N, Winchester E, Spencer J, Kruglyak L, Stein L, Hsie L, Topaloglou T, Hubbell E, Robinson E, Mittmann M, Morris MS, Shen N, Kilburn D, Rioux J, Nusbaum C, Rozen S, Hudson TJ, Lander ES et al. Large-scale identification, mapping, and genotyping of single-nucleotide polymorphisms in the human genome. Science 1998; 280: 1077–82.
13. Kozal MJ, Shah N, Shen N, Yang R, Fucini R, Merigan TC, Richman DD, Morris D, Hubbell E, Chee M, Gingeras TR. Extensive polymorphisms observed in HIV-1 B protease gene using high-density oligonucleotide arrays. Nat Med 1996; 2: 753–9.
14. Gunthard HF, Wong JK, Ignacio CC, Havlir DV, Richman DD. Comparative performance of high-density oligonucleotide sequencing and dideoxynucleotide sequencing of HIV type 1 pol from clinical samples. AIDS Res Hum Retroviruses 1998; 14: 869–76.
15. Ono K, Tanaka T, Tsunoda T, Kitahara O, Kihara C, Okamoto A, Ochiai K, Takagi T, Nakamura Y. Identification by cDNA microarray of genes involved in ovarian carcinogenesis. Cancer Res 2000; 60: 5007–11.
16. Hong TM, Yang PC, Peck K, Chen JJ, Yang SC, Chen YC, Wu CW. Profiling the downstream genes of tumor suppressor PTEN in lung cancer cells by complementary DNA microarray. Am J Respir Cell Mol Biol 2000; 23: 355–63.
17. Wang T, Hopkins D, Schmidt C, Silva S, Houghton R, Takita H, Repasky E, Reed SG. Identification of genes differentially over-expressed in lung squamous cell carcinoma using a combination of cDNA subtraction and microarray analysis. Oncogene 2000; 19: 1519–28.
18. Forozan F, Mahlamaki EH, Monni O, Chen Y, Veldman R, Jiang Y, Gooden GC, Ethier SP, Kallioniemi A, Kallioniemi OP. Comparative genomic hybridization analysis of 38 breast cancer cell lines: a basis for interpreting complementary DNA microarray data. Cancer Res 2000; 60: 4519–25.
19. Barlund M, Forozan F, Kononen J, Bubendorf L, Chen Y, Bittner ML, Torhorst J, Haas P, Bucher C, Sauter G, Kallioniemi OP, Kallioniemi A. Detecting activation of ribosomal protein S6 kinase by complementary DNA and tissue microarray analysis. J Natl Cancer Inst 2000; 92: 1252–9.
20. Perou CM, Sorlie T, Eisen MB, van de Rijn M, Jeffrey SS, Rees CA, Pollack JR, Ross DT, Johnsen H, Akslen LA, Fluge O, Pergamenschikov A, Williams C, Zhu SX, Lonning PE, Borresen-Dale AL, Brown PO, Botstein D. Molecular portraits of human breast tumours. Nature 2000; 406: 747–52.
21. Hernandez A, Smith F, Wang Q, Wang X, Evers BM. Assessment of differential gene expression patterns in human colon cancers [In Process Citation]. Ann Surg 2000; 232: 576–85.
22. Vaarala MH, Porvari K, Kyllonen A, Vihko P. Differentially expressed genes in two LNCaP prostate cancer cell lines reflecting changes during prostate cancer progression. Lab Invest 2000; 80: 1259–68.
23. Elek J, Park KH, Narayanan R. Microarray-based expression profiling in prostate tumors. In Vivo 2000; 14: 173–82.
24. Xu J, Stolk JA, Zhang X, Silva SJ, Houghton RL, Matsumura M, Vedvick TS, Leslie KB, Badaro R, Reed SG. Identification of differentially expressed genes in human prostate cancer using subtraction and microarray. Cancer Res 2000; 60: 1677–82.

25. Pandita A, Zielenska M, Thorner P, Bayani J, Godbout R, Greenberg M, Squire JA. Application of comparative genomic hybridization, spectral karyotyping, and microarray analysis in the identification of subtype-specific patterns of genomic changes in rhabdomyosarcoma. Neoplasia 1999; 1: 262–75.
26. Su YA, Bittner ML, Chen Y, Tao L, Jiang Y, Zhang Y, Stephan DA, Trent JM. Identification of tumor-suppressor genes using human melanoma cell lines UACC903, UACC903(+6), and SRS3 by comparison of expression profiles. Mol Carcinog 2000; 28: 119–27.
27. Villaret DB, Wang T, Dillon D, Xu J, Sivam D, Cheever MA, Reed SG. Identification of genes overexpressed in head and neck squamous cell carcinoma using a combination of complementary DNA subtraction and microarray analysis. Laryngoscope 2000; 110: 374–81.
28. Fung LF, Lo AK, Yuen PW, Liu Y, Wang XH, Tsao SW. Differential gene expression in nasopharyngeal carcinoma cells. Life Sci 2000; 67: 923–36.
29. Clark EA, Golub TR, Lander ES, Hynes RO. Genomic analysis of metastasis reveals an essential role for RhoC. Nature 2000; 406: 532–5.
30. Kudoh K, Ramanna M, Ravatn R, Elkahloun AG, Bittner ML, Meltzer PS, Trent JM, Dalton WS, Chin KV. Monitoring the expression profiles of doxorubicin-induced and doxorubicin-resistant cancer cells by cDNA microarray. Cancer Res 2000; 60: 4161–6.
31. Sarles H, Bernard JP, Johnson C. Pathogenesis and epidemiology of chronic pancreatitis. Annu Rev Med 1989; 40: 453–68.
32. DiMagno EP. A short, eclectic history of exocrine pancreatic insufficiency and chronic pancreatitis. Gastroenterology 1993; 104: 1255–62.
33. Adler G, Schmid RM. Chronic pancreatitis: still puzzling? [editorial; comment]. Gastroenterology 1997; 112: 1762–5.
34. Steer ML, Waxman I, Freedman S. Chronic pancreatitis. N Engl J Med 1995; 332: 1482–90.
35. Braganza JM. A framework for the aetiogenesis of chronic pancreatitis. Digestion 1998; 59: 1–12.
36. Ravnik-Glavac M, Dean M, di Sant'Agnese P, Chernick M, Kozelj M, Krizman I, Glavac D. Evidence that hereditary pancreatitis is a genetically heterogeneous disorder. Pflugers Arch 2000; 439: R50–2.
37. Okazaki K, Uchida K, Ohana M, Nakase H, Uose S, Inai M, Matsushima Y, Katamura K, Ohmori K, Chiba T. Autoimmune-related pancreatitis is associated with autoantibodies and a Th1/Th2-type cellular immune response. Gastroenterology 2000; 118: 573–81.
38. Friess H, Büchler MW, Mueller C, Malfertheiner P. Immunopathogenesis of chronic pancreatitis [editorial]. Gastroenterology 1998; 115: 1018–22.
39. Wodicka L, Dong H, Mittmann M, Ho MH, Lockhart DJ. Genome-wide expression monitoring in Saccharomyces cerevisiae. Nat Biotechnol 1997; 15: 1359–67.
40. Friess H, Ding J, Kleeff J, Liao Q, Berberat PO, Hammer J, Büchler MW. Identification of disease-specific genes in chronic pancreatitis using DNA array technology. Ann Surgery 2001; in press.

3 Pathogenesis of chronic pancreatitis: Current state and trends

3.1 Alcohol and pancreatitis

F. S. Gorelick, G. Robles-Diaz

Introduction

It is generally held that alcohol abuse can lead to acute pancreatitis, acute pancreatitis superimposed on chronic disease, and chronic pancreatitis. Studies of the pathophysiologic effects of ethanol and the epidemiologic studies support a probable relationship between alcohol abuse and pancreatic disease. However, the precise mechanism of such injury remains an issue of discussion.

Clinical evidence that alcohol abuse may cause pancreatitis

The natural history of those who abuse alcohol may follow several patterns. Based on the classifications of pancreatic diseases as established in the Marseilles-Rome 1988 Classification [74], the Cambridge International Workshop in 1983, and the Atlanta Symposium on Acute Pancreatitis in 1992 [14], alcoholic pancreatitis most often presents with chronic pancreatitis (chronic pain and/or permanent loss of pancreatic function due to destruction of gland associated with chronic inflammation and fibrosis). Less often acute pancreatitis (acute onset of abdominal pain associated with increased pancreatic enzymes in the blood or urine, pancreatic inflammation that resolves with a return to normal pancreatic function) may occur in the apparent absence of chronic disease. Patients with chronic pancreatitis may have bouts of acute disease. The development of acute pancreatitis after a short period (days or weeks) of alcohol abuse in a non-alcoholic is rare.

Several factors have made it difficult to establish a firm relationship between alcohol ingestion and the development of pancreatitis. First, quantitation of alcohol intake is unreliable. Second, the "gold-standard" of tissue histology is rarely available. As a result, subtle forms of disease may be easily overlooked. Despite these reservations, reasonable epidemiologic studies provide a strong link between alcohol ingestion and pancreatitis.

It appears that less than 5% of alcoholics develop pancreatitis related to the ethanol consumption, but subclinical pancreatic injury may be much more common than overt clinical disease [60, 81]. In a series of autopsies on chronic alcoholics without a clinical history of pancreatitis, about one third demonstrated perilobular fibrosis typical of chronic alcoholic injury [81]. If the findings of fibrosis are considered to be equivalent to chronic pancreatitis, the incidence of disease is higher than 5%.

The mean ethanol intake and duration of consumption affect the risk of developing acute and chronic alcoholic pancreatitis [75, 82]. In several series, patients with either acute or chronic alcoholic pancreatitis had consumed excessive amounts of alcohol for 13 to 18 years [21, 77, 82]. In United States servicemen hospitalized for chronic alcoholism, the relative risk of death from pancreatitis was about 7 times greater than controls [68]. The daily level of alcohol consumption also affects the risk of developing disease. In a Swedish study of 50,000 subjects, the relative risk of death due to alcoholic pancreatitis or

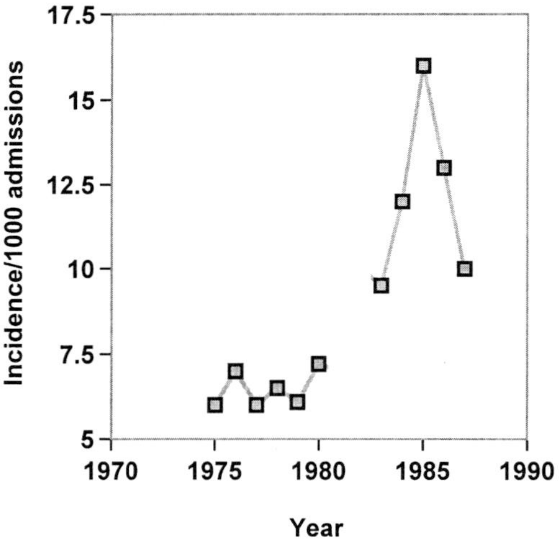

Figure 3.1-1. Hospital admissions for alcoholic pancreatitis are increasing (modified from [70]).

cirrhosis increased from 1.5 in those consuming between 101–250 g/week to 11.0 in those ingesting > 250 g/week [4]. The daily alcohol intake in patients who develop either acute or chronic alcoholic pancreatitis seems to be similar: both groups ingest 100 to 200 g of ethanol per day [82]. Increases in alcohol consumption over the past 20 years have been reported in a number of countries. In Mexico, this increase has correlated with an increased number of hospital admissions for chronic pancreatitis (Fig. 3.1-1 and ref. [69]). Other factors, such as improvements in diagnostic techniques, are likely to have contributed to the apparent increased incidence of disease. However, these studies support a time-dependent relationship between alcohol abuse and the development of pancreatitis.

Whether there is a direct relationship between the amount of alcohol intake and the risk of disease is a topic of discussion. There appears to be no precise threshold of toxicity above which alcoholic pancreatitis is inevitable, but a spectrum of sensitivities. Some

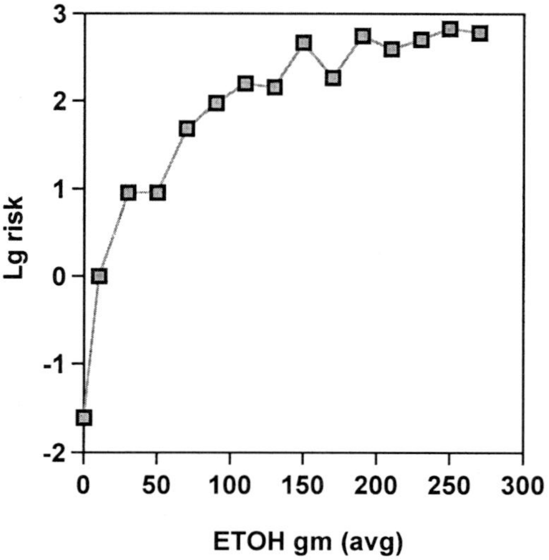

Figure 3.1-2. The risk of developing alcoholic pancreatitis is related to intake. (Calculated from [21].

appear to get disease with intakes of 20 g alcohol/day while others may drink 10 times that amount but do not develop pancreatitis. Only one study has found a direct relationship between alcohol intake and disease risks [22]; this was demonstrated for ingestion between 50 g and 150 g per day (Fig. 3.1-2). In general, the broad range of individual susceptibilities has made it difficult to correlate levels of alcohol ingestion with disease risk. The most important criteria for estimating the risk of alcoholic pancreatitis may be the total alcohol consumption (duration times average daily intake).

Susceptibility to alcoholic pancreatitis

Factors. The low incidence of pancreatic disease among alcohol abusers suggests that other factors must influence the development of disease. Genetic factors such as blood groups, HLA determinants, and a1-antitrypsin phenotypes have been examined, but not linked to disease. Similarly, polymorphisms of the ethanol-metabolizing enzyme, alcohol dehydrogenase isoenzyme, did not appear to affect disease development (reviewed in [36]). Mutations in the trypsinogen gene cause hereditary pancreatitis and alcohol may accelerate the course of this autosomal dominant disease [30]. However, the natural history of hereditary pancreatitis and rarity of trypsinogen mutations suggest that it will account for few patients with alcoholic pancreatitis. Mutations in the pancreatic trypsin inhibitor, SPINK-1, do not cause pancreatitis, but appear to increase the risk of developing disease [59, 88]. Whether SPINK-1 might sensitize the pancreas to the damaging effects of alcohol is unknown. Mutations in the cystic fibrosis transmembrane regulator, CFTR, have been linked to chronic pancreatitis [17, 78]. Notably, these patients do not have the classic symptoms of cystic fibrosis, and lack pulmonary disease. Preliminary studies have suggested that CFTR mutations might predispose to alcoholic pancreatitis. Cytokines appear to play an essential role in the pathogenesis of acute pancreatitis. Polymorphisms in the genes that generate TNF and IL-1 may lead to over-production of these potentially harmful cytokines and constitute a risk factor for developing severe pancreatitis. Similar effects have been reported with leptin. Though a number of genetic factors have been shown to cause pancreatitis or affect the severity of pancreatitis, none has been clearly demonstrated to predispose to alcoholic disease.

Other factors. In addition, factors such as diet and nutritional status, tobacco smoking, and coexisting conditions as hypertriglyceridemia, reduction of pancreatic blood flow, and the anatomic relationship between the distal biliary and pancreatic ducts may affect the development of disease [89].

A relationship between the risks of developing pancreatitis from ethanol in the presence of hypertriglyceridemia has not been demonstrated: Serum triglycerides and cholesterol levels are normal at the time of admission in most patients with alcoholic acute pancreatitis [20]. In two groups of alcoholics with similar ethanol consumption, triglyceride levels were equivalent in the absence or presence of pancreatitis [35].

Gender may affect the risk of developing alcoholic pancreatitis; the mean alcohol intake for men who develop pancreatitis is about twice that of women (Berger and Pap 1991). The patient's gender may also influence the target for ethanol-induced injury; the male/female ratio is greater in patients with alcoholic pancreatitis than in alcoholic cirrhosis [70, 87].

The role of cigarette smoking has been a topic of discussion. Most, but not all, studies have found that smoking affects the development of chronic pancreatitis [39, 43, 51]. The risk of developing alcoholic pancreatitis may be increased 2- to 12-fold by cigarette smoking. Not all elements of disease are equally affected; smoking seems to increase risks for fibrosis and calcification, but not to affect the development of endocrine or exocrine insufficiency. These effects of smoking might be linked to its effect on ethanol-dependent TNF release [45].

Acute pancreatitis in patients with chronic alcoholic pancreatitis

There is uniform agreement that patients with established chronic alcoholic pancreatitis can develop acute disease. Further, it is estimated that 85% of patients with acute alcoholic pancreatitis will have underlying chronic disease. A retrospective series of 21 patients with acute alcoholic pancreatitis found them to have chronic pancreatitis within an average 5.5 years (range 1–19 years) [32]. Once alcoholic pancreatitis has been established, the natural history may follow several patterns. In most, the intensity and frequency of the acute recurrent painful attacks will decrease over time as the patients develop functional or morphological deterioration [9, 16, 40, 70]. About 10% of patients will experience progressive decline in pancreatic function in the absence of painful crises. The course of alcoholic pancreatitis is improved by abstinence; conversely, those who continue to imbibe are more likely to experience functional deterioration and to respond poorly to pain control measures [2, 31].

Acute pancreatitis in patients without chronic alcoholic pancreatitis

It is estimated that about 15% of alcoholics will develop acute alcoholic pancreatitis in the absence of chronic disease. Functional and histologic studies support this contention. Assessments of pancreatic function after an acute attack, using direct measures of pancreatic exocrine secretion [5] or the stool chymotrypsin [3], reported that more than 20% of patients have normal function when tested between 6 months and 11 years later.

The greatest support for alcoholic acute pancreatitis occurring in the absence of underlying chronic disease comes from autopsy studies. In a cohort of 314 patients hospitalized with acute pancreatitis, 61 underwent an autopsy over the next 5 years [77]. In 47 of the 61 patients, alcohol was thought to be the cause of the pancreatitis. Acute and/or chronic pancreatitis was diagnosed in 33 autopsy cases. In this group with histologic acute and/or chronic pancreatitis, 27 were alcoholics. Notably, the pancreas demonstrated no findings of chronic pancreatitis in 28 patients; 20 of these were alcoholics. Another retrospective autopsy study examined 405 patients who died with acute pancreatitis [47, 65]. Alcohol was thought to be the etiology of the pancreatitis in 60.9% (247/405) and histologic evidence of chronic pancreatitis was found in only 47% (116/247). Since patients without chronic pancreatitis are said to be more likely to die from an attack of acute alcoholic pancreatitis, the later study may have systematically excluded patients with chronic alcoholic pancreatitis who did not die from an acute attack. However, these functional and histopathological studies strongly support the hypothesis that patients may develop acute alcoholic pancreatitis in the absence of chronic disease.

Does acute alcoholic AP lead to chronic pancreatitis?

Acute inflammatory conditions may lead to chronic inflammation and fibrosis. It has been suggested that the natural history of alcoholic pancreatitis may follow two pathways: Either patients may have recurrent bouts of acute pancreatitis but not progress to chronic pancreatitis or acute pancreatitis may lead to chronic disease. Kloppel and Maillet have hypothesized that recurrent episodes of pancreatic necrosis may lead to fibrosis [47]. Amman and co-workers have suggested that this progression may depend on the severity and site of pancreatic necrosis; patients that have less severe bouts of acute pancreatitis and localization of the inflammation to the distal pancreas appear to have a reduced risk of developing chronic disease [1].

Other observations suggest that chronic pancreatitis may arise independent of acute disease. Angelini and coworkers described 14 alcoholic patients with a *first attack of* severe pancreatitis [5]. In a four year follow-up, all but one patient had normal exocrine function. This suggests that severe acute pancreatitis does not always lead to chronic disease. On the other hand, patients may develop chronic pancreatitis without bouts of severe acute disease [70, 74]. In a study of 21 patients with an initial bout of alcoholic pancreatitis, four had the severe disease [33]. Although only one was found to have evidence of chronic pancreatitis at the time of presentation, all 21 patients developed chronic disease when examined on average 5.5 years after the initial attack. Thus, the risk of developing chronic disease may not be related to the severity of the initial attack or to the number of subsequent attacks. Further, the observation that the age of patients with alcoholic acute and chronic pancreatitis is similar is consistent with the lack of progression from acute to chronic disease [77, 82]. Thus, the causal relationship between acute alcoholic disease with severe necrosis and chronic pancreatitis remains unclear.

Mechanisms of ethanol-induced pancreatic injury

A number of pathologic effects of ethanol have been related to the development of pancreatitis; the various mechanisms are summarized in Figures 3.1-3 and 3.1-4 (see page 90). Its effects on pancreatic duct pressures are complex and may result in both the reflux of noxious substances and increased ductal pressure. The effect of ethanol on blood flow may predispose to ischemia and its enhancement of ductal permeability may permit the movement of pancreatic duct contents into the interstitial space. Ethanol also may be directly toxic to the acinar cell or have metabolic effects that promote acinar cell injury and pancreatic inflammation. Since it is difficult to study many of the potential effects of ethanol in humans, animal models have been frequently used. However, there is no animal model that fully recapitulates the effects of ethanol on the human pancreas.

Pancreatic duct pressure

Pancreatic duct pressure is a function of the viscosity of pancreatic fluid, the rate of secretion, and the resistance to outflow within the duct caused by Sphincter of Oddi dysfunction, pancreatic duct stones or strictures. Ethanol has been found to induce changes in the Sphincter of Oddi that may predispose to the development of acute pancreatitis by at least three potential mechanisms: a) contraction of the Sphincter may cause bile reflux into the pancreatic duct when there is a common opening, b) contraction of the Sphincter may cause obstruction of pancreatic duct when the ducts open separately, c) pathologic relaxation of the Sphincter may result in reflux of duodenal contents into the pancreatic duct [29, 57]. Two recent studies demonstrated increased basal Sphincter of Oddi and pancreatic duct pressures in patients with chronic alcoholic pancreatitis compared to controls [29, 57]. However, these studies involved few subjects. The relationship between sphincter dysfunction and alcoholic pancreatitis is unclear.

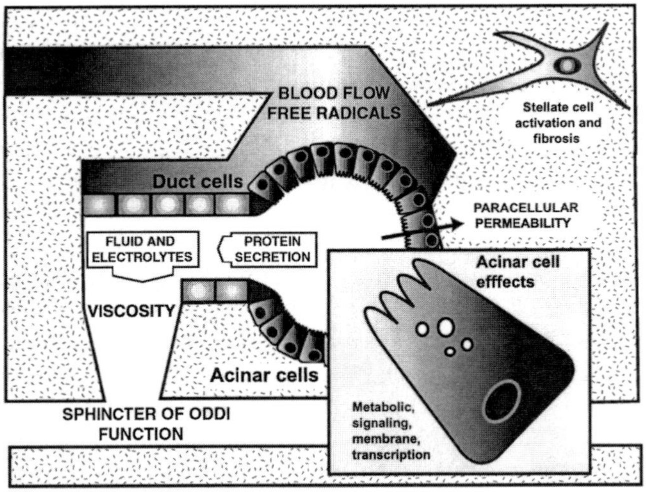

Figure 3.1-3. Some potential mechanisms of acute ethanol toxicity in the pancreas.

Based on experimental and pathologic studies, a number of mechanisms may play a role in ethanol-induced pancreatic injury. Changes in pancreatic blood flow may predispose to ischemia and reperfusion injury and oxidant stress. Other factors include the release of cytokines that induce inflammation and cell death, the pathologic activation of zymogens within the acinar cell or the interstitial space as well as other direct toxic effects on the acinar cell, increased pancreatic secretion, and dysfunction of the Sphincter of Oddi that might lead to obstruction or the reflux of duodenal contents (see text for additional details). Ethanol increases paracellular permeability and may allow access of digestive enzymes into the interstitial space. The stellate cell plays a role in pancreatic fibrosis – ethanol stimulates its production of collagen.

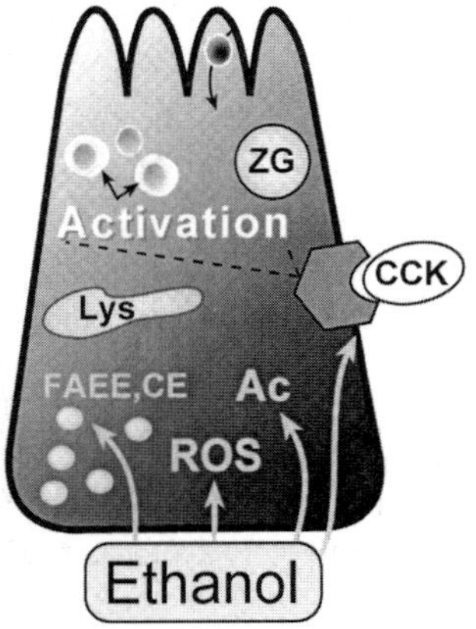

Figure 3.1-4. Potential mechanisms of ethanol toxicity on the acinar cell. Ethanol may act directly or be metabolized by the pancreatic acinar cell through oxidative or non-oxidative pathways. Ethanol may sensitize the CCK receptor and enhance the ability of the hormone to cause zymogen activation within the acinar cell. Ethanol may cause changes in membrane lipid composition and cause lysosome membranes to become fragile. It may also inhibit endocytosis. Not shown on the diagram are the effects of ethanol on protein synthesis. Ac = acetaldehyde, CCK = cholecystokinin, FAEE = fatty acid ethyl esters, CE = cholesterol esters, Lys = lysosome, ROS = reactive oxygen species, ZG = zymogen granule.

Pancreatic duct permeability

The epithelial lining of the pancreatic duct is a barrier that prevents the movement of pancreatic juice into the interstitial space. Pancreatic zymogens that escape into the interstitial space may be activated and play a role in the development of pancreatitis [25]. Two pathologic mechanisms might allow the movement of secretory products into the interstitium: a) The paracellular barrier may be disrupted by increased intraductal pressure or by pathologic cellular signaling that leads to disassembly of the tight junction [23], and

b) zymogens may be aberrantly released from the basolateral pole of the acinar cell [76]. Movement of ductal contents through the paracellular barrier is likely to be the most important mechanism. The effects of ethanol on pancreatic ductal pressure and permeability have been examined after its intragastric and intravenous administration or after using duct perfusion. Studies performed in dogs and humans have demonstrated that oral and intravenous ethanol result in similar ethanol concentrations in pancreatic juice and blood [11, 28]. Thus, studies that examine the effects of perfusion of the duct with ethanol are relevant.

Though the effects of ethanol on human duct permeability are unknown, perfusion of the cat pancreatic duct with ethanol, aspirin, or bile increases its permeability [63]. Intragastric ethanol was associated with an increase in the permeability of pancreatic ducts to moderate size (20,000) molecules [83]. However, changes in permeability alone do not cause pancreatitis.

Pancreatic secretion

The levels of various exocrine pancreatic secretory products in serum and in duodenal or pure pancreatic juice have been used in clinical assessment of acute and chronic pancreatic injury. Although ethanol may have acute effects on the secretory activity and synthetic function of the pancreas, the relationship of these changes to pancreatic injury is unknown.

Ethanol has been reported to both stimulate and suppress pancreatic secretion in animal models. The variability may be due to distinct responses among species and differences in the state of consciousness and concentration of ethanol. In human studies, the acute effects of ethanol on exocrine secretion may vary depending on the history of its use and the type of beverage. In non-alcoholics, ethanol tends to inhibit pancreatic secretion [38]. When administered with a meal, ethanol decreased pancreatic trypsin secretion by about 50% compared to a glucose-fed control. When compared to similar amounts of ethanol in beer or gin, wine was a much less potent suppressant of food-stimulated pancreatic secretion [38]. However, ethanol may have different effects in chronic alcoholics. Intravenous ethanol suppressed meal-stimulated pancreatic secretion in normal subjects, but it did not reduce secretion in chronic alcoholics [61]. The relatively enhanced secretory response observed in chronic alcoholics has been attributed to alcohol stimulation of cholinergic reflexes [44].

In summary, the effect of alcohol on pancreatic secretion, ductal pressure and/or permeability may vary according to the dose employed, species studied, diet, mode of ethanol administration, the secretory state of the pancreas, and whether ethanol was administered acutely or acutely on a background of chronic alcohol consumption. The variations among study designs, potential differences in the species responses, and paucity of studies in human subjects make it difficult to conclude that acute ethanol ingestion has a predictable effect on the human exocrine pancreas.

Viscosity

An increased concentration of proteins in pancreatic juice has been found in chronic alcoholics without chronic pancreatitis in the resting and stimulated states [13]. These changes have been attributed to increased protein secretion and decreased bicarbonate and water. The increased viscosity of pancreatic juice may contribute to increased intraductal pressures observed in some patients with chronic pancreatitis. These changes may be related to the formation of intraductal protein-plugs that obstruct small pancreatic ducts [34]. The effect of short-term alcohol ingestion on the viscosity of pancreatic juice or plug formation remains unknown.

Relative amounts of pancreatic enzymes

Pancreatic juice from rats chronically fed alcohol demonstrated an increase in trypsinogen and chymotrypsinogen and decreased trypsin inhibitor levels compared to controls fed a standard diet. There was a corresponding increase in pancreatic trypsinogen and chymotrypsinogen content and increased trypsin activity in ethanol-fed animals [79]. A similar study demonstrated that chronic ethanol feeding was associated with increased pancreatic levels of trypsinogen, chymotrypsinogen, and lipase [62]. Chronic ethanol feeding has also been associated with increased pancreatic cathepsin B activities [64, 66, 67] and increased pancreatic levels of trypsinogen and chymotrypsinogen mRNA and decreased amylase mRNA [58]. Some of the effects of ethanol on pancreatic enzyme content may be at the transcriptional level.

The effects of chronic ethanol consumption on the composition of pancreatic secretory proteins have been studied in juice obtained from human subjects. In two studies, the relative levels of trypsinogen increased in pancreatic juice, as did the ratio of trypsinogen to trypsin inhibitor [66]. It is estimated that the levels of trypsin inhibitor present in the pancreas are sufficient to quench only about 10% of pancreatic trypsin activity. Therefore, an increase in the trypsinogen to trypsin inhibitor ratio would favor the expression of trypsin activity. Increased levels of cathepsin B has also been found in pancreatic juice from chronic alcoholic patients. Since cathepsin B can activate trypsinogen, it has been implicated in the pathogenesis of pancreatitis [80]. Thus, the effects of chronic ethanol feeding on pancreatic enzyme composition in animal models are similar to those reported in humans. These studies suggest that chronic alcohol use results in changes in pancreatic secretory protein synthesis and generates conditions that may increase the risk of premature zymogen activation.

Pancreatic blood flow and oxidants

Experimental and clinical evidence supports a relationship between pancreatic ischemia, oxygen-derived free radicals, and the pathogenesis of acute pancreatitis [73]. Reduced pancreatic blood flow and tissue acidosis has been found in chronic pancreatitis, but is probably not specific to alcohol [8].

Acute ethanol administration reduced pancreatic blood flow *in vivo* in several experimental animal models [27]. In the cat, the reduced pancreatic blood flow was accompanied by increases in both interstitial pressure and vascular resistance and accentuated by partial pancreatic duct ligation [85]. In addition to causing anoxic tissue damage, pancreatic ischemia has also been associated with the activation of trypsinogen [53].

In some systems, ethanol is a potent stimulant of free radical generation. There are a variety of cellular mechanisms that may contribute to the generation of this oxidant stress including: a) microsomal metabolism of ethanol to acetaldehyde, b) ethanol stimulation of hypoxanthine and xanthine oxidase reaction, c) ethanol-dependent activation of NAD(P)H oxidase, and d) ethanol-dependent generation of an arachidonic acid metabolite that then stimulates generation of superoxide anions (reviewed in [56]).

Several mechanisms may contribute to ethanol-induced oxidative stress. Perfusion of acetaldehyde, a metabolite of ethanol, on a background of ischemia in isolated *ex vivo* canine pancreas resulted in pancreatic edema and increased amylase activity in the perfusate [55]. The injury may result from the additive effects of two conditions that are known to generate O_2-: a) Acetaldehyde is oxidized by xanthine oxidase which leads to reduction of O_2 and the release of O_2- and H_2O_2, b) Hypoxic tissue accumulates hypoxanthine due to catabolism of ATP and accumulates lactic acid from the glycolysis of glucose and glycogen. The low pH of hypoxic tissues, the Bohr effect, reactive hyperemia, and the presence of acetaldehyde may result in excessive high tissue concentrations of O_2 during reperfusion. Ethanol has been found to synergize with oxidants and trypsin cells in culture. Although ethanol has not been found to add to oxidant stress in one experimental model of pancreatitis [52], additional studies are required to determine whether it may increase damage in other models of pancreatitis.

Free radicals can lead to depletion of intracellular antioxidants such as glutathione and to subsequent oxidant damage of lipids, proteins, and nucleic acids. Notably, the oxidized forms of many proteins are dramatically more sensitive to proteolysis than non-oxidized forms [18]. This fact may contribute to the zymogen activation associated with acute pancreatitis. Although the effects of ethanol on blood flow and oxidant stress in humans has not been examined, experimental models suggest that alcohol ingestion may predispose the pancreas to various forms of ischemic injury including oxidant stress.

Direct effects of ethanol on the pancreatic acinar cell

Ethanol and its metabolites may have short-term and long-term affects on acinar cell physiology and cause changes in the composition of cell membranes and membrane movement and cell signaling that may contribute to its toxic effects.

Ethanol affects cell membranes and trafficking

Ethanol may affect membrane integrity and permit the breakdown of cellular organelles. Leakage of lysosomal enzymes from lysosomes has been reported to occur in experimental pancreatitis and attributed to increased membrane fragility [71]. Similar increases in fragility of lysosomal membranes have been reported in ethanol-fed rats [86]. This effect appears not to be due to ethanol or its metabolite, acetaldehyde, but may be the result of ethanol-induced cholesterol ester accumulation [37] or ethanol-enhanced phospholipase A_2 activity [50]. The acute effects of ethanol on membrane integrity have not been examined.

Physiologic studies relevant to the membrane effects of ethanol are limited. However, ethanol has been found to affect the trafficking of cell surface proteins through endocytic pathways. Reduced endocytosis of the epidermal growth factor (EGF) receptor by ethanol [100 mM] in hepatocytes may be related to changes in membrane fluidity and the disruption of the clatharin coat required for endocytosis [10]. Ethanol [50 mM] reduces endocytosis of the insulin receptor from the hepatocyte [24]. Whether ethanol affects endocytic pathways or other trafficking events in the acinar cell is unknown.

Ethanol affects intracellular signaling

Ethanol has been found to influence both cyclic nucleotide and calcium messenger systems. In many systems ethanol stimulates adenylate cyclase (AC) activity; pathologic stimulation of AC activity requires very high concentrations [> 500 mM] of ethanol in most systems, including the pancreas (reviewed in [41]). However, when added in the presence of ligands that activate AC, low doses of ethanol [< 25 mM] often dramatically enhance AC activation [42]. Although the mechanism of ethanol sensitization of AC activity is unclear, it may act by decreasing the activity of G_i [54] by increasing the efficacy of G_{as} in activating AC and thereby enhancing nucleotide exchange.

In many cell systems, very high concentrations of ethanol can affect intracellular calcium levels in the absence of receptor occupancy. The most common effect is a transient increase in intracellular calcium that has been linked to G protein-dependent phospholipase C activation. The increase in intracellular calcium as well as 1,4,5, inositol triphosphate generation associated with ethanol treatment is more short-lived than that generated by natural ligands [19]. However, physiologically relevant concentrations of ethanol probably have little effect on acinar cell signaling but it could have important effects on cell signaling when it is combined with neurohumoral agents.

Effects of ethanol on zymogen activation

The pathologic activation of pancreatic zymogens within the acinar cell is thought to play a role in the initiation of some forms of pancreatitis. Animals treated with high concentrations of CCK or cholinergic agonists develop pancreatitis; treatment of isolated pancreatic acini with similar concentrations of these agents results in the intracellular activation of pancreatic enzymes [48]. Ethanol dramatically sensitizes the acinar cell to the effects of cholecystokinin on zymogen activation; 25 mM ethanol, a physiologically relevant concentration, shifts the concentration-dependence for CCK two orders of magnitude to the left [46]. These findings suggest that a combination of ethanol and increased CCK levels might lead to the pathologic activation of zymogens within the acinar cell (Fig. 3.1-5).

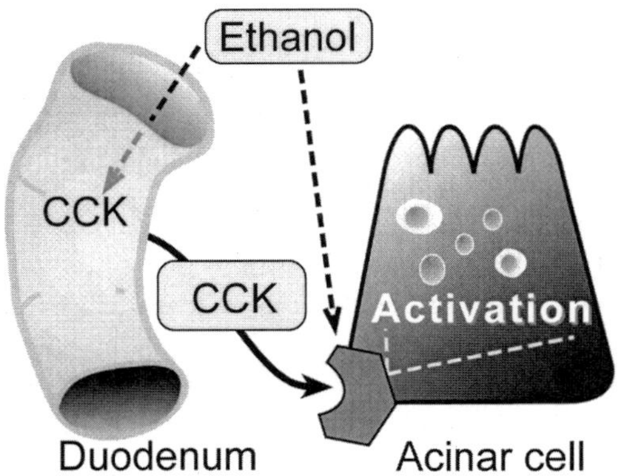

Figure 3.1-5. Ethanol may affect CCK-dependent zymogen processing by at least 2 mechanisms. Ethanol both enhances CCK release from the specialized cells in the duodenum and can sensitize the CCK receptor to the effects of CCK on zymogen activation within the acinar cell.

Mechanisms of pancreatic fibrosis

Stellate cells are found in a number of tissues such as the liver, where they play a central role in fibrogenesis. More recently they have been identified in the pancreas [7]. Under normal conditions, these cells exist in a quiescent state and can be identified by the presence of vitamin A-containing lipid droplets in the cytoplasm. In pancreatic injury, stellate cells are activated and exhibit increased proliferation, transform into myofibroblast-like cells and synthesize increased amounts of extracellular proteins that form fibrous tissue

[6]. *In vitro*, pancreatic stellate cells are activated when exposed to ethanol and its metabolite acetaldehyde or to oxidant stress. Also, acetaldehyde significantly increased collagen synthesis. These changes were prevented by treatment of antioxidant vitamin E [6]. Cytokines also activated stellate cells *in vitro* [7]. These data suggest that fibrosis may develop in the pancreas as a result of alcohol abuse by two fibrogenic pathways (acting in parallel): the necroinflammatory and the non-necroinflammatory pathway. Activation of pancreatic stellate cells by cytokines released during ethanol-induced acinar cell necrosis would represent the necroinflammatory pathway of pancreatic fibrogenesis, whereas direct activation of stellate cells by ethanol via acetaldehyde and/or oxidant stress would represent the non-inflammatory pathway [6].

Generation of pancreatitis in experimental models

It has been difficult to generate acute alcoholic pancreatitis in experimental models. Although ethanol alone does not appear to cause pancreatic injury, it may have a synergetic effect when combined with other insults. The acute administration of ethanol in the rat resulted in increased injury when pancreatitis was induced by a combination of pancreatic duct obstruction and hyperstimulation [26, 49]. Rats chronically fed ethanol also demonstrated more severe pancreatitis in this model. Ethanol alone does not cause pancreatitis in the cat, but it can enhance pancreatic injury under specific conditions. Perfusion of the duct with pancreatic enzymes or stimulation of secretion in the presence of partial duct obstruction does not cause pancreatitis, but pretreatment with intragastric ethanol results in pancreatitis under both treatment conditions. These results suggest that ethanol contributes to the development of acute pancreatitis when there are active enzymes in the pancreatic duct or when secretion is stimulated in the setting of obstruction to pancreatic outflow.

Some of the toxic effects of ethanol may be secondary to its effects on lipid metabolism and other metabolic pathways. Ethanol can lead to increased serum triglyceride levels, a condition known to cause pancreatitis. Pancreatic fatty acid ethyl ester (FAEE) levels are elevated during acute pancreatitis; this increase is associated with high pancreatic FAEE-synthase levels. Ethanol enhances pancreatic FAEE synthase activity. Further, FAEE have been shown to sensitize the rat to CCK-induced pancreatic injury [84].

Supraphysiologic concentrations of CCK are known to cause pancreatitis. Alcohol may act through two mechanisms to promote injury by this physiologic regulator. Chronic ethanol feeding has been shown to enhance the sensitivity of rats to CCK-induced pancreatitis. The animals also exhibited an enhanced inflammatory response. Notably, rats developed pancreatitis when receiving physiologic concentrations of CCK only when they had been chronically treated with high doses of intragastric ethanol. Others have found that acute ethanol administration results in CCK release from the duodenum [72]. A combination of sensitization of the acinar cell to CCK and ethanol-induced CCK release from the duodenum may play a important role in regulating its acute effects on pancreatic zymogen activation.

The inactivation and clearance of active enzymes from the systemic circulation may play a role in determining the severity of pancreatitis. In chronic alcoholic patients, the inhibition and clearance of circulating pancreatic enzymes may be decreased. Although the mechanism of this decrease is not well described, acetaldehyde has been reported to decrease the antitryptic activity of α_1-proteinase inhibitor [15].

Summary

The pancreatic injury induced by ethanol exposure is likely to be multifactorial. Proposed mechanisms include: a) ductal hypertension induced by increased viscosity of secretions in combination with obstruction secondary to sphincter of Oddi dysfunction, stimulation of secretion, and increased duct permeability, b) decreased pancreatic blood flow, c) inflammation and oxidant stress, d) direct acinar cell toxicity, e) changes in protein synthesis, f) an enhanced inflammatory response, and g) stimulation of pancreatic fibrosis. A growing body of evidence suggests that alcohol can cause acute injury even in the absence of underlying chronic disease. Future studies should define the factors that result in patients developing either acute bouts of disease or chronic pancreatitis. Since only a fraction of patients that abuse alcohol develop pancreatic disease, elucidation of the determinants that increase an individual's susceptibility to alcohol is an important topic for study.

References

1. Ammann RW, Muelhaupt B. Progression of alcoholic acute to chronic pancreatitis. Gut 1994; 35: 552–6.
2. Ammann RW, Akovbiantz A, Largiader F, Schueler G. Course and outcome of chronic pancreatitis. Longitudinal study of a mixed medial-surgical series of 245 patients. Gastroenterology 1984; 86: 820–8.
3. Ammann RW, Buehler H, Bruehlmann W, Kehl O, Muench R, Stamm B. Acute (nonprogressive) alcoholic pancreatitis: prospective longitudinal study of 144 patients with recurrent alcoholic pancreatitis. Pancreas 1986; 1: 195–203.
4. Andreasson S, Romelsjo A, Allebeck P. Alcohol, social factors and mortality among young men. British Journal of Addiction 1991; 86: 877–87.
5. Angelini G, Pederzoli P, Caliari S, Fratton S, Brocco G, Marzoli G, Bovo P, Cavallini G, Scuro LA. Long-term outcome of acute necrohemorrhagic pancreatitis. A 4-year follow-up. Digestion 1984; 30: 131–7.
6. Apte MV, Phillips PA, Fahmy RG, Darby SJ, Rodgers SC, McCaughan GW, Korsten MA, Pirola RC, Naidoo D, Wilson JS. Does alcohol directly stimulate pancreatic fibrogenesis? Studies with rat pancreatic stellate cells. Gastroenterology 2000 Apr; 118(4): 780–94.
7. Apte MV, Haber PS, Applegate TL, Norton ID, McCaughan GW, Korsten MA, Pirola RC, Wilson JS. Periacinar stellate shaped cells in rat pancreas: identification, isolation, and culture. Gut 1998; 43: 128–33.
8. Ashley SW, Schwarz M, Alvarez C, Nguyen TN, Vdovenko A, Reber HA. Pancreatic interstitial pH regulation: effects of secretory stimulation. Surgery 1994; 115: 503–9.
9. Bank S. Chronic pancreatitis: clinical features and medical management. Am J Gastroenterol 1986; 81: 153–67.
10. Baskin G. Ethanol and regulation of receptor-mediated endocytosis. Hepatology 1990; 12: 1240–5.
11. Beck IT, Paloshi GB, Dinda PK, Beck M. Effect of intragastric administration of alcohol on the ethanol concentrations and osmolality of pancreatic juice, bile and portal and peripheral blood. Gastroenterology 1974; 67: 484–9.
12. Berger Z, Pap A. Chronic pancreatitis in Hungary. In: Sarles H, Johnson CD, Sauniere JF, eds. Pancreatitis. New data and geographical distribution. Paris: Arnette-Blackwell, 1991: 185–90.
13. Boustiere C, Sarles H, Lohse J, Durbec JP, Sahel J. Citrate and calcium secretion in the pure human pancreatic juice of alcoholic and non alcoholic men and of chronic pancreatitis patients. Digestion 1985; 32: 1–9.

14. Bradley EL. A clinically based classification system for acute pancreatitis. Arch Surg 1993; 128: 586–90.
15. Brecher AS, Pavlock JL. Acetaldehyde decreases the antitryptic activity of alpha 1-proteinase inhibitor. Alcohol 1992; 9: 181–4.
16. Chari ST, Singer MV. The problem of classification and staging of chronic pancreatitis. Proposals based on current knowledge of its natural history. Scand J Gastroenterol 1994; 29: 949–60.
17. Cohn JA, Friedman KJ, Noone PG, Knowles MR, Silverman LM, Jowell PS. Relation between mutations of the cystic fibrosis gene and idiopathic pancreatitis. New Eng J of Med 1998; 339: 653–8.
18. Davies KJA, Goldberg AL. Proteins damaged by oxygen radicals are rapidly degraded in extracts of red blood cells. J Bio Chem 1987; 262: 8227–34.
19. De Petrillo PB, Swift RM. Ethanol exposure results in a transient decrease in human platelet cAMP levels: evidence for a protein kinase C mediated process. Alcohol Clin Exp Res 1992; 16: 290–4.
20. Dickson AP, O'Neill J, Imrie CW. Hyperlidaemia, alcohol abuse and acute pancreatitis. Br J Surg 1984; 71: 685–8.
21. Durbec J, Sarles H. Multicenter study of the epidemiology of pancreatic disorders. Relationship between the relative risk of developing chronic pancreatitis and alcohol, protein and lipid consumption. Digestion 1978; 18: 337.
22. Durbec JP, Sarles H. Epidemiology of chronic pancreatitis. Alcohol and dietary habits. Pancreatitis – Concepts and Classification 1984; 351–3.
23. Fallon M, Gorelick F, Anderson J, Mennone A, Saluja A, Steer, M. Effect of cerulein hyperstimulation on the paracellular barrier of rat exocrine pancreas. Gastroenterology 1995; 108: 1863–72.
24. Fawcett J, Hammond B, Smith GD. Acute effects of ethanol on hepatic endocytosis and processing of insulin in perfused rat liver. Am J Physiol 1993; 264: E420–7.
25. Fernandez-del Castillo C, Schmidt J, Warshaw AL, Rattner DW. Interstitial protease activation is the central event in progression to necrotizing pancreatitis. Surgery 1994; 116: 497–504.
26. Foitzik T, Lewandrowski KB, Castillo CF, Rattner DW, Klar E, Warshaw AW. Exocrine hyperstimulation but not pancreatic duct obstruction increases the susceptibility to alcohol-related pancreatic injury. Arch Surg 1994; 129: 1081–5.
27. Friedman HS, Lowery R, Shaughnessy E, Scorza J. The effects of ethanol on pancreatic blood flow in awake and anesthetized dogs. Proc Soc Exp Biol Med 1983; 174: 377–82.
28. Gjorup I, Dueholm S, Andersen B, Burcharth F. Ethanol in pancreatic juice after oral and intravenous administration. Gut 1990; 31: 1411–3.
29. Goff JS. The effect of ethanol on the pancreatic duct sphincter of Oddi. Am J Gastroenterol 1993; 88: 656–60.
30. Gorry MC, Gabbaizedeh D, Furey W, Gates LK Jr, Preston RA, Aston CE, Zhang Y, Ulrich C, Ehrlich GD, Whitcomb DC. Mutations in the cationic trypsinogen gene are associated with recurrent acute and chronic pancreatitis. Gastroenterology 1997; 113: 1063–8.
31. Gullo L, Barbara L, Labo G. Effect of cessation of alcohol use on the course of pancreatic dysfunction in alcoholic pancreatitis. Gastroenterology 1988; 95: 1063–8.
32. Gullo L, Durbec J. Pancreatitis: concepts and classification. In: Gyr K, Singer M, Sarles H, eds. Epidemiology and etiology of pancreatitis. Amsterdam: Excerpta Medica, 1984a: 371–6.
33. Gullo L, Durbec JP. Epidemiology and etiology of pancreatitis. Summary. In: Gyr KE, Singer MV, Sarles H, eds. Pancreatitis: Concepts and classification. Amsterdam: Elsevier Science Publishers B.V., 1984b: 371–6.
34. Guy O, Robles-Diaz G, Adrich Z, Sahel J, Sarles H. Protein content of precipitates present in pancreatic juice of alcoholic subjects and patients with chronic calcifying pancreatitis. Gastroenterology 1983; 84: 102–7.
35. Haber P, Wilson J, Apte M, Hall W, Goumas K, Pirola R. Lipid intolerance does not account for susceptibility to alcoholic and gallstone pancreatitis. Gastroenterology 1994; 106: 742–8.

36. Haber P, Wilson J, Apte M, Korsten M, Pirola R. Individual susceptibility to alcoholic pancreatitis: still an enigma [see comments]. J Lab Clin Med 1995; 125: 305–12.
37. Haber PS, Wilson JS, Apte MV, Pirola RC. Fatty acid ethyl esters increase rat pancreatic lysosomal fragility. J Lab Clin Med 1993; 121: 759–64.
38. Hajnal F, Flores M, Radley S, Valenzuela J. Effect of alcohol and alcoholic beverages on meal-stimulated pancreatic secretions in humans. Gastroenterology 1990; 98: 191–6.
39. Hartwig W, Werner J, Ryschich E, Mayer H, Schmidt J, Gebhard MM, Herfarth C, Klar E. Cigarette smoke enhances ethanol-induced pancreatic injury [In Process Citation]. Pancreas 2000 Oct; 21(3): 272–8.
40. Hayakawa T, Kondo T, Shibata T, Sugimoto Y, Kitagawa M. Chronic alcoholism and evolution of pain and prognosis in chronic pancreatitis. Dig Dis Sci 1989; 34: 33–8.
41. Hoek JB, Higashi K. Effects of alcohol on polyphosphoinositide-mediated intracellular signaling. Ann N Y Acad Sci 1991; 625: 375–87.
42. Hoffman P, Tabakoff B. Ethanol and guanine nucleotide binding proteins: a selective interaction. FASEB Journal 1990; 4: 2612–22.
43. Imoto M, DiMagno EP. Cigarette smoking increases the risk of pancreatic calcification in late-onset but not early-onset idiopathic chronic pancreatitis [In Process Citation]. Pancreas 2000 Aug; 21(2): 115–9.
44. Johnson CD. Alcohol and the neural regulation of pancreatic secretion. In: Sarles H, Johnson CD, Sauniere JF, eds. Pancreatitis: New data and geographical distribution. 1 ed. Paris: Arnette-Blackwell, 1991: 53–65. Notes: Chapter Num: 6.
45. Kamimura S, Tsukamoto H. Cytokine gene expression by Kupffer cells in experimental alcoholic liver disease. Hepatology 1995; 22: 1304–9.
46. Katz M, Carangelo R, Miller LJ, Gorelick F. Effect of ethanol on cholecystokinin-stimulated zymogen conversion in pancreatic acinar cells. Am J Physiol 1996; 270: G171–5.
47. Kloppel G, Maillet B. Ultrastructural observations on cytotoxic effector cells infiltrating pancreatic islets of low-dose streptozocin treated mice. Virchows Arch A Path Anat 1992; 420: 1–4.
48. Leach SD, Modlin IM, Scheele GA, Gorelick FS. Intracellular activation of digestive zymogens in rat pancreatic acini. Stimulation by high doses of cholecystokinin. J Clin Invest 1991; 87: 362–6.
49. Letko G, Nosofsky T, Lessel W, Siech M. Transition of rat pancreatic juice edema into acute pancreatitis by single ethanol administration. Path Res Pract 1991; 187: 247–50.
50. Letko G, Siech M. Effect of phospholipase A2 and ethanol on the survival of acinar cells isolated from the rat pancreas. Digestion 1992; 51: 193–7.
51. Lin Y, Tamakoshi A, Hayakawa T, Ogawa M, Ohno Y. Cigarette smoking as a risk factor for chronic pancreatitis: a case-control study in Japan. Research Committee on Intractable Pancreatic Diseases [In Process Citation]. Pancreas 2000 Aug; 21(2): 109–14.
52. Luthen R, Niederau C, Grendell JH. Intrapancreatic zymogen activation and levels of ATP and glutathione during caerulein pancreatitis in rats. Am J Physio 1995; 268: G592–604.
53. Mithofer K, Fernandez-del Castillo C, Frick TW, Foitzik T, Bassi DG, Lewandrowski KB, Ratter DW. Increased intrapancreatic trypsinogen activation in ischemia-induced experimental pancreatitis. Ann Surg 1995; 221: 364–71.
54. Nagy LE, De Silva SE. Ethanol increases receptor-dependent cyclic AMP production in cultured hepatocytes by decreasing G(i)-mediated inhibition. Biochem J 1992; 286: 681–6.
55. Neuschwander-Tetri BA, Barnidge M, Janney CG. Cerulein-induced pancreatic cysteine depletion: prevention does not diminish acute pancreatitis in the mouse [see comments]. Gastroenterology 1994; 107: 824–30.
56. Nordmann R, Ribiere C, Rouach H. Implication of free radical mechanisms in ethanol-induced cellular injury. Free Radical Bio & Med 1992; 12: 219–40.
57. Okazaki K, Yamamoto Y, Kagiyama S, Tamura S, Sakamoto Y, Morita M. Pressure of papillary sphincter zone and pancreatic main duct patients with alcoholic and idiopathic chronic pancreatitis. Int J Pancreatol 1988; 3: 457–68.
58. Perkins PS, Rutherford RE, Pandol SJ. Effect of chronic ethanol feeding on digestive enzyme synthesis and mRNA content in rat pancreas. Pancreas 1995; 10: 14–21.

59. Pfutzer RH, Barmada MM, Brunskill AP, Finch R, Hart PS, Neoptolemos J, Furey WF, Whitcomb DC. SPINK1/PSTI polymorphisms act as disease modifiers in familial and idiopathic chronic pancreatitis. Gastroenterology 2000 Sep; 119(3): 615–23.
60. Pitchmoni CS, Glasser M, Saran RM, Panchacharam P, Thelmo W. Pancreatic fibrosis in chronic alcoholics and nonalcoholics without clinical pancreatitis. Am J Gastroenterol 1984; 79: 382–8.
61. Planche N, Palasciano G, Meullenet J, Laugier R, Sarles H. Effects of intravenous alcohol on pancreatic and biliary secretion in man. Dig Dis Sci 1982; 27: 449–53.
62. Ponnappa B, Hoek J, Jubinski L, Rubin E. Effect of chronic ethanol ingestion on pancreatic protein synthesis. Biochim Biophys Acta 1988; 966: 390–402.
63. Reber HA, Tweedie JH. Effects of aspirin plus ethanol on the pancreatic duct to macromolecules. Surg Forum 1981; 32: 219–21.
64. Renner IG, Rinderknecht H, Valenzuela JE, Douglas AP. Studies of pure pancretic secretions in chronic alcoholic subjects without pancreatic insufficiency. Scand J Gastroenterol 1980; 15: 241–4.
65. Renner IG, Savage WE, Pantoja JL, Renner VJ. Death due to acute pancreatitis. A retrospective analysis of 405 autopsy cases. Dig Dis Sci 1985; 30: 1005–18.
66. Rinderknecht H, Renner IG, Carmack C. Trypsinogen variants in pancreatic juice of healthy volunteers, chronic alcoholics, and patients with pancreatitis and cancer of the pancreas. Gut 1979a; 20: 886–91.
67. Rinderknecht H, Renner IG, Koyama HH. Lysosomal enzymes in pure pancreatic juice from normal healthy volunteers and chronic alcoholics. Dig Dis Sci 1979b; 24: 180–6.
68. Robinette C, Hrubec Z, Fraumeni JF. Chronic alcoholism and subsequent mortality in World War II veterans. Am J Epidemiol 1979; 109: 786–800.
69. Robles-Diaz G, Garcia-Tsao G. Chronic pancreatitis in Mexico City: comparison with chronic liver disease. In: Sarles H, Johnson CD, Sauniere JF, eds. Pancreatitis. New data and geographical distribution. Paris: Arnette-Blackwell, 1991: 197–202.
70. Robles-Diaz G, Vargas F, Uscanga L, Fernandez-del Castillo C. Chronic pancreatitis in Mexico City. Pancreas 1990; 5: 479–83.
71. Saluja A, Saluja M, Villa A, Leili U, Turledge P, Meldolesi J, Steer M. Pancreatic duct obstruction in rabbits causes digestive zymogen and lysosomal enzyme colocalization. J Clin Invest 1989; 84: 1260–6.
72. Saluja AK, Lu L, Yamaguchi Y, Hofbauer B, Runzi M, Dawra R, Bhatia M, Steer ML. A cholecystokinin-releasing factor mediates ethanol-induced stimulation of rat pancreatic secretion. J Clin Invest 1997; 99: 506–12.
73. Sanfey H, Bulkley GB, Cameron JL. The pathogenesis of acute pancreatitis: The source and role of oxygen-derived free radicals in three different experimental models. Ann Surg 1985; 201: 633–8.
74. Sarles H, Adler G, Dani R, Frey C, Gullo L, Harada H, Martin E, Norohna M, Scuro LA. The pancreatitis classification of Marseilles–Rome. Scand J Gastroenterol 1989; 24: 641–2.
75. Sarles H, Sarles J, Camatte R, Muratore R, Gaini M, Guien C, Pastor J, LeRoy F. Observations on 205 confirmed cases of acute pancreatitis, recurring pancreatitis, and chronic pancreatitis. Gut 1965; 6: 545–59.
76. Scheele G, Adler G, Kern H. Exocytosis occurs at the lateral plasma membrane of the pancreatic acinar cell during supramaximal secretagogue stimulation. Gastroenterology 1987; 92: 345–53.
77. Seligson U, Cho JW, Ihre T, Lundh G. Clinical course and autopsy findings in acute and chronic pancreatitis. Acta Chir Scand 1982; 148: 269–74.
78. Sharer N, Schwarz M, Malone G, Howarth A, Painter J, Super M, Braganza J. Mutations of the cystic fibrosis gene in patients with chronic pancreatitis [see comments]. N Engl J Med 1998; 339(10): 645–52.
79. Singh M. Effect of chronic ethanol feeding on factors leading to inappropriate intrapancreatic activation of zymogens in the rat pancreas. Digestion 1992; 53: 114–20.

80. Steer ML, Meldolesi J. The cell biology of experimental pancreatitis. N Engl J Med 1987; 316: 144–50.
81. Suda K, Shiotsu H, Nakamura T, Akai J, Nakamura T. Pancreatic fibrosis in patients with chronic alcohol abuse: correlation with alcoholic pancreatitis. Am J Gastroenterol 1994; 89: 2060–2.
82. Talamini G, DiFrancesco V, Frulloni L, Tebaldi M, Falconi M, Vaona B, Bovo P, Casarini M, Andreaus M, Pederzoli P, Cavallini G. Acute and chronic alcoholic pancreatitis: are there any clinico-epidemiological characteristics distinguishing between these entities? Gut 1995; 37: A60.
83. Wedgwood K, Adler G, Kern H, Reber H. Effects of oral agents on pancreatic duct permeability. Dig Dis Sci 1986; 31: 1081–8.
84. Werner J, Laposata C, Fernandez-del Castillo C, Saghir M, Iozzo V, Lewandrowski KB, Warshaw AL. Pancreatic injury in rats induced by fatty acid ethyl ester, a nonoxidative metabolite of alcohol. Gastroenterology 1997; 113: 286–95.
85. Widdison AL, Alvarez C, Schwarz M, Reber HA. The influence of ethanol on pancreatic blood flow in cats with chronic pancreatitis. Surgery 1992; 112: 202–10.
86. Wilson JS, Apte MV, Thomas MC, Haber PS, Pirola RC. Effects of ethanol, acetaldehyde and cholesteryl esters on pancreatic lysosomes. Gut 1992; 33: 1099–1104.
87. Wilson JS, Bernstein L, McDonald C, Tait A, McNeil D, Pirola RC. Diet and drinking habits in relation to the development of alcoholic pancreatitis. Gut 1985; 26: 882–7.
88. Witt H, Luck W, Hennies HC, Classen M, Kage A, Lass U, Landt O, Becker M. Mutations in the gene encoding the serine protease inhibitor, Kazal type 1 are associated with chronic pancreatitis. Nat Genet 2000 Jun; 25(2): 213–6.
89. Yatto R, Siegel J. The role of pancreatobiliary duct anatomy in the etiology of alcoholic pancreatitis. J Clin Gastroenterol 1984; 6: 419–23.

3.2 Chronic pancreatitis: Development from acute pancreatitis?*)

P. G. Lankisch

Abstract

Whether or not acute pancreatitis may progress to the chronic form is subject to controversy. Equally debatable is whether acute pancreatitis due to alcohol abuse develops in a chronically diseased gland or in a normal pancreas. As for the state of the gland, several postmortem studies have shown that acute pancreatitis may occur after acute alcohol abuse in the normal pancreas. As for progression from acute to chronic pancreatitis, a number of experimental studies have demonstrated signs of the chronic form of the disease in animals, but these signs were reversible. Some clinical studies have shown that alcohol-induced acute pancreatitis may progress to chronic pancreatitis. However, there are presently no predictive parameters indicating when such a progression will occur or not.

Introduction

Alcohol abuse is the dominant cause of acute and chronic pancreatitis. The relationship between alcohol-induced acute and chronic pancreatitis, however, is disputed [1]. Whether these two diseases are two different types or whether chronic pancreatitis is the result of several attacks of alcohol-induced acute pancreatitis and whether the first alcohol-induced acute episode develops in an already chronically diseased pancreas are especially unclear. To answer the question of whether alcohol-induced chronic pancreatitis involving chronic fibrotic lesions and pancreaticolithiasis precedes acute pancreatitis and – if not – when and after how many attacks an initial episode of acute pancreatitis progresses to the chronic form, some other preliminary questions should be answered:

- Does alcohol-induced acute pancreatitis occur in patients with a normal pancreas?
- Does chronic pancreatitis develop in animals that survive experimentally induced acute pancreatitis?
- Do follow-up studies in previously asymptomatic patients with alcohol-induced acute pancreatitis show an eventual progression to chronic pancreatitis?

Before answering these questions, chronic pancreatitis, as well as which criteria are necessary to diagnose the disease, must be defined.

Definition and diagnosis of chronic pancreatitis

During past decades, several attempts to give a clear-cut definition of acute and chronic pancreatitis have been made. Major attempts are the first classification of Marseilles [2], the Cambridge classification [3, 4], the second classification of Marseilles [5], and the classification of Marseilles-Rome 1988 [6].

* Taken from Surgical Clinics of North America 1999; 79: 815–27 with permission.

The first classification of Marseilles in 1963 [2] defines acute and chronic pancreatitis primarily on the basis of morphological criteria. The definition differentiates between acute pancreatitis, acute relapsing pancreatitis, chronic relapsing pancreatitis, and chronic pancreatitis. Chronic pancreatitis takes a primarily painless course. The classification states that it is unusual for acute pancreatitis to develop into chronic pancreatitis, but it may occur.

The Cambridge classification of 1984 [3, 4] differentiates only between acute and chronic pancreatitis. Acute pancreatitis may relapse, but when and how frequently acute pancreatitis progresses to the chronic form of the disease is not clearly defined. The definition states that a single episode of acute pancreatitis may have implications for pancreatic function and pancreatic morphology and that follow-up examinations have to clarify whether reduced pancreatic function or altered morphology returns to normal. A patient with silent underlying disease may present for the first time with an acute attack but, in fact, have chronic disease.

The second Marseilles classification of 1984 [5] again stated that acute pancreatitis rarely leads to chronic pancreatitis. The participants of the meeting agreed that it was not

Table 3.2-1. Diagnosis of chronic pancreatitis according to the scoring systems of the Mayo Clinic and the Lüneburg Clinic.

Parameter	**Mayo Clinic score***	**Lüneburg score****
Morphologic examinations		
– Postmortem diagnosis of chronic pancreatitis	4	4
– Histologic diagnosis obtained intraoperatively	4	4
– Characteristic intraoperative findings, no histology	n. m.	4
– Pancreatic calcifications, obtained histologically or by an imaging procedure	4	4
Abnormal pancreatic function tests		
– Secretin-pancreozymin test (SPT)	2***	3
– Pancreolauryl test	n. m.	2
– Fecal chymotrypsin estimation	n. m.	2
– Fecal elastase-1 estimation	n. m.	2
– Steatorrhea	2***	1
Abnormal imaging procedures		
– Ultrasonography	n. m.	3
– Endoscopic ultrasonography	n. m.	3
– Computed tomography	n. m.	3
– Endoscopic retrograde cholangiopancreatography	3	3

* ≥ 4 Defines proven chronic pancreatitis
** ≥ 4 Defines proven chronic pancreatitis; 3, probably chronic pancreatitis
*** Exocrine pancreatic insufficiency was considered to be present by the Mayo Clinic when steatorrhea was qualitatively or quantitatively (> 7 g/d) demonstrated or cholecystokinin (pancreozymin) test was abnormal.
n. m. = not mentioned
Data *from* The Mayo Clinic, Rochester, MN, USA; and the Lüneburg Clinic, Lüneburg, Germany.

unusual to have patients present with chronic pain and abnormal function tests of the pancreas, but the endoscopic retrograde cholangiopancreatography (ERCP) in those patients could be perfectly normal. They also agreed that the opposite may also occur occasionally. These investigators concluded that pancreatic function tests and imaging procedures complement each other and that the grading system based on both test procedures may provide an important diagnostic advance and should be investigated prospectively.

The 1988 Marseilles-Rome classification [6] states that the morphologic changes of acute pancreatitis are, as a rule, reversible; however, if the necrosis involves a segment of the main duct, stenosis may result and lead to duct obstruction and chronic pancreatitis caudal to the stenosis. This was very likely based on the results obtained in animal experiments by Sarles' group [7].

Diagnostic criteria using a scoring system have been developed only by the Mayo Clinic [8] (Table 3.2-1), the Japan Pancreas Society [9] (Table 3.2-2), and the author's department at Lüneburg; the author's criteria were developed largely on the basis of those of the Mayo Clinic (see Table 3.2-1).

Table 3.2-2. Diagnostic criteria for chronic pancreatitis.

Definite chronic pancreatitis

1. (a) Ultrasonography: Pancreatic stones, evident by intrapancreatic hyperreflective echoes with acoustic shadows behind.
   (b) CT: Pancreatic stones evident by intrapancreatic calcifications.
2. ERCP: (i) Irregular dilatation of pancreatic duct branches of variable intensity with scattered distribution throughout the entire pancreas or (ii) irregular dilatation of the main pancreatic duct and branches proximal to complete or incomplete obstruction of the main pancreatic duct (with pancreatic stones or protein plugs).
3. Secretin test: Abnormally low bicarbonate concentration combined with either decreased enzyme outputs or decreased secretory volume.
4. Histologic examination: Irregular fibrosis with destruction and loss of exocrine parenchyma in tissue specimens obtained at biopsy, surgery, or autopsy. The fibrosis has an irregular and patchy distribution in the interlobular spaces. Intralobular fibrosis alone is not specific for chronic pancreatitis.
5. Additionally, protein plugs, pancreatic stones, dilatation of the pancreatic duct, hyperplasia and metaplasia of ductal epithelium, and cyst formation are observed.

Probable chronic pancreatitis

1. (a) Ultrasonography: Intrapancreatic coarse hyperreflectivities, irregular dilatation of pancreatic ducts, or pancreatic deformity with irregular contour.
   (b) CT: Pancreatic deformity with irregular contour.
2. ECRP: Irregular dilatation of the main pancreatic duct alone, intraductal filling defects suggestive of noncalcified pancreatic stones or protein plugs.
3. (a) Secretin test: (i) Abnormally low bicarbonate concentration alone or (ii) decreased enzyme outputs plus decreased secretory volume.
   (b) Tubeless tests: Simultaneous abnormalities in the BT-para-amino benzoic acid test and fecal chymotrypsin test, observed at two points in time several months apart.
4. Histologic examination: Intralobular fibrosis with one of the following findings: loss of exocrine parenchyma, isolated islets of Langerhans, or pseudocysts.

ERCP = endoscopic retrograde cholangiopancreatography.
From Homma T, Harada H, Koizumi M. Diagnostic criteria for chronic pancreatitis by the Japan Pancreas Society. Pancreas 1997; 15: 14; with permission.

The Mayo Clinic and the Lüneburg scoring systems have some criteria in common but differ in others. Both give up to 4 points for the result of single investigations. Both consider chronic pancreatitis to be established if 4 points or more are reached. The Lüneburg score also gives the diagnosis of probable chronic pancreatitis if these patients have 3 points with either an abnormal imaging procedure or an abnormal secretin-pancreozymin-test (SPT), the gold standard test for exocrine pancreatic function. As a rule, these patients failed to turn up for the complimentary follow-up investigation so that neither a pancreatic function test nor an imaging procedure could be performed.

Both scoring systems place a high value on morphologic findings to prove chronic pancreatitis. These objective findings include histology obtained at postmortem examination or during operation and pancreatic calcifications. In addition, the author believes that the diagnosis of chronic pancreatitis may be made on the basis of intraoperative findings, which may help surgeons avoid the risks of a pancreatic biopsy to prove the diagnosis in case they are performing a drainage operation and not a partial resection of the pancreas.

Finally, the histologic assessment of chronic pancreatitis at postmortem examination may be difficult. In one study, when pancreases were diagnosed by general pathologists as "chronically diseased" and reevaluated by an experienced gastrointestinal pathologist, only 47% had chronic pancreatitis, 9% showed a repair stage of acute pancreatitis, and the remainder had other conditions. Thus, the histologic diagnosis of chronic pancreatitis may be an overdiagnosis [10].

Imaging procedures are given higher scores than for the direct pancreatic function test at the Mayo Clinic [8], but not so at Lüneburg (Mayo Clinic, 3 versus 3 points; Lüneburg Clinic, 3 versus 3 points; see Table 3.2-1). To use only the result of an imaging procedure to diagnose chronic pancreatitis is problematic for three reasons:

1. Pancreatic duct changes may persist after acute pancreatitis, whereas exocrine pancreatic insufficiency returns to normal during recovery [11, 12]. Thus, ductal abnormalities may represent persistent scarring after the acute attack and not represent chronic pancreatitis.
2. Comparisons of the results of the SPT and ERCP [13, 14] have shown that, in the majority of the patients, the results of both examinations agree; however, some patients have exocrine pancreatic insufficiency and normal ductal systems, and vice versa. As a rule, patients with abnormal ductal systems but normal pancreatic functioning do not tend to develop chronic pancreatitis even after a longer follow-up. The majority of patients seem to have experienced earlier acute pancreatitis, and the duct changes are scars rather than signs of chronic disease [14]. In contrast, late development of duct changes in patients with abnormal function tests and initially normal duct system may reflect chronic pancreatitis [13, 14].
3. Comparisons of ERCP and the secretin-cholecystokinin (CCK) test with histology show that the secretin-CCK test better reflects the presence of histopathologically confirmed chronic pancreatitis than does the ERCP [15, 16].

The Mayo Clinic and the Lüneburg Clinic scores also differ concerning pancreatic function tests. The Mayo Clinic gives equal points for an abnormal direct pancreatic function test and for the qualitative and quantitative demonstration of steatorrhea (2 points for each test). Because the SPT is much more specific and sensitive than the presence of steatorrhea, a direct pancreatic function test, if abnormal, is given 3 points in the Lüneburg score. Steatorrhea may be secondary to several nonpancreatic causes [17], and the author does not consider qualitative demonstration of steatorrhea to be helpful. Thus, the qualitative demonstration of steatorrhea is not mentioned in the Lüneburg scoring system, and the presence of steatorrhea is given only 1 point. Furthermore, the Mayo Clinic does not mention indirect pancreatic function tests, in large part because they have never been widely accepted in the United States. Because these tests are frequently used in Europe, they are mentioned in the Lüneburg scoring system, but because they are less sensitive [18] than direct tests, they get less points in the Lüneburg score than do the direct tests.

The diagnostic criteria of chronic pancreatitis in Japan resemble those of the scoring systems of the Mayo and Lüneburg clinics. Similar to the Lüneburg scoring system, the Japanese classification differentiates between proven and probable chronic pancreatitis (see Table 3.2-2) [19]. Divergent from the Mayo Clinic and Lüneburg scores, however, chronic pancreatitis is considered to be proven or probable when only one test, that is, an imaging procedure or a function test, shows an abnormal result or when the diagnosis is proven histologically. In the European experience, indirect pancreatic function tests are deemed inferior to direct pancreatic function tests, and their results, if abnormal, indicate only probable chronic pancreatitis, a diagnosis that is more likely when the indirect pancreatic function test is abnormal when repeated and is abnormal several months later.

Postmortem examinations

To prove whether alcohol-induced acute pancreatitis develops in a normal pancreas, early postmortem examinations must be considered. Weiner and Tennant [20] reviewed 4000 postmortem examinations and found that 38 (1%) patients had acute necrotizing pancreatitis and 97 (2,4%) had chronic pancreatitis. Death occured after acute alcohol abuse in 51 patients of whom 27 (53%) showed pancreatic lesions and 24 (47%) did not. Of these 27 patients, 25 (93%) had acute pancreatitis and only 2 (7%) had chronic pancreatitis. In 41 patients, death was caused by long-term alcohol abuse; only 19 (47%) patients had the histologic changes of chronic pancreatitis, whereas 22 (53%) had a normal pancreas.

- Clark [21] reported that only 10 of 15 patients with alcohol-induced acute pancreatitis and chronic alcohol abuse showed fibrosis of the pancreas, which was severe in 3 patients, moderate in 2, and mild in 5; 5 had no pancreatic fibrosis. Thus alcohol-induced acute pancreatitis in these patients occured in a normal pancreas.

Table 3.2-3. Histological signs of chronic pancreatitis in 405 patients who died of acute pancreatitis (postmortem examinations).

Etiology	Patients (n)	Signs of chronic pancreatitis Present	Absent
Chronic alcoholic	247	116 (47%)	131 (53%)
Common duct stone	25	8 (32%)	17 (68%)
Postoperative	37	12 (32%)	25 (68%)
Miscellaneous	18	8 (44%)	10 (56%)
Idiopathic	78	11 (14%)	67 (86%)
Total	405	155 (38%)	250 (62%)

From Renner IG, Savage WT III, Pantoja JL, et al. Death due to acute pancreatitis: A retrospective analysis of 405 autopsy cases. Dig Dis Sci 1985; 30: 1005; with permission.

- Seligson et al. [22] reported 11 patients who died of acute necrotizing pancreatitis. A few patients died after a first acute attack of pancreatitis following severe alcohol abuse for 7 to 14 days.
- Klöppel et al. [23] retrospectively studied the pancreas of 367 patients at postmortem examination and 3 patients at operation for acute pancreatitis; they did not find signs of chronic disease in all patients with alcohol-induced acute pancreatitis.
- Renner et al. [24] reported on 50,227 postmortem examinations, with acute pancreatitis being the main cause for death in 405. Etiologic subgroups were long-term alcohol abuse, common duct stones, surgical procedures, other causes, and an idiopathic group (i.e., of unknown cause) (Table 3.2-3). Despite chronic alcohol abuse, the majority of patients with acute pancreatitis had no histologic signs of chronic pancreatitis. In all other etiologic subgroups, the percentage of patients with a normal pancreas who developed acute pancreatitis was even higher. Patients with idiopathic pancreatitis had significantly less frequent chronic pancreatitis than all other groups together ($p < 0.001$).
- Finally, Schulz and Wruck [25] studied 106 patients in whom acute pancreatitis was the cause of death. Acute pancreatitis as a consequence of chronic alcohol abuse was present in eight (8%) patients, but no signs of chronic pancreatitis were present in any of these patients.

Conclusions concerning postmortem examinations

Acute pancreatitis may develop after alcohol abuse in the normal pancreas; however, postmortem examinations obviously cannot answer the question of why acute pancreatitis develops in some patients in a normal and in others in the diseased pancreas.

Animal experiments

Several experimental studies have been performed in animals to investigate whether animals surviving the experimental acute pancreatitis or related pancreatic injury go on to develop chronic pancreatitis, that is, whether their pancreas shows macroscopic or microscopic criteria of this disease. Of special interest was the question of whether pancreatic fibrosis could be demonstrated (Table 3.2-4):

- Sarles' group induced acute pancreatitis in rats [26, 27] and rabbits [28] by injecting trypsin into the pancreas of the animals. Rats at 4 days [26, 27], and rabbits at 4 weeks [28] developed pancreatic fibrosis and interlobular and intralobular degeneration of acini and tubular complexes that have been described during the development of chronic pancreatitis in humans [29–31]. All histologic signs of chronic pancreatitis, however, disappeared in rats after 9 to14 days [26, 27] and in rabbits after 12 weeks [28].
- Elsässer and colleagues [32, 33] induced acute pancreatitis using the cerulein-stimulation model in rats. In the pancreas, collagen biosynthesis was markedly increased in comparison with healthy controls; however, after 10 to 11 days, no differences were evident between the two groups [23]. In a subsequent experiment, acute pancreatitis was induced 9 times within 20 days by repetitive cerulein stimulation. Signs suggestive of chronic pancreatitis were found initially but disappeared after 6 weeks [33].
- Riaz et al. [34] induced acute pancreatitis in rats with the ethionine-supplemented, choline-deficient diet. A moderate to severe intralobular and perilobular fibrosis and

Table 3.2-4. Animal experiments to clarify the question of whether there are signs of chronic pancreatitis in animals surviving acute pancreatitis.

Study	Model	Animal	Demonstration of morphologic criteria	Persistance of criteria of chronic pancreatitits
Odaira et al. [26]	Intrapancreatic injection of trypsin	Rat	+	–
Iovanna et al. [28]	Intrapancreatic injection of trypsin	Rabbit	+	–
Lechenne de la Porte et al. [27]	Intrapancreatic injection of trypsin	Rat	+	–
Elsässer et al. [32]	Cerulein hyperstimulation	Rat	+	–
Elsässer et al. [33]	Cerulein hyperstimulation	Rat	+	–
Riaz et al. [34]	Ethionine-supplemented choline-deficient diet	Rat	+	–
Freiburghaus et al. [35]	Ischemia model	Rabbit	+	Tendency to decrease with time
Svensson et al. [36]	Duct model	Rat	+	–
Sarles et al. [7]	Duct model	Rat	+	+

other histologic changes indicating chronic pancreatitis that lasted a maximum of 8 weeks after onset of the disease were demonstrated in surviving animals; however, also in this study, all morphologic changes disappeared within 16 weeks [34].

- Freiburghaus et al. [35] used a model of microvascular pancreatitis in rabbits by injecting polystyrene microspheres into the pancreatic branches of the splenic artery. One week later, histologic signs of chronic pancreatitis, especially interstitial fibrosis, were evident; however, these changes tended to decrease. Long-term follow-up investigations were not performed, unfortunately, in this study [35].
- In two other studies, acute pancreatitis was induced by retrograde bile injections into the pancreatic ducts of rats. Divergent results were found. Svensson et al. [36] found an extensive atrophy of the pancreas and only mild fibrosis in surviving animals. Protein plugs in the pancreatic ducts typical of chronic pancreatitis were not detected. An additional administration of alcohol to surviving animals also did not lead to chronic pancreatitis [36]. In the second study [7], intensive microscopic examinations of the pancreas of the surviving animals 6 days after acute pancreatitis showed that the largest ducts draining pathologic areas were obstructed by fibrosis. Distal to this obstruction, intralobular ducts were dilated and their epithelium flattened or atrophied. Acini were atrophied and replaced by perilobular and intralobular fibrosis. Lesions were limited to areas drained by obstructed ducts, with the rest of the pancreas being normal. The investigators concluded that chronic lesions that persist after acute pancreatitis in humans are caused by duct obstruction and not pancreatic necrosis.

Conclusions concerning animal experiments

On the whole, several investigators with different experimental models of acute pancreatitis have demonstrated in surviving animals short-lived "criteria" of chronic pancreatitis, especially pancreatic fibrosis; however, all changes were reversible [26–28, 32–36]. Only Sarles et al. [7] obtained different results with persistence of chronic changes. Repeating this experimental model using other animals, with special attention to the pancreas distal to duct strictures, would be of interest.

Clinical studies

Only a few studies that show an eventual progression to chronic pancreatitis exist with long-term follow-up in previously asymptomatic patients with alcohol-induced acute pancreatitis. In 1946, Comfort et al. [37, 38] proposed that chronic pancreatitis develops on the basis of several relapsing attacks of acute pancreatitis. This hypothesis was based on long-term studies on 29 patients with alcohol-induced acute pancreatitis. In the 1960s, Sarles and colleagues [39, 40] postulated that acute pancreatitis rarely progresses to the chronic form; however, in their investigations, patients with mainly biliary and not alcohol-induced pancreatitis were studied.

To clarify whether chronic alcohol abuse alone, without previous attacks of pancreatitis, leads to pancreatic fibrosis, Pitchumoni et al. [41] examined the pancreas of 101 patients with chronic alcohol abuse who had never had an attack of acute pancreatitis during their lives. Diffuse fibrosis was found in 47% of alcoholics, but only in 29% of nonalcoholics. The fibrosis of nonalcoholics seemed to increase with age. On the basis of these results, these investigators concluded that pancreatic lesions in chronic alcoholics increase before acute pancreatitis occurs.

- Ammann et al. [42–44] have repeatedly addressed the question of what happens to the pancreatic parenchyma after alcohol-induced acute pancreatitis: In 1986, they reported 144 consecutive patients with alcohol-induced relapsing pancreatitis in whom pancreatic function tests and imaging procedures were performed prospectively at regular intervals [42]. They focused on whether pancreatic calcifications, pancreatic ductal changes, or histologic changes of the pancreas had developed and whether exocrine pancreatic function had deteriorated. In 95 (66%) of the patients, chronic pancreatitis developed after a median follow-up of 9.7 years, whereas in 49 (34%) patients, no progress to chronic pancreatitis occurred during median follow-up of 8.3 years. The authors differentiated between progressive alcohol-induced and nonprogressive alcohol-induced acute pancreatitis. The reason why the disease progressed in one group of patients and not in the other could not be elicited.
- Some time later, this group [43] reported the histologic changes in the pancreas of 73 patients, 37 of whom had been operated on for chronic pancreatitis and 46 of whom had undergone postmortem examination. All patients had suffered at the beginning of the disease from alcohol-induced acute pancreatitis. Morphologically, pancreatic pseudocysts, necrosis, pancreatic calcifications, or a perilobular or intralobular fibrosis were sought in the pancreas. Postmortem examinations were performed a mean of 12 years after the first attack of acute pancreatitis. The pancreas showed severe perilobular and intralobular fibrosis (85%) and pancreatic calcifications (74%), but rarely necrosis (4%). In 10 patients, fibrosis was correlated with a progressing exocrine pan-

creatic insufficiency. Surgery was performed a mean of 4.1 years after the first attack of acute pancreatitis. Focal necrosis was demonstrated in 49% and a mild perilobular fibrosis in 54% of these patients. Pancreatic pseudocysts were present in 88% of patients 6 years after the first acute attack. These findings supported the theory that the chronic form of the disease may develop after severe alcohol-induced acute pancreatitis.

- Furthermore, Ammann and colleagues [44] reported 254 patients in whom, after a first attack of alcohol-induced acute pancreatitis, extensive yearly controls were performed prospectively. These control investigations included a clinical evaluation of signs and symptoms, routine laboratory diagnostics, pancreatic function tests (especially analysis of fecal chymotrypsin), postprandial blood glucose investigations or an oral glucose tolerance test, and radiographic examinations of the pancreas in three projections. In addition, ultrasonography, CT and ERCP examinations as well as fecal fat analyses were performed when indicated. According to the long-term course, the patients were divided into three groups: (1) those with pancreatic calcifications (n = 185), (2) those without pancreatic calcifications (n = 30), and (3) those with a non-progressive disease (n = 39). The incidence of relapsing pancreatitis was significantly higher in groups (1) and (2) than in group (3). The progression to advanced chronic pancreatitis in groups (1) and (2) correlated with severity of the pancreatitis attacks; however, a clear definition of *severity* was not given. Pancreatic pseudocysts were mostly found in the head of the pancreas in groups (1) and (2) (58–71%), and in the tail of the pancreas in group (3) (61%). These findings correlated with the necrosis-fibrosis sequence proposed by Klöppel and Maillet [45, 46]. On the basis of pathologic-anatomical findings, the investigators concluded that chronic pancreatitis may be a sequela of necrotizing acute pancreatitis.

In contrast to the investigations of Ammann's group [42], a French study [47] showed a more rapid and more frequent progression from acute to chronic pancreatitis in alcoholics. In 101 (89%) of 114 patients, signs of chronic pancreatitis were found within 2 years of follow-up (pancreatic calcifications in 71 patients and mild to moderate duct changes in 19). The disease was diagnosed microscopically in eight and perioperatively in three patients. In 61 (54%) patients, the diagnosis of chronic pancreatitis was made during the first year of follow-up, whereas in the remaining 40 (56%), diagnosis was made during the second year of follow-up. The percentage of patients with chronic pancreatitis is possibly falsely high because, as discussed earlier, pancreatic duct changes alone are not necessarily diagnostic of chronic pancreatitis.

The German and other international health systems do not allow as extensive prospective investigations as do the Swiss [42, 44]. Asymptomatic patients are certainly not sent to a hospital for extensive investigations at regular intervals. To perform radiologic examinations in three projections for follow-up would be especially difficult unless in a research setting. Follow-up examinations at the author's clinic in Lüneburg are restricted as follows: At regular intervals, general practitioners who take care of the patients after an attack of acute pancreatitis or the patients themselves are interviewed by phone or questionnaires, and only symptomatic patients are investigated and scored (see Table 3.2-1) on whether or not chronic pancreatitis may be proven or may be probable. In accordance with the 1984 Marseilles classification [5], the diagnosis of chronic pancreatitis should be based on a combination of pancreatic function tests and imaging procedures. In the author's experience, acute pancreatitis progresses to symptomatic chronic pancreatitis in approximately 10% of these patients within 4 to 6 years; however, at variance with the studies of Ammann and Muellhaupt [44], this progression seems to be independent of the severity of the first acute attack; that is, patients with a higher Balthazar score (necrotizing pancreatitis) do not develop more frequently chronic pancreatitis than those with the interstitial form of the disease [48, 49].

Conclusions concerning clinical studies

In conclusion, several studies [42–44, 47–49] have shown that acute pancreatitis may progress to chronic pancreatitis. This observation is well established in alcoholics, but in other etiologic subgroups, data are insufficient to answer the question reliably. What factors cause progression from acute to chronic pancreatitis, and especially whether it will take place only after a severe attack of acute pancreatitis, are unclear. Establishing parameters for predicting the progression from acute to chronic pancreatitis will be not only of great interest from the scientific point of view, but also financially, because in this subgroup it may be beneficial to follow up these patients more intensively than other patients with acute pancreatitis. Furthermore, such a follow-up could show how the progression to chronic pancreatitis could be prevented. Such studies will require a large number of patients and therefore be impossible for one center alone; however, before undertaking such a multi-institutional study, a consensus on defining the criteria for a diagnosis of chronic pancreatitis and what examinations are necessary for follow-up will be required.

References

1. Hanck C, Singer MV. Does acute alcoholic pancreatitis exist without preexisting chronic pancreatitis? Scand J Gastroenterol 1997; 32: 625–6.
2. Sarles H. Proposal adopted unanimously by the participants of the Symposium, Marseilles 1963. In: Sarles H, ed. Pancreatitis. Bibl Gastroenterol 7. Basel–New York: Karger, 1965: VII–VIII.
3. Sarner M, Cotton PB. Classification of pancreatitis. Gut 1984; 25: 756–9.
4. Sarner M, Cotton PB. Definitions of acute and chronic pancreatitis. Clin Gastroenterol 1984; 13: 865–70.
5. Singer MV, Gyr K, Sarles H. Revised classification of pancreatitis. Report of the Second International Symposium on the Classification of Pancreatitis in Marseille, France, March 28–30, 1984. Gastroenterology 1985; 89: 683–5.
6. Sarles H, Adler G, Dani R, Frey C, Gullo L, Harada H, Martin E, Norohna M, Scuro LA. The pancreatitis classification of Marseilles–Rome 1988. Scand J Gastroenterol 1989; 24: 641–2.
7. Sarles H, Camarena-Trabous J, Gomez-Santana C, Choux R, Iovanna J. Acute pancreatitis is not a cause of chronic pancreatitis in the absence of residual duct strictures. Pancreas 1993; 8: 354–7.
8. Layer P, Yamamoto H, Kalthoff L, Clain JE, Bakken LJ, DiMagno EP. The different courses of early- and late-onset idiopathic and alcoholic chronic pancreatitis. Gastroenterology 1994; 107: 1481–7.
9. Wallraven M, Schiling D, Adamek HE, Weitz M, Lankisch PG, Riemann JF. Main pancreatic duct stricture due to pancreatic carcinoma mimicking post-acute pancreatitis – lessons to be learned. Pancreas 1997; 15: 460 (abstr).
10. Shimizu M, Hirokawa M, Manabe T. Histological assessment of chronic pancreatitis at necropsy. J Clin Pathol 1996; 49: 913–5.

11. Angelini G, Pederzoli P, Caliari S, Fratton S, Brocco G, Marzoli G, Bovo P, Cavallini G, Scuro LA. Long-term outcome of acute necrohemorrhagic pancreatitis. A 4-year follow-up. Digestion 1984; 30: 131–7.
12. Seidensticker F, Otto J, Lankisch PG. Recovery of the pancreas after acute pancreatitis is not necessarily complete. Int J Pancreatol 1995; 17: 225–9.
13. Lambiase L, Forsmark CE, Albert C, Toskes PP. Secretin test diagnoses chronic pancreatitis earlier than ERCP. Gastroenterology 1993; 104: A315 (abstr).
14. Lankisch PG, Seidensticker F, Otto J, Lübbers H, Mahlke R, Stöckmann F, Fölsch UR, Creutzfeldt W. Secretin-pancreozymin test (SPT) and endoscopic retrograde cholangiopancreatography (ERCP): both are necessary for diagnosing or excluding chronic pancreatitis. Pancreas 1996; 12: 149–52.
15. Heij HA, Obertop H, van Blankenstein M, ten Kate FW, Westbroek DL. Relationship between functional and histological changes in chronic pancreatitis. Dig Dis Sci 1986; 31: 1009–13.
16. Heij HA, Obertop H, van Blankenstein M, Nix GAJJ, Westbroek DL. Comparison of endoscopic retrograde pancreatography with functional and histologic changes in chronic pancreatitis. Acta Radiol 1987; 28: 289–93.
17. Lankisch PG, Lembcke B. Indirect pancreatic function tests: chemical and radioisotope methods. Clin Gastroenterol 1984; 13: 717–37.
18. Lankisch PG. Progress report: exocrine pancreatic function tests. Gut 1982; 23: 777–98.
19. Homma T, Harada H, Koizumi M. Diagnostic criteria for chronic pancreatitis by the Japan Pancreas Society. Pancreas 1997; 15: 14–5.
20. Weiner HA, Tennant RA. A statistical study of acute hemorrhagic pancreatitis (hemorrhagic necrosis of pancreas). Am J Med Sci 1938; 196: 167–76.
21. Clark E. Pancreatitis in acute and chronic alcoholism. Am J Dig Dis 1942; 9: 428–31.
22. Seligson U, Cho JW, Ihre T, Lundh G. Clinical course and autopsy findings in acute and chronic pancreatitis. Acta Chir Scand 1982; 148: 269–74.
23. Klöppel G, Gerkan R v, Dreyer T. Pathomorphology of acute pancreatitis. Analysis of 367 autopsy cases and 3 surgical specimens. In: Gyr KE, Singer MV, Sarles H, eds. Pancreatitis. Concepts and classification. Proc. 2nd Int. Symp. on the Classification of Pancreatitis, Marseilles, France, 1984. Amsterdam–New York–Oxford: Excerpta Medica, 1984: 29–35.
24. Renner IG, Savage III WT, Pantoja JL, Renner VJ. Death due to acute pancreatitis. A retrospective analysis of 405 autopsy cases. Dig Dis Sci 1985; 30: 1005–18.
25. Schulz HJ, Wruck U. Zu Todesursachen und einigen ätiologischen Aspekten der akuten und chronischen Pankreatitis. Dtsch Z Verdau Stoffwechselkr 1987; 47: 33–8.
26. Odaira C, Berger Z, Iovanna JL, Sarles H. Localized necrohemorrhagic pancreatitis in the rat after pancreatic interstitial trypsin injection. Regressive pseudochronic lesions. Digestion 1986; 34: 68–77.
27. Lechene de la Porte P, Iovanna J, Odaira C, Choux R, Sarles H, Berger Z. Involvement of tubular complexes in pancreatic regeneration after acute necrohemorrhagic pancreatitis. Pancreas 1991; 6: 298–306.
28. Iovanna JL, Odaira C, Berger Z, Sarles H. Temporary pseudochronic lesions during the recovery of acute necrohemorrhagic pancreatitis in rabbits. Pancreas 1988; 3: 433–8.
29. Payan H, Sarles H, Demirdjian M, Gauthier AP, Cros RC, Durbec JP. Study of the histological features of chronic pancreatitis by correspondence analysis. Identification of chronic calcifying pancreatitis as an entity. Rev Eur Etudes Clin Biol 1972; 17: 663–70.
30. Tasso F, Stemmelin N, Sarles H, Clop J, Durbec JP, Cros RC, Cornée J. Comparative morphometric study of the human pancreas in its normal state and in primary chronic calcifying pancreatitis. Biomedicine 1973; 18: 134–44.
31. Bockman DE, Boydston WR, Anderson MC. Origin of tubular complexes in human chronic pancreatitis. Am J Surg 1982; 144: 243–9.
32. Elsässer HP, Adler G, Kern HF. Fibroblast structure and function during regeneration from hormone-induced acute pancreatitis in the rat. Pancreas 1989; 4: 169–78.

33. Elsässer HP, Haake T, Grimmig M, Adler G, Kern HF. Repetitive cerulein-induced pancreatitis and pancreatic fibrosis in the rat. Pancreas 1992; 7: 385–90.
34. Riaz C, Ochi K, Tanaka J, Harada H, Ichimura M, Miki H. Does recurrent acute pancreatitis lead to chronic pancreatitis? Sequential morphological and biochemical studies. Pancreas 1997; 14: 334–41.
35. Freiburghaus AU, Redha F, Ammann RW. Does acute pancreatitis progress to chronic pancreatitis? A microvascular pancreatitis model in rat. Pancreas 1995; 11: 374–81.
36. Svensson C, Franzén L, Klöppel G, Sjödahl R, Ihse I. Pancreatic atrophy follows bile-induced acute pancreatitis in the rat. Scand J Gastroenterol 1988; 23: 321–6.
37. Comfort MW, Gambill EE, Baggenstoss AH. Chronic relapsing pancreatitis. A study of twenty-nine cases without associated disease of the biliary or gastro-intestinal tract. Gastroenterology 1946; 6: 239–85.
38. Comfort MW, Gambill EE, Baggenstoss AH. Chronic relapsing pancreatitis. A study of twenty-nine cases without associated disease of the biliary or gastro-intestinal tract (continued). Gastroenterology 1946; 6: 376–408.
39. Sarles H, Sarles JC, Camatte R, Muratore R, Gaini M, Guien C, Pastor J, Le Roy F. Observations on 205 confirmed cases of acute pancreatitis, recurring pancreatitis, and chronic pancreatitis. Gut 1965; 6: 545–59.
40. Sarles H, Muratore R, Sarles JC, Gaini M, Camatte R, Pastor J, Guien C. Aetiology and pathology of chronic pancreatitis. Bibl Gastroenterol 1965; 7: 75–120.
41. Pitchumoni CS, Glasser M, Saran RM, Panchacharam P, Thelmo W. Pancreatic fibrosis in chronic alcoholics and nonalcoholics without clinical pancreatitis. Am J Gastroenterol 1984; 79: 382–8.
42. Ammann RW, Buehler H, Bruehlmann W, Kehl O, Muench R, Stamm B. Acute (nonprogressive) alcoholic pancreatitis: prospective longitudinal study of 144 patients with recurrent alcoholic pancreatitis. Pancreas 1986; 1: 195–203.
43. Ammann RW, Heitz PU, Klöppel G. Course of alcoholic chronic pancreatitis: a prospective clinicomorphological long-term study. Gastroenterology 1996; 111: 224–31.
44. Ammann RW, Muellhaupt B. Progression of alcoholic acute to chronic pancreatitis. Gut 1994; 35: 552–6.
45. Klöppel G, Maillet B. Chronic pancreatitis: evolution of the disease. Hepatogastroenterology 1991; 38: 408–12.
46. Klöppel G, Maillet B. The morphological basis for the evolution of acute pancreatitis into chronic pancreatitis. Virchows Arch [Pathol Anat] 1992; 420: 1–4.
47. Skinazi F, Lévy P, Bernades P. Les pancréatites aiguës alcooliques révèlent-elles toujours une pancréatite chronique? Gastroenterol Clin Biol 1995; 19: 266–9.
48. Assmus C. Die Prognose der akuten Pankreatitis. Eine epidemiologische Untersuchung. Medical Dissertation, University of Göttingen, 1999.
49. Lankisch PG, Assmus C, Petersen M, Gottesleben F, Dröge M. Acute pancreatitis (AP): How many patients progress to chronic pancreatitis (CP)? Gastroenterology 1997; 112: A455 (abstr).

3.3 Experimental models of pancreatic fibrogenesis and the role of stellate cells

M. V. Apte, J. S. Wilson

Introduction

Pancreatic fibrosis is a key pathological feature of chronic pancreatitis [1], but its pathogenesis remains to be fully elucidated. In recent years, research into pancreatic fibrogenesis has gained considerable momentum, largely due to the identification and characterization of stellate shaped cells in the pancreas [2, 3] which are morphologically similar to the hepatic stellate cells known to play a central role in liver fibrosis [4].

Pancreatic stellate cells (PSCs) are situated at the base of pancreatic acini, with their extended cytoplasmic processes encircling the basal aspect of acinar cells [2, 3, 5] (Fig. 3.3-1). They can be identified in normal pancreatic sections by positive immunostaining for the cytoskeletal intermediate filament protein desmin (a stellate cell selective marker) and for other marker proteins such as glial fibrillary acidic protein (GFAP). The cells store vitamin A (as evidenced by the characteristic, rapidly fading blue-green fluorescence emitted by the cells on exposure to UV light) in the form of lipid droplets in the cytoplasm. Electron microscopy reveals a prominent rough endoplasmic reticulum, collagen fibrils and vacuoles (lipid droplets) surrounding a central nucleus [2, 5].

Methods have now been developed to isolate and culture pancreatic stellate cells [2, 3, 5], providing a valuable *in vitro* tool to study their biology. Phase contrast micrographs of

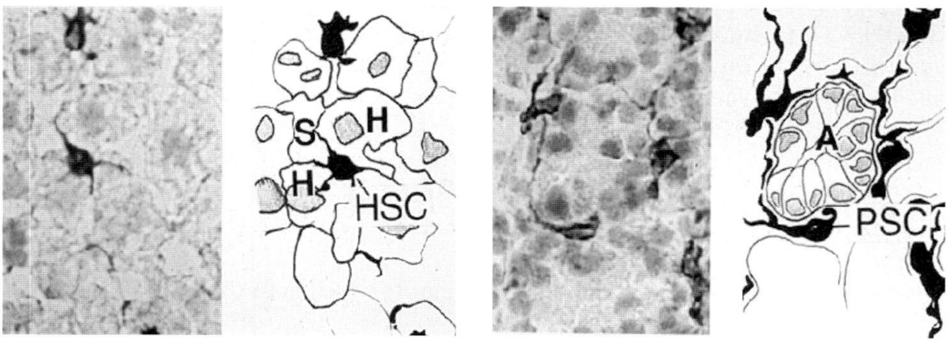

Liver *Pancreas*

Figure 3.3-1. Immunostaining for desmin in liver and pancreatic tissue sections (× 40 objective). The Figure shows a photomicrograph of a section of the liver on the left and the pancreas on the right with corresponding line diagrams adjacent to each picture. Hepatic stellate cells (HSC) were stained brown and were located in the perisinusoidal space between hepatocytes (H) and hepatic sinusoids (S). Desmin positive stellate shaped cells (PSC) were also observed in the pancreas located in the interstitium between acini (A). The cells had elongated cytoplasmic processes extending around the basal aspect of adjacent acinar cells.

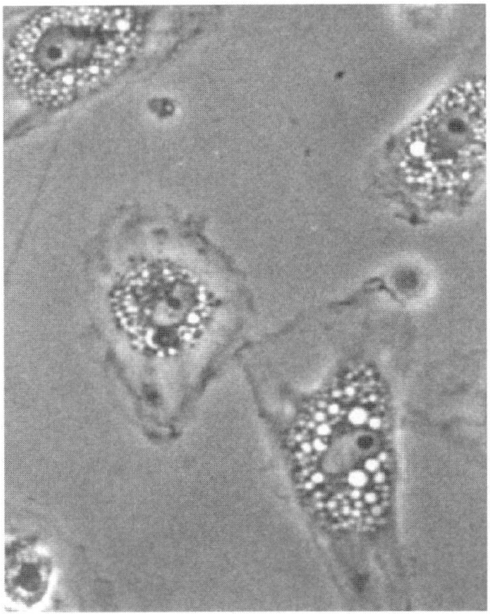

Phase Contrast Microscopy

Figure 3.3-2. Phase contrast microscopy of pancreatic stellate cells after 24 hours in culture (× 20 objective). The cells assume a flattened, angular appearance and show abundant lipid droplets in the cytoplasm.

PSCs in early culture (24–48 hours) demonstrate flattened polygonal cells with prominent lipid droplets in the cytoplasm (Fig. 3.3-2). Cultured PSCs exhibit positive staining for desmin and glial fibrillary acidic protein (GFAP) in a pattern typical of cytoskeletal proteins. The cells are activated when cultured on plastic for more than 48 hours, as indicated by positive staining for alpha smooth muscle actin (α-SMA) and by the loss of cytoplasmic lipid droplets. This phenomenon has been well described in hepatic stellate cells (HSCs) [4]. Immunocytochemistry has demonstrated that cultured pancreatic stellate cells have the capacity to synthesize extracellular matrix proteins such as collagens I and III, fibronectin and laminin [6]. Recent preliminary work by our group indicates that PSCs also secrete the enzymes known to degrade extracellular matrix (MMPs – matrix metalloproteinases) and their inhibitors (TIMPs – tissue inhibitors of matrix metalloproteinases) [7]. This capacity of PSCs to not only synthesize but also degrade ECM proteins suggests that PSCs may play a role in the maintenance of normal tissue architecture by regulating extracellular matrix turnover.

With respect to the possible role of PSCs in the production of pancreatic fibrosis, it is hypothesized that the cells are activated during pancreatic injury (in a manner analogous to hepatic stellate cells), so that they i) proliferate, ii) lose their vitamin A-containing lipid droplets and transform into myofibroblast-like cells that stain positive for α-SMA, iii) become responsive to proliferative and profibrogenic growth factors such as platelet-derived growth factor (PDGF) and transforming growth factor β (TGF-β) and proinflammatory cytokines and iv) synthesize and secrete increased amounts of the extracellular matrix proteins that comprise fibrous tissue. This hypothesis has been examined using both *in vivo* and *in vitro* approaches.

In vivo studies

Methodology

The *in vivo* approach has involved the use of pancreatic sections from patients with chronic pancreatitis [8] and from experimental models of pancreatic fibrosis [8, 9].

Experimental models of pancreatic fibrosis
Two different rat models of pancreatic fibrosis have been used to date for pancreatic stellate cell studies.

TNBS-induced pancreatic fibrosis. This well-described model involves infusion of a chemical toxin, trinitrobenzene sulfonic acid (TNBS), into the pancreatic duct of rats. TNBS infusion produces pancreatic necroinflammation followed by fibrosis within 4 weeks [10]. The pattern of fibrosis produced in this model closely resembles that seen in human chronic pancreatitis, i.e. prominent periductal fibrosis accompanied by intralobular (particularly peri-acinar) fibrosis. The presence of fibrosis in the peri-acinar region is in keeping with the concept that PSCs play an important role in fibrogenesis since these cells have been shown (by desmin staining and electron microscopy) to be located in the peri-acinar region in the normal pancreas.

Dibutyltin chloride(DBTC)-induced pancreatic fibrosis. This model involves the administration of a single intravenous dose of DBTC (6 to 8 mg/kg body weight) to rats [11]. The animals develop moderate to severe pancreatitis within one week of injection, followed by fibrosis in the gland within 4 weeks after DBTC injection.

Analysis of human and rat pancreatic sections
The methodology used to examine PSCs in human and rat pancreatic sections is detailed in the following paragraphs:

Human pancreas. Paraffin sections obtained from patients with chronic alcoholic pancreatitis were stained with hematoxylin and eosin and for collagen using Sirius Red [12]. Immunohistochemistry was performed for α-SMA and for the pro-fibrogenic cytokine transforming growth factor β (TGF-β). The relationship between pancreatic fibrosis and pancreatic stellate cell activation was studied by (i) staining of serial sections for α-SMA and collagen; and (ii) dual-staining of sections for α-SMA plus Sirius Red for collagen protein or α-SMA plus *in situ* hybridization for procollagen α_1 (I) mRNA.

Rat pancreas. Paraffin sections of rat pancreatic tissue were stained by hematoxylin and eosin and Sirius Red. Immunohistochemistry was performed for collagen type I, α-SMA and TGF-β using paraffin sections, and for desmin, glial fibrillary acidic protein (GFAP) and platelet-derived growth factor receptor β (PDGFR-β) using frozen sections. Serial frozen sections were stained for collagen, desmin and PDGFR-β. Dual-staining of sections (for α-SMA plus collagen protein or α-SMA plus procollagen α_1 (I) mRNA) was also performed as described for human tissue.

Immunohistochemistry of human and rat pancreatic sections
In preparation for immunostaining, paraffin sections of the pancreas were rehydrated and washed in TBS for 5 minutes three times, while frozen sections were fixed with acetone at 4°C for 10 minutes, air dried for 10 minutes and washed in TBS as above. Sections were incubated with 1% H_2O_2 for 30 minutes to block endogenous peroxidases and

washed. To prevent non-specific binding of antibody, sections were incubated for 30 minutes at room temperature with a blocking solution containing TBS, 1% bovine serum albumin (BSA), and 10% goat serum.

α-SMA. Paraffin sections of the pancreas were prepared for immunostaining as described above and then incubated at room temperature for 30 minutes with the anti-α-SMA primary antibody (mouse monoclonal antibody, clone 1A4; Sigma), diluted 1:100 in the blocking solution. After further washes, the secondary antibody (horseradish peroxidase conjugated goat anti-mouse IgG; Sigma) was applied in a dilution of 1:100 for 30 minutes at room temperature. After further washes, the color was developed using the DAKO 3,3-diaminobenzidine tetrahydrochloride (DAB) substrate-chromogen system (DAKO, Botany, Australia). Sections were counterstained with Mayer's hematoxylin (Sigma) for 5 minutes. Sections incubated with an isotype control monoclonal IgG served as negative controls.

Desmin. Immunohistochemistry for desmin was performed using frozen sections of the pancreas. The primary antibody used was a mouse monoclonal antibody (clone de-u-10; Sigma) and the same types of negative controls were used as described for α-SMA above. Color was developed using the DAKO 3,3-diaminobenzidine tetrahydrochloride (DAB) substrate-chromogen system (DAKO, Botany, Australia) and sections were subsequently counterstained with Mayer's hematoxylin (Sigma).

PDGFR-β. Frozen sections of the pancreas were used for PDGFR-b immunostaining. The primary anti-PDGFR-β was a rabbit polyclonal antibody (1:50; Santa Cruz Biotechnology Inc, Santa Cruz, California). which was prepared in 10% swine serum in 1% BSA and TBS and applied overnight at 4°C. The secondary antibody was alkaline phosphatase-conjugated swine anti-rabbit IgG diluted 1:100 in the appropriate blocking solution. After TBS washes, the color was developed using the Sigma Fast Red naphthol substrate system according to the manufacturer's instructions. Sections incubated with pre-immune host serum were used as negative controls.

Collagen type I. The collagen type I antibody was a rabbit polyclonal antibody (specific for rat collagen type I, no cross reactivity with collagen types III or IV; Amrad Pharmacia Biotech, Victoria, Australia) which was diluted 1:50 in 10% swine serum in TBS containing 1% BSA and incubated overnight at 4°C. The secondary antibody was alkaline phosphatase-conjugated swine anti-rabbit IgG and the chromogen was the Sigma Fast Red naphthol substrate system.

TGF-β. Paraffin sections of the pancreas were subjected to antigen retrieval by heating in a microwave oven on high power for 8 minutes in 0.01M citrate buffer (pH 6.0), then incubated with a mouse monoclonal anti-TGF-β primary antibody to active TGF-β (150 μg/mL; Genzyme Diagnostics, Cambridge, MA) for the cellular localization of TGF-β protein as previously described. The DAKO StreptAB Complex/horseradish peroxidase kit was used as the detection system with DAB as the chromogenic substrate.

In situ hybridization for detection of procollagen α_1 (I) mRNA

In situ hybridization for procollagen α_1 (I) mRNA was performed on both rat and human pancreas sections using previously described methods [13, 14]. Briefly, a 1500 bp fragment of human procollagen α_1 (I) cDNA was subcloned into pGEM 11Z vector and then subjected to alkaline hydrolysis to produce a 300bp fragment for use in *in situ* hybridization. Digoxigenin-labeled riboprobes, for sense (control) and antisense, were produced by *in vitro* transcription with SP6 and T7 polymerases. *In situ* hybridization was performed on 5 μm rat and human paraffin-embedded pancreas sections. After hybridization, sections were washed to remove unbound probe, and incubated with alkaline phosphatase conjugated anti-digoxigenin polyclonal sera (1:200) at room temperature for two hours. Unbound antibody was removed by washes prior to color visualization with nitroblue tetrazolium chloride/5-bromo-4-chloro-3-indolyl phosphate in the dark at room temperature for 16 hrs. Unbound complex was removed by washing and sections were subjected to immunohistochemistry for α-SMA to determine whether procollagen α_1(I) mRNA co-localized with α-SMA positive PSCs.

Results (*in vivo* studies)

Human pancreatic fibrosis

With respect to human chronic pancreatitis, the above studies [8] have demonstrated that:

- Collagen is the predominant extracellular matrix protein in areas of fibrosis, as indicated by the Sirius Red stain for collagen.
- Areas that stain positive for collagen (by Sirius Red) also exhibit positive immunostaining for α-SMA, suggesting the presence of activated pancreatic stellate cells in the fibrotic areas.
- α-SMA positive cells in fibrotic areas are the only cells that exhibit positive staining for messenger RNA for collagen (Fig. 3.3-3), indicating that activated PSCs may be the principal source of the collagen deposited in fibrotic pancreas.
- Pancreatic acinar cells adjacent to areas of fibrosis exhibit strongly positive staining for TGF-β (a known profibrogenic growth factor for stellate cells), while such staining is absent in acinar cells remote from bands of fibrosis. These observations suggest that TGF-β secreted by pancreatic acinar cells may have a paracrine effect on PSCs, leading to increased collagen synthesis by the cells. TGF-β staining is also apparent in spindle-shaped cells in the fibrotic bands.

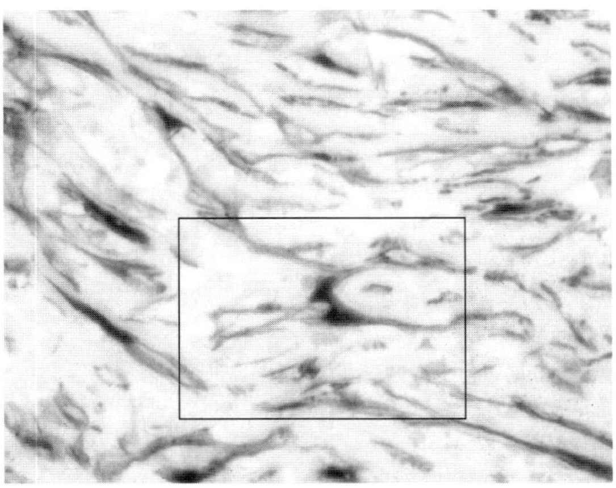

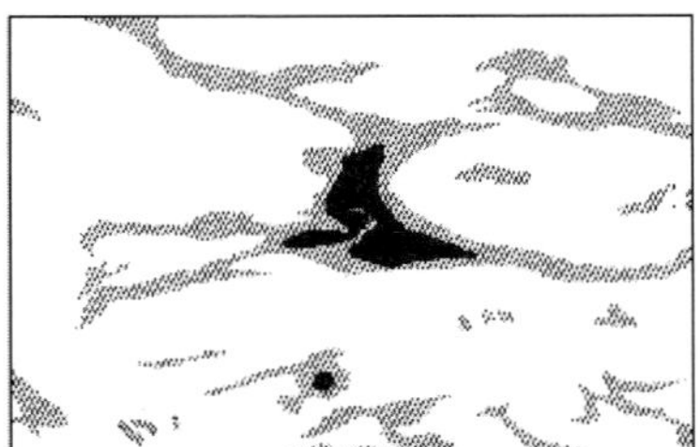

In-line diagram:
Black area – positive stain for procollagen mRNA
Hatched area – positive stain for α-SMA

Figure 3.3-3. Colocalization of α-SMA and procollagen α_1 (I) mRNA expression of fibrotic areas in human pancreas. On the left is a photomicrograph of an area of pancreatic fibrosis stained for α-SMA (by immunostaining) and procollagen mRNA (by *in situ* hybridization). On the right is a line diagram of the box outlined on the micrograph, representing positive staining for α-SMA as hatched areas and positive staining for procollagen α_1 (I) mRNA as black areas in the cell.

Rat pancreatic fibrosis

Using the TNBS model of experimental pancreatic fibrosis it has been demonstrated that [9]:

- Areas of fibrosis in the pancreas stain positive for both collagen protein (Sirius Red) and α-SMA (indicating the presence of activated PSCs).
- Dual staining for α-SMA (by immunochemistry) and for procollagen α_1I mRNA (by *in situ* hybridization) demonstrates colocalization of the two stains in the same cells (as observed with human chronic pancreatitis), suggesting that activated PSCs are the principal source of collagen in rat pancreatic fibrosis.
- Serial sections of the pancreas demonstrate that areas of fibrosis show increased staining for collagen (Sirius Red), desmin and PDGF receptor. Increased desmin staining is an indicator of stellate cell proliferation in fibrotic areas. Since PDGF is a potent proliferative growth factor for a variety of cells, it is possible that an increase in PDGF receptor expression on the surface of PSCs mediates the proliferative response of these cells to pancreatic injury.

Changes (pertaining to PSCs) described in the DBTC model include [9]:

- Increased desmin positivity in the first week during the acute necroinflammatory phase (in the absence of overt fibrosis), indicating PSC proliferation in response to pancreatic injury.
- Increased α-SMA expression during the first two weeks with levels remaining elevated for the duration of the experiment (8 weeks). This observation suggests that PSC activation occurs early in pancreatic injury and this activation can be sustained for prolonged periods.
- Raised levels of the profibrogenic growth factor TGF-β associated with increased collagen I expression, as assessed by western blotting analysis of pancreatic tissue homogenates. The upregulation of TGF-β and collagen levels occurred within 2 weeks of DBTC injection and remained so throughout the development of chronic pancreatitis and fibrosis in the model.

In vitro studies

Methodology

The mechanisms responsible for the observed in vivo activation of PSCs during pancreatic injury have not yet been fully elucidated, but, in recent years, *in vitro* studies have characterized the response of cultured PSCs to a number of putative activating factors. Candidate activating factors that have been examined include:

- Proinflammatory cytokines and growth factors known to be upregulated during pancreatic necroinflammation, such as tumor necrosis factor α (TNF-α), interleukin-6 (IL-6), interleukin-1 (IL-1), TGF-β and PDGF.
- Oxidant stress: The generation of reactive oxygen species and depletion of intracellular anti-oxidant defenses has been well described in both human and experimental pancreatitis 15–17]. The resultant oxidant stress within the pancreas may activate PSCs.
- Alcohol and its metabolite acetaldehyde: Alcohol (ethanol) abuse is a major association of pancreatitis. It is now known that ethanol can be metabolized by pancreatic

acinar cells to generate acetaldehyde [18]. Recent work by our group has also demonstrated that pancreatic stellate cells themselves exhibit alcohol dehydrogenase (ADH) activity (ADH is known to be the predominant alcohol metabolizing enzyme in the liver), suggesting that PSCs also have the capacity for metabolizing ethanol to acetaldehyde [19]. Activation of PSCs during chronic ethanol consumption may therefore occur in response to alcohol itself or to its metabolite acetaldehyde.

Incubation of PSCs with activating factors

To assess PSC response to the above factors, cultured PSCs (between 1st and 3rd passage) were incubated with varying concentrations of candidate factors (detailed below), at 37°C in a 5% CO_2-air humidified atmosphere. Triplicate wells of cells were used for each concentration of the factors under consideration.

Effect of proinflammatory cytokines

PDGF. PSCs were exposed to the PDGF isoform PDGF BB in increasing concentrations (1, 5 and 10 ng/ml culture medium) for 48 hours. Cells incubated in medium without PDGF BB served as controls. The rate of cell proliferation after exposure to PDGF BB was assessed using two parameters – cell counts per well and rate of DNA synthesis as measured by the incorporation of ^{3}H-thymidine into TCA precipitable material.

TGF-β1. Cells were incubated with TGF-β1 at concentrations of 0.25, 0.5 and 1 ng/ml culture medium for 48 hours. PSCs incubated without TGF-β1 were used as controls. Cell activation was assessed by determination of expression of α-SMA and by measurement of collagen synthesis.

TNF-α, IL-1 and IL-6. Triplicate wells of cells were incubated with culture medium containing increasing concentrations of TNF-α (2.5, 5, 10, 25 and 50 units/ml) or IL-1 or IL-6 (0.001, 0.01, 0.1, 1 and 10 ng/ml) for 24 hours. Cells incubated in culture medium without the relevant cytokine were used as controls. The concentrations of cytokines were selected on the basis of tissue levels reported in pancreatitis [20].

Effect of oxidant stress

To determine whether intracellular oxidant stress leads to activation of pancreatic stellate cells, cultured cells were exposed to a pro-oxidant compound (10 μM $FeSO_4$/100 μM ascorbic acid) or culture medium alone (controls) according to the method of Poli et al. [21]. The generation of oxidant stress was confirmed by measuring the production of malondialdehyde (a lipid peroxidation product) in the cells after incubation with the pro-oxidant complex for 3 hours and 24 hours at 37°C. The earlier (3 hour) time point was selected since it is known that generation of MDA is an early event in conditions of oxidant stress; indeed Poli et al. have demonstrated that MDA levels in hepatic stellate cells exposed to a pro-oxidant compound show an early peak, then fall steadily, approaching control levels at 6 hours of incubation [21].

Assessment of MDA levels. Pancreatic stellate cells incubated with and without the pro-oxidant complex were harvested by trypsinization and lysed in 5% trichloroacteic acid. MDA levels in cell lysates were detected as described previously, via the formation of adducts with thiobarbituric acid (TBA) which were then quantified using reverse phase HPLC and fluorescence detection. Typically, the reaction mixture consisted of 50 μl sample, 300 μl 0.2M phosphoric acid, and 50 μl 0.11M TBA in glass vials. The mixture was heated at 100°C for one hour, then allowed to cool to room temperature. It was neutralized by the addition of 200 μl 0.1N NaOH and proteins were precipitated by the addition of 2 ml methanol. Samples were centrifuged and MDA-TBA adducts in the supernatant assayed by reverse-phase HPLC according to the method of Young and Trimble [22]. Briefly, sample was injected with the use of a BAS-200 pump (Bioanalytical Systems) in an isocratic mobile phase composed of 20% acetonitrile, 50% 25 mM phosphate buffer, pH 6.5 and 30% methanol, at a flow rate of 1.2 ml/minute. A 250 × 4.6 mm ALLTIMA™ C18 5U column (Alltech) was used. Detection was performed using a Waters 470 scanning fluorescence detector (Millipore, Sydney, Australia) with an excitation wavelength of 532 nm and an emission wavelength of 553 nm. Results were expressed as nmols MDA produced per milligram cellular protein.

Influence of vitamin E on oxidant stress induced activation of stellate cells. In order to determine whether the presence of an antioxidant such as vitamin E in the culture medium could alter the effect of the pro-oxidant compound on collagen synthesis by stellate cells, cultured cells were incubated for 24 hours at 37°C as follows: i) culture medium alone (control); ii) 10 μM FeSO4/100 μM ascorbic acid; iii) 100 μM vitamin E and iv) 10 μM $FeSO_4$/100 μM ascorbic acid + 100 μM vitamin E. It is to be noted that there was a preincubation period of 45 minutes with vitamin E alone for cells in groups (iii) and (iv), before the addition of fresh medium containing vitamin E (group iii) or medium containing 10 μM $FeSO_4$/100 μM ascorbic acid + vitamin E (group iv). Collagen synthesis was measured in the above cell groups as detailed below.

Effect of ethanol and acetaldehyde

For incubations with ethanol and acetaldehyde, air-tight culture plates were used. Cultured stellate cells that had been harvested and replated at equal seeding densities (passages 2 or 3) were incubated (in triplicate wells) with ethanol (final concentration of 10 mM and 50 mM) or acetaldehyde (final concentration 150 μM and 200 μM) in Iscove Dulbecco's modified culture medium containing 10% fetal calf serum. The medium was changed at 24 hours to fresh medium with ethanol and acetaldehyde at the concentrations mentioned above and the cells were incubated for a further 24 hours. Cells incubated with culture medium alone served as controls. At the end of 48 hours, cells were harvested by trypsinization, counted using a hemocytometer, and lysed. Aliquots of cell lysates were set aside for protein and DNA determinations. Cell proliferation, α-SMA expression and collagen synthesis in response to exposure to ethanol or acetaldehyde were then assessed.

As indicated, the above experiments used passaged stellate cells. It has been established that pancreatic stellate cells are activated (express α-SMA) after approximately 48 hours of culture on uncoated plastic. In order to determine the response of pancreatic stellate cells in early culture (i.e. non-activated cells) to ethanol, additional experiments were performed whereby cells, within 18 hours of isolation and culture, were exposed to 50 mM ethanol or culture medium alone for a further 24 hours. At the end of the incubation period, cells were harvested, lysed and cell lysates assessed for α-SMA expression. In order to obtain visible signals for α-SMA in early culture cells, a minimum of 40 μg protein had to be loaded per lane and the blots exposed to x-ray film for one hour (in contrast to 15 μg protein loading per lane and an exposure time of only 15 seconds for passaged cells). It was expected that the results of these studies would indicate whether prior activation of cells was required for ethanol to exert its stimulatory effects.

Effect of inhibitors of ethanol and acetaldehyde metabolism. To determine whether any observed effects of ethanol or acetaldehyde on collagen synthesis could be attributable to the metabolism of these compounds by pancreatic stellate cells, the above experiments were repeated using 4-methyl pyrazole (4MP), an inhibitor of ethanol oxidation via inhibition of the major ethanol oxidizing enzyme alcohol dehydrogenase. Thus triplicate wells of cells were incubated as follows: i) Control – culture medium alone; ii) Ethanol 50 mM; iii) 4 methylpyrazole 2 mM; iv) Ethanol 50 mM + 4MP 2 mM. Collagen synthesis was assessed as a marker of cell activation.

Oxidant stress in pancreatic stellate cells exposed to ethanol or acetaldehyde. To determine whether exposure to ethanol or acetaldehyde produced oxidant stress within stellate cells, MDA levels were assessed at 3 hours of incubation with the two compounds, as described earlier. The influence of oxidant stress or any observed effects of ethanol or acetaldehyde on pancreatic stellate cell activation was further studied by assessing collagen synthesis in the presence or absence of the antioxidant vitamin E. For these experiments, cells were incubated as follows: i) culture medium alone; ii) ethanol 50 mM or acetaldehyde 200 μM; iii) vitamin E (a-tocopherol) 100 μM and iv) ethanol 50 mM + vitamin E 100 μM or acetaldehyde 200 μM + vitamin E 100 μM. There was a preincubation period of 45 minutes with vitamin E alone for cells in groups (iii) and (iv), before the addition of fresh medium containing vitamin E (group iii) or medium containing ethanol + vitamin E or acetaldehyde + vitamin E (group iv). At the end of the incubation period of 48 hours at 37°C, cells were harvested by trypsinization and counted. Samples were then processed for collagen synthesis assays.

Assessment of PSC activation

Following exposure to the factors described above, PSC activation was assessed using one or more of three activation indices – cell proliferation, α-SMA expression and collagen synthesis. The methodologies used for these assays are described below.

Cell proliferation

Cell counts. Cells were washed twice in HBSS, harvested by trypsinization using 0.5% trypsin-0.2% EDTA, resuspended in 200 μl culture medium and counted using a hemocytometer.

DNA synthesis (incorporation of ^{3}H-thymidine). For the last 16 hours of incubation with candidate factors, cells were pulsed with ^{3}H-thymidine at a concentration of 5 μCi per well. The reaction was stopped by aspirating the medium and cells were washed twice with HBSS. Ice-cold 10% TCA was then added to the wells and cells incubated for 10 minutes at 4°C. This was followed by a further two incubations with 5% TCA for 10 minutes each at 4°C. Five hundred μl of 1N NaOH was then added to the wells which were shaken on a rotary shaker at room temperature for 30 minutes. The reaction was stopped by adding 500 μl of 1N HCl. The mixture was then transferred to scintillation vials and radioactivity of the samples was measured using a liquid scintillation counter (Tricarb 4000 Series, Canberra Packard, Five Dock, NSW, Australia).

α-SMA expression

Levels of α-SMA in PSCs were estimated by western blotting of cell lysate proteins, using a monoclonal mouse antibody to α-SMA. Briefly, cells were harvested by trypsinization, and cell lysates were obtained by incubating the cells overnight in lysis buffer [50 mM Tris

HCl (pH 7.5), 150 mM NaCl, 1% Triton X-100, 0.5% deoxycholate, 1% SDS, 1 mM Na orthovanadate, 2 mM EDTA, 10 mM NaF, 10 μg/ml aprotinin, 10 μg/ml leupeptin, 1 mM phenylmethylsulfonyl fluoride]. Samples were then centrifuged at 2200g for 10 minutes and the supernatant was harvested for measurement of a-SMA levels.

Protein levels in cell lysates were measured by the method of Lowry et al. [23] using bovine serum albumin as the standard. Proteins (15 μg) from each sample were separated by gel electrophoresis using a 15% SDS-polyacrylamide gel. Known molecular weight protein standards were run alongside the samples. Separated proteins were transferred onto nitrocellulose membrane using a commercial semi-dry blotting apparatus (Biorad, Richmond, CA, USA). The nitrocellulose membrane was then incubated at room temperature with 5% skim milk powder in Tris buffered saline (pH 7.6) for one hour to prevent non-specific binding of antibody. This was followed by an overnight incubation at 4°C with the primary antibody (monoclonal mouse anti-a-SMA antibody 1:200) in fresh blocking solution. The filter was then washed and incubated with the secondary antibody (goat anti-mouse IgG 1:500; Amersham International, Buckinghamshire, UK) for 60 minutes at room temperature. α-SMA bands were detected by the enhanced chemiluminescence technique using the Amersham ECL kit and quantified by densitometry of scanned autoradiographs (Scanalytics One-D Scan, Boston, MA). Densitometry readings were expressed as integrated optical densities (arbitrary densitometer units calculated from the density as well as the size of each band) per μg protein loaded on the membranes.

Collagen synthesis

Collagen synthesis was assessed by measuring the incorporation of radiolabeled proline into collagenase-sensitive protein, using a modification of the method of Agelli and Wahl [24]. Briefly, cells were incubated for one hour in proline-free medium and then labeled for 16 hours with 2 μCi/ml ^{14}C-proline in Dulbecco's medium containing 1% fetal bovine serum, 50 μg/ml ascorbic acid (freshly made), and 75 μg/ml β-aminoproprionitrile. At the end of the incubation period, culture medium in the wells was aspirated and kept aside. Cells were harvested by trypsinization, washed and added to the reserved medium. The samples were sonicated for 90 seconds and proteins were precipitated with 10% TCA (final concentration). TCA-treated samples were centrifuged at 1000 g for 10 minutes and the pellet (comprising precipitated protein) was solubilized in 200 μl of 0.2N NaOH. After neutralization with 0.2N HCl, samples were divided into two equal aliquots. One aliquot was incubated with collagenase solution [containing 6.25 mM $CaCl_2$, 70 mM Tris (pH 7.4), 30 mM NEM (N-ethylmaleimide) and 360 units/ml collagenase Type III] while the other aliquot was incubated with the above solution in the absence of collagenase for 120 minutes at 37°C. Incorporation of ^{14}C-proline into collagen and non-collagen protein was determined following precipitation with TCA. Collagen-incorporated radioactivity was recovered in the TCA-soluble fraction while non-collagen radioactivity was found in the TCA precipitate. Collagen production was determined using formulae derived by Peterkofsky et al. [25] and was expressed as counts per minute (cpm) per μg DNA.

To determine whether any observed alteration of collagen synthesis by pancreatic stellate cells is regulated at the transcriptional level, mRNA levels for procollagen α_1(I) were assayed by Northern and dot blot analysis of total cellular RNA, using radiolabeled cDNA probes for rat procollagen (a kind gift from G Sparmann, University of Rostock, Germany) and for GAPDH (internal control). Collagen I is the major fibrillary collagen found in fibrous tissue. Although the assay used for collagen synthesis (described above) does not identify the subtypes of collagen synthesized, previous studies (albeit on hepatic stellate cells) have shown that activated cells produce more collagen I than any other types of collagen (particularly III and IV) [26]. It is possible therefore that any observed change in collagen synthesis in pancreatic stellate cells may be regulated, at least in part, by changes in mRNA for procollagen α_1(I).

Protein and DNA determinations

Protein content of cell lysates was measured by the method of Lowry et al. [23] using bovine serum albumin as the standard. Pancreatic DNA was assayed by a modified fluorimetric microassay as described by Kapuscinski and Skoczylas [27] using calf thymus DNA as the standard.

Statistical analysis

Results were expressed as means ± SEM. Data were analyzed using repeated measures analysis of variance (ANOVA) [28]. Fisher's protected least significant difference (PLSD) was used for comparison of individual groups provided the F-test was significant [28]. The analyses were run on a Macintosh personal computer using the Statview II statistical program.

Results (*in vitro* studies)

Effect of proinflammatory cytokines

PDGF BB significantly increased the rate of proliferation of pancreatic stellate cells (Fig. 3.3-4A). TGF-β1 increased -SMA expression and collagen synthesis in PSCs (Figs. 3.3-4B and 3.3-4C). The observed TGF-β-induced increase in collagen synthesis was likely mediated at the mRNA level as evidenced by the significant increase in mRNA levels for procollagen α_1(I) in PSCs exposed to TGF-β. TNF-α, IL-1 and IL-6 all increased α-SMA expression in the PSCs, but their effects on cell proliferation and collagen synthesis varied. The responses of PSCs to the cytokines examined are summarized in Table 3.3-1.

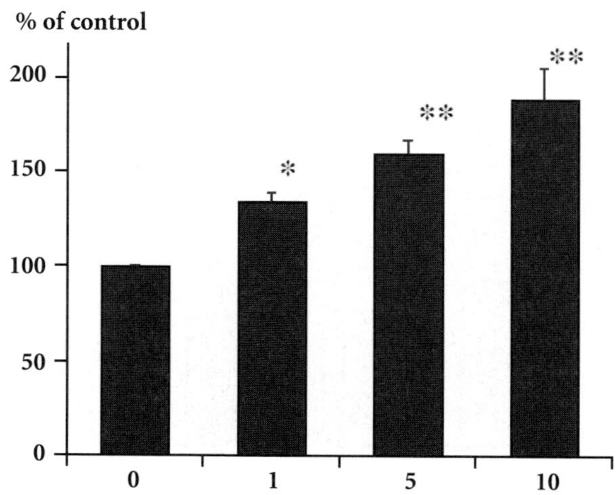

Figure 3.3-4A. Effect of PDGF on DNA synthesis (n = 5 separate cell preparations). DNA synthesis was estimated by measuring the incorporation of ^{3}H-thymidine into TCA precipitable material. Results are expressed as a percent of control values observed in cells not incubated with PDGF. A dose-dependent increase in ^{3}H-thymidine incorporation was observed with increasing concentrations of PDGF.

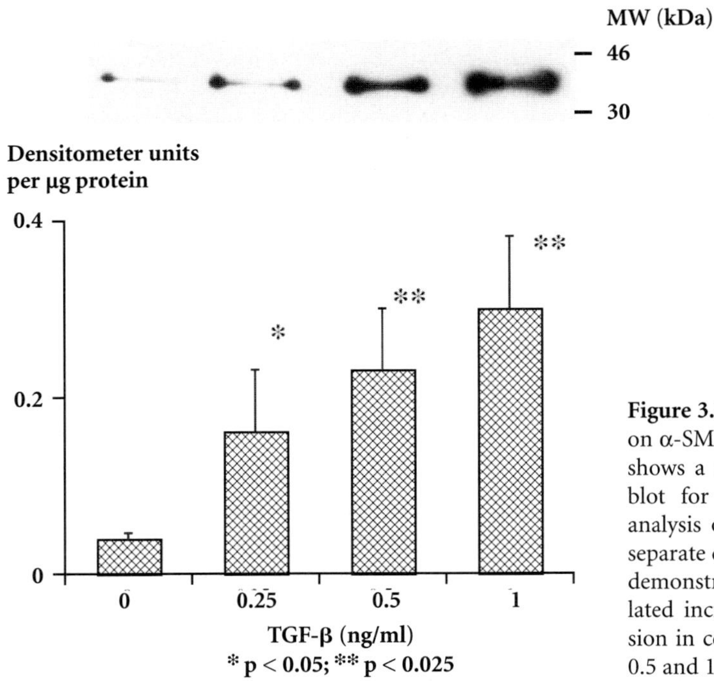

Figure 3.3-4B. Effect of TGF-β on α-SMA expression. The figure shows a representative immunoblot for a-SMA. Densitometric analysis of immunoblots from 5 separate cell preparations (graph) demonstrates a marked dose-related increase in α-SMA expression in cells incubated with 0.25, 0.5 and 1 ng/ml TGF-β1.

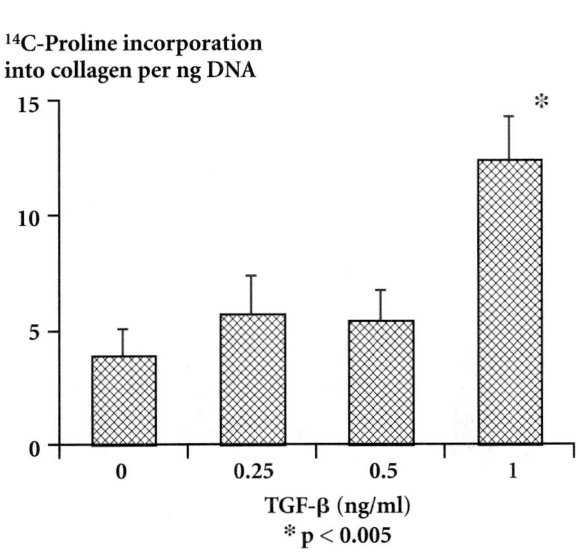

Figure 3.3-4C. Effect of TGF-β1 on collagen synthesis (n = 5 separate cell preparations). Results are expressed as cpm of ^{14}C-proline incorporated into collagen per ng DNA. At concentrations of 0.25 and 0.5 ng/ml TGF-β1 induced modest increases in collagen synthesis, while a marked statistically significant increase in collagen synthesis was observed at a concentration of 1 ng/ml TGF-β1.

Table 3.3-1. Effects of cytokines on pancreatic stellate cells.

CYTOKINE	PSC RESPONSE
• PDGF	↑ Cell proliferation
• TGF-β	↑ α-SMA expression ↑ collagen synthesis
• TNF-α	↑ α-SMA expression ↑ collagen synthesis
• IL-1, IL-6	↑ α-SMA expression

Effect of oxidant stress

Incubation of PSCs with the pro-oxidant compound produced oxidant stress within the cells as indicated by the increase in MDA (a lipid peroxidation product) levels as early as after 3 hours of incubation. PSCs incubated with the pro-oxidant complex for 24 hours demonstrated increased α-SMA expression as well as collagen protein synthesis (accompanied by increased mRNA levels for procollagen). The activation of PSCs by the pro-oxidant complex was completely prevented in the presence of the anti-oxidant vitamin E.

Effect of ethanol and acetaldehyde

Both ethanol and acetaldehyde activated PSCs as demonstrated by increased SMA expression (Fig. 3.3-5A) and increased collagen protein synthesis (Fig. 3.3-5B) associated with increased procollagen mRNA levels. The ethanol-induced increase in α-SMA expression was also observed in (non-activated) cells in early culture suggesting that prior activation of PSCs is not essential for ethanol to exert its stimulatory effects on these cells.

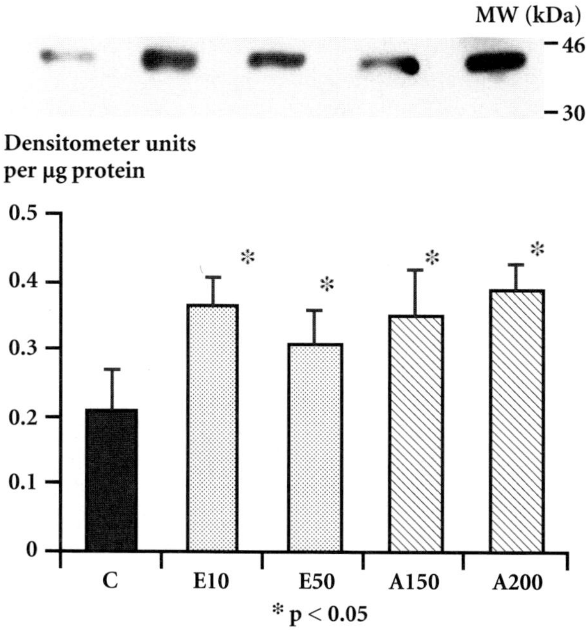

Figure 3.3-5A. Effect of ethanol and acetaldehyde on α-SMA expression in stellate cells. The figure shows a representative immunoblot for α-SMA expression in cells incubated with either culture medium alone (controls; C), or ethanol (10 mM and 50 mM; E10 and E50 respectively) or acetaldehyde (150 μM and 200 μM; A150 and A200 respectively). Densitometric analysis of immunoblots from 5 separate cell preparations (graph) demonstrates a significant increase in α-SMA expression in cells exposed to ethanol or acetaldehyde compared to controls.

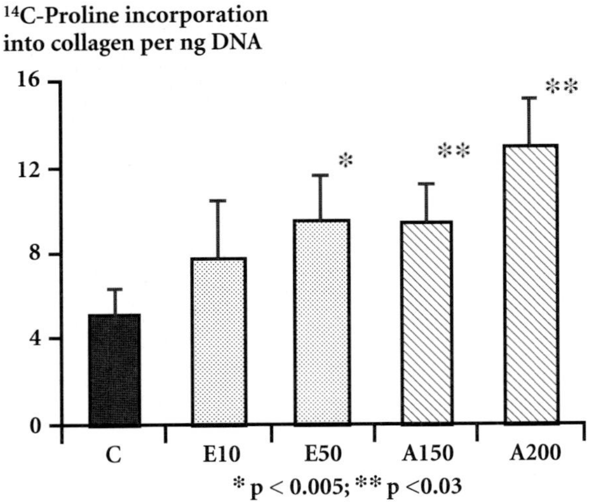

Figure 3.3-5B. Effect of ethanol and acetaldehyde on collagen synthesis (n = 5 separate cell preparations). Results are expressed as cpm of ^{14}C-proline incorporated into collagen per ng DNA. 10 mM ethanol (E10) induced a modest increase in collagen synthesis, while 50mM (E50) ethanol produced a marked, statistically significant increase in collagen synthesis. Acetaldehyde at both 150 μM (A150) and 200 μM (A200) significantly increased collagen synthesis in pancreatic stellate cells.

The ethanol-induced increase in collagen synthesis by PSCs was prevented in the presence of 4-methylpyrazole (an inhibitor of the major ethanol metabolizing enzyme alcohol dehydrogenase) suggesting that the effect of ethanol on PSCs was mediated by its metabolism within the cells to acetaldehyde. The activation of PSCs by acetaldehyde in turn appears to be mediated by oxidant stress, as demonstrated by the findings that: i) MDA levels were increased in PSCs incubated with ethanol or acetaldehyde, indicating the generation of oxidant stress within the cells; ii) in the presence of the antioxidant vitamin E, the ethanol- or acetaldehyde-induced increase in MDA levels in PSCs was prevented, as was the increase in collagen synthesis.

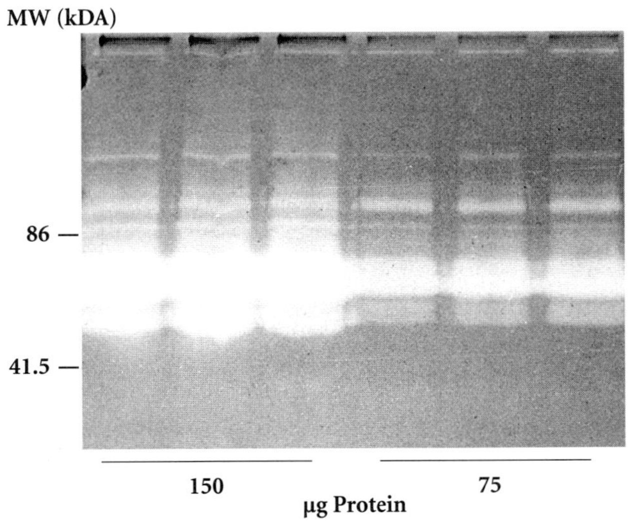

Figure 3.3-6A. Zymography analysis of serum-free conditioned media (150 μg and 75 μg protein) from 3 separate stellate cell preparations. Samples were separated on a SDS-polyacrylamide gel containing gelatin (a substrate for MMPs). Coomassie blue staining of gels after overnight incubation in activating buffer reveals the presence of MMPs as opaque bands on a dark background. This zymogram demonstrates the presence of numerous MMPs in secretions from pancreatic stellate cells.

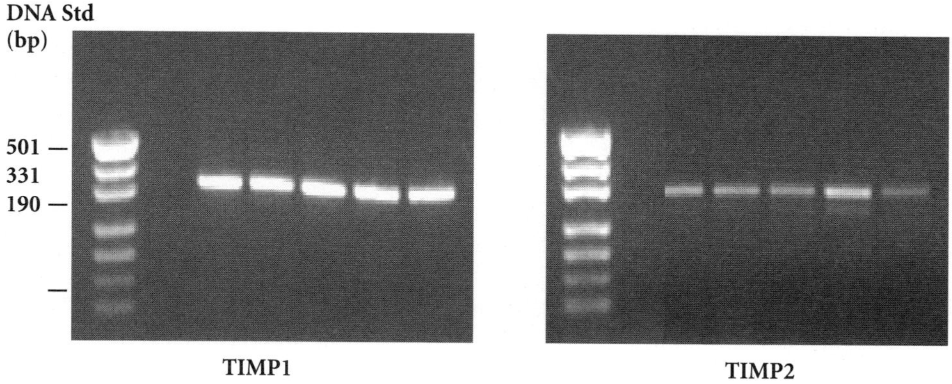

Figure 3.3-6B. Expression of TIMP1 and TIMP2 mRNA by PSCs using RT-PCR. Cellular RNA samples extracted from 4 separate cell preparations were reverse transcribed. The resultant cDNA products were amplified using specific primers for TIMP1 and TIMP2. Amplified products were separated by agarose gel electrophoresis to reveal distinct bands corresponding to the expected product sizes of TIMP1 and TIMP2.

Additional preliminary *in vitro* studies

Most recently we have performed preliminary experiments to determine whether PSCs have the capacity to i) synthesize and secrete MMPs (enzymes that degrade extracellular matrix) and TIMPs (inhibitors of MMPs); and ii) express the cytokines TGF-β and IL-1. Zymography was used to assess MMP secretion by PSCs while RT-PCR techniques were employed to examine expression of TIMP1 and TIMP2 (two of the four known subtypes of TIMPs), TGF-β and IL-1.

Zymography for MMPs

This technique was developed on the basis of the known gelatinolytic activity of MMPs [29]. To determine whether PSCs secrete MMPs, cells were first incubated overnight in serum-free culture medium. The medium was then removed and proteins in the medium concentrated by lyophilization. The concentrated samples were subjected to electrophoresis in a 7% SDS-polyacrylamide gel containing 1 mg/ml gelatin. Following electrophoresis, SDS was extracted from the gel by extensive washing with Triton X-100. The gel was then incubated at 37°C overnight in 50 mM Tris HCl (pH 7.4) containing 5 mM CaCl2 and 5 µM ZnCl2 (activating buffer) and subsequently stained with Coomassie brilliant blue G250. Using this technique, MMPs can be detected as opaque white bands against a blue background.

RT-PCR for TIMP1, TIMP2, TGF-β and IL-1

Total RNA was extracted from cultured stellate cells by a modification of the method described by Chomczynski and Sacchi [30] using the Tri-reagent kit (Sigma Chemical Co, USA). The A_{260}/A_{280} of the RNA samples was routinely in the range of 1.6–1.7. Agarose gel electrophoresis of extracted RNA confirmed that the RNA samples were not degraded. Two µg of extracted RNA was then reverse transcribed using the Gibco Superscript RNase H- enzyme kit. The resulting cDNA was then used for amplification with specific primers (constructed from published sequences) for TGF-b, IL-1, TIMP1 and TIMP2, as detailed below:

TGF-β: 5'-TGAGTGGCTGTCTTTTGACG-3' and 5'-TGGGACTGATCCCATTGATT-3'
35 cycles – 1 minute at 94°C, 1 minute at 55°C, and 2.5 minutes at 72°C
Extension – 8 minutes at 72°C.

IL-1: 5'-CAGGATGAGGACATGGAGACC-3'
and 5'-CTCTGCAGACTCAAACTCCAC-3'
35 cycles – 1 minute at 94°C, 1 minute at 55°C, and 2.5 minutes at 72°C
Extension – 8 minutes at 72°C.

TIMP1: 5'-ACAGCTTTCTGCAACTCG-3' and 5'-CTATAGGTCTTTACGAAGGCC-3'
35 cycles – 1 minute at 94°C, 1 minute at 55°C, and 2.5 minutes at 72°C
Extension – 8 minutes at 72°C.

TIMP2: 5'-ATTTATCTACACGGCCCC-3' and 5'-CAAGAACCATCACTTCTCTTG-3'
40 cycles – 0.5 minutes at 94°C, 1 minute at 60°C, 2 minutes at 68°C
Extension – 7 minutes at 68°C

GAPDH (control): 5'-AATCCCATCACCATCTTCCA-3'
and 5'-GGCAGTGGCATGGACTG-3'
35 cycles – 1 minute at 94°C, 1 minute at 55°C, and 2.5 minutes at 72°C
Extension – 8 minutes at 72°C.

PCR performed without cDNA or without added specific primers served as the negative control for each PCR reaction. PCR products were analyzed by agarose gel electrophoresis. Predicted product sizes for TGF-β, IL-1, TIMP1, TIMP2 and GAPDH were 146bp, 447bp, 400bp, 335bp, 342bp and 370bp respectively.

Results (preliminary *in vitro* studies)

Zymography (Fig. 3.3-6A) demonstrated that PSCs have the ability to secrete a number of matrix metalloproteinases as indicated by the multiple distinct opaque bands observed on the zymogram after Coomassie staining. The expression of TIMP1 and TIMP2 in PSCs was evident on RT-PCR (Fig. 3.3-6B). RT-PCR also demonstrated that PSCs have the capacity to synthesize both TGF-β and IL-1 (Figs 3.3-7A and 3.3-7B).

Discussion

The identification and characterization of pancreatic stellate cells in recent years has significantly stimulated research efforts into elucidating the mechanisms responsible for the development of fibrosis in the pancreas. Pancreatic fibrosis is a characteristic feature of chronic pancreatic injury from various causes, including alcohol abuse, recurrent and/or persistent inflammation, malnutrition and trauma. In general, fibrosis represents a pathological change in the composition and amount of extracellular matrix in tissues. It would be reasonable to hypothesize therefore that cells that have the capacity to regulate ECM turnover in tissues play an important role in the fibrogenic process.

There is increasing evidence to suggest that in the pancreas, ECM turnover may be regulated by pancreatic stellate cells. It is now well established that these cells have the capacity to synthesize ECM proteins. Furthermore, our recent preliminary studies have demonstrated that PSCs also synthesize the enzymes that degrade ECM proteins, namely matrix metalloproteinases (MMPs). Thus, in health, PSCs may be responsible for main-

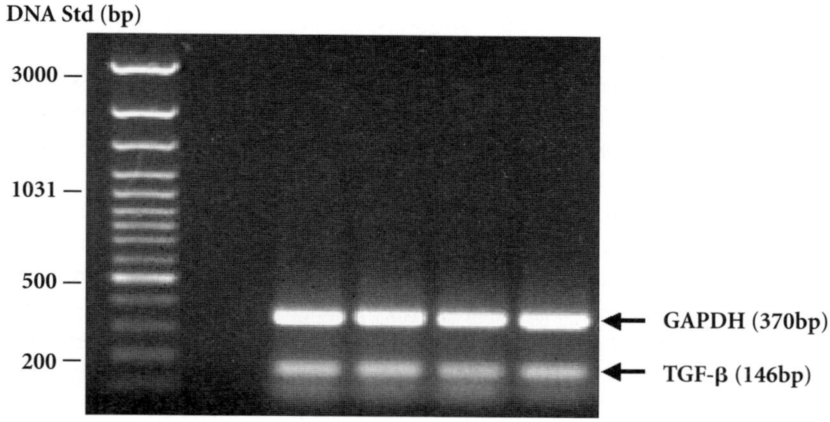

Figure 3.3-7A. Expression of TGF-β mRNA by PSCs using RT-PCR. Cellular RNA samples extracted from 4 separate cell preparations were reverse transcribed. The resultant cDNA products were amplified using specific primers for TGF-β (as detailed in text) and GAPDH. Amplified products were separated by agarose gel electrophoresis to reveal distinct bands corresponding to the expected product sizes of GAPDH and TGF-β.

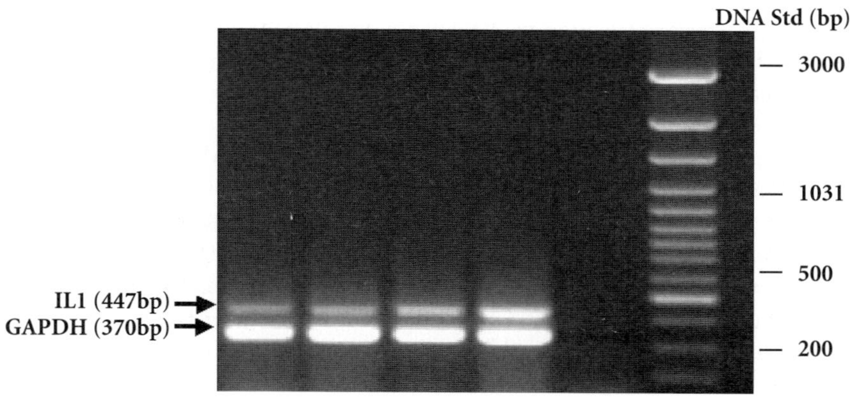

Figure 3.3-7B. Expression of IL-1 mRNA by PSCs using RT-PCR. Cellular RNA samples extracted from 4 separate cell preparations were reverse transcribed. The resultant cDNA products were amplified using specific primers for IL-1 and GAPDH. Amplified products were separated by agarose gel electrophoresis to reveal distinct bands corresponding to the expected product sizes of GAPDH and IL-1.

taining normal tissue architecture. On the other hand, during pancreatic injury, PSCs may undergo morphological and functional alterations (a process known as activation) leading to excessive deposition of ECM proteins and the consequent development of fibrosis in the gland. This notion is supported by the results of the *in vivo* studies described in this chapter. Pancreatic sections from patients with chronic pancreatitis as well as from rats with experimental pancreatic fibrosis demonstrate the presence of α-SMA positive cells (indicating activated PSCs) in close association with fibrotic areas. Serial sections of fibrotic pancreas demonstrate that areas of fibrosis show increased staining for the stellate cell selective marker desmin (suggesting PSC proliferation) as well as increased staining for PDGF receptor β (suggesting that the observed increase in PSC proliferation may be mediated by enhanced responsiveness of the cells to PDGF). *In situ* hybridization in combination with immunostaining studies provide evidence that the α-SMA positive cells in fibrotic areas also exhibit positive staining for procollagen mRNA, suggesting that activated PSCs may be the primary source of collagen in the fibrotic gland.

In order to identify the factors that may activate PSCs during pancreatic injury, *in vitro* studies have been performed using cultured pancreatic stellate cells. Cell proliferation, α-SMA expression and collagen synthesis have been examined in cultured PSCs after exposure to a variety of putative activating agents, including alcohol and its metabolite acetaldehyde, oxidant stress, growth factors and cytokines. As noted earlier in this chapter, ethanol and its metabolite acetaldehyde were found to cause activation of PSCs *in vitro.* The prevention of ethanol-induced cell activation in the presence of 4-methyl pyrazole (a compound that inhibits the activity of the ethanol metabolizing enzyme alcohol dehydrogenase) suggests that the effect of ethanol on PSC activation may be mediated by its metabolism to acetaldehyde within the cells. The effect of acetaldehyde, in turn, on PSC activation may be mediated by oxidant stress, given the observations that exposure to ethanol or acetaldehyde generates oxidant stress within the cells and that the antioxidant vitamin E inhibits activation of PSCs by ethanol or acetaldehyde. The finding that ethanol activates PSCs even at very early stages of culture (non-activated cells) is important because it indicates that prior activation of PSCs is not essential for ethanol to exert its effect on the cells.

Additional factors that may activate PSCs include growth factors and proinflammatory cytokines known to be upregulated during pancreatitis. As noted earlier in this chapter, cultured PSCs have been found to be activated by PDGF and TGF-β and by TNF-α, IL-1 and IL-6. Our preliminary experiments demonstrating that PSCs themselves have the capacity to secrete IL-1 and TGF-β suggest that autocrine loops may also be involved in cytokine-mediated PSC activation. It is possible that persistent/repeated exposure to cytokines leads to a sustained activation of PSCs, causing a "permanent" phenotypic change in the cells and preventing reversion to the quiescent state, thereby leading to excessive synthesis and deposition of extracellular matrix proteins and the development of pancreatic fibrosis. This idea is supported by a recent *in vivo* study which showed that the persistence of elevated TGF-β levels in the pancreas (caused by injection of cyclosporin A) caused caerulein-induced acute pancreatitis to be converted into a chronic condition with pancreatic scarring [31].

Based on the *in vivo* and *in vitro* studies discussed in this chapter, there is strong evidence in support of a central role for pancreatic stellate cells in pancreatic fibrogenesis. A major cause of pancreatic fibrosis and chronic pancreatitis is alcohol abuse. On the basis of observations that PSCs are activated directly by alcohol as well as by proinflammatory cytokines, it may be postulated that there are two fibrogenic pathways (acting in parallel) in alcoholic pancreatitis: the necroinflammatory pathway and the non-necroinflammatory pathway (Fig. 3.3-8). Activation of pancreatic stellate cells by cytokines released during alcohol-induced acinar cell necrosis would represent the necroinflammatory pathway of pancreatic fibrogenesis, while the direct activation of stellate cells by alcohol via acetaldehyde and/or oxidant stress would represent the non-necroinflammatory pathway. The identification of non-necroinflammatory mediators of stellate cell activation raises an interesting point. It suggests that tissue necrosis or inflammation may not be an absolute

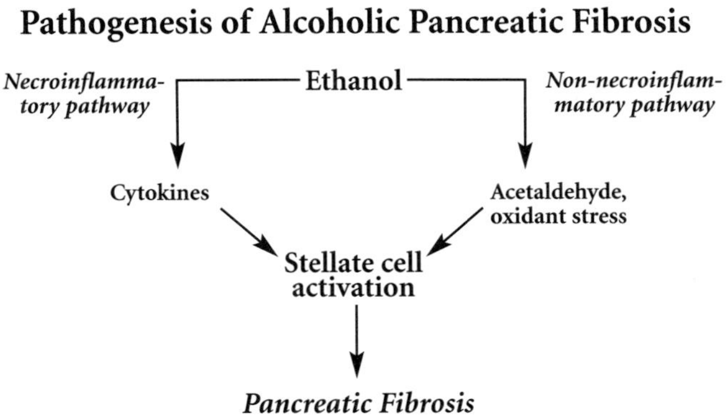

Figure 3.3-8. Postulated fibrogenic pathways in alcoholic pancreatitis – i) the necroinflammatory pathway involving activation of PSCs by cytokines released during pancreatic necroinflammation; ii) the non-necroinflammatory pathway involving activation of PSCs by ethanol itself (via factors generated during its metabolism).

prerequisite for the stimulation of fibrogenesis in the pancreas during alcohol abuse. In this regard, it is of interest to note that a postmortem study by Pitchumoni et al. [32] has demonstrated the presence of pancreatic fibrosis in alcoholics in the absence of any clinical history of pancreatitis during life. The concept of a "non-necroinflammatory" pathway of fibrosis is also supported by a recent study on alcoholic liver disease, where hepatic stellate cell activation was observed in the absence of hepatitis in liver biopsies from alcoholic patients [33]. It is possible therefore, that pancreatic stellate cell activation occurs early in chronic ethanol consumption; perpetuation of this activation with subsequent development of pathological fibrosis may depend on the dose and duration of ethanol exposure and/or the presence of other "activating" stimuli in the gland.

In conclusion, studies to date into the biology of PSCs have provided important insights into the process of fibrogenesis in the pancreas. However, there is much that remains unknown. Future directions of research in this area would be expected to build on current observations to include i) detailed characterization of the preliminary observations demonstrating that PSCs secrete ECM degrading enzymes and their inhibitors; ii) studies into the significance of the endogenous expression of cytokines in PSCs; iii) examination of the interaction of PSCs with neighboring acinar cells; iv) characterization of cell signaling pathways mediating PSC activation. The ultimate goal of such research would of course be to develop therapeutic strategies to modulate PSC function so as to prevent or retard the progression of pancreatic fibrosis.

Acknowledgement

Supported by grants from the National Health and Medical Research Council of Australia, Australian Brewers' Foundation and the Gastroenterological Society of Australia.

References

1. DiMagno EP, Layer P, Clain JE. Chronic Pancreatitis. In: Go VLW, DiMagno EP, Gardner JD, Lebenthal E, Reber HA, Scheele GA, eds. The Pancreas: Biology, Pathobiology and Disease. New York: Raven Press, 1993: 665–706.
2. Apte MV, Haber PS, Applegate TL, Norton ID, McCaughan GW, Korsten MA, Pirola RC, Wilson JS. Periacinar stellate-shaped cells in rat pancreas: identification, isolation and culture. Gut 1998; 42: 128–33.

3. Bachem MG, Schneider E, Gross H, Weidenbach H, Schmid RM, Menke A, Siech M, Beger H et al. Identification, culture, and characterization of pancreatic stellate cells in rats and humans. Gastroenterology 1998; 115: 421–32.
4. Friedman SD. The cellular basis of hepatic fibrosis. New Engl J Med 1993; 328: 1828–35.
5. Watari N, Hotta Y, Mabuchi Y. Morphological studies on a vitamin A-storing cell and its complex with macrophage observed in mouse pancreatic tissues following excess vitamin A administration. Okajimas Folia Anat Jpn 1982; 58: 837–58.
6. Apte MV, Haber PS, Darby SJ, Rodgers SC, McCaughan GW, Korsten MA, Pirola RC, Wilson JS. Pancreatic stellate cells are activated by proinflammatory cytokines: implications for pancreatic fibrogenesis. Gut 1999; 44: 534–41.
7. Phillips P, Pirola R, McCaughan G, Korsten M, Wilson J, Apte M. Pancreatic stellate cells secrete matrix metalloproteinases – implications for extracellular matrix turnover. (Abstr). Pancreas 2000. (in press.)
8. Haber P, Keogh G, Apte M, Moran C, Pirola R, McCaughan G, Korsten M, Wilson J. Activation of pancreatic stellate cells in human and experimental pancreatic fibrosis. Am J Pathol 1999; 155: 1087–95.
9. Emmrich J, Weber I, Sparmann GH, Liebe S. Activation of pancreatic stellate cells in experimental chronic pancreatitis in rats. Gastroenterology 2000; 118: A166.
10. Puig-Divi V, Molero X, Salas A, Guarner F, Guarner L, Malagelada JR. Induction of chronic pancreatic disease by trinitrobenzene sulfonic acid infusion into rat pancreatic ducts. Pancreas 1996; 13: 417–24.
11. Sparmann G, Merkord J, Jaschke A, Nizze H, Jonas L, Lohr M, Liebe S, Emmrich J. Pancreatic fibrosis in experimental pancreatitis induced by dibutyltin dichloride. Gastroenterology 1997; 112: 1664–72.
12. Ma X, Zhao J, Lieber CS. Polyvenylphosphatidylcholine attenuates non-alcoholic hepatic fibrosis and accelerates its regression. Journal of Hepatology 1996; 24: 604–13.
13. Ramm GA, Nair VG, Bridle KR, Shepherd RW, Crawford DH. Contribution of hepatic parenchymal and nonparenchymal cells to hepatic fibrogenesis in biliary atresia. Am J Pathol 1998; 153: 527–35.
14. Rex M, Scotting PJ. Simultaneous detection of RNA and protein in tissue sections by nonradioactive in situ hybridisation followed by immunohistochemistry. Biochemica 1994; 3: 24–6.
15. Nonaka A, Manabe T, Asano N, Kyogoku T, Imanishi K, Tamura K, Tobe T, Sugiura Y et al. Direct ESR measurement of free radicals in mouse pancreatic lesions. International Journal of Pancreatology 1989; 5: 203–11.
16. Gough DB, Boyle B, Joyce WP, Delaney CP, McGeeney KF, Gorey TF, Fitzpatrick JM. Free radical inhibition and serial chemiluminescence in evolving experimental pancreatitis. Br J Surg 1990; 77: 1256–9.
17. Guyan PM, Uden S, Braganza JM. Heightened free radical activity in pancreatitis. Free Radical Biology & Medicine 1990; 8: 347–54.
18. Haber PS, Apte MV, TL A, Norton ID, Korsten MA, Pirola RC, Wilson JS. Metabolism of ethanol by rat pancreatic acinar cells. J Lab Clin Med 1998; 132: 294–302.
19. Apte MV, Phillips PA, Fahmy RG, Darby SJ, Rodgers RC, McCaughan GW, Korsten MA, Pirola RC, Naidoo D, Wilson JS. Does alcohol directly stimulate pancreatic fibrogenesis? Studies with rat pancreatic stellate cells? Gastroenterology 2000; 118: 780–94.
20. Norman J. The role of cytokines in the pathogenesis of acute pancreatitis. Am J Surg 1998; 175: 76–83.
21. Poli G, Parola M, Leonarduzzi G, Pinzani M. Modulation of hepatic fibrogenesis by antioxidants. Molecular Aspects of Medicine 1993; 14: 259–64.
22. Young IS, Trimble ER. Measurement of malondialdehyde in plasma by high performance liquid chromatography with fluorimetric detection. Ann Clin Biochem 1991; 28: 504–8.
23. Lowry OH, Rosebrough NJ, Farr AL, Randall RJ. Protein measurement with the folin phenol reagent. J Biol Chem 1951; 193: 265–75.

24. Agelli M, Wahl SM. Collagen production by fibroblasts. Methods in Enzymology 1988; 163: 643–56.
25. Peterkofsky B, Chojkier M, Bateman J, eds. Determination of collagen synthesis in tissue and cell culture systems. Boca Raton, Florida: CRC, 1981. (Furthmayer H, ed. Immunochemistry of the Extracellular Matrix; vol II).
26. Geerts A, Vrijsen R, Rauterberg J, Burt A, Schellinck P, Wisse E. In vitro differentiation of fat-storing cells parallels marked increase of collagen synthesis and secretion. Journal of Hepatology 1989; 9: 59–68.
27. Kapuscinski J, Skoczylas B. Simple and rapid fluorimetric method for DNA microassay. Analytical Biochemistry 1977; 83: 252–7.
28. Snedecor GW, Cochran WG. Statistical Methods. (8 ed.) Ames, Iowa: Iowa State University Press, 1989.
29. Musso O, Theret N, Campion JP, Turlin B, Milani S, Grappone C, Clement B. In situ detection of matrix metalloproteinase-2 (MMP2) and the metalloproteinase inhibitor TIMP2 transcripts in human primary hepatocellular carcinoma and in liver metastasis. Journal of Hepatology 1997; 26: 593–605.
30. Chomczynski P, Sacchi N. Single-step method of RNA isolation by acid guanidinium thiocyanate-phenol-chloroform extraction. Analytical Biochemistry 1987; 162: 156–9.
31. Vaquero E, Molero X, Tian X, Salas A, Malagaleda JR. Myofibroblast proliferation, fibrosis, and defective repair induced by cyclosporin in rats. Gut 1999; 45: 269–77.
32. Pitchumoni CS, Glasser M, Saran RM, Panchacharam P, Thelmo W. Pancreatic fibrosis in chronic alcoholics and nonalcoholics without clinical pancreatitis. Am J Gastroenterol 1984; 79: 382–8.
33. Reeves HL, Burt AD, Wood S, Day CP. Hepatic stellate cell activation occurs in the absence of hepatitis in alcoholic liver disease and correlates with the severity of steatosis. Journal of Hepatology 1996; 25: 677–83.

3.4 Pancreatic stellate cells and their role in human pancreatic fibrogenesis

M. G. Bachem, A. Schmid-Kotsas, H.-J. Gross, E. Schneider, A. Menke, H. Weidenbach, G. Adler, M. Siech, H. Beger, A. Grünert

Introduction

Chronic pancreatitis is defined by the presence of chronic inflammation, destruction of acinar and ductal cells, intra- and perilobular fibrosis and finally by the irreversible scarring of parenchyma [1]. Until recently the molecular mechanisms and cell-cell interactions resulting in pancreas fibrosis were largely unknown. However, the progressive appearance of fibrotic tissue is regardless of the initiating triggers a result of an increased deposition and a reduced degradation of extracellular matrix [2, 3]. In contrast to fibrogenesis in the pancreas, liver fibrogenesis has been studied extensively during the past 2 decades. It is now generally accepted that hepatic stellate cells (HSC), formerly named perisinusoidal fat-storing cells and Ito-cells, which are located in the space of Disse, play a central role in liver fibrogenesis. In experimental and human liver injury HSC change their phenotype from a quiescent retinoid storing cell to a highly active and "synthetic" myofibroblast-like cell producing the majority of extracellular matrix [4, 5, 6] including collagen types I and III, fibronectin, and proteoglycans. Years ago the presence of retinoid containing fat-storing cells was demonstrated in the pancreas of mice [7], rats and humans [8]. While a potential role of these cells in pancreas remodeling and fibrosis was already discussed by Ikejiri et al. [8], it took another 8 years to isolate and characterize these cells [9, 10]. We detected retinoid-containing fat-storing cells in low numbers on cross sections of pancreatic tissue from humans, rats, and mice [10]. Because these cells show similarities in their retinoid metabolism and morphology to hepatic stellate cells, e.g. numerous retinoid containing perinuclear fat droplets, cytoplasmic extensions, stellate shape morphology, expression of the cytoskeletal filaments vimentin, desmin, and α-smooth muscle actin, we named them pancreatic stellate cells (PSC). On untreated plastics cultured PSC are activated, their retinoid content deceases and the cells acquire a highly proliferative and "synthetic" phenotype [10]. Furthermore, within 4–8 days after seeding the number and size of the fat droplets decrease, the diameter of the cells increases, the cells develop a prominent endoplasmic reticulum, and the cells express α-smooth muscle actin in increasing amounts [10]. The same changes have been found using cultured hepatic stellate cells.

Results and discussion

Characterization of pancreatic stellate cells

In earlier studies the cells producing extracellular matrix in the pancreas were described as "fibroblast-like" cells showing characteristics of myofibroblast, e.g. expression of α-smooth muscle actin, synthesis of collagens and fibronectin, and the formation of dense bodies (microfilaments) [11–13]. It has been discussed that retinoid-containing fat-storing cells in the pancreas might originate from 2 cell lineages; the first being the fibroblast, and the second being the pericyte of the blood capillaries [7]. Fat-storing cells, which were thought to originate from fibroblasts, were distributed in the interlobular and intralobular connective tissue. Cells which originated from pericytes adhered to endothelial cells and were surrounded by a thin basal lamina [7]. In rats the number of desmin and smooth-muscle-alpha-actin positive PSC increases with the age of the animals [10]. Also in alcoholic chronic pancreatitis in man high numbers of PSC have been described [14, 15].

During primary culture of PSC the number and size of retinoid-containing fat droplets decrease in parallel to the increase in a-sm-actin-expression and extracellular matrix synthesis [10]. Measurement of retinoids by HPLC demonstrated that with the change in the cells phenotype the cellular content of retinol and retinyl-palmitate decreased significantly [10]. The characteristics of the "fat-storing" and the "myofibroblast-like" phenotype of PSC are summarized in Figure 3.4-1. The "myofibroblast-like" phenotype of PSC synthesize and secrete high amounts of collagen types I and III and fibronectin. By quantitative measurement of the procollagen peptides it was shown that the

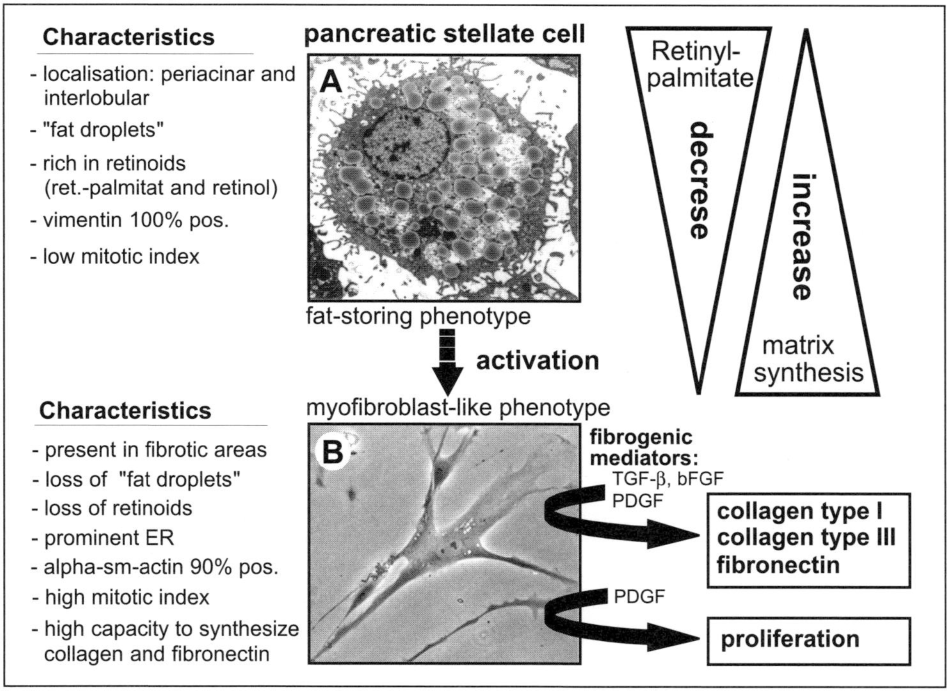

Figure 3.4-1A, B. Characterization of the *fat-storing* and *myofibroblast-like* phenotype of pancreatic stellate cells. During pancreatitis and also in primary culture the number and size of retinoid-containing fat droplets decrease parallel to the increase in a-sm-actin-expression and extracellular matrix synthesis. The *myofibroblast-like* phenotype of PSC synthesize and secrete high amounts of collagen types I and III and fibronectin. TGF-β1, bFGF and PDGF, respectively, act as fibrogenic mediators stimulating extracellular matrix synthesis and PDGF represents the most important mitogen-stimulating PSC proliferation. Insert **A:** transmission electron micrograph of PSC with the *fat-storing phenotype.* Insert **B:** secondary cultured PSC 48 hours after passage *(myofibroblast-like phenotype).*

"myofibroblast-like" phenotype of human PSC synthesize 25–40fold more collagen type I than collagen type III. Regarding the steady state levels of mRNA the difference between the expression of the collagen types I and III was highly significant.

Identification of fibrogenic mediators

As shown on protein and mRNA level human serum stimulates proliferation (Fig. 3.4-2) and the synthesis of collagen types I and III and fibronectin in cultured human PSC (Fig. 3.4-3). According to (i) published data in other cell types [1 20], (ii) the histopathological appearance of certain growth factors in chronic pancreatitis [21–23], and (iii) data obtained in transgenic mice overexpressing transforming growth factor β (TGF-β1) and transforming growth factor alpha (TGF-α) in the pancreas [24, 25], we studied the effects of the polypeptide growth factors basic fibroblast growth factor (bFGF), TGF-α, TGF-β1, platelet-derived growth factor (PDGF), insulin-like growth factor 1 (IGF1), insulin-like growth factor 2 (IGF2), and tumor necrosis factor alpha (TNF-α), respectively, on proliferation and matrix synthesis of cultured PSC. As shown in Figure 3.4-4 in the absence of serum TGF-β1, TGF-α, bFGF and PDGF, respectively, stimulate c-fibronectin synthesis of cultured human PSC, whereas in the presence of serum only TGF-β1 displayed significant stimulation. Identical growth factors stimulated cell associated matrix synthesis in cultured rat PSC (Fig. 3.4-5A–J). TNF-α, IFG1, and IGF2, respectively, were without significant effect on extracellular matrix synthesis of cultured PSC (data not shown). However, in all experiments PDGF represented the most effective mitogen both in human and rat PSC (data not shown).

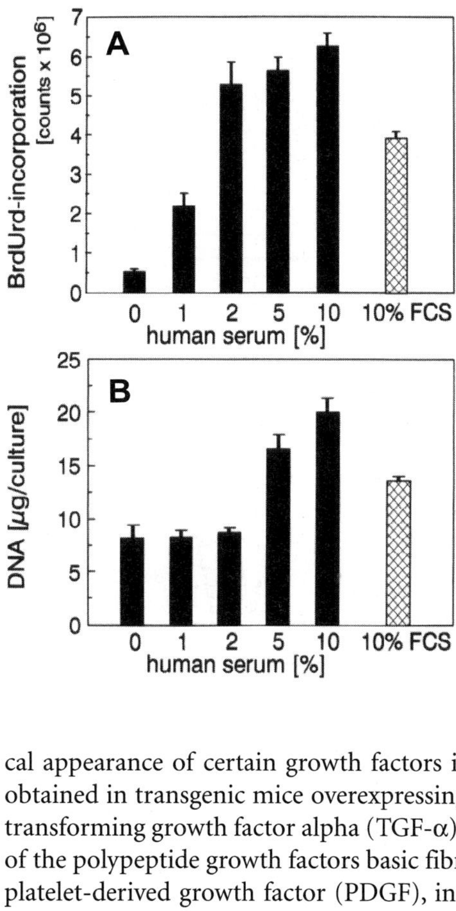

Figure 3.4-2A, B. Effect of increasing serum concentrations on proliferation of human pancreatic stellate cells in culture. **A:** Proliferation-measured bromodeoxyuridine incorporation. Bromodeoxyuridine was quantified by time-resolved fluorescence of a Europium chelate. **B:** DNA was quantified by fluorometry using Bisbenzimide and calf thymus DNA as a standard. FCS, fetal calf serum.

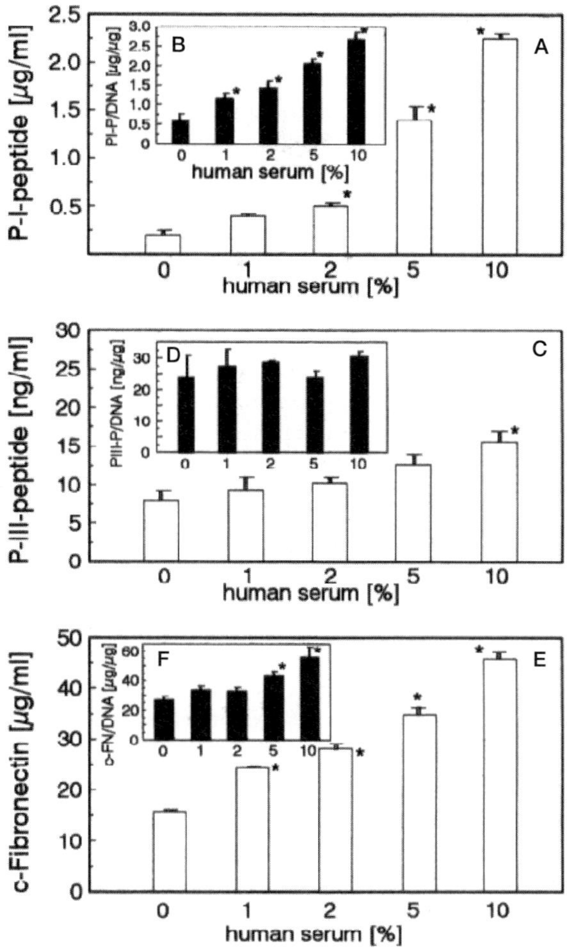

Figure 3.4-3A–F. Effect of serum on the synthesis of collagen type I (**A, B**), collagen type III (**C, D**) and fibronectin (**E, F**) of cultured human pancreatic stellate cells. Serum was added in concentrations of 1, 2, 5, and 10% to secondary cultured human pancreatic stellate cells. After 36 hours cultures were stopped. Procollagen I peptide, procollagen III peptide and fibronectin were measured in the cell supernatants; DNA was measured in the cell layer. Figures **A, C** and **E** express the procollagen peptides and fibronectin concentration; Inserts **B, D,** and **F** express the procollagen peptides and fibronectin concentration on the basis of DNA. Mean +/– SD of 3 cultures each with 3 wells. *, $p < 0.05$.

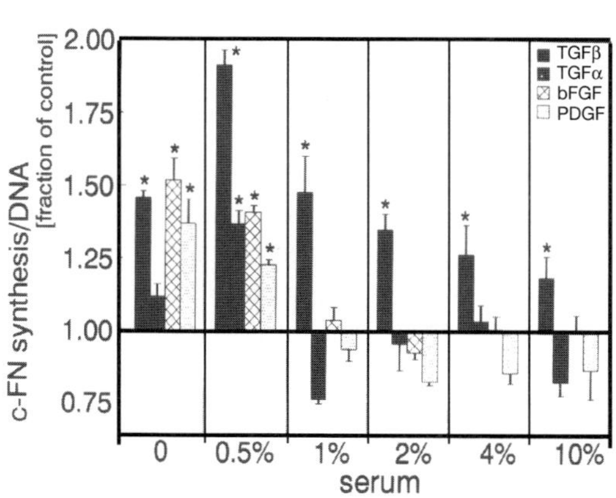

Figure 3.4-4. Effect of TGFβ1, TGFα, bFGF and PDGF on the synthesis of c-fibronectin by cultured human pancreatic stellate cells. The growth factors (TGF-β1 2ng/ml; TGF-α 20ng/ml; bFGF 20ng/ml and PDGF 20ng/ml) were added in the presence of 0, 0.5%, 1%, 2%, 4% and 10% serum to secondary cultured human pancreatic stellate cells. 24 hours later cultures were stopped and c-fibronectin was measured in the cell supernatants; DNA was measured in the cell layer. The columns represent fractions of control (without growth factors). Mean +/– SD of 3 cultures each with 3 wells. *, $p < 0.05$.

Paracrine stimulation of pancreatic stellate cells

Pancreas fibrosis is commonly associated with chronic inflammation [26]. In chronic pancreatitis infiltrating mononuclear cells [27] might potentiate fibrogenesis by (i) the release of cytokines stimulating stromal cells [28] and (ii) by their cytotoxic effects [29]. Furthermore, because macrophages are sometimes located in close proximity to PSC [10] the capacity of macrophages to release fibrogenic mediators is of particular interest. Therefore we studied paracrine stimulation of PSC by activated macrophages. The decreased intestinal motility during pancreatitis causes a bacterial translocation to the peritoneal fluid, lymph, blood, liver and pancreas [30]. In chronic pancreatitis, the TGF-β precursor was detected mainly in mononuclear cells located in fibrotic areas [31]. Also the latent TGF-β-binding protein (LTBP) is predominantly present in mononuclear cells and in the extracellular matrix around them. The presence of both pro-TGF-β and LTBP in monocytes and/or macrophages in areas of fibrosis strongly suggests that this cytokine is involved in the pathophysiology of chronic pancreatitis [31]. To demonstrate paracrine stimulation of PSC by soluble mediators produced by macrophages, we measured proliferation and extracellular matrix synthesis of PSC after addition of macrophage conditioned media or during coculture experiments. The media had been conditioned for 24 hours by unstimulated and LPS-stimulated macrophages in the absence of fetal calf serum. Immunofluorescence staining of cell-associated collagen types I and III and fibronectin, Northern-blot analyses of collagen type I and fibronectin and quantitative immunoassay for collagen type I and c-fibronectin in cell culture supernatants were employed to examine the effects of macrophages on extracellular matrix synthesis of cultured human PSC. The results obtained by the different methods were corresponding. In particular transiently acidified media from LPS-activated macrophages significantly upregulated extracellular matrix synthesis of cultured PSC (Fig. 3.4-6). To demonstrate the effects of macrophage supernatants on cell-associated collagens and fibronectin secondary cultured human PSC grown on glass coverslips were incubated with transiently acidified macrophage supernatant and after 38 hours cultures were fixed and immunostained. Intensive staining patterns of collagen type I and III and fibronectin were observed in cultures receiving supernatants of LPS-activated macrophages (data not shown). There was no significant difference in staining patterns between untreated cells and PSC incubated with conditioned media of unstimulated macrophages. To demonstrate that TGF-β1 represents the fibrogenic mediator produced by activated macrophages, TGF-β1 concentration was measured in supernatants of unstimulated and LPS-stimulated macrophages by time-resolved fluorescence-immunoassay. As expected, LPS-activated macrophages produced 3.4fold more TGF-β (6.61 pg/μg DNA) compared to unstimulated macrophages (1.97 pg/μg DNA) in 24 hours. To investigate the effect of macrophage supernatants on proliferation of cultured PSC BrdU-incorporation was measured. Neither native nor acidified supernatants of unstimulated and LPS-stimulated macrophages showed any inhibitory or stimulatory effect on PSC proliferation.

Furthermore, because platelet aggregates had been detected in capillaries of human pancreatitis tissue [32], we studied the effects of platelet-derived growth factors on proliferation and matrix synthesis of cultured human PSC. Native platelet lysate (nPL) and to an even higher extent acidified platelet lysate (aPL) significantly stimulated cell proliferation measured by DNA (Fig. 3.4-7A) and the incorporation of bromodeoxy-uridine (Fig. 3.4-7B). Furthermore, platelet lysate significantly stimulated the synthesis of colla-

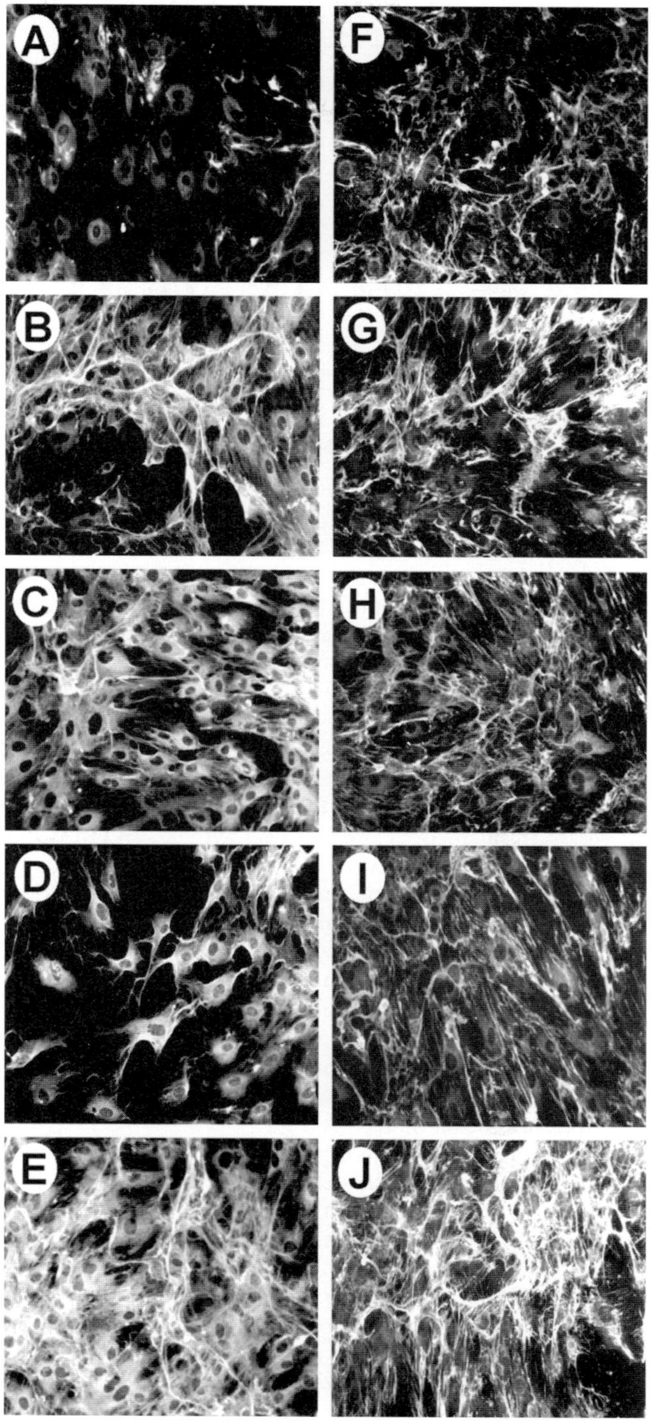

Figure 3.4-5A–J. Fluorescence micrographs showing the immunoreactivity of collagen type I and fibronectin in cultured rat PSC stimulated with TGF-β1, PDGF(AB), TGF-α, and bFGF. Cultured rat PSC (4th passage) grown on glass coverslips were stimulated for 24 hours with TGF-β1, PDGF(AB), TGFα, and bFGF. Thereafter the cultures were washed and fixed in acetone and immunostaining was performed. **A, B, C, D, E:** collagen type I; **F, G, H, I, J:** fibronectin; **A, F:** control 0.5% fetal calf serum; **B, G:** 5 ng/ml TGF-β1; C, H, 50 ng/ml PDGF(AB); **D, I:** 20 ng/ml TGF-α; **E, J:** 50 ng/ml bFGF. To compare staining intensities all micrographs were taken using the same exposure time. Original magnification × 400.

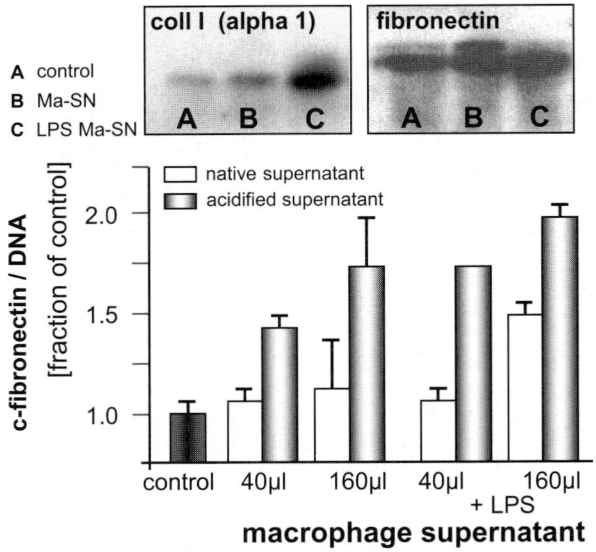

Figure 3.4-6. Stimulation of extracellular matrix synthesis in cultured PSC by macrophage supernatants. Northern blot hybridisation of the collagen α1(I)- and fibronectin-mRNA. Transiently acidified macrophage supernatants were added to secondary cultured human PSC. Ten hours later cultures were stopped and RNA was isolated. Hybridizations were performed by standard procedures. Lane A: RNA isolated from unstimulated PSC (control); lane B: RNA isolated from PSC stimulated with supernatant of macrophages; lane C: RNA isolated from PSC stimulated with supernatant of LPS-activated macrophages.

The column diagram demonstrates the effect of macrophage supernatants on fibronectin synthesis of cultured pancreatic stellate cells. Native and acidified macrophage supernatants (40 and 160 µl/ml medium) were added to secondary cultured pancreatic stellate cells. After 24 hours cultures were stopped and fibronectin was measured in PSC supernatants; DNA was measured in the cell layer. Values are expressed as means ± SD of three independent experiments, each condition performed in triplicate culture wells.*, $p < 0.05$.

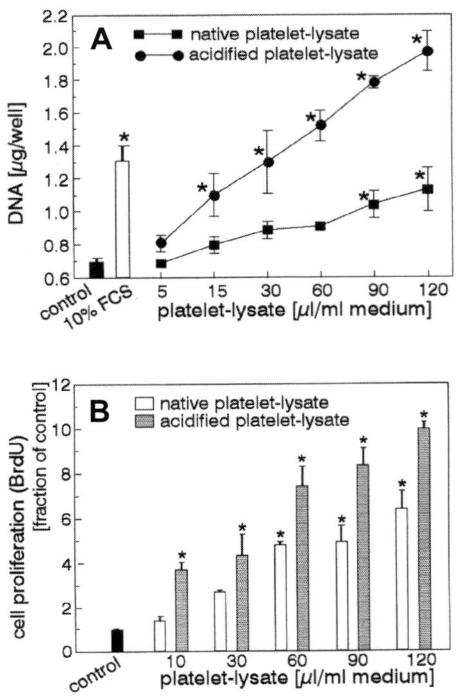

Figure 3.4-7A, B. Effect of platelet lysate on proliferation of cultured human PSC.

A: Measurement of DNA. Human PSC were seeded with a density of 105 cells/cm^2 and cultured in the presence of 0.5% fetal calf serum. 72 h after addition of native and transiently acidified platelet lysates (5, 15, 30, 60, 90, and 120 µl/ml medium) the medium was changed and cell cultures were stimulated for another 72 h. Thereafter cultures were stopped and DNA was measured by fluorometry using bisbenzimide. Mean values +/– SD of three independent experiments, each with n = 3.

B: Measurement of BrdU incorporation. Human PSC were cultured in the presence of 0.5% fetal calf serum. 4h after addition of native and transiently acidified platelet lysates (10, 30, 60, 90, and 120 µl/ml medium) BrdU (final concentration 10^{-5}M) was added. Cultures were stopped 16h later. BrdU incorporation was measured quantitatively by time-resolved fluorescence. Mean values +/– SD of three independent experiments, each with n = 3.

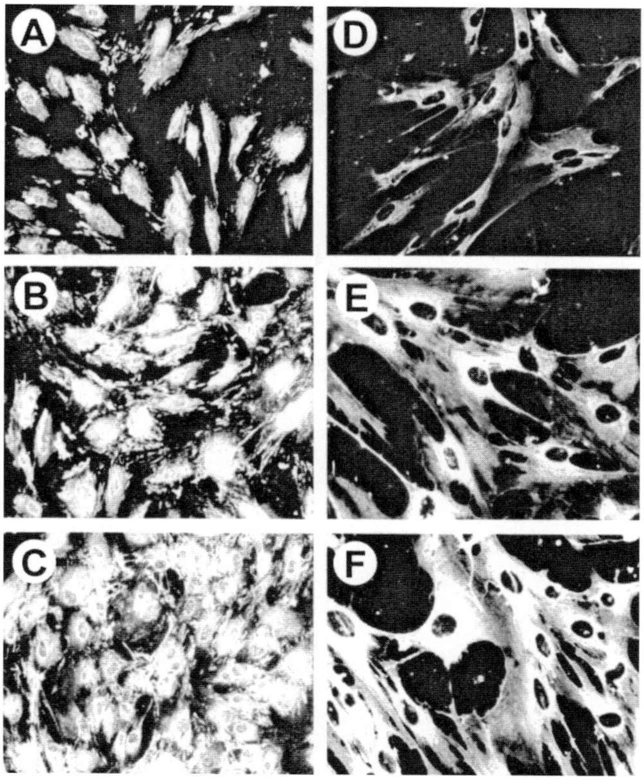

Figure 3.4-8A–F. Fluorescence micrographs showing the immunoreactivity of collagen type I and fibronectin in cultured human PSC stimulated with platelet lysate.

Cultured human PSC (4th passage) grown on glass coverslips were stimulated for 36 hours with 120 µl/ml native and acidified platelet lysate. Thereafter the cultures were washed and fixed in acetone and immunostaining was performed. **A, B, C:** collagen type I; **D, E, F:** fibronectin; **A, D:** control 0.5% FCS; **B, E:** 120 µl/ml native PL; **C, F:** 120 µl/ml acidified PL. To compare staining intensities all micrographs were taken using the same exposure time. **A, B, C:** original magnification × 200; **D, E, F:** original magnification × 400.

gen type I and fibronectin (Fig. 3.4-8). By preincubation of aPL with TGF-β1- and PDGF-neutralizing antibodies and the TGF-β-latency associated peptide, respectively, TGF-β1 was identified as the main mediator stimulating matrix synthesis and PDGF as the responsible mitogen (data not shown). From these data we suggest that platelets and PSC cooperate in the development of human pancreas fibrosis.

Autocrine stimulation of PSC

As shown by real-time RT-PCR during the spontaneous change of the fat-storing phenotype to the myofibrobalst-like phenotype in primary culture on plastic the expression of the TGF-β1-mRNA increased in parallel to the alpha-sm-actin-mRNA (Fig. 3.4-9) and the cells secrete latent TGF-β1. Since (i) human PSC express type II TGF-β-receptors on their cell surface (Fig. 3-410A and B), cultured PSC respond to added TGF-β1 by an increased matrix synthesis (Fig. 3.4-4 and Fig. 3.4-5), and PSC synthesized by itself TGF-β1, autocrine stimulatory mechanisms were suggested. To prove this hypothesis the growth factor scavenger alpha-2-macroglobulin, TGF-β-neutralizing antibodies, and the TGF-ß-latency associated peptide, respectively, were added to PSC growing in dense culture in the absence of serum. Alpha-2-macroglobulin dose dependently reduced fibronectin synthesis (Fig. 3.4-11A) and proliferation (Fig. 3.4-11B) of cultured PSC. TGF-β-neutralizing antibodies and the TGF-β-latency-associated peptide also reduced extracellular matrix synthesis by 20–30% but did not influence proliferation (data not shown). Because alpha-2-macroglobulin binds in addition to TGF-β1 also mitogens (e.g. PDGF, IGFs, FGF,

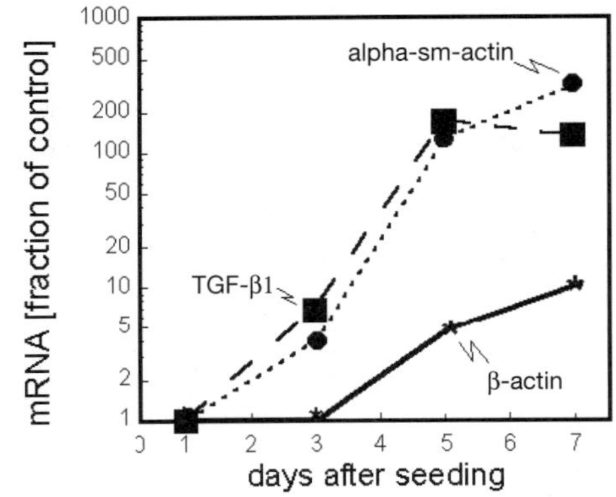

Figure 3.4-9. Real-time quantitative RT-PCR for TGF-β1, alpha-smooth-muscle-actin and β-actin during primary culture of rat pancreatic stellate cells. RNA was isolated from cultured PSC at day 1, 3, 5, and 7 after seeding. RT-PCR was performed using specific primers with the Light-Cycler of Roche (Basel, Swizerland).

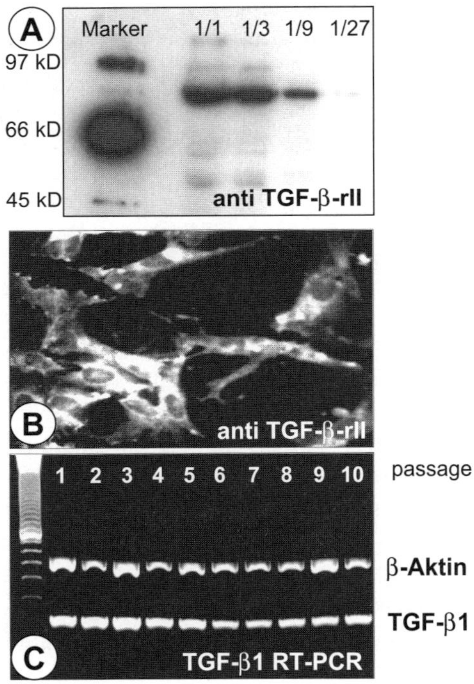

Figure 3.4-10A–C. Demonstration of the TGF-β-receptor-II and TGF-β1-expression in cultured human pancreatic stellate cells. **A:** Western-blot of TGF-β-receptor II using different concentrations of solubilized PSC cell membrane proteins. **B:** immunofluorescence staining of TGF-β-receptor II in cultured human PSC. **C:** RT-PCR showing the expression of the TGF-β1-mRNA in cultured human PSC of passage 1–10.

TGF-alpha) we suggest autocrine stimulation of matrix synthesis via TGF-β1 and autocrine stimulation of PSC proliferation via presently unidentified mitogen(s). Another proof of autocrine-stimulated matrix synthesis via TGF-β1 was obtained using TGF-β1-antisense oligonucleotides. Antisense approaches have been succesfully used to study autocrine-negative growth regulation of TGF-β1 in tumor cells and hepatopoetic cells. We used the transfection reagent DOSPER (Roche, Basel) to transport the TGF-β1-antisense oligonucleotides into the cells. Fluorescein-labeled antisense oligonucleotides were detected in cytoplasm and in cell nucleus 6 h after addition. Collagen type I and fibronectin synthesis was significantly reduced after addition of the antisense oligonucleotide (data

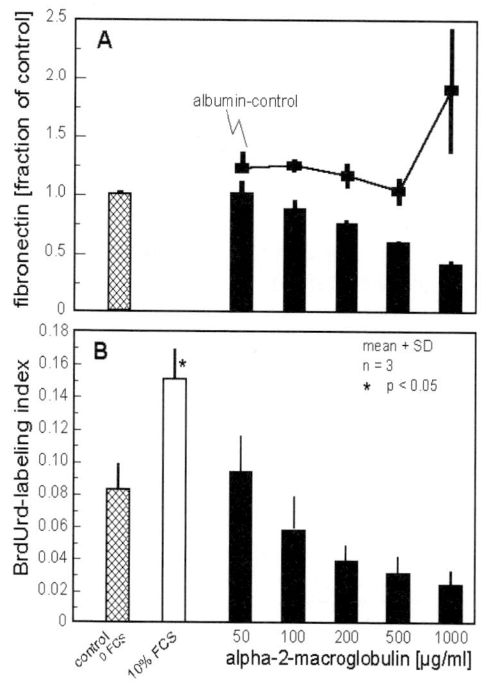

Figure 3.4-11A, B. Dose-dependent inhibition of autocrine-stimulated fibronectin-synthesis (A) and proliferation (B) of cultured human PSC by the growth factor scavenger alpha-2-macroglobulin. 50–1000 µg/ml alpha-2-macroglobulin was added to PSC growing in dense culture in the absence of fetal calf serum. Six hours later BrdU was added and 18 hours later cultures were stopped. Fibronectin was measured in cell culture supernatants and incorporated BrdU was measured quantitatifely by time-resolved fluorescence using a Europium chelate. Mean values +/– SD of three independent experiments, each with n = 3.

not shown). Appropriate concentrations of sense oligonucleotides and a scrambled oligonucleotide did not influence extracellular matrix synthesis. These data strongly support the conclusion of an autocrine stimulatory loop of extracellular matrix synthesis in cultured human PSC via TGF-β1.

Summary and conclusion

Fibrogenesis in pancreatitis is the result of a dynamic cascade of mechanisms beginning with acinar cell injury and necrosis and followed by inflammation, activation of macrophages [33], aggregation of platelets [32], release of growth factors and reactive oxygen species, activation of pancreatic stellate cells (PSC), stimulated synthesis of extracellular matrix and reduced matrix degradation with the consequence of a net matrix acumulation (Fig. 3.4-12). Pancreatic stellate cells represent the main cellular source of extracellular matrix in chronic pancreatitis [14, 15, 34, 35]. PSC share homologies with hepatic stellate cells including storage of retinyl palmitate, retinol esterification, expression of the cytofilaments vimentin and desmin and phenotypic transition to an active matrix producing myofibroblast-like cell. The change in the cells phenotype includes the disappearance of fat droplets and retinyl-esters, the development of a prominent endoplasmatic reticulum, the expression of iso-a-smooth muscle actin, an increased cell proliferation, and a stimulated production of collagen types I and III and fibronectin.

Preliminary data obtained after addition of cultured acinar cell supernatants to cultured PSC suggest paracrine stimulation of PSC by injured acinar cells (data not shown). In this line are recently published data demonstrating the sequence of acinar-cell-induced lipid-peroxidation phenomena in chronic aethanol-induced pancreatitis and active collagen synthesis by activated PSC [14]. In human and experimental chronic pancreatitis high numbers of iso-a-smooth muscle actin positive PSC are located in and around fibrotic areas (in the neighborhood of injured acinar cells). Supernatants of activated macrophages and platelet lysates stimulate extracellular matrix synthesis and proliferation of cultured PSC. The growth factors TGF-β, bFGF, PDGF, and TGF-α (which are released by activated macrophages and aggregating platelets) were identified as stimulating extracellular matrix synthesis of PSC. In particular PDGF acts as a mitogen for PSC. Furthermore, cultured PSC have the ability to stimulate their own matrix synthesis via production of TGF-β1. Addition of alpha-2-macroglobulin, TGF-β-LAP and neutralizing anti-TGF-β1 to cultured PSC significantly reduced collagen and fibronectin synthesis. Furthermore, TGF-β1-antisense-oligonucleotides inhibiting the synthesis of TGF-β1 in PSC also significantly reduced extracellular matrix synthesis. From these data it is suggested that pancreas fibrosis might accelerate also in the absence of further injury and inflammation if the number of activated PSC is high enough to undergo paracrine and autocrine stimulation. A simplified model demonstrating cell-cell interaction via polypeptide growth factors in acute and chronic pancreatitis (and pancreas cancer) is presented

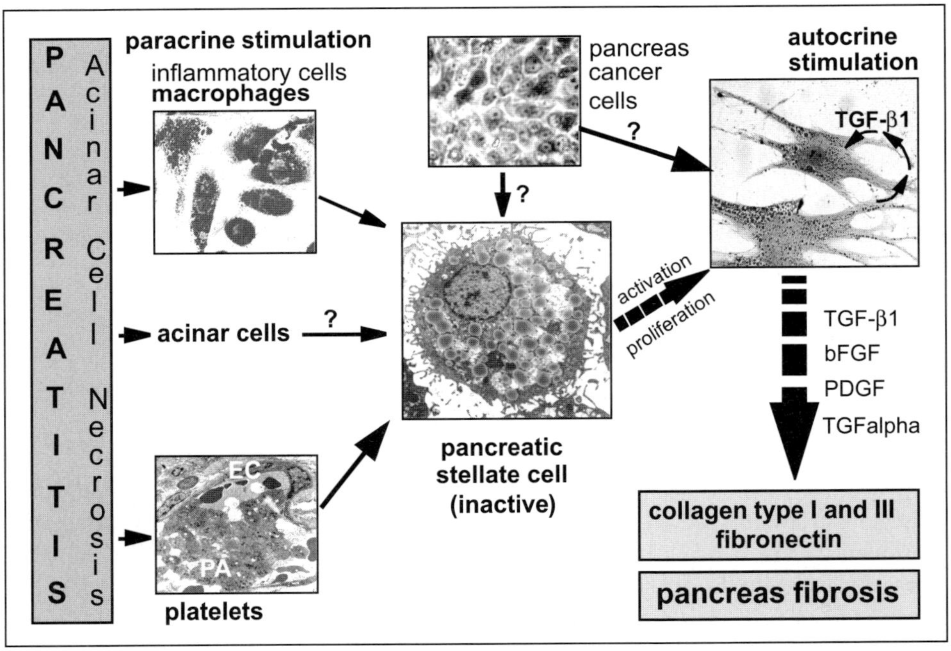

Figure 3.4-12. Simplified model demonstrating cell-cell interactions via soluble mediators in pancreatitis. Activated macrophages and aggregating platelets (probably also injured acinar cells and cancer cells) release fibrogenic mediators stimulating proliferation of pancreatic stellate cells and a change in the cells phenotype to a *myofibroblast-like cell.* The *myofibroblast-like phenotype* synthesizes high amounts of extracellular matrix including collagen types I and III and fibronectin. Activated PSC are also able to stimulate themselves by production of TGF-β1 (and probably other growth factors). The result of these mechanisms is an increased matrix synthesis leading to pancreas fibrosis. The role of a reduced matrix degradation in fibrogenesis will be the subject of further studies.

in Figure 3.4-12. Presently only preliminary data are available demonstrating paracrine stimulation of PSC by pancreas cancer cells.

Taken together, valuable insights into the pathogenesis of pancreas fibrogenesis have been obtained in recent years. Future studies will further analyze the cell-cell interactions and molecular mechanisms leading to pancreas fibrogenesis. *In vivo* and *in vitro* data have demonstrated that PSC play a central role in fibrogenesis but the highly complicated cascade of interacting cell types and molecular mediators require experimental designs which provide better images of the *in situ* situation. Only if our knowledge on these mechanisms expands can adequate therapies to reduce the enhanced extracellular matrix deposition be developed.

References

1. DiMagno EP, Layer P, Clain JE. Chronic pancreatitis. In: Go VLW, DiMagno EP, Gardner JD, eds. The pancreas. 21st ed. New York: Raven Press, 1993: 655–706.
2. Uscanga L, Kennedy RH, Choux R, Druguet M, Grimaud RM, Sarles H. Sequential connective matrix changes in experimental acute pancreatitis. An immunohistochemical and biochemical assessment in the rat. Int J Pancreatol 1987; 2: 33–45.
3. Gress TM, Menke A, Bachem MG, Müller-Pillasch F, Ellenrieder V, Weidenbach H, Wagner M, Adler G. Role of extracellular matrix in pancreatic diseases. Digestion 1998; 59: 625–37.
4. Bachem MG, Meyer D, Melchior R, Sell KM, Gressner AM. Activation of rat liver perisinusoidal lipocytes by transforming growth factors derived from myofibroblastlike cells. J Clin Invest 1992; 89: 19–27.
5. Friedman SL, Roll FJ, Boyles J, Bissel DM. Hepatic lipocytes. The principal collagen-producing cells of normal rat liver. Proc Natl Acad Sci USA 1985; 82: 8681–85.
6. Gressner AM, Bachem MG. Cellular sources of noncollagenous matrix proteins: role of fat-storing in fibrogenesis. Sem Liv Dis 1990; 10: 30–46.
7. Watari N, Hotta Y, Mabuchi Y. Morphological studies on a vitamin A-storing cell and its complex with macrophage observed in mouse pancreatic tissues following excess vitamin A administration. Okajimas Folia Anat Jpn 1982; 58: 837–58.
8. Ikejiri N. The vitamin A-storing cells in the human and rat pancreas. Kurume Med J 1990; 37: 67–81.
9. Apte MV, Haber PS, Applegate TL, Norton ID, McCaughan GW, Korsten MA, Pirola RC, Wilson JS. Periacinar stellate shaped cells in rat pancreas: identification, isolation, and culture. Gut 1998; 43: 128–33.
10. Bachem MG, Schneider E, Gross H, Weidenbach H, Schmid RM, Menke A, Siech M, Beger H, Grünert A, Adler G. Identification, culture, and characterization of pancreatic stellate cells in rats and humans. Gastroenterology 1998; 115: 421–32.
11. Saotome T, Inoue H, Fujimiya M, Fujiyama Y, Bamba T. Morphological and immunocytochemical identification of periacinar fibroblast-like cells derived from human pancreatic acini. Pancreas 1997; 14: 373–82.
12. Kato Y, Inoue H, Fujiyama Y, Bamba T. Morphological identification of and collagen synthesis by periacinar fibroblastoid cells cultured from isolated rat pancreatic acini. J Gastroenterol 1996; 31: 565–71.
13. Okumura Y, Shintani Y, Kato Y, Tamba J, Inoue H, Fujiyama Y, Bamba T. Proliferative effect of phospholipase A2 on rat periacinar fibroblastoid cells of the pancreas. Pancreas 1998; 16: 505–10.
14. Casini A, Galli A, Pignalosa P, Frulloni L, Grappone C, Milani S, Pederzoli P, Cavallini G, Surrenti C. Collagen type I synthesized by pancreatic periacinar stellate cells (PSC) co-localizes with lipid peroxidation-derived aldehydes in chronic alcoholic pancreatitis. J Pathol 2000; 192: 81–9.

15. Haber PS, Keogh GW, Apte MV, Moran CS, Stewart NL, Crawford DH, Pirola RC, McCaughan GW, Ramm GA, Wilson JS. Activation of pancreatic stellate cells in human and experimental pancreatic fibrosis. Am J Pathol 1999; 155: 1087–95.
16. Bachem MG, Sell KM, Melchior R, Kropf J, Eller T, Gressner AM. Tumor necrosis factor a and transforming growth factor b1 stimulate fibronectin synthesis and the transdifferentiation of fat-storing cells into myofibroblasts. Virchows Arch Cell Pathol 1993; 63: 123–30.
17. Bachem MG, Meyer D, Melchior R, Sell KM, Gressner AM. Activation of rat liver perisinusoidal lipocytes by transforming growth factors derived from myofibroblastlike cells. J Clin Invest 1992; 89: 19–27.
18. Czaja MJ, Weiner FR, Flanders CH, Giambrone HA, Wino R, Biempica L, Zern MA. In vitro and in vivo association of transforming growth factor beta with hepatic fibrosis. J Cell Biol 1989; 108: 2477–82.
19. Matsuoka M, Pham NG, Tsukamoto H. Differential effects of interleukin-1 a, tumor necrosis factor a and transforming growth factor b1 on cell proliferation and collagen formation by cultured fat-storing cells. Liver 1989; 9: 71–8.
20. Pinzani M, Gesualdo L, Sabbah GM, Abboud HE. Effects of platelet-derived growth factor and other polypeptide mitogens on DNA synthesis and growth of cultured rat liver fat-storing cells. J Clin Invest 1989; 84: 1786–93.
21. Friess H, Yamanaka Y, Buechler M, Beger HG, Do DA, Kobrin MS, Korc M. Increased expression of acidic and basic fibroblast growth factors in chronic pancreatitis. Am J Pathol 1994; 144: 117–28.
22. Kimura Y, Torimura T, Ueno T, Inuzuka S, Tanikawa K. Transforming growth factor b1, extracellular matrix and inflammatory cells in wound repair using a closed duodenal loop pancreatitis model in rat. Scand J Gastroenterol 1995; 30: 707–14.
23. Ebert M, Kasper HU, Hernberg S, Friess H, Büchler MW, Roessner A, Korc M, Malfertheiner P. Overexpression of platelet-derived growth factor (PDGF) B chain and type beta PDGF receptor in human chronic pancreatitis. Dig Dis Sci 1998; 43: 567–74.
24. Bockman DE, Merlino G. Cytological changes in the pancreas of transgenic mice overexpressing transforming growth factor a. Gastroenterology 1992; 103: 1883–92.
25. Lee MS, Gu D, Feng L, Curriden S, Arnush M, Krahl T, Gurushanthaiah D, Wilson C, Loskutoff DS, Fox H, Sarvetnick N. Accumulation of extracellular matrix and developmental dysregulation in the pancreas by transgenic production of transforming growth factor b1. Am J Pathol 1995; 147: 42–52.
26. Emmerich J, Weber I, Nausch M, Sparmann G, Koch K, Seyfarth M, Löhr M, Liebe S. Immunohistochemical characterization of the pancreatic cellular infiltrate in normal pancreas, chronic pancreatitis and pancreatic carcinoma. Digestion 1998; 59: 192–98.
27. Bockmann DE, Büchler MW, Beger HG. Ultrastructure of human acute pancreatitis: Int J Pancreatol 1986; 1: 141–53.
28. Wahl SM, McCartney-Francis N, Mergenhagen SE. Inflammatory and immunoregulatory roles of TGF b. Immunol Today 1989; 10: 258–61.
29. Rabinovitch A, Suarez-Pinzon WL. Cytokines and their role in pancreatic islet beta-cell destruction and insulin-dependent diabetes mellitus. Biochem Pharmacol 1998; 55: 1139–49.
30. Gianotti L, Munda R, Alexander JW, Tchervenkov JI, Babcock GF. Bacterial translocation: a potent source for infection in acute pancreatitis. Pancreas 1993; 8: 551–8.
31. Van Laethem JL, Deviere J, Resibois A, Rickaert F, Vertongen P, Ohtani H, Cremer M, Miyazono K, Robberecht P. Localization of transforming growth factor b1 and its latent binding protein in human chronic pancreatitis. Gastroenterology 1995; 108: 1873–81.
32. Luttenberger T, Schmid-Kotsas A, Menke A, Siech M, Beger H, Adler G, Grünert A, Bachem MG. Platelet-derived growth factors stimulate proliferation and extracellular matrix synthesis of pancreatic stellate cells: implications in pathogenesis of pancreas fibrosis. Lab Invest 2000; 80: 47–55.
33. Schmid-Kotsas A, Gross J, Menke A, Weidenbach H, Adler G, Siech M, Beger H, Grünert A, Bachem MG. LPS-activated macrophages stimulate the synthesis of collagen type I and c-fibronectin in cultured pancreatic stellate cells. Am J Pathol 1999; 155: 1749–58.

34. Apte MV, Phillips PA, Fahmy RG, Darby SJ, Rodgers SC, McCaughan GW, Korsten MA, Pirola RC, Naidoo D, Wilson JS. Does alcohol directly stimulate pancreatic fibrogenesis? Studies with rat pancreatic stellate cells. Gastroenterology 2000; 118: 780–94.
35. Neuschwander-Tetri BA, Burton FR, Presti ME, Britton RS, Janney CG, Garvin PR, Brunt EM, Galvin NJ, Poulos JE. Repetitive self-limited acute pancreatitis induces pancreatic fibrogenesis in the mouse. Dig Dis Sci 2000; 45: 665–74.
36. Neuschwander-Tetri BA, Bridle KR, Wells LD, Marcu M, Ramm GA. Repetitive acute pancreatic injury in the mouse induces procollagen alpha 1 (I) expression colocalized to pancreatic stellate cells. Lab Invest 2000; 80: 143–50.

3.5 Pancreatic fibrosis, tubular complexes and tumor development in TGF-α transgenic mice

R. M. Schmid , M. Wagner, F. R. Greten, Ch. K. Weber, G. Adler

Fibrosis and tubular complex formation

Pancreatic cancer and chronic pancreatitis are characterized by profound alterations in the formation and composition of the extracellular matrix. However, the underlying molecular events are poorly defined. Studies in humans are descriptive and offer few insights into regulatory and functional aspects. Animal models are required to understand the complex process of pancreatic fibrogenesis, in addition to *in vitro* studies. Mice overexpressing TGF-α in the pancreas display an aggregation of intralobular iso-alpha-smooth muscle actin positive cells starting early after birth. Progressive fibrosis and accumulation of extracellular matrix is evident as TGF-α transgenic mice age. The extracellular matrix producing cells in this model are most likely activated pancreatic stellate cells (PSC). Bachem and coworkers have shown that pancreatic stellate cells (PSCs) are located in interlobular areas and in interacinar regions of the pancreas [1]. During primary culture, these cells change from a quiescent fat-storing phenotype to highly synthetic myofibroblast-like cell expressing iso-alpha-smooth muscle actin (> 90%) and desmin (20%–40%). Furthermore, these cells strongly express collagen types I and III, fibronectin, and laminin. Pancreatic PSC share similarities with hepatic stellate cells, suggesting that PSCs participate in the development of pancreatic fibrosis. However, PSCs in the liver seem to require different polypeptide growth factors for activation as compared to pancreatic PSCs. Mice overexpressing TGF-α under the control of a metallothionin promoter develop fibrosis selectively in the pancreas although this promoter is active in the liver [2, 3].

In addition to the progressive fibrosis, acinar cells display profound alterations over time in TGF-α transgenic mice. Early changes of acinar cells are observed already 14 days after birth and progress to the formation of tubular complexes in adult mice. The process of tubular complex formation is characterized by a loss of acinar cell characteristics and a gain of a ductal phenotype. These duct cells form branches and anastomosing tubules. The changes are not equally distributed throughout the pancreas. Areas with tubular structures are mixed with areas with normal-appearing acinar cells. Acinar cells loose their height and acinar markers, but gain characteristics of duct cells including basal tight junctions and mucin granules. This seems to be a slow process, since "intermediate" cell types can be detected which express amylase and carbonic anhydrase activity simultaneously [4]. It is a matter of debate whether this process represents a transdifferentiation process or rather a combination of dedifferentation and redifferentiation. Recently, Song and coworkers have shown that overexpression of TGF-α induces an expansion of Pdx1-expressing epithelium cells in the pancreas [5]. The Pdx1 homeodomain transcription factor is involved in the formation of differentiated cell types from ductal progenitor cells during pancreatic development. In addition to Pdx1 gene activation, TGF-α induced epithelial changes demonstrated a pluripotent differentiation capacity, as evidenced by focal expression of Pax6 and initiation of islet cell neogenesis. The majority of Pdx1-positive epithelial cells showed no expression of insulin, similar to the pattern observed during embryonic development [5]. These findings suggest that TGF-α stimulation may recapitulate a developmental program active during embryogenesis.

Tumor development

We have previously shown that mice overexpressing TGF-α under the control of the elastase promoter develop pancreatic tumors originating from cells within tubular complexes after one year of age [4]. These data suggest the premalignant nature of cells within tubular structures. Persistent stimulation of the EGF-receptor by TGF-α increases GTP loading of Ras and phosphorylation of Erk1/2 selectively in cells within tubular structures but not in acinar cells [6]. Almost all of these cells forming tubular complexes show nuclear accumulation of cyclin D1. Neither acinar cells nor fibroblasts are positive for cyclin D1 or Cdk4, suggesting that increased cyclin D/Cdk4 activity is restricted to duct cells. In comparison to 28 days with few cells positive for cyclin E, nuclear accumulation of cyclin E is even less frequently observed in the pancreas at 180 days. Moreover, no induction of other S-phase proteins like PCNA is detectable, indicating that TGF-α is able to promote progression through G1, but not S phase. These data indicate that at 28 days ductal cells within developing tubular complexes divide, whereas later, at 180 days, most of these cells become growth arrested.

These findings recapitulate previous *in vitro* data that *ras* is not only a transforming oncogene but can also exert a negative effect on cell growth. Furthermore, it was observed that these negative effects of Ras could be overcome, in some cases, by simultaneous expression of a co-operating oncogene [7]. Some more recent data provide a possible explanation for these earlier results. Introduction of oncogenic Ras into mouse fibroblasts leads to cell-cycle arrest, through induction of Cdk inhibitors $p16^{Ink4a}$ and $p21^{Cip1}$ as well as $p19^{Arf}$ and p53 [8–10]. In contrast to $p16^{Ink4a}$, which is not upregulated in the pancreas of TGF-α transgenic mice, $p21^{Cip1}$ is induced several-fold [6]. Increased expression of $p21^{Cip1}$ would provide a logical explanation for the G1 arrest [11]. The molecular basis for the induction of $p21^{Cip1}$ is complex. In addition to activation through Raf/MEK/ Erk, $p21^{Cip1}$ is subject to transcriptional induction by p53 [8, 12]. Nuclear accumulation of p53 is present in ductal cells in the tubular complexes, suggesting that p53 represents a candidate for mediating growth arrest in these premaligant lesions. The protein levels of p53 are determined primarily by ubiquitination and subsequent proteolytic degradation. The main ubiquitin ligase for p53 is the oncogene Mdm2. $p19^{Arf}$ appears to protect p53 from degradation by binding directly to Mdm2 [13, 14]. Although it is clear from *in vitro* studies that overexpression of Ras leads to the induction of $p19^{Arf}$, we cannot detect an upregulation of $p19^{Arf}$ in the pancras of TGF-a transgenic mice [6]. Fibroblasts derived from $p53^{-/-}$ mice were able to overcome the G1 arrest mediated by Ras and form transformed foci [9]. In mating experiments we show a dramatically accelerated tumor formation in TGF-α/$p53^{-/-}$ mice resulting in pancreatic cancer development before the age of 120 days. TGF-α transgenic mice, hemizygous for p53-deficiency, display accelerated disease and almost all of these tumors segregate the wild-type p53 allele. Loss of p53 accelerates tumor formation; however, it takes 45 days to develop cancerous lesions in TGF-α transgenic mice null for p53. In the pancreas of these mice persistent activation of Ras and cyclin D1/Cdk4 is observed shortly after birth. This suggests inactivation of additional genes coding for growth arrest proteins to be required during tumorigenesis. LOH analysis revealed frequent homozygous losses of the *Ink4a/Arf* locus in TGF-α/p53$^{+/-}$ mice. The deletion also includes *Ink4b*. The *Ink4a/Arf* locus encodes the two related, putative tumor suppressors, p16^{Ink4a} and p19^{Arf} [15]. p16^{Ink4a} represents a potent tumor suppressor in humans and is frequently inactivated in pancreatic neoplasms [16]. In addition, inherited mutations of exon 1a implicate p16^{Ink4a} in familial tumor susceptibility [17]. However, the final proof of p16^{Ink4a} as a tumor suppressor in mice awaits the specific inactivation of the p16^{Ink4a} gene. The loss of function approach strongly suggested that p19^{Arf} is the major tumor suppressor in mice [15, 18]. Deletions of the *Ink4a/Arf* locus occurred in six of fifteen tumors in TGF-α/p53$^{+/-}$ and TGF-α/p53$^{-/-}$ mice. This result was unexpected from previous findings, indicating a mutually exclusive manner of p53 and p19^{Arf} inactivation in c-myc-induced lymphomagenesis [19]. All tumors retained other polymorphic markers showing that the effect cannot be simply explained due to chromosomal instability. These data therefore suggest that the *Ink4a/Arf* locus is synergistic to p53 in tumor suppression in TGF-α transgenic mice. Similarly, human pancreatic cancer involves homozygous deletion of the region 9p21–p22, resulting in inactivation of the p14^{ARF} and the p15^{INK4b} genes [20]. Similar to human pancreatic cancer, LOH of the *SMAD4/DPC4* locus occurred only with a lower frequency in our tumor model [21]. Recent data suggest functional inactivation of the TGF-β-Smad4 pathway in the presence of activated Ras, which might explain a reduced selection pressure for LOH at the *Smad4* locus [22]. Furthermore, the *Rb1* locus was infrequently affected by LOH. This is consistent with the low number of Rb mutations in human pancreatic cancer.

Carcinogenesis is a multistep process. The malignant phenotype requires multiple alterations affecting several levels of growth control. TGF-α transgenic mice represent a murine pancreatic cancer model that recapitulates pathomorphological features and genetic alterations of human pancreatic cancer.

References

1. Bachem MG, Schneider E, Gross H, Weidenbach H, Schmid RM, Menke A, Siech M, Beger H, Grünert A, Adler G. Identification, culture, and characterization of pancreatic stellate cells in rats and humans. Gastroenterology 1998; 115: 421–32.
2. Jhappan C, Stahle C, Harkins RN, Fausto N, Smith GH, Merlino GT. TGF alpha overexpression in transgenic mice induces liver neoplasia and abnormal development of the mammary gland and pancreas. Cell 1990; 61: 1137–46.
3. Sandgren EP, Luetteke NC, Palmiter RD, Brinster RL, Lee DC. Overexpression of TGF alpha in transgenic mice: induction of epithelial hyperplasia, pancreatic metaplasia, and carcinoma of the breast. Cell 1990; 61: 1121–35.
4. Wagner M, Luhrs H, Kloppel G, Adler G, Schmid RM. Malignant transformation of duct-like cells originating from acini in transforming growth factor transgenic mice. Gastroenterology 1998; 115: 1254–62.
5. Song SY, Gannon M, Washington MK, Scoggins CR, Meszoely IM, Goldenring JR, Marino CR, Sandgren EP, Coffey RJ, Wright CV, Leach SD. Expansion of Pdx1-expressing pancreatic epithelium and islet neogenesis in transgenic mice overexpressing transforming growth factor alpha. Gastroenterology 1999; 117: 1416–26.
6. Wagner M, Greten FR, Weber CK, Koschnick S, Mattfeldt T, Deppert W, Kern H, Adler G, Schmid RM. A murine tumor progression model for pancreatic cancer recapitulating the genetic alterations of the human disease. Genes Dev 2001; 15: 286–93.
7. Franza BR, Maruyama K, Garrels JI, Ruley HE. In vitro establishment is not a sufficient prerequisite for transformation by activated ras oncogenes. Cell 1986; 44: 409–18.

8. Macleod KF, Sherry N, Hannon G, Beach D, Tokino T, Kinzler K, Vogelstein B, Jacks T. p53-dependent and independent expression of p21 during cell growth, differentiation, and DNA damage. Genes Dev 1995, 9: 935–44.
9. Serrano M, Lin AW, McCurrach ME, Beach D, Lowe SW. Oncogenic ras provokes premature cell senescence associated with accumulation of p53 and p16INK4a. Cell 1997; 88: 593–602.
10. Palmero I, Pantoja C, Serrano M. p19ARF links the tumour suppressor p53 to Ras. Nature 1998; 395: 125–6.
11. Sherr CJ, Roberts JM. CDK inhibitors: positive and negative regulators of G1-phase progression. Genes Dev 1999; 13: 1501–12.
12. El-Deiry WS, Tokino T, Velculescu VE, Levy DB, Parsons R, Trent JM, Lin D, Mercer WE, Kinzler KW, Vogelstein B. WAF1, a potential mediator of p53 tumor suppression. Cell 1993; 75: 817–25.
13. Pomerantz J, Schreiber AN, Liegeois NJ, Silverman A, Alland L, Chin L, Potes J, Chen K, Orlow I, Lee HW, Cordon CC, DePinho RA. The Ink4a tumor suppressor gene product, p19Arf, interacts with MDM2 and neutralizes MDM2's inhibition of p53. Cell 1998; 92: 713–23.
14. Furuya N, Kawa S, Akamatsu T, Furihata K. Long-term follow-up of patients with chronic pancreatitis and K-ras gene mutation detected in pancreatic juice. Gastroenterology 1997; 113: 593–8.
15. Serrano M, Lee H, Chin L, Cordon CC, Beach D, DePinho RA. Role of the INK4a locus in tumor suppression and cell mortality. Cell 1996, 85: 27–37.
16. Caldas C, Hahn SA, da Costa LT, Redston MS, Schutte M, Seymour AB, Weinstein CL, Hruban RH, Yeo CJ, Kern SE. Frequent somatic mutations and homozygous deletions of the p16 (MTS1) gene in pancreatic adenocarcinoma. Nat Genet 1994; 8: 27–32.
17. Gruis NA, #van d, V?#, Sandkuijl LA, Prins DE, Weaver FJ, Kamb A, Bergman W, Frants RR. Homozygotes for CDKN2 (p16) germline mutation in Dutch familial melanoma kindreds. Nat Genet 1995; 10: 351–3.
18. Kamijo T, Zindy F, Roussel MF, Quelle DE, Downing JR, Ashmun RA, Grosveld G, Sherr CJ. Tumor suppression at the mouse INK4a locus mediated by the alternative reading frame product p19ARF. Cell 1997; 91: 649–59.
19. Eischen CM, Weber JD, Roussel MF, Sherr CJ, Cleveland JL. Disruption of the ARF-Mdm2-p53 tumor suppressor pathway in Myc-induced lymphomagenesis. Genes Dev 1999; 13: 2658–69.
20. Naumann M, Savitskaia N, Eilert C, Schramm A, Kalthoff H, Schmiegel W. Frequent codeletion of p16/MTS1 and p15/MTS2 and genetic alterations in p16/MTS1 in pancreatic tumors. Gastroenterology 1996; 110: 1215–24.
21. Hahn SA, Schutte M, Hoque AT, Moskaluk CA, da Costa LT, Rozenblum E, Weinstein CL, Fischer A, Yeo CJ, Hruban RH, Kern SE. DPC4, a candidate tumor suppressor gene at human chromosome 18q21.1. Science 1996; 350–3.
22. Kretzschmar M, Doody J, Timokhina I, Massague J. A mechanism of repression of TGF beta/ Smad signaling by oncogenic Ras. Genes Dev 1999; 13: 804–16.

3.6. Chronic pancreatitis: Molecular alterations and clinical implications

M. P. A. Ebert

Summary

Chronic pancreatitis is an inflammatory disease of the pancreas leading to exocrine and endocrine insufficiency. In recent years our knowledge of the disease has improved. Some molecular and genetic alterations underlying the pathogenesis of this disease have been revealed. The main clinical problem, i.e. differentiating chronic inflammation from cancer of the pancreas, however, remains a challenge for clinicians and scientists. This review will highlight the present knowledge of the molecular pathogenesis of chronic pancreatitis, the potential role of molecular changes for the diagnosis and clinical management of the disease and the role of molecular markers for differentiating chronic pancreatitis from pancreatic cancer.

Introduction

Chronic pancreatitis is characterized by a progressive destruction of the exocrine and endocrine pancreas, leading to exocrine and later to endocrine insufficiency. The incidence of the disease is estimated to be around 3 to 5 patients per 100,000 individuals [1]. The most important risk factor for the development of chronic pancreatitis in Europe is increased ethanol consumption. In approximately 20% of the cases a definite etiological factor cannot be identified and the disease is classified as idiopathic chronic pancreatitis [1, 2]. Other underlying conditions such as hyperthyroidism, trauma or pathoanatomical variations such as pancreas anulare or tumors of the pancreas are rare causes of a chron-

Table 3.6-1. Etiology of chronic pancreatitis.

Chronic Pancreatitis	
1. Ethanol (> 70%)	
2. Idiopathic (20%)	juvenile form senile form
3. Rare causes	hypercalcemia uremia hypoproteinemia drugs hereditary
Additional types	
1. Chronic obstructive pancreatitis	pancreas divisum pancreas anulare stenosis of papilla tumors
2. Tropical pancreatitis	

ic inflammation of the pancreas (Table 3.6-1). Increased ethanol consumption is the most important etiological factor. The amount of ethanol intake correlates with the risk of developing chronic pancreatitis [3]. Yet the molecular alterations underlying the pathogenesis of alcoholic chronic pancreatitis remain largely unknown. Besides alcoholic chronic pancreatitis a small group of other forms of chronic pancreatitis exist. Thus, tropical pancreatitis exists in Asia and Africa which develops independent of ethanol intake and which is characterized by the development of endocrine insufficiency in young years [1–3]. Obstructive chronic pancreatitis may develop due to tumors or anatomical variations of the pancreatic duct system [2]. All forms of chronic pancreatitis are characterized by abdominal pain and weight loss. In cases with enlargement of the pancreatic head and obstruction of the biliary duct system jaundice may also develop.

Pathogenesis of chronic pancreatitis

Chronic pancreatitis is a chronic inflammatory disease of the exocrine pancreas leading to destruction of the pancreatic parenchyma and the generation of pancreatic fibrosis [4, 5]. Histologically the pancreas in chronic pancreatitis exhibits ductal hyperplasia, dedifferentiation of acinar cells, proliferation of fibroblasts and atrophy. The fibrosis is classified in 4 degrees [6,7]. Interstitial fibrosis, grade I, leads to the reduction of zymogen granula; however, the cellular architecture is preserved. In grade II fibrosis, the periductal fibrosis is thickened, lymphocytes infiltrate the pancreas and acinar cells contain large vacuoles. In grade III fibrosis, fibrotic scars occur in the pancreas and acinar cells diminish, until finally in end stage fibrosis, the gland is transformed into fibrotic tissue in association with acinar cell atrophy. The molecular alterations underlying the histological changes of the pancreas are largely unknown. Several theories have been developed. The alteration of lithostatin as well as the development of fibrosis as a result of recurrent attacks of acute pancreatitis with necrotic changes have been implicated in the development of a chronic inflammatory reaction of the pancreas [2, 8]. Furthermore, oxygen free radicals and a direct toxic effect of ethanol have been discussed as well (Table 3.6-2) [9, 10]. Lithostatins are a family of glycoproteins that prevent precipitation of calcium carbonate. Alterations in the synthesis and secretion of lithostatins with the development of pancreatic duct obstruction have been described in the pancreas in chronic pancreatitis. In addition, the pancreas of patients with chronic pancreatitis exhibits decreased expression of its mRNA moieties [8, 11]. Animal experiments have shown that oxidative stress may activate transcription factors such as AP1 and NF-kB, which in turn may activate other cytokines [12]. Apart from these models, recently molecular analysis has revealed that cy-

Table 3.6-2. Models of chronic pancreatitis pathogenesis.

Hypothesis	Reference
Accumulation of lithostatin	Sarles 1990
Toxic effect of oxygen free radicals	Beger 1990
Direct toxic effect of ethanol	Apte 2000
Necrosis-fibrosis theory	Klöppel 1993
Cytokines, growth factors	Saurer 2000
T-cell mediated autotoxicity	Hunger 1997
Mutation of CFTR	Sharer 1998

Table 3.6-3. Transgenic models of pancreatic fibrosis.

Gene	Phenotype	Reference
TGF-α	fibrosis, ductal metaplasia dysplasia, tumors	Bockmann 1992 Wagner 1998
TGF-β1	fibrosis, lymphocytic infiltration	Lee, Sanvito 1995
IL-6	islet cell hyperplasia, lymphocytic infiltration	Campbell 1994
Oncostatin M	fibrosis, lymphocytic infiltration	Bamber 1998
MHCII knock out	atrophy, lymphocytic infiltration	Vallance 1998

tokines and other mediators may be produced and secreted by inflammatory cells which infiltrate the pancreas in chronic pancreatitis [13, 14]. In fact, the overexpression of these cytokines and growth factors in transgenic models leads to the development of pancreatic fibrosis and a massive lymphocytic infiltration which resembles the histomorphological alterations that are present in human chronic pancreatitis [15, 16] (Table 3.6-3).

Molecular alterations in chronic pancreatitis

The molecular alterations underlying pancreatic fibrogenesis and the pathogenesis of chronic pancreatitis are still under investigation. Through linkage-analysis the genetic cause of hereditary pancreatitis has been identified. Hereditary pancreatitis is characterized by recurrent attacks of acute pancreatitis from early ages leading to fibrosis of the pancreas. Whitcomb et al. identified mutations in the trypsinogen-gene which lead to an exchange of arginine by histidine or asparagine by isoleucine [17]. Through these mutations the hydrolysis of trypsin is inhibited which goes on to activate further proteases. This disease is associated with a 40% risk of developing pancreatic cancer at age 70 and older. In addition this disease demonstrates that recurrent attacks of necrotizing pancreatitis may lead to pancreatic fibrosis and eventually cancer of the pancreas [9]. Mutations of the cystic fibrosis transmembrane regulator gene have been identified in 18 of 134 patients with chronic pancreatitis [18]. However, the genetic and molecular alterations underlying the vast majority of alcoholic chronic pancreatitis cases are unknown. From the comparative analysis of gene expression in chronic pancreatitis and pancreatic cancer, several factors have been identified which may be overexpressed in both diseases or – more importantly – only in one of the two diseases. While pancreatic cancers frequently harbor p53 gene mutations, several studies failed to identify p53 mutations in the pancreas of patients with chronic pancreatitis [19, 20]. Furthermore, MDM2, which binds and inactivates wildtype p53, is overexpressed in pancreatic cancer, but not in chronic pancreatitis [21]. Mutations of the K-ras oncogene are frequent in pancreatic cancer; however, the frequency of K-ras mutations in the non-malignant pancreatic parenchyma varies greatly [22–24]. In recent studies K-ras mutations were identified not only in pancreatic cancer cells but also in papillary hyperplasia, mucinous hypertrophy and squamous cell metaplasia. In addition, K-ras mutations can also be found in the normal duct epithelium in chronic pancreatitis and pancreatic cancer [24]. Thus, K-ras mutations may be an early event in pancreatic carcinogenesis; however, it may not be useful to differentiate chronic inflammation of the pancreas from pancreatic malignancy.

Recently several studies have analyzed the expression of growth factors and cytokines in chronic pancreatitis and pancreatic cancer. While many pancreatic cancers overexpress growth factors of the PDGF, EGF, HGF, FGF and TGF-β family, several groups have also identified overexpression of TGF-β1, PDGFs and TGF-α in chronic pancreatitis and preneoplastic lesions of the exocrine pancreas [25–27]. TGF-β1 plays a central role in the pathogenesis of pancreatic fibrogenesis. Enhanced expression of TGF-β1 was reported in acute and chronic pancreatitis [28]. Furthermore, repeated injection of TGF-β1 in the pancreas of mice with acute pancreatitis leads to pancreatic fibrosis [29]. In addition, TGF-β1 antibodies inhibit the production of components of the extracellular matrix [30]. The generation of transgenic mice overexpressing various growth factors, such as TGF-α and TGF-β1 has contributed to our understanding of the development of pancreatic fibrosis. These mice develop pancreatic fibrosis after overexpression of these growth factors in the pancreas [15, 16, 31].

Recently, stellate cells have been identified in the pancreas of patients with chronic pancreatitis. These stellate cells transform to myofibroblasts after activation by PDGF and TGF-β1 [32]. Furthermore, after activation of these cells by various growth factors, stellate cells produce several components of the extracellular matrix [33]. Besides the exocrine pancreas and its contribution to the process of pancreatic fibrosis in chronic pancreatitis, lymphocytes may also infiltrate the pancreas in chronic pancreatitis. Besides the induction of MHC-class-I and -II molecules in chronic pancreatitis, cytotoxic T-cells infiltrate the pancreas [34, 35]. These T-cells express perforin, which induces T-cell mediated autotoxicity of the pancreas in chronic pancreatitis. Furthermore, the degree of lymphocytic infiltration of the pancreas correlates with the severity of pain in patients with chronic pancreatitis. Apart from these T-cells, other cytokines may also be expressed in the pancreas. Thus, chemokines of the C-X-C family, such as IL-8, and of the C-C-chemokine family, such as MCP-1, can be identified in chronic pancreatitis [14, 36, 37]. Apart from these cytokines, growth factors play an important role in the pathogenesis of pancreatic fibrosis. Besides the activation of stellate cells, the overexpression of growth factors of the EGF and TGF-β-family in transgenic mice leads to pancreatic fibrosis and lymphocytic infiltration [15, 16]. Furthermore, in the model of TGF-α transgenic mice, the development of pancreatic fibrosis is associated with the development of dysplasia and cancer of the exocrine pancreas. Interestingly, these tumors exhibit increased EGF-receptor and p53 expression. In contrast, K-ras mutations could not be identified in these lesions [31]. Apart from these models, the overexpression of IL-6 or oncostatin M also leads to fibrosis and lymphocytic infiltration of the pancreas, pointing to a role for several cytokines and growth factors in the initiation and promotion of pancreatic fibrosis [38–41] (Table 3.6-3).

Molecular diagnosis of chronic pancreatitis

Epidemiological studies have revealed an increased risk of developing pancreatic cancer in patients with chronic pancreatitis. In a large study by Lowenfels et al. a 16-fold increased risk was reported for patients with a long history of chronic pancreatitis [42]. However, in an analysis by Karlson et al. the risk of developing pancreatic cancer in patients admitted to Swedish hospitals with the diagnosis pancreatitis was estimated to be only twofold increased [43]. However, most epidemiological studies are hampered by the missing histological verification of the disease. Nonetheless the epidemiological association seems to be well established and patients with chronic pancreatitis should undergo regular clinical follow-up to detect pancreatic cancer early.

The molecular analysis of pancreatic cancers has revealed a number of genetic and molecular alterations which occur in and contribute to the process of pancreatic carcinogenesis. Thus, pancreatic cancers frequently harbour mutations of the K-ras oncogene and overexpress a wide variety of growth factors and growth factor receptors [44, 45]. In addition, inactivation of several tumor suppressor genes, such as p53, p16 and Smad4, has been identified in the majority of pancreatic cancers [19, 46–48]. In contrast, inactivation of DNA repair enzymes and microsatellite instability seem to be less frequent in this type of malignancy. The analysis of the pancreatic parenchyma in chronic pancreatitis has revealed a number of molecular alterations which are also present in pancreatic cancer cells. The high frequency of K-ras gene mutations in pancreatic cancer cells has raised the hypothesis that this genetic marker might be useful to detect early pancreatic cancer in chronic pancreatitis. However, K-ras mutations are also present in preneoplastic lesions of the exocrine pancreas, and – even more important – in the normal ductal epithelium in pancreatic cancers [22–24]. Thus, K-ras gene mutations can be detected in papillary hyperplasia, mucinous hypertrophy, squamous metaplasia, and normal ducts [24]. Thus, the identification of K-ras gene mutations is of little help in the differentiation of pancreatic cancer in chronic pancreatitis. K-ras gene mutations have also been detected in the stool, serum and pancreatic juice of individuals with pancreatic cancer [49–52]. However, the high incidence of K-ras mutations in the samples obtained from patients with chronic pancreatitis along with the present data demonstrating a high frequency of K-ras gene mutations in non-malignant lesions of the exocrine pancreas indicate that K-ras gene mutations may not be a suitable marker for the differentiation of pancreatic cancer from chronic pancreatitis (Table 3.6-4).

The p53 tumor suppressor gene is mutated in the majority of epithelial cancers of the GI tract. Mutant p53 has an increased half-life which makes it suitable as a target for immunohistochemical analysis [19]. The p53 protein is important for regulation of the cell cycle and induction of apoptosis [53]. However, inactivation of the gene by point mutation leads to accumulation of an inactive protein in the nucleus. Loss of the remaining al-

Table 3.6-4. Clinical value of detection of molecular alterations in chronic pancreatitis.

Sample	CP	PaCa	Reference
Brush cytology			
Oxygen insensitivity test	0/11	28/28	Van Driel 1999
Pancreatic juice			
p53 overexpression	16/27	10/15	Maacke 1997
Duodenal juice			
K-ras mutations	20/54 (no cancer in follow-up)		Furuya 1997
K-ras mutations	1/29	10/19	Iguchi 1996
Serum			
p53 antibodies	0/11	8/29	Laurent 1995
increase in circulating p53	0/15	23/104	Suwa 1997
K-ras mutations	0/6	14/20	Theodor 1999
Stool			
K-ras mutations	2/5	7/36	Wenger 1999
K-ras mutations	1/3	6/11	Caldas 1994

lele has been detected in several cancer cell lines [54]. In pancreatic cancers p53 gene mutations are present in approximately 50% of cancers [19]. Mutations of the p53 gene are less frequent in chronic pancreatitis. Thus, in a series of 24 cases of chronic pancreatitis, no p53 gene mutation was detected [19], whereas in a series of 80 cases of chronic pancreatitis 8 genetic alterations of the p53 gene were detected [20]. Thus, this gene might be more valuable for the molecular differentiation of chronic pancreatitis from pancreatic cancer. Therefore, p53 alterations have been studied in various biological samples obtained from patients with chronic pancreatitis or pancreatic cancer. Thus, in pancreatic juice p53 gene mutations were identified in 11 of 26 pancreatic cancers, however in none of the chronic pancreatitis patients [52]. Furthermore, brush cytology was obtained from 53 patients with benign or malignant disease of the pancreas or associated regions. Using p53 immunocytology, alterations of the p53 gene were found in approximately 50% of the cancers, whereas none of the 3 chronic pancreatitis patients exhibited p53 gene mutations in the brush cytology obtained by ERCP [55]. Apart from pancreatic juice or cytology obtained directly from the pancreatic duct, p53 alterations have also been analyzed in the serum of patients with pancreatic cancer or chronic pancreatitis. In a study analyzing the circulating p53 protein in the serum of patients with pancreatic cancer, none of 15 patients with chronic pancreatitis exhibited increased values, in contrast to 23 of 104 pancreatic cancer patients [56]. Furthermore, p53 antibodies were detected only in patients with pancreatic cancer, but not in patients with chronic pancreatitis [57] (Table 3.6-4). Thus, from these analyses, identifying p53 gene alterations in tissue samples or fluids from patients with chronic pancreatitis may be more suitable for the exclusion of pancreatic cancer than analyzing K-ras gene mutations.

Recently other markers have also been evaluated. Thus, the tumor suppressor gene p16 is inactivated in the majority of pancreatic cancers [46], whereas in chronic pancreatitis only 1 of 20 cases harboured a p16 gene alteration [58]. In addition, measuring the oxygen insensitivity of brush cytology specimens in patients with chronic pancreatitis or pancreatic cancer has proven to be a valuable tool for the differentiation of chronic pancreatitis from pancreatic cancer [59] (Table 3.6-4).

Conclusion

The molecular analysis of pancreatic cancers has revealed a number of genetic and molecular alterations which are present in pancreatic carcinogenesis. In recent years K-ras gene mutations have also been identified in the pancreatic parenchyma in patients with chronic pancreatitis and pancreatic preneoplastic lesions. Thus, the detection of K-ras gene mutations is not suitable for the differentiation of chronic pancreatitis from pancreatic cancer. However, recent studies point to a major role for p53 as a molecular marker for pancreatic cancer. Several small studies have indicated that it may be helpful to analyse the p53 gene in fluids taken from patients with suspected pancreatic cancer or chronic pancreatitis. In addition, new data also support a role for the oxygen insensitivity assay for the differentation of benign inflammatory from malignant disease of the pancreas.

Acknowledgements

Supported in part by DFG, DAAD, Rudolf-Bartling-Stiftung, Pinguin-Stiftung and Matthias-Lackas-Stiftung.

References

1. Beger HG, Büchler MW, Ditschuneit H, Malfertheiner P. Chronic Pancreatitis. Berlin: Springer-Verlag, 1990.
2. DiMagno EP, Layer P, Clain JE. Chronic Pancreatitis. In: Go VLW, ed. The Pancreas, Pathology and Disease. New York: Raven Press, 1993: 665–706.
3. Lankisch PG, Lohr-Happe A, Otto J, Creutzfeldt W. Natural course in chronic pancreatitis. Digestion 1993; 54: 145–55.
4. Oertel JE, Heffess CS, Oertel YC. Pancreas. In: Sternberg SS, ed. Diagnostic surgical pathology. New York: Raven Press, 1993: 57–93.
5. Elsässer HP, Adler G, Kern HF. Fibroblast structure and function during regeneration from hormone-induced acute pancreatitis in the rat. Pancreas 1989; 4: 169–78.
6. Morgenroth K. Pathologie der chronischen Pankreatitis. In: Mössner J, Adler G, Fölsch UR, Singer MV, eds. Erkrankungen des exkretorischen Pankreas. Jena: Gustav-Fischer-Verlag, 1995: 325–33.
7. Stolte M. Chronische Pankreatitis. Verh Dtsch Ges Path 1987; 71: 24–33.
8. Sarles H, Bernard JP, Gullo L. Pathogenesis of chronic pancreatitis. Gut 1990; 31: 629–32.
9. Mössner J, Adler G, Fölsch UR, Singer MV, eds. Erkrankungen des exkretorischen Pankreas. Jena: Gustav-Fischer-Verlag, 1995.
10. Steer ML, Waxman I, Freedman S. Chronic pancreatitis. N Engl J Med 1995; 332: 1482–90.
11. Giorgi D, Bernard JP, Rouquier S, Iovanna J, Sarles H, Dagorn JC. Secretory pancreatic stone protein messenger RNA. Nucleotide sequence and expression in chronic calcifying pancreatitis. J Clin Invest 1989; 84: 100–6.
12. Adler G, Schmid RM. Chronic pancreatitis: still puzzling? Gastroenterology 1997; 112: 1762–5.
13. Ebert M, Kasper HU, Hernberg S, Friess H, Büchler MW, Roessner A, Korc M, Malfertheiner P. Overexpression of platelet-derived growth factor (PDGF) B chain and type b PDGF receptor in human chronic pancreatitis. Dig Dis Sci 1998; 43: 567–74.
14. Saurer L, Reber P, Schaffner T, Büchler MW, Buri C, Kappeler A, Walz A, Friess H, Müller C. Differential expression of chemokines in normal pancreas and in chronic pancreatitis. Gastroenterology 2000; 118: 356–67.
15. Bockman DE, Merlino G. Cytological changes in the pancreas of transgenic mice overexpressing transforming growth factor-alpha. Gastroenterology 1992; 103: 1883–92.
16. Sanvito F, Nichols A, Herrera PL, Huarte J, Wohlwend A, Vassalli JD, Orci L. TGF-b1 overexpression in murine pancreas induces chronic pancreatitis and, together with TNF-alpha, triggers insulin-dependent diabetes. Biochem Biophys Res Comm 1995; 217: 1279–86.
17. Whitcomb DC. Hereditary pancreatitis: new insights into acute and chronic pancreatitis. Gut 1999; 45: 317–22.
18. Sharer N, Schwarz M, Malone G, Howarth A, Painter J, Super M, Braganza J. Mutations of the cystic fibrosis gene in patients with chronic pancreatitis. N Engl J Med 1998; 339: 645–52.
19. Casey G, Kobrin MS, Yamanaka Y, Friess H, Kobrin MS, Lopez ME, Büchler MW, Beger HG, Korc M. p53 mutations are common in pancreatic cancer and are absent in chronic pancreatitis. Cancer Lett 1993; 69: 151–60.
20. Gansauge S, Schmid RM, Muller J, Adler G, Mattfeldt T, Beger HG. Genetic alterations in chronic pancreatitis: evidence for early occurence of p53 but not K-ras mutations. Br J Surg 1998; 85: 337–40.
21. Ebert M, Yokoyama M, Kobrin MS, Friess H, Büchler MW, Korc M. Increased MDM2 expression and immunoreactivity in human pancreatic ductal adenocarcinoma. Int J Oncol 1994; 5: 1279–84.
22. Furuya N, Kawa S, Akamatsu T, Furihata K. Long-term follow-up of patients with chronic pancreatitis and K-ras gene mutation detected in pancreatic juice. Gastroenterology 1997; 113: 593–8.
23. Tada M, Ohashi M, Shiratori Y, Okudaira T, Komatsu Y, Kawabe T, Yoshida H, Machinami R, Kishi K, Omata M. Analysis of K-ras gene mutation in hyperplastic duct cells of the pancreas without pancreatic disease. Gastroenterology 1996; 110: 227–31.

24. Lüttges J, Schlehe B, Menke MA, Vogel I, Henne-Bruns D, Kloppel G. The K-ras mutation pattern in pancreatic ductal adenocarcinoma usually is identical to that in associated normal, hyperplastic, and metaplastic ductal epithelium. Cancer 1999; 85: 1703–10.
25. Ebert M, Yokoyama M, Kobrin MS, Friess H, Lopez ME, Büchler MW, Johnson GR, Korc M. Induction and expression of amphiregulin in human pancreatic cancer. Cancer Res 1994; 54: 3959–62.
26. Ebert M, Yokoyama M, Friess H, Büchler MW, Korc M. Coexpression of the c-met protooncogene and hepatocyte growth factor in human pancreatic cancer. Cancer Res 1994; 54: 5775–8.
27. Ebert M, Yokoyama M, Friess H, Kobrin MS, Büchler MW, Korc M. Induction of platelet-derived growth factor A and B chains and overexpression of their receptors in human pancreatic cancer. Int J Cancer 1995; 62: 529–35.
28. Van Laethem JL, Deviere J, Resibois A, Rickaert F, Vertongen P, Ohtani H, Cremer M, Miyazono K, Robberecht P. Localisation of transforming growth factor β1 and its latent binding protein in human chronic pancreatitis. Gastroenterology 1995; 108: 1873–81.
29. Van Laethem JL, Robberecht P, Resibois A, Deviere J. Transforming growth factor promotes development of fibrosis after repeated courses of acute pancreatitis. Gastroenterology 1996; 110: 576–82.
30. Menke A, Yamaguchi H, Gress TM, Adler G. Extracellular matrix is reduced by inhibition of transforming growth factor β1 in pancreatitis in the rat. Gastroenterology 1997; 113: 295–303.
31. Wagner M, Lührs H, Klöppel G, Adler G, Schmid RM. Malignant transformation of duct-like cells originating from acini in transforming growth factor alpha transgenic mice. Gastroenterology 1998; 115: 1254–62.
32. Apte MV, Haber PS, Darby SJ, Rodgers SC, McCaughan GW, Korsten MA, Pirola RC, Wilson JS. Pancreatic stellate cells are activated by proinflammatory cytokines: implications for pancreatic fibrogenesis. Gut 1999; 44: 534–41.
33. Lüttenberger T, Schmid-Kotsas A, Menke A, Siech M, Beger H, Adler G, Grünert A, Bachem MG. Platelet-derived growth factors stimulate proliferation and extracellular matrix synthesis of pancreatic stellate cells: implications in pathogenesis of pancreatic fibrosis. Lab Invest 2000; 80: 47–55.
34. Jalleh RP, Gilbertson JA, Williamson RCN, Slater SD, Foster CD. Expression of major histocompatibility antigens in human chronic pancreatitis. Gut 1993; 34: 1452–7.
35. Ebert MPA, Ademmer K, Müller-Ostermeyer F, Friess H, Büchler MW, Schubert W, Malfertheiner P. CD8+CD103+ T cell analogous to intestinal intraepithelial lymphocytes infiltrate the pancreas in chronic pancreatitis. Am J Gastroenterol 1998; 93: 2141–7.
36. Hunger RE, Mueller C, Zgraggen K, Friess H, Büchler MW. Cytotoxic cells are activated in cellular infiltrates of alcoholic chronic pancreatitis. Gastroenterology 1997; 112: 1656–63.
37. Di Sebastiano P, Fink T, Weihe E, Friess H, Innocenti P, Beger HG, Büchler MW. Immune cell infiltration and growth-associated protein 43 expression correlate with pain in chronic pancreatitis. Gastroenterology 1997; 112: 1648–55.
38. Lee MS, Gu D, Feng L, Curriden S, Arnush M, Krahl T, Gurushanthaiah D, Wilson C, Loskutoff DL, Fox H, Sarvetnick N. Accumulation of extracellular matrix and developmental dysregulation in the pancreas by transgenic production of transforming growth factor b1. Am J Pathol 1995; 147: 42–52.
39. Bamber B, Reife RA, Haugen HS, Clegg CH. Oncostatin M stimulates excessive extracellular matrix accumulation in a transgenic mouse model of connective tissue disease. J Mol Med 1998; 76: 61–9.
40. Campbell IL, Hobbs MV, Dockter J, Oldstone MBA, Allison J. Islet inflammation and hyperplasia induced by the pancreatic islet-specific overexpression of interleukin-6 in transgenic mice. Am J Pathol 1994; 145: 157–66.
41. Vallance BA, Hewlett BR, Snider DP, Collins SM. T cell-mediated exocrine pancreatic damage in major histocompatibility complex class II-deficient mice. Gastroenterology 1998; 115: 978–87.

42. Lowenfels AB, Maisonneuve P, Cavallini G, Ammann RW, Lankisch PG, Andersen JR, DiMagno EP, Andren-Sandberg A, Domellof L. Pancreatitis and the risk of pancreatic cancer. International Pancreatitis Study Group. N Engl J Med 1993; 328: 1433–7.
43. Karlsson BM, Ekbom A, Josefsson S, McLaughlin JK, Fraumeni JF, Nyren O. The risk of pancreatic cancer following pancreatitis: an association due to confounding? Gastroenterology 1997; 113: 587–92.
44. Almoguera C, Shibata D, Forrester K, Martin J, Perucho M. Most human carcinomas of the exocrine pancreas contain mutant c-K-ras genes. Cell 1988; 53: 549–54.
45. Korc M. Role of growth factors in pancreatic cancer. Surg Oncol Clin NA 1998; 7: 25–41.
46. Caldas C, Hahn SA, da Costa LT, Redston MS, Schutte M, Seymour AB, Weinstein CL, Hruban RH, Yeo CJ, Kern SE. Frequent somatic mutations and homozygous deletions of the p16 (MTS1) gene in pancreatic adenocarcinoma. Nat Genet 1994; 8: 27–32.
47. Simon B, Weinel R, Höhne M, Watz J, Schmidt J, Körtner G, Arnold R. Frequent alterations of the tumor suppressor genes p53 and DCC in human pancreatic carcinoma. Gastroenterology 1994; 106: 1645–51.
48. Hahn SA, Schutte M, Shansul Hoque ATM, Moskoluk CA, da Costa LI, Rozenblum E, Weinstein CL, Fischer A, Yeo CJ, Hruban RH, Kern SE. DPC4, a candidate tumor suppressor gene at human chromosome 18q21.1. Science 1996; 271: 350–3.
49. Caldas C, Hahn SA; Hruban RH, Redston MS, Yeo CJ, Kern SE. Detection of K-ras mutations in the stool of patients with pancreatic adenocarcinoma and pancreatic ductal hyperplasia. Cancer Res.1994; 54: 3568–73.
50. Theodor L, Melzer E, Sologov M, Idelmann G, Friedman E, Bar-Meir S. Detection of pancreatic carcinoma: diagnostic value of K-ras mutations in circulating DNA from serum. Dig Dis Sci 1999; 44: 2014–9.
51. Wenger FA, Zieren J, Peter FJ, Jacobi CA, Muller JM. K-ras mutations in tissue and stool samples from patients with pancreatic cancer and chronic pancreatitis. Langenbecks Arch Surg 1999; 384: 181–6.
52. Yamaguchi Y, Watanabe H, Yrdiran S, Ohtsubo K, Motoo Y, Okai T, Sawabu N. Detection of mutations of p53 tumor suppressor gene in pancreatic juice and its application to diagnosis of patients with pancreatic cancer: comparison with K-ras mutations. Clin Cancer Res 1999; 5: 1147–53.
53. Lane DP. Cancer, p53, guardian of the genome? Nature 1992; 358: 15–6.
54. Kalthoff H, Schmiegel W, Roeder C, Kasche D, Schmidt A, Lauer G, Thiele HG, Honold G, Pantel K, Riethmüller G, Scherer E, Maurer J, Maacke H, Deppert W. P53 and K-ras alterations in pancreatic epithelial cell lesions. Oncogene 1993; 8: 289–93.
55. Tascilar M, Surm PD, Caspers E, Smit M, Polak MM, Huibregtse K, Noordyn LA, Offerhaus GJ. Diagnostic p53 immunostaining of endobiliary brush cytology: preoperative cytology compared with the surgical specimen. Cancer 1999; 87: 306–11.
56. Suwa H, Ohshio G, Okada N, Wang Z, Fukumoto M, Imamura T, Imamura M. Clinical significance of serum p53 antigen in patients with pancreatic carcinomas. Gut 1997; 40: 647–53.
57. Laurent-Puig P, Lubin R, Semhoun-Ducloux S, Pelletier G, Fourre C, Ducreux M, Briantais MJ, Buffet C, Soussi T. Antibodies against p53 protein in serum of patients with benign or malignant pancreatic and biliary diseases. Gut 1995; 36: 455–8.
58. Hu YX, Watanabe H, Ohtsubo K, Yamaguchi Y, Ha A, Okai T, Swabu N. Frequent loss of p16 expression and its correlation with clinicopathological parameters in pancreatic carcinoma. Clin Cancer Res 1997; 3: 1473–7.
59. Van Driel BEM, Van Gulik TM, Sturm PDJ, Johan G, Offerhaus JA, Gouma DJ, Van Noorden CJF. Differential diagnosis of chronic pancreatitis and pancreatic cancer in brush cytology specimens. Cancer Res 1999; 59: 5732–6.

4 Chronic pancreatitis: The role of nerves and neuroimmune interaction

4.1 Morphology of pancreatic nerves in health and disease

D. E. Bockman

Introduction

The pancreas is well innervated. Nervous control is exerted over the smooth muscle in the blood vessels of the pancreas. Nerves participate in the control of secretion of digestive enzymes. Furthermore, they are positioned to be involved in the control of the endocrine pancreas.

Under normal conditions, activity in the pancreas does not enter consciousness. Although there are afferent nerves associated with the pancreas, they are said to remain silent because their activity is not perceived. It takes different or greatly increased stimulation to bring about firing of the nerves sufficient to cause sensation. Pancreatic diseases are capable of achieving this level of stimulation, and the result is perceived as pain.

Nerves are affected by different pancreatic diseases including diabetes, acute and chronic pancreatitis, and pancreatic cancer. The mechanisms by which nerves are affected by these diseases are varied, and are poorly understood. An attempt is made in this chapter to outline the nature and organization of the nerves serving the pancreas, and to suggest some ways that different disease states affect them.

Organization of pancreatic nerves

The pancreas is served by motor and sensory nerve fibers that travel in the splanchnic and vagus nerves. Nerves serving the pancreas pass through the celiac plexus, but only one set of nerve fibers forms synapses there. Motor nerve fibers (sympathetic fibers) originating from the intermediolateral cell column of the spinal cord synapse in the celiac ganglia. Postsynaptic fibers enter the pancreas. A significant proportion of the nerve endings from this source is found in association with the smooth muscle cells of blood vessels.

The other nerve fibers, motor fibers in the vagus (parasympathetic), and afferent fibers in both the splanchnic and vagus nerves, pass through the celiac ganglion without synapse. The parasympathetic fibers synapse on the cell bodies of ganglia within the pancreas. Fibers extending from these intrinsic ganglia terminate within the pancreas in the neighborhood of acinar cells and islet cells.

Afferent fibers traveling in the vagus nerve reach from pancreas to brain. Their cell bodies are located in the jugular or nodose ganglia of the vagus.

Afferent fibers traveling in the splanchnic nerves reach from the pancreas to the dorsal horn of the spinal cord. They traverse the sympathetic chain. Their cell bodies are in the dorsal root ganglia at thoracic levels five through nine. It is these fibers that are thought to carry the nervous impulses that are interpreted as pain originating in the pancreas. Nerve tracts within the central nervous system conduct the impulses to a region of the brain where the pain is perceived. Synaptic transmission from pain receptors to dorsal horn neurons is mediated by glutamate and peptide transmitters, including substance P.

It is the dorsal root ganglion neurons with bare nerve endings that mediate painful sensations. The terminals of the peripheral branch of these axons are sensitive to noxious or tissue-damaging stimuli.

Distribution to the pancreas is from both right and left sides. Approaching the pancreas from the celiac plexus, pancreatic nerves come into intimate contact with the celiac and superior mesenteric arteries. They are distributed along these arteries and along the smaller arteries that branch from them to supply the pancreas. Nerves that supply the pancreatic parenchyma separate from arterioles to distribute in the connective tissue and terminate as free nerve endings.

Nerves within the pancreas are microscopic, in contrast to the large nerves that supply, for example, the muscles of the extremities. Nerves within the pancreas are mainly unmyelinated, while the large nerves have mainly myelinated fibers. Afferent impulses are transmitted from the pancreas through the splanchnic nerves via small myelinated and unmyelinated fibers.

Intrapancreatic nerves, although mainly unmyelinated, are not without protection during most of their course. The nerve fibers are surrounded singly or in groups by Schwann cells. The collections of nerve fibers that form a nerve are surrounded by a sheath of flattened epithelioid cells that form the perineurium. The perineurium commonly is formed by two or three layers of perineurial cells. The cells in each layer are connected to each other at their periphery by tight junctions. A basal lamina frequently is present immediately outside and inside each layer of perineurial cells. Thus a perineurium consisting of three layers of cells would also have six basal laminae. Material exchanged between the interior of the nerve and the surrounding extracellular matrix would traverse three layers of cells, six basal laminae, plus intermediate layers of connective tissue. This arrangement provides a formidable barrier capable of maintaining a specialized microenvironment around the nerve fibers contained within the pancreatic nerves.

Generation of pain signals in the nerves

Persistent pain can be described as nociceptive or neuropathic. Nociceptive pain results from the direct activation of nociceptors (pain receptors) in response to tissue injury. Accompanying inflammation can contribute to the generation of pain. For example, a tumor that invades soft tissue may cause damage that results in severe nociceptive pain. The pain that accompanies arthritis would be described as nociceptive.

Neuropathic pains result from direct injury to nerves. An example of a neuropathic pain is postherpetic neuralgia, a severe pain that occurs in some patients after a bout of herpes zoster (shingles) in which there is inflammation of ganglia and dorsal nerve roots as a result of varicella-zoster virus.

Tissue damage, leakage and hemorrhage, and products of inflammatory cells likely cause extreme stimulation of visceral afferent fibers. Substance P is released from small, unmyelinated fibers in response to tissue injury or to intense stimulation of nerves. Calcitonin gene-related peptide similarly is released from sensory endings in response to injury. Both substance P and calcitonin gene-related peptide may contribute to the spread of edema by acting directly on venules to produce vasodilation. Inflammation mediated by neural activity is referred to as neurogenic inflammation. The sensitization of nociceptors after injury or inflammation results from the release of a variety of chemicals by the damaged cells and tissues in the vicinity of the injury. These substances include bradykinin, histamine, prostaglandins, leukotrienes, acetylcholine, serotonin, and substance P. The substances act to decrease the threshold for activation of nociceptors. Some activate nociceptors.

It is not known precisely how noxious stimuli generate action potentials. However, they must be able to cause a depolarizing electrical potential through interaction with the membrane of the afferent neuron.

The nociceptors in the pancreas are said to be silent. They normally are not activated by noxious stimulation. However, inflammation can make them more susceptible to the generation of action potentials.

Firing in pain fibers may be initiated by distention, stretching, noxious stimuli, hypoxia and changes in pH [10, 11, 15]. Elevated pressures, which would lead to some of these stimuli, have been demonstrated in the ducts and tissue of patients with chronic pancreatitis [3, 7]. Experimental studies confirm the relationship of ductal pressure with tissue pressure [9, 13] and procedures that relieve ductal pressure frequently are followed by improvement in pain. However, a study indicated that pancreatic parenchymal pressure, although correlated with ductal changes, is not closely related to the pain score in chronic pancreatitis [12].

Alteration of nerves in diabetes

Common complications of diabetes mellitus include alterations of blood vessels and of nerves. The latter complication, diabetic neuropathy, is characterized by changes in larger, myelinated nerves. Nerve degeneration is common in the extremities. Both sensory and motor fibers may be affected. Pain and numbness as well as motor deficits can result. Autonomic fibers may be involved.

Vascular changes include marked thickening and duplication of the basal lamina. In the larger nerves, these vascular changes are observed in the blood vessels in the connective tissue epineurium and in some of the vessels that penetrate into the nerve.

Thickening of the basal laminae of the perineurium also has been described in patients with peripheral neuropathy [8]. Interchange of material between the interior of nerves and the surrounding extracellular matrix takes place through the perineurial cells and the basal laminae that lie on each side of each layer of cells. Thickened basal laminae could therefore affect this transmission. Moreover, transmission between the nerve and the bloodstream would be affected by the thickened and duplicated basal lamina of the blood vessels.

The situation in acute pancreatitis

The nature and extent of changes in the pancreas differs with the change from mild to severe acute pancreatitis. Mild pancreatitis may involve mainly alteration of the vascular system with the development of edema, increasing pressure, and some infiltration of acute inflammatory cells. With severe disease, there is considerable breakdown of pancreatic tissue accompanied by necrosis, marked inflammation and hemorrhage. The increased pressure due to edema is thus accompanied by a multitude of biologically active molecules that are added to the extracellular matrix, setting the stage for generation of nociceptive pain.

While acute pancreatitis is present, the free endings of pancreatic nerves are susceptible to the noxious substances present in their environment. Action potentials could be generated in sensory fibers traveling in the splanchnic nerves as a result of the attack by these substances. This activity is in addition to the action potentials that might be initiated by stretching due to increased pressure and ischemia due to decreased blood flow resulting from the pressure.

Alteration of nerves in chronic pancreatitis

Foci of chronic inflammatory cells sometimes are intimately associated with nerves in chronic pancreatitis, as illustrated in Figure 4.1-1. The affinity of lymphoid cells is not limited to nerves proper, but also extends to the cell bodies in pancreatic ganglia (Fig. 4.1-2). Lymphoid cells and macrophages are most numerous in these foci, but polymorphonuclear neutrophils and other granulocytes may be present.

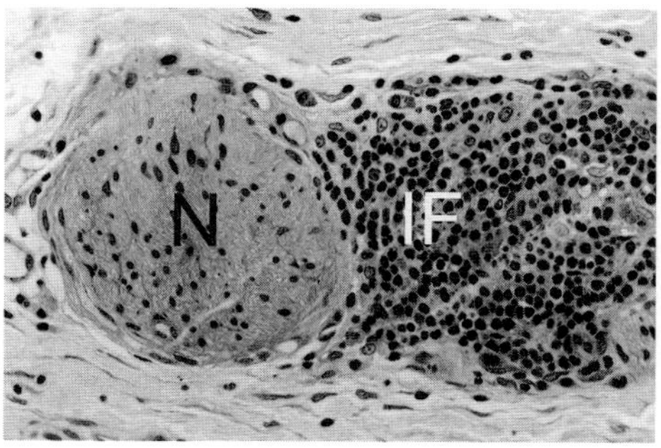

Figure 4.1-1. A histological section from the wall of the main pancreatic duct from a patient with chronic pancreatitis illustrates the intimate association of an inflammatory focus (IF) with a nerve (N).

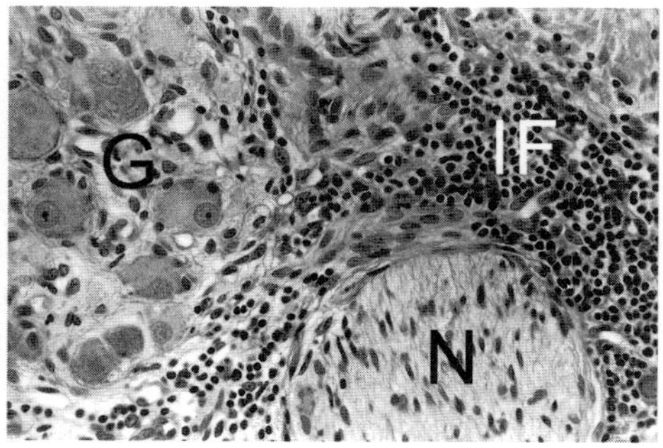

Figure 4.1-2. An inflammatory focus (IF) in the pancreas from a patient with chronic pancreatitis. The inflammatory cells are associated with a nerve (N) and with a pancreatic ganglion (G).

Lymphoid cells in foci include T cells [5, 6] and natural killer cells. Different subpopulations of T cells are found, including those positive for CD4 (indicating helper T cells) and CD8 (indicating cytotoxic T cells). A population of natural killer cells is positive for CD57. Antibody to CD57 was used to localize the cells in Figure 4.1-3, which reveals a large population of cells that are positive for this antigen. It is interesting that natural killer cells are a good source of transforming growth factor beta, which induces fibrosis. The accumulation of these cells suggests cell-mediated cytotoxicity is involved in chronic pancreatitis, including the effect on nerves.

Study of the relationship of chronic inflammatory foci and nerves in tissue from patients with chronic pancreatitis has revealed that the perineurium, which normally forms a barrier between the nerve proper and the external environment, may be damaged [1]. There may be neural edema and damage to nerve fibers and Schwann cells. The lack of the perineurial barrier renders the nerves susceptible to stimulation by any of the noxious

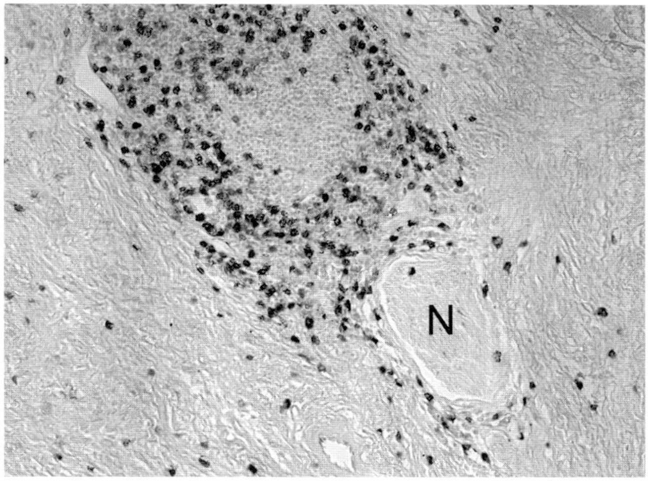

Figure 4.1-3. An inflammatory focus adjacent to a nerve (N). A population of natural killer cells is positive for CD57. The section has been treated with antibody to CD57. The darkly stained cells are positive for this antigen.

substances that are present in the extracellular matrix. Because there is direct damage to the nerve, pain resulting from this process is described as neuropathic.

Thus it may be seen that direct nerve damage may be added to the other possible mechanisms for generation of pain during chronic pancreatitis, including ischemia, increased pressure, and nociceptive pain due to tissue destruction and intense stimulation of free nerve endings by noxious substances.

It is also possible, since pancreatic nerves are mixed motor and sensory, that the neuropathic mechanisms can cause increased stimulation of motor nerves, thus causing hyperstimulation of the cells affected by the motor fibers.

Interaction of pancreatic cancer with nerves

Pancreatic adenocarcinoma has an affinity for nerves in and around the pancreas. A common pathway taken by pancreatic cancer out of the pancreas is along nerves that supply the organ. Previous assumptions about the cancer growing through lymphatic vessels located around nerves have proven not to be true. The cancer may to some extent follow a path of least resistance in the interval around nerves. However, this is by no means the extent of the relationship between pancreatic cancer and nerves.

Examination of sections of the pancreas from patients with pancreatic cancer frequently will reveal not only an intimate relationship between adenocarcinoma and nerves (Fig. 4.1-4), but also a distortion and alteration of the nerves themselves. Extensions from the adenocarcinoma approach nerves, damage the perineurium surrounding them, then replace the perineurium to lie adjacent to the nerve fibers with no cellular layers intervening [2]. The cancer may extend into the nerve proper, distorting and damaging it. There may be simultaneous appearance of chronic inflammation (Fig. 4.1-5), adding all of the possible pain-causing stimuli discussed for chronic pancreatitis to the damage caused by the cancer.

It is likely that numerous cell-signaling mechanisms are involved in the attraction between pancreatic nerves and pancreatic cancer. One that has been suggested is an interaction of transforming growth factor alpha and epidermal growth factor receptor [2].

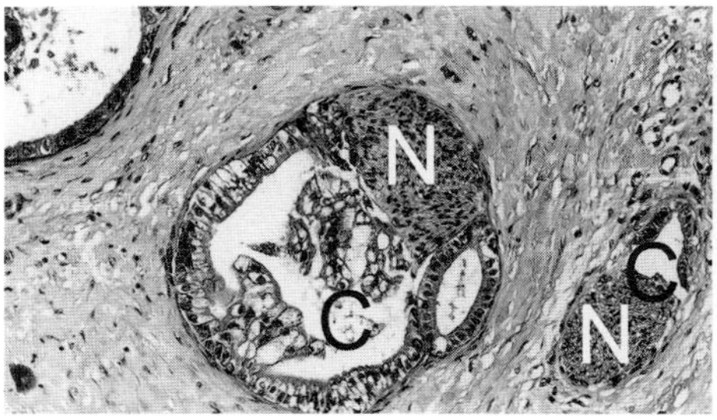

Figure 4.1-4. Section from a patient with pancreatic cancer. The cancer (C) is in intimate association with pancreatic nerves (N).

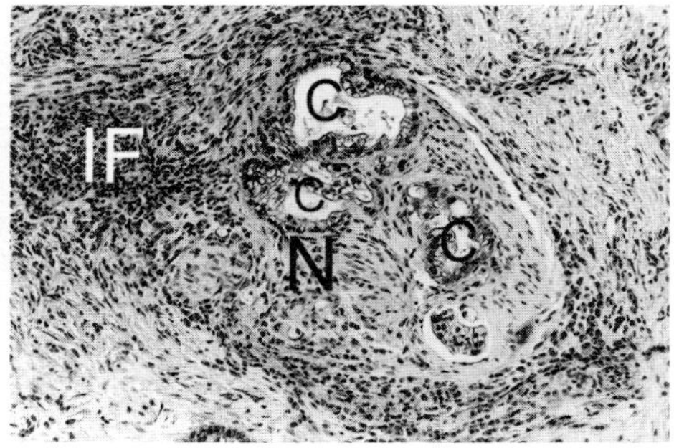

Figure 4.1-5. In this section a pancreatic nerve (N) has been invaded by pancreatic cancer (C). In addition, the nerve is associated with and partially surrounded by an inflammatory focus (IF).

Pancreatic cancer cells overexpress the receptor for epidermal growth factor, which is the receptor activated by transforming growth factor alpha. Pancreatic nerves were shown to be a source of transforming growth factor alpha. It was suggested, therefore, that the nerves supply a factor that provides a growth advantage for the cancer, thus encouraging growth along and into the nerves. As this happens, the perineurium and nerve fibers are damaged, a process that would seem to be an obvious way to initiate and sustain pain.

Conclusion

The pancreas is served by a network of microscopic nerves that, under conditions of health, silently regulate the circulation of blood as well as the secretion by exocrine and endocrine cells. Both sensory and motor fibers are contained within the nerves. The nerves are resistant to damage, due in part to a protective layer, the perineurium. They have been demonstrated to remain and even increase while other pancreatic elements are degenerating. However, under the conditions of pancreatic disease, including acute and chronic pancreatitis, and pancreatic cancer, the silent sensory nerves are stimulated to produce action potentials that are relayed to the central nervous system and interpreted as pain. Noxious substances derived from tissue breakdown and inflammation in the extracellular matrix act on free nerve endings to initiate these impulses. Pressure due to edema and changes in pH due to ischemia can lead to the same result. In addition, the nerves may be damaged directly by chronic inflammation and through the invasion by cancer cells. These neuropathic mechanisms must be included in the explanation of chronic pain generation resulting from pancreatic disease.

References

1. Bockman DE, Büchler MW, Malfertheiner P, Beger HG. Analysis of nerves in chronic pancreatitis. Gastroenterology 1988; 94: 1459–69.
2. Bockman DE, Büchler MW, Beger HG. Interaction of pancreatic ductal carcinoma with nerves leads to nerve damage. Gastroenterology 1994; 107: 219–30.
3. Bradley EL III. Pancreatic duct pressure in chronic pancreatitis. Am J Surg 1982; 144: 313–6.

4. Ebbehöj N, Borly L, Bülow J, Rasmussen SG, Madsen P, Matzen P, Owre A. Pancreatic tissue fluid pressure in chronic pancreatitis. Relation to pain, morphology, and function. Scand J Gastroenterol 1990; 25: 1046–51.
5. Ebert MP, Ademmer K, Müller-Ostermeyer F, Friess H, Büchler MW, Schubert W, Malfertheiner P. $CD8^+CD103^+$ T cells analogous to intestinal intraepithelial lymphocytes infiltrate the pancreas in chronic pancreatitis. Am J Gastroenterol 1998; 93: 2141–7.
6. Emmrich J, Weber I, Nausch M, Sparmann G, Koch K, Seyfarth M, Lohr M, Liebe S. Immunohistochemical characterization of the pancreatic cellular infiltrate in normal pancreas, chronic pancreatitis and pancreatic carcinoma. Digestion 1998; 59: 192–8.
7. Jalleh RP, Aslam M, Williamson RC. Pancreatic tissue and ductal pressures in chronic pancreatitis. Br J Surg 1991; 78: 1235–7.
8. Johnson PC, Brendel K, Meezan E. Human diabetic perineurial cell basement membrane thickening. Lab Invest 1981; 44: 265–70.
9. Karanjia ND, Singh SM, Widdison AL, Lutrin FJ, Reber HA. Pancreatic ductal and interstitial pressures in cats with chronic pancreatitis. Dig Dis Sci 1992; 37: 268–73.
10. Klöppel G. Pathology of chronic pancreatitis and pancreatic pain. Acta Chir Scand 1990; 156: 261–5.
11. Longhurst JC, Dittman LE. Hypoxia, bradykinin and prostaglandins stimulate ischemically sensitive visceral afferents. Am J Physiol 1987; 253: H556–67.
12. Manes G, Büchler MW, Pieramico O, DiSebastiano P, Malfertheiner P. Is increased pancreatic pressure related to pain in chronic pancreatitis? Int J Pancreatol 1994; 15: 113–7.
13. Patel AG, Toyama MT, Ashley SW, Benjamin IS, Reber HA. Duct decompression in chronic pancreatitis: effects on blood flow and interstitial pH. Brit J Surg 1994; 81: 1816.
14. Raddawi HM, Geenen JE, Hogan WJ, Dodds WJ, Venu RP, Johnson GK. Pressure measurements from biliary and pancreatic segments of sphincter of Oddi: comparison between patients with functional abdominal pain, biliary, or pancreatic disease. Dig Dis Sci 1991; 36: 71–4.
15. Stahl GL, Longhurst JC. Ischemically sensitive visceral afferents: importance of H^+ derived from lactic acid and hypercapnia. Am J Physiol 1992; 262: H748–53.

4.2 Neurotransmitters and nerve growth factors in chronic pancreatitis

H. Friess, S. Shrikhande, M. W. Büchler

Introduction

The typical histomorphological features of chronic pancreatitis (CP) are fibrosis replacing the exocrine pancreatic parenchyma and various degrees of pancreatic calcification [1–3]. Other common features include various inflammatory cell infiltrates, acinar cell degeneration and some degree of ductal cell proliferation [2, 4, 5]. The ongoing pancreatic destruction leads to varying degrees of maldigestion and in advanced stages even to endocrine deficiency. The other clinically relevant feature of CP is abdominal pain that is usually recurrent and occurs in 80–90% of patients [1].

Pathogenesis of pain in CP

Increased intraductal pressure as a result of single or multiple strictures and/or calculi is believed to be a common cause of pain in patients with a dilated main pancreatic duct disease and relief from pain by drainage of a dilated main pancreatic duct is often seen [6, 7]. The other suggested causes of pain have been duodenal and common bile duct stenosis due to ongoing pancreatic inflammation and subsequent scarring [8]. Additionally, pancreatic fibrosis, interstitial hypertension and pancreatic ischemia have all been implicated either as sole or as additional factors involved in the pathogenesis of pain [9, 10].

Molecular pathogenesis of pain

The most recent concept of pathogenesis of pain in CP postulates alterations in pancreatic nerves and neuroimmune interactions as crucial factors in the development of the pain syndrome [11, 12]. Pancreatic nerves are preferentially retained while the pancreatic parenchyma degenerates and is replaced by fibrotic tissue. The innervation area per nerve is reduced, the diameter of nerves is increased, their perineurium damaged and inflammatory cells are concentrated around intrapancreatic nerves [13]. Growth-associated protein-43 (GAP-43) is up-regulated in pancreatic nerves, suggesting that pancreatic nerves grow actively in the chronically inflamed pancreas. Furthermore, active nerve growth in CP has been correlated with the severity of abdominal pain in CP patients. This is considered to be indirect evidence for the high activation state of both the intrinsic and extrinsic nervous system in the course of painful CP [11]. Concomitantly, along with the nerve changes, pain neurotransmitters such as substance P (SP) and calcitonin gene-related peptide (CGRP) are also increased in the enlarged nerve fibers of CP patients [14]. While these observations appear to indicate that alterations in neural structures contribute significantly to the pain syndrome of patients with CP, they raise important questions regarding factors promoting nerve growth in CP and the targets for neurotransmitters in the chronically inflamed pancreas.

Nerve growth factor (NGF) and its receptor (TrkA) in CP

Nerve growth factor belongs to the neurotrophin (NT) family, which also includes brain-derived neurotrophic factor and NT-3, -4, -5, and -6 [15–18]. NGF plays a role in neuroblast proliferation and neuronal maturation, affecting the neuronal phenotype and maintaining neuronal survival [15–18]. Since it has been suggested that NGF and TrkA might augment chronic pain and the inflammatory reaction in certain chronic inflammatory conditions, and in view of the pronounced neural changes in CP, our group sought to investigate the expression of NGF and TrkA in CP and correlate the molecular findings with clinical parameters [19]. By a combination of modern molecular biology techniques, it was observed that NGF and TrkA mRNA expression was significantly ($p < 0.01$) increased in CP [19]. *In situ* hybridization revealed enhanced NGF mRNA signals in ductal complexes, degenerating acinar cells and acinar cells de-differentiating into tubular structures (Fig. 4.2-1C). Enhanced TrkA mRNA expression was noted in the perineurium of enlarged pancreatic nerves of CP patients (Fig. 4.2-1F). Concomitant increased NGF and TrkA mRNA expression was also observed in the intrapancreatic ganglia and in blood vessels of CP patients.

Immunohistochemical analysis (Figure 4.2-2) showed findings similar to those of *in situ* hybridization. These interesting molecular findings were correlated with clinical data (Table 4.2-1). While there was a positive correlation between NGF mRNA expression levels and the degree of pancreatic fibrosis, the degree of acinar cell damage and the degree of ductal metaplasia, TrkA mRNA expression levels correlated with the intensity of pain [19]. Thus it appears that nerve growth and other morphological changes of CP might be influenced by activation of the NGF/TrkA pathway through autocrine and paracrine mechanisms. NGF released from degenerating acinar and metaplastic ductal cells possibly interacts with TrkA localized in the perineurium of enlarged pancreatic nerves of CP to promote these neural changes and also influence the pain syndrome. This hypothesis is already supported by recent research in rats, where it has been shown that NGF interacts with its receptor to play a crucial role in nerve growth and repair [20]. The significance of the NGF/TrkA pathway for the generation and modulation of pain has also been described in various previous studies.

Animal models using gene-targeted mutant mice demonstrated an important role for NGF and the TrkA receptor in the maturation and function of nociceptive sensory neurons. The loss of both NGF and TrkA in NGF/Trk-A null mutant mice resulted in a dramatic loss of small-diameter sensory neurons, combined with an insensitivity to pain stimuli [21]. The importance of NGF/TrkA signaling in pain could also be demonstrated in patients with a mutation in the TrkA gene which resulted in the absence of high-affin-

Table 4.2-1. Relationship of molecular findings with clinical parameters [19].

Clinical parameter	NGF mRNA	Trk-A mRNA
Fibrosis	r = 0.64 ($p < 0.05$)	r = 0.27 (n. s.)*
Acinar cell damage	r = 0.74 ($p < 0.05$)	r = 0.18 (n. s.)*
Duct metaplasia	r = 0.64 ($p < 0.05$)	r = 0.32 (n. s.)*
Intensity of pain	r = 0.03 (n. s.)*	r = 0.84 ($p < 0.05$)
Frequency of pain	r = 0.18 (n. s.)*	r = 0.15 (n. s.)*

* n. s. = not significant

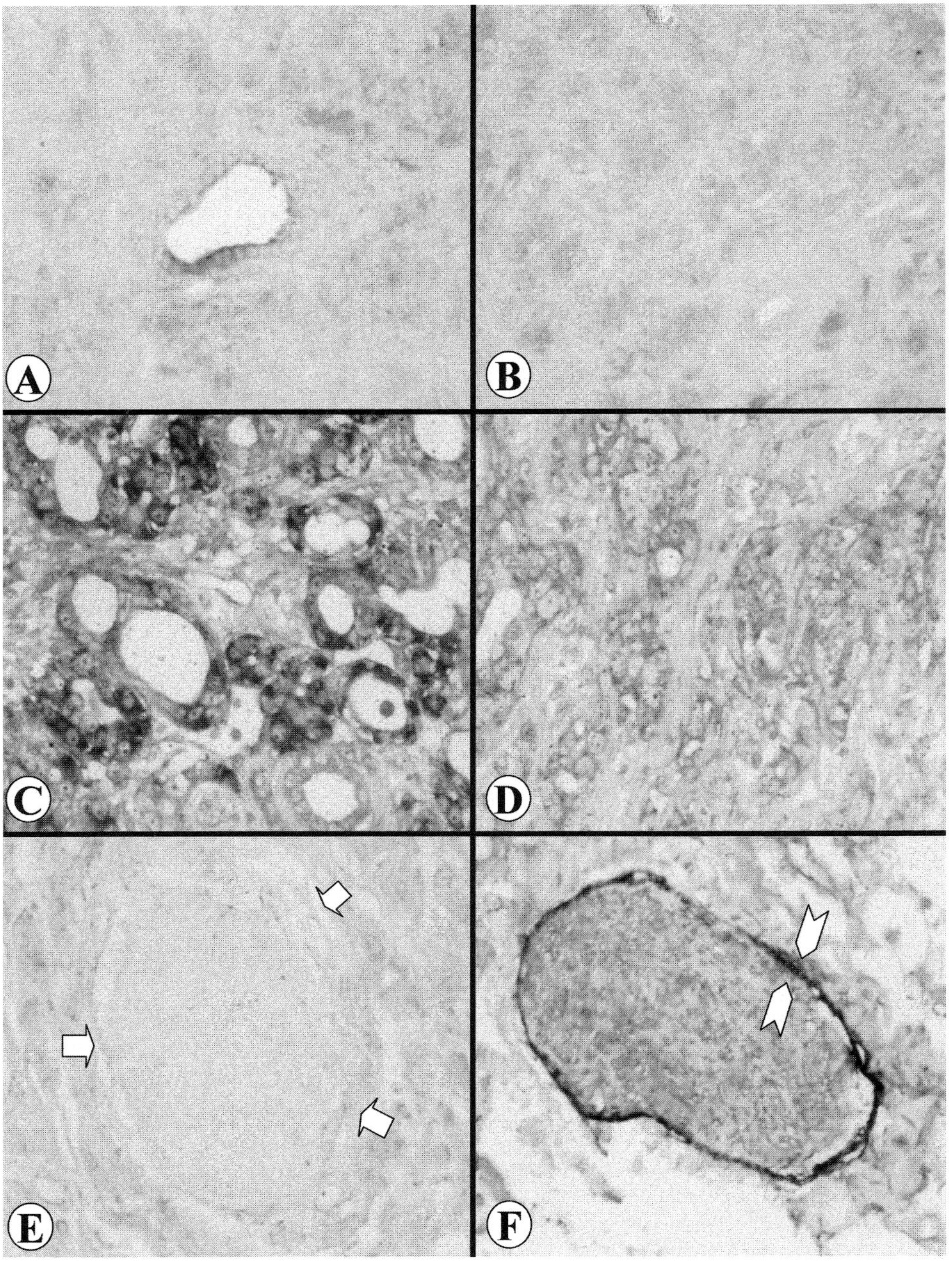

Figure 4.2-1A–F. *In situ* hybridization of NGF (**A, C, E**) and TrkA (**B, D, F**) in normal pancreas and chronic pancreatitis. In normal pancreas, NGF mRNA signal was weakly present in pancreatic ductal cells and absent in acinar cells (**A**). TrkA mRNA signal was absent in ductal and acinar cells (**B**). In chronic pancreatitis, NGF mRNA signal was strongly present in ductular complexes and degenerating acinar cells (**C**) and absent in pancreatic nerves (**E,** arrows: nerve fiber). TrkA mRNA signals were absent in ductular complexes and degenerating acinar cells (**D**) and moderately or strongly present in the perineurium (**F**), (arrow head: perineurium). The original magnifications (**A–F**) are ×200.

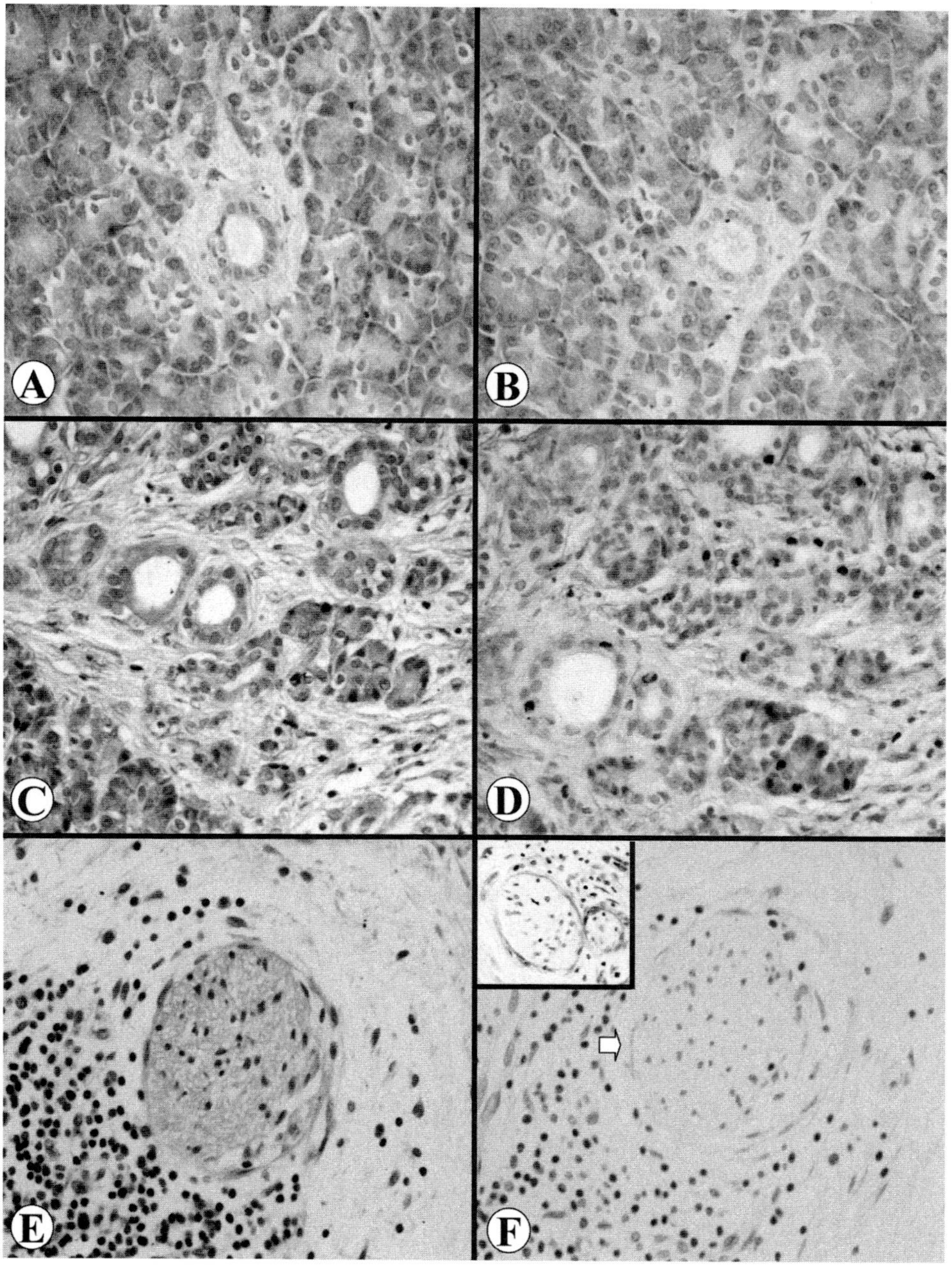

Figure 4.2-2A–F. Immunostaining of NGF (**A, C, E**) and TrkA (**B, D, F**) in normal pancreas and chronic pancreatitis. In normal pancreas, NGF immunoreactivity was weakly present in pancreatic ductal cells and absent in acinar cells (**A**). TrkA immunoreactivity was absent in ductal and acinar cells (**B**). In chronic pancreatitis, NGF immunoreactivity was strongly present in ductular complexes and degenerating acinar cells (**C**) and moderately present in pancreatic nerves (**F**). TrkA immunoreactivity was absent in ductular complexes and degenerating acinar cells (**D**) and moderately or strongly present in the perineurium (**F**), (arrow: perineurium). The original magnifications (**A–F**) are ×200.

ity NGF receptors and a chronic insensitivity to pain [22]. NGF also alters pain thresholds by modulating the sensitivity of adult, NGF-independent primary sensory neurons [23]. Another mechanism by which NGF might influence chronic pain is the regulation of transcription and the synthesis of substance P (SP) and calcitonin gene-related peptide (CGRP), as well as through the release of histamine [24, 25]. Blocking of NGF by specific anti-NGF antibodies produced a sustained thermal and chemical hypoalgesia and a down-regulation of SP and CGRP in animal experiments [26]. Inasmuch as the sensory neurotransmitters SP and CGRP are increased in enlarged pancreatic nerves in CP, these observations indicate a potential regulatory interaction between both mediator systems in pain generation [14].

Substance P and NK-1 receptor in CP (SP and NK-1R)

Neurotransmitters are major players in pain transmission. Our group previously demonstrated [14] that the potential pain neurotransmitter substance P (SP) is increased in intra-pancreatic nerve fibers in CP. Also, there is increasing evidence in CP of an interaction between pancreatic nerves and inflammatory cells [12]. However, mechanisms and mediators that are involved in the interaction between inflammatory cells, nerves and ganglia – the "neuroimmune cross-talk" – are not yet fully clarified. However, SP functions via its specific receptor NK-1 (NK-1R), and therefore the determination of the presence of the NK-1R and the localization of the site of NK-1R expression would provide further insight into SP-mediated pathways [27]. Therefore, to investigate the role of SP in CP and the potential routes and sites of its action, the expression of NK-1R mRNA was quantitatively studied and the site of its mRNA and protein expression localized. Furthermore, an evaluation was performed whether a relationship exists between the presence of NK-1R mRNA levels and pain and inflammation in CP. NK-1R was localized in enlarged intrapancreatic nerves, ganglia, blood vessels and inflammatory cells. The NK-1R mRNA levels obtained by quantitative PCR were also correlated with clinical parameters. This analysis revealed that levels of NK-1R mRNA expression correlated significantly with the intensity, duration and frequency of pain, but not with the severity of pancreatic inflammation [27].

Conclusion

Our findings suggest that the NGF/Trk-A pathway is activated in CP and this activation influences nerve growth and the pain syndrome of CP by various direct but also indirect pathways [23, 25, 28, 29]. Furthermore, NGF might be regulating the transcription and synthesis of substance P and CGRP, thereby influencing pain and the inflammatory reaction indirectly [24, 25].

The expression of NK-1R in CP provides further confirmatory evidence that neuroimmune interactions seem to be of crucial importance in CP. It thus appears that expression of NK-1R in various neuronal and other structures of the chronically inflammed pancreas influences both the pain syndrome and morphological changes characteristic of this disease. The potential regulatory interactions between both mediator systems involved in pain in CP are summarized in Figure 4.2-3.

In view of our findings, future research should be directed towards NK-1R and NGF/Trk-A antagonists that might hold the potential to influence the course of pain and

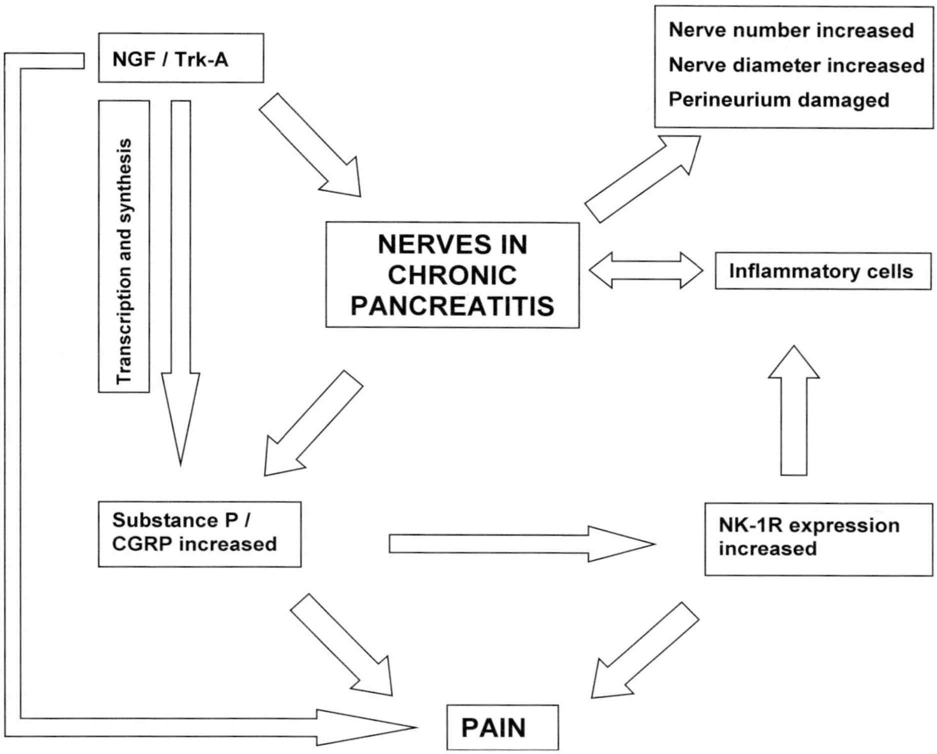

Figure 4.2-3. Nerves in chronic pancreatitis and their interactions with neurotransmitters, growth factors and inflammatory cells.

morphologial changes of CP. Simultaneously, efforts should be directed towards developing a relevant experimental model of CP that mimics the clinical picture of human chronic pancreatitis. If a clinically relevant experimental CP model can be set up, it will allow further evaluation of the effects of NGF/TrkA and SP/NK-1R pathway antagonists on pain and inflammation in this disorder.

References

1. DiMagno EP: A short, eclectic history of exocrine pancreatic insufficiency and chronic pancreatitis. Gastroenterology 1993; 104: 1255–62.
2. Oertel JE, Heffess CS, Oertel YC. Pancreas. In: Sternberg SS, ed. Diagnostic surgical pathology. New York: Raven Press, 1989: 1057–93.
3. DiMagno EP, Layer P, Clain JE. Chronic pancreatitis. In: Go VLW, DiMagno EP, Gardner JD, Lebenthal E, Reber HA, Scheele GA, eds. The exocrine pancreas: Biology, Pathobiology and Diseases. New York: Raven Press, 1993: 665–706.
4. Kennedy RH, Bockman DE, Uscanga L, Choux R, Grimaud JA, Sarles H. Pancreatic extracellular matrix alterations in chronic pancreatitis. Pancreas 1987; 2: 61–72.
5. Hunger RE, Mueller C, Z'graggen K, Friess H, Buchler MW. Cytotoxic cells are activated in cellular infiltrates of alcoholic chronic pancreatitis. Gastroenterology 1997; 112: 1656–63.
6. Warshaw AL, Popp JW, Jr., Schapiro RH. Long-term patency, pancreatic function, and pain relief after lateral pancreaticojejunostomy for chronic pancreatitis. Gastroenterology 1980; 79: 289–93.

7. Bradley EL, III: Long-term results of pancreatojejunostomy in patients with chronic pancreatitis. Am J Surg 1987; 153: 207–13.
8. Manes G, Pieramico O, Uomo G. Pain in chronic pancreatitis: recent pathogenetic findings. Minerva Gastroenterol Dietol 1992; 38: 137–43.
9. Reber HA, Karanjia ND, Alvarez C, Widdison AL, Leung FW, Ashley SW, Lutrin FJ. Pancreatic blood flow in cats with chronic pancreatitis. Gastroenterology 1992; 103: 652–9.
10. Karanjia ND, Widdison AL, Leung F, Alvarez C, Lutrin FJ, Reber HA. Compartment syndrome in experimental chronic obstructive pancreatitis: effect of decompressing the main pancreatic duct. Br J Surg 1994; 81: 259–64.
11. Di Sebastiano P, Fink T, Weihe E, Friess H, Innocenti P, Beger HG, Buchler MW. Immune cell infiltration and growth-associated protein 43 expression correlate with pain in chronic pancreatitis. Gastroenterology 1997; 112: 1648–55.
12. Weihe E, Nohr D, Muller S, Buchler M, Friess H, Zentel HJ. The tachykinin neuroimmune connection in inflammatory pain. Ann NY Acad Sci 1991; 632: 283–95.
13. Bockman DE, Buchler MW, Malfertheiner P, Beger HG. Analysis of nerves in chronic pancreatitis. Gastroenterology 1988; 94: 1459–69.
14. Buchler MW, Weihe E, Friess H, Malfertheiner P, Bockman E, Muller S, Nohr D, Beger HG. Changes in peptidergic innervation in chronic pancreatitis. Pancreas 1992; 7: 183–92.
15. Levi-Montalcini R, Skaper SD, Dal Toso R, Petrelli L, Leon A. Nerve growth factor: from neurotrophin to neurokine. Trends Neurosci 1996; 19: 514–20.
16. Levi-Montalcini R, Dal Toso R, della VF, Skaper SD, Leon A. Update of the NGF saga. J Neurol Sci 1995; 130: 119–27.
17. Barbacid M: Neurotrophic factors and their receptors. Curr Opin Cell Biol 1995; 7: 148–55.
18. Levi-Montalcini R: The nerve growth factor 35 years later. Science 1987; 237: 1154–62.
19. Friess H, Zhu ZW, di Mola FF, Kulli C, Graber HU, Andren-Sandberg A, Zimmermann A, Korc M, Reinshagen M, Buchler MW. Nerve growth factor and its high-affinity receptor in chronic pancreatitis. Ann Surg 1999; 230: 615–24.
20. Yamamoto M, Iseki S. Nerve growth factor receptor (NGFR)-like immunoreactivity in the perineurial cells of the adult rat peripheral nerves: normal appearance and response to nerve section. Kaibogaku Zasshi 1992; 67: 642–9.
21. Smeyne RJ, Klein R, Schnapp A, Long LK, Bryant S, Lewin A, Lira SA, Barbacid M. Severe sensory and sympathetic neuropathies in mice carrying a disrupted Trk/NGF receptor gene. Nature 1994; 368: 246–9.
22. Indo Y, Tsuruta M, Hayashida Y, Karim MA, Ohta K, Kawano T, Mitsubuchi H, Tonoki H, Awaya Y, Matsuda I. Mutations in the TRKA/NGF receptor gene in patients with congenital insensitivity to pain with anhidrosis. Nat Genet 1996; 13: 485–8.
23. Joseph A, Markerson MD. Mechanism of Pain. Am J Med 1996; 101: 6–18.
24. McMahon SB, Bennett DL, Priestley JV, Shelton DL. The biological effects of endogenous nerve growth factor on adult sensory neurons revealed by a TRKA-IgG fusion molecule [see comments]. Nat Med 1995; 1: 774–80.
25. McMahon SB: NGF as a mediator of inflammatory pain. Philos Trans R Soc Lond B Biol Sci 1996; 351: 431–40.
26. Aloe L, Probert L, Kollias G, Micera A, Tirassa P. Effect of NGF antibodies on mast cell distribution, histamine and substance P levels in the knee joint of TNF-arthritic transgenic mice. Rheumatol Int 1995; 14: 249–52.
27. Shrikhande SV, Friess H, Di Mola F, Tempia A, Conejio Garcia JR, Zhu Z, Zimmermann A, Buchler MW. NK-1 receptor gene expression is related to pain in chronic pancreatitis. Pain 2000. (in press.)
28. Woolf CJ. Phenotypic modification of primary sensory neurons: the role of nerve growth factor in the production of persistent pain. Philos Trans R Soc Lond B Biol Sci 1996; 351: 441–8.
29. Lewin GR, Mendell LM. Nerve growth factor and nociception. Trends Neurosci 1993; 16: 353–9.

4.3 Correlation of pain, neural growth and inflammation in chronic pancreatitis

P. Di Sebastiano, F. F. di Mola, H. Friess, M. W. Büchler

Introduction

Chronic pancreatitis (CP) is characterized histologically by atrophy of the exocrine pancreatic tissue, increase in the local fibrosis and modification of the nerves in the area of inflammation. These histological changes are accompanied by chronic inflammation and upper abdominal pain. However, the leading symptom of CP is abdominal pain. Surgical management is often indicated in cases with medically intractable pain and this has repercussions on the economic management of these patients [1].

Up to this point in time the etiology of pain is still unclear and several hypotheses have been postulated.

Multifactorial elements are involved and this may explain why all patients do not respond to the same treatment modality. Extrapancreatic and pancreatic causes have been implicated in the development of pain [2]. Potential extrapancreatic causes are common bile duct stenosis by continued inflammation of the head of the pancreas and duodenal stenosis caused by extensive fibrosis that envelops the wall of the duodenum. The pancreatic causes may be resembled in acute inflammation of the pancreas, increased intrapancreatic pressure and neurogenic inflammation.

Considering this latter hypothesis, recent concepts in neurobiology indicate the possible role of the enteric nervous system (ENS) [3, 4].

During the last few decades much information has been accumulated on the occurrence and distribution of neuropeptides in the gastro-entero-pancreatic system. Alterations of the enteric nervous system in the regulation of gut functions have been postulated for different pathological conditions [5, 6].

Supporting this hypothesis Keith et al. [7] postulated that neural and perineural alteration might be important in pain pathogenesis in CP.

In a further study [8], an increase both in number and diameter of pancreatic nerve fibers has been reported. In addition, "foci" of inflammatory cells are often found surrounding pancreatic nerves, which exhibit a damaged perineurium and invasion by eosinophile granulocytes. In addition, in these enlarged nerve fibers [9] we demonstrated that the pattern of intrinsic and possibly extrinsic innervation is changed in CP, leading to an increased expression of neuropeptides such as substance P and VIP that are known to be proinflammatory and pronociceptive mediators. The increasing evidence for profound changes in the innervation pattern of the human pancreas under inflammatory conditions suggests the involvement of neuronal plasticity in the inflamed pancreatic tissue.

Neuronal activation in chronic pancreatitis

Recently, we supplied evidence for neuronal activation in CP using growth-associated protein-43 (GAP-43), a well-established marker for neuronal plasticity [10]. GAP-43 is known to be involved in the development of axonal growth cones and presynaptic terminals. More recent studies revealed a modulation of GAP-43 expression after injuries of peripheral nerves [11]. In these experimental models, GAP-43 was re-expressed in high levels, reflecting neuronal contribution in inflammation and postlesional repair. In the chronically inflamed human pancreas, using enzymatic and double fluorescence immunocytochemistry, we were able to demonstrate a highly significant re-expression of GAP-43 in the majority of pancreatic nerve fibers and a significantly intensified immunostaining for GAP-43 in intrinsic neurons compared to generally low-level expression of GAP-43 in the normal human pancreas (Fig. 4.3-1).

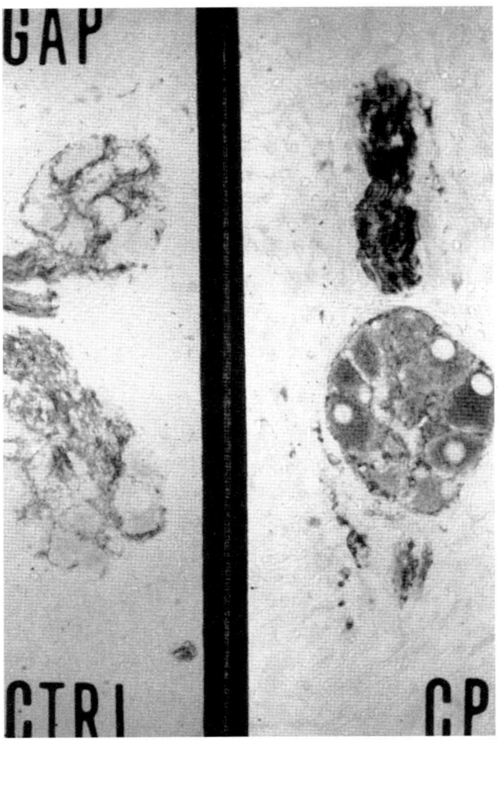

Figure 4.3-1. GAP-43 immunohistochemical expression in human pancreas.
GAP-43 is significantly re-expressed at high levels in pancreatic tissue specimens of chronic pancreatitis (CP): the vast majority of nerve fibers and intrinsic neurons shows strong GAP-43 immunoreactivity. In normal pancreatic tissue (CTRL), the presence of GAP-43 immunoreactive fibers is reduced to a basic expression.

Clinical correlation with immunohistochemical findings

In another study [12], the possible relationship between immunocytochemical results and clinical data as pain history and preoperative pain scores was investigated. In addition, we correlated individual pain scores with the degree of pancreatic fibrosis and addressed the question of whether perineural infiltration of pancreatic nerves by immune cells correlates with abdominal pain in CP.

To evaluate possible relations between clinical symptoms and immunocytochemical findings, the clinical data, obtained with the symptom questionnaire, the degree of perineural inflammation, as expressed in the infiltration score, and GAP-43 immunocytochemical expression were analyzed. There was a significant relation between the infiltration score and the intensity of pain (Fig. 4.3-2). In contrast, no relation was found between degree of fibrosis and intensity of pain ($p > 0.05$). Patients with higher pain intensity exhibited a significantly stronger GAP-43 immunoreactivity in intrinsic neurons (Fig. 4.3-3). Furthermore, there was a significant relation between GAP-43 immunoreactivity in nerve fibers and the intensity of pain (Fig. 4.3-4). In addition, the infiltration score correlated with the intensity of GAP-43 immunoreactivity in intrinsic neurons ($p < 0.05$). The duration of the disease correlated linearly with the intensity of GAP-43 immunostaining in nerve fibers ($p < 0.05$) and the expression of GAP-43 in intrinsic neurons ($p < 0.05$). Thus, patients with longstanding CP showed a strong up-regulation of GAP-43 immunoreactivity in both neurons and nerve fibers. An association between duration of the disease and intensity of pain, however, was not detected.

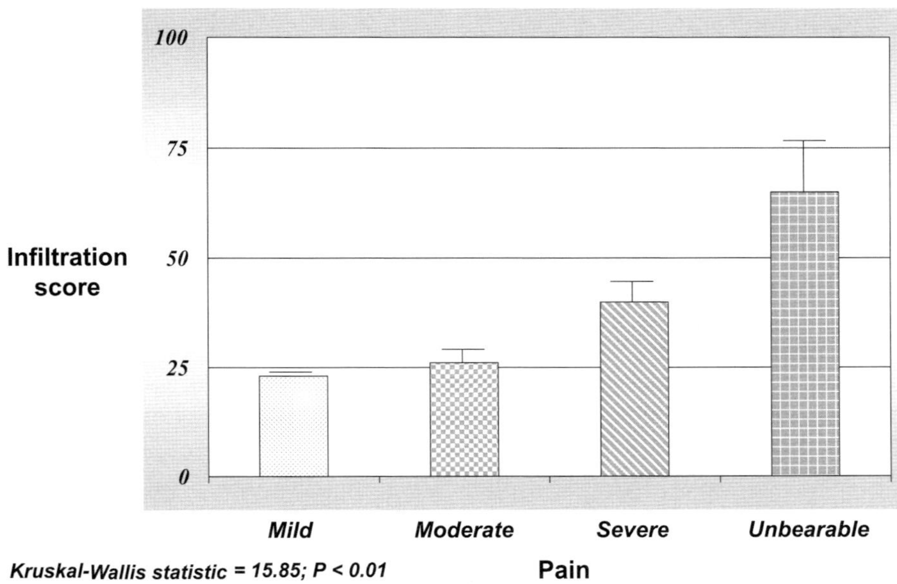

Figure 4.3-2. Relationship between intensity of pain and infiltration score was present in patients suffering from chronic pancreatitis. Patients suffering from severe pain also exhibited a higher infiltration score.

This study provided evidence for a direct correlation of histological changes and pain in human CP.

Our observation of neuronal changes in the chronically inflamed pancreas is in line with former reports [8] and demonstrates for the first time a direct correlation between the degree of perineural inflammation and clinical pain symptoms, which strongly supports the hypothesis of a neuro-immune interaction as an important if not predominant factor in pain generation in CP.

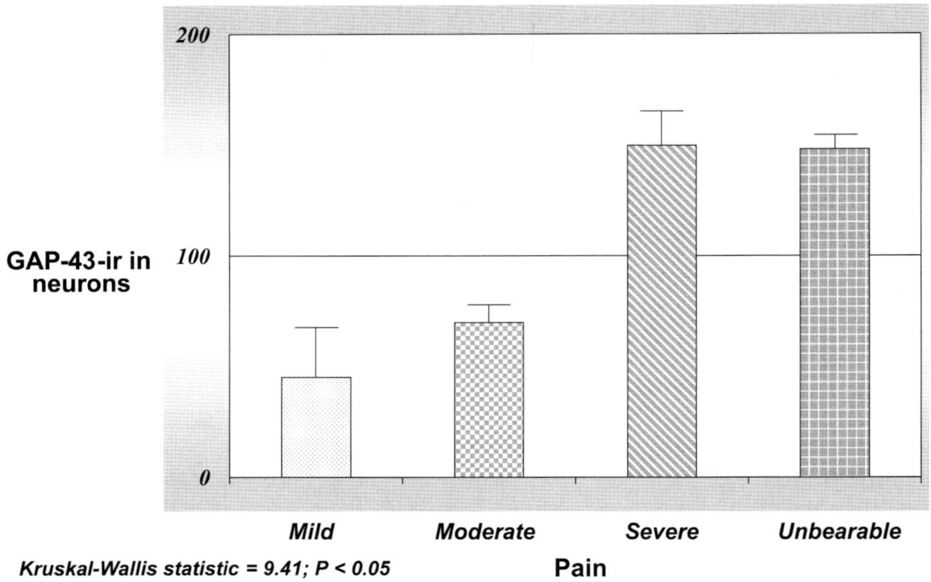

Figure 4.3-3. Relationship between GAP-43 immunoreactivity in intrinsic neurons and intensity of pain in chronic pancreatitis. Patients with higher pain intensity showed stronger GAP-43 immunoreactivity in intrinsic neurons.

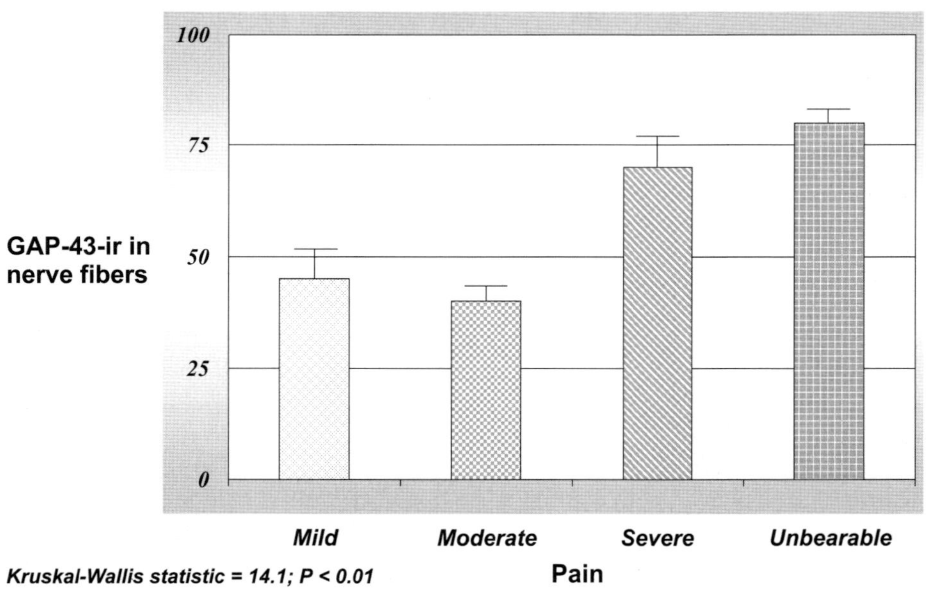

Figure 4.3-4. Relationship between GAP-43 immunoreactivity in nerve fibers and intensity of pain in chronic pancreatitis. Patients with higher pain intensity showed stronger GAP-43 immunoreactivity in intrapancreatic nerve fibers.

The neuroimmune connection

Neuropeptides such as SP have also been implicated in local immune response. SP has also been shown to increase activated lymphocyte proliferation and immunoglobulin synthesis both *in vivo* and *in vitro*. Furthermore, cytokines, a class of glycoprotein immunoregulators, have been shown to interact with SP in various paradigms for pain and inflammation. These observations strongly suggest that neuropeptides and cytokines might be involved in the pathophysiology of chronic inflammation in CP.

Several studies have emphasized a possible link between neuropeptides and inflammatory mediators, suggesting that immunological and inflammatory responses might be regulated by signals deriving from the nervous system. In the example, interleukin 8 (IL-8) release from inflammatory cells is mediated in part from different neuropeptides such as SP during the inflammatory response [13].

Therefore, we investigated the mRNA gene expression of preprotachykinin-A (PPT-A), the gene encoding substance P and IL-8, a proinflammatory and hyperalgesic mediator whose release is co-regulated by substance P [14].

In pancreatic tissue specimens obtained from 21 patients with CP, the gene expression of preprotachykinin-A and IL-8 was studied by Northern blot analysis. Their respective proteins were localized using immunohistochemistry.

Northern blot analysis showed that preprotachykinin-A mRNA expression levels were present at comparable levels in normal and chronic pancreatitis tissue samples. In contrast, IL-8 mRNA was expressed at very low levels in normal controls and 25-fold increased in CP tissue samples (Fig. 4.3-5). By immunohistochemistry, IL-8 protein was localized mainly in immune cells often found around enlarged pancreatic nerves. In addition, in CP intense IL-8 immunostaining was present in metaplastic ductal cells of the atrophic pancreatic parenchyma.

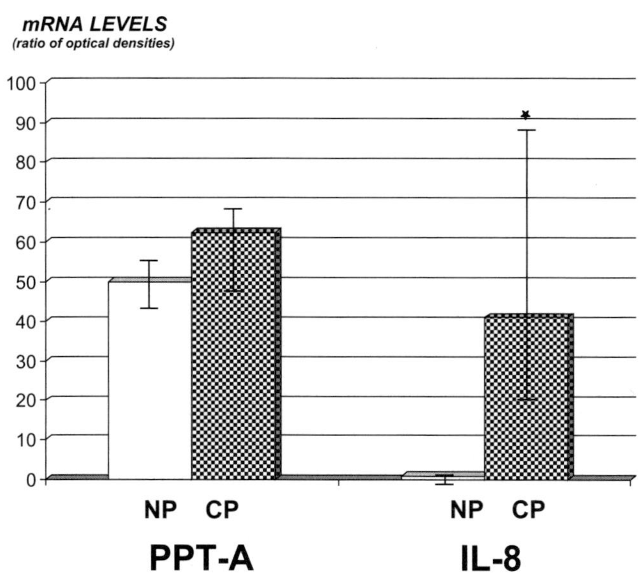

Figure 4.3-5. Preprotachykinin-A and interleukin-8 mRNA gene expression in chronic pancreatitis [14]. The densitometric analysis revealed that IL-8 mRNA levels were dramatically increased in chronic pancreatitis compared to normal pancreas. No differences in PPT-A mRNA expression were detected between normal and chronically inflamed pancreas.

These data indicate that in CP the increase in SP-immunoreactivity in enlarged pancreatic nerves is not caused by enhanced intrapancreatic preprotachykinin-A mRNA expression, suggesting that the location of SP synthesis is outside of the pancreas. In addition, the close localization of IL-8 positive immune cells around pancreatic nerves further supports the existence of neuroimmune interactions as a pathophysiological mechanism in CP.

Conclusions

There is still disagreement regarding the mechanisms that contribute to the generation of pain and regarding the best method of managing pain in chronic pancreatitis.

Earlier pain hypotheses, for example increased intraductal and intraparenchymal pressure or post-prandial pancreatic hyperstimulation caused by decreased enzyme secretion and the insufficient functioning of the so-called *"negative feedback mechanism"*, are more and more often questioned as reliable explanations of abdominal pain in patients with CP.

Alterations of the ENS in the regulation of the gut functions have been postulated for a number of pathological conditions, including achalasia, inflammatory bowel diseases, irritable bowel diseases etc.

In our studies we supplied evidence for neuronal activation in CP, using GAP-43, a well-established marker for neuronal plasticity. In addition, a correlation between GAP-43 expression in intrapancreatic nerves and abdominal pain was found.

These findings led to the hypothesis that alterations of pancreatic nerves, possibly interrelated with the immunological response, could be involved in the pathogenesis of pain and also in the inflammation of the pancreas.

Damage to the perineural sheath in CP, as we have shown previously, might allow for free access of tissue mediators to the surrounding tissue, including the inflammatory cells, and thus provide the basis for local bi-directional communication between the nervous and the immune system.

The involvement of neuropeptides released from enteric nerves and their functional interaction with inflammatory cells confirm the concept of "neurogenic inflammation", as already discussed in disorders of the eye, skin and respiratory and gastrointestinal tract.

The direct correlation between the immunohistochemical findings and clinical symptoms provides evidence for *"neuroimmune cross-talk"* in the pathogenesis of pain in CP.

Our results provide new insights into the role played by the nervous system in the modulation of inflammatory response. These data suggest that local neuroimmune mechanisms are involved in the pathophysiology of pain and inflammation in CP.

References

1. Büchler MW, Friess H, Müller M, Wheatley AM, Beger HG. Randomized trial of duodenum-preserving pancreatic head resection versus pylorus-preserving Whipple in chronic pancreatitis. Am J Surg 1995; 169: 65–9.
2. Klöppel G. Pathology of chronic pancreatitis and pancreatic pain. Acta Chir Scand 1990; 156: 261–5.
3. Holzer P. Local effector functions of capsaicin-sensitive sensory nerve endings: involvement of tachykinins, calcitonin gene-related peptide and other neuropeptides. Neuroscience 1988; 24: 739–68.

4. Mantyh PW, Catton MD, Boehmer CG et al. Receptors for sensory neuropeptides in human inflammatory diseases: implications for the effector role of sensory neurons. Peptides 1989; 10: 627–45.
5. Bishop AE, Polak JM, Bryant MG, Bloom SR, Hamilton S. Abnormalities of vasoactive intestinal polypeptide-containing nerves in Crohn's disease. Gastroenterology 1980; 79: 853–60.
6. Di Sebastiano P, Fink T, di Mola FF, Weihe E, Innocenti P, Friess H, Büchler MW. Neuroimmune appendicitis. The Lancet 1999; 354: 461–6.
7. Keith RG, Keshavjee SH, Kerenyi NR. Neuropathology of chronic pancreatitis in humans. Can J Surg 1985; 28: 207–11.
8. Bockman DE, Büchler M, Malfertheiner P, Beger HG. Analysis of nerves in chronic pancreatitis. Gastroenterology 1988; 94: 1459–69.
9. Büchler M, Weihe E, Friess H, Malfertheiner P, Bockman DE, Müller S, Nohr D, Beger HG. Changes in peptidergic innervation in chronic pancreatitis. Pancreas 1992; 7: 183–92.
10. Fink T, Di Sebastiano P, Büchler MW, Beger HG, Weihe E. Growth-associated protein-43 and Protein gene product 9.5 innervation in human pancreas: changes in chronic pancreatitis. Neuroscience 1994; 63: 249–66.
11. Chong MS, Fitzgerald M, Winter J, Hu-Tsai M, Emson PC, Wiese U, Woolf CJ. GAP-43 mRNA in rat spinal cord and dorsal root ganglia neurons: developmental changes and re-expression following peripheral nerve injury. Eur J Neurosci 1992; 4: 883–95.
12. Di Sebastiano P, Fink T, Weihe E et al. Immune cell infiltration and growth associated protein-43 correlate with pain in chronic pancreatitis. Gastroenterology 1997; 112: 1648–55.
13. Serra MC, Calzetti F, Ceska M et al. Effect of substance P on superoxide anion and IL-8 production by human PMNL. Immunology 1994; 82: 63–9.
14. Di Sebastiano P, di Mila FF, di Febbo C, Baccante G, Porreca E, Innocenti P, Friess H, Büchler MW. Expression of interleukin-8 (IL-8) and substance P in human chronic pancreatitis. Gut 2000; 47: 423–8.

4.4 Cellular immune reactions in chronic pancreatitis

C. Mueller, L. Saurer

Introduction

Despite numerous hypotheses on the etiopathogenesis of chronic pancreatitis, the precise pathogenetic steps of this disease still remain enigmatic. In particular, the question whether chronic pancreatitis arises *de novo* or is closely linked to recurrent episodes of acute pancreatitis has yet to be answered. Indications for a possible involvement of the immune system in the pathogenesis of chronic pancreatitis are the observed local up-regulation of MHC class I and II antigens on pancreatic ductal and ductular (interlobular and intralobular) epithelium [1] and the regular observation of macrophages, T and B lymphocytes in affected pancreatic lobuli of patients with chronic pancreatitis. When tissue sections from patients with alcoholic chronic pancreatitis are subjected to immunostainings for the specific localization of CD3 T cells, CD79a positive B cells and CD68 positive macrophages distinct distribution patterns are observed: T lymphocytes are either loosely scattered within the fibrotic tissue; present as more dense aggregates around residual lobules and ducts; or present in small lymphoid clusters. Frequently, nerves are also surrounded by focal aggregates of T cells. In normal pancreatic tissue T lymphocytes are virtually absent. The pattern of B cell distribution resembles the one seen for T cells, although in affected pancreatic tissues B cells more frequently tend to form small clusters. Macrophages are scattered throughout the fibrotic parts of the tissue or are present as small clusters of large foamy cells. Typically, this cell population is often found to surround remaining pancreatic tissue and even to infiltrate the lobules. Low numbers of macrophages are occasionally detected on tissue sections from normal pancreas. Typical distribution patterns of the inflammatory infiltrates are given in Figure 4.4-1.

Recruitment of leukocytes to sites of inflammation

Recruitment of inflammatory cells to the site of inflammation is one of the key steps in the initiation and progression of inflammatory reactions. Recent evidence clearly demonstrated that extravasation of inflammatory cells is not random but rather involves multiple sequential steps [2]. Initially, leukocytes become attached to the vascular endothelium but are still allowed to roll along the vessel wall. Attachment and rolling are promoted by vasodilation and by expression of the selectin family of adhesion molecules. L-selectin is expressed constitutively on the majority of circulating leukocytes whereas P-selectin and E-selectin expression on endothelial cells is rapidly induced by a variety of stimuli, including lipopolysaccharide and cytokines such as tumor necrosis factor (TNF) and interleukin(IL)-1. In a second step, leukocytes spread and firmly attach to the endothelial layer through interaction of integrins expressed on the surface of leukocytes with ligands on the endothelium such as ICAM-1 and VCAM-1. The integrins are not expressed constitutively but must be activated in order to become competent adhesion molecules. Cy-

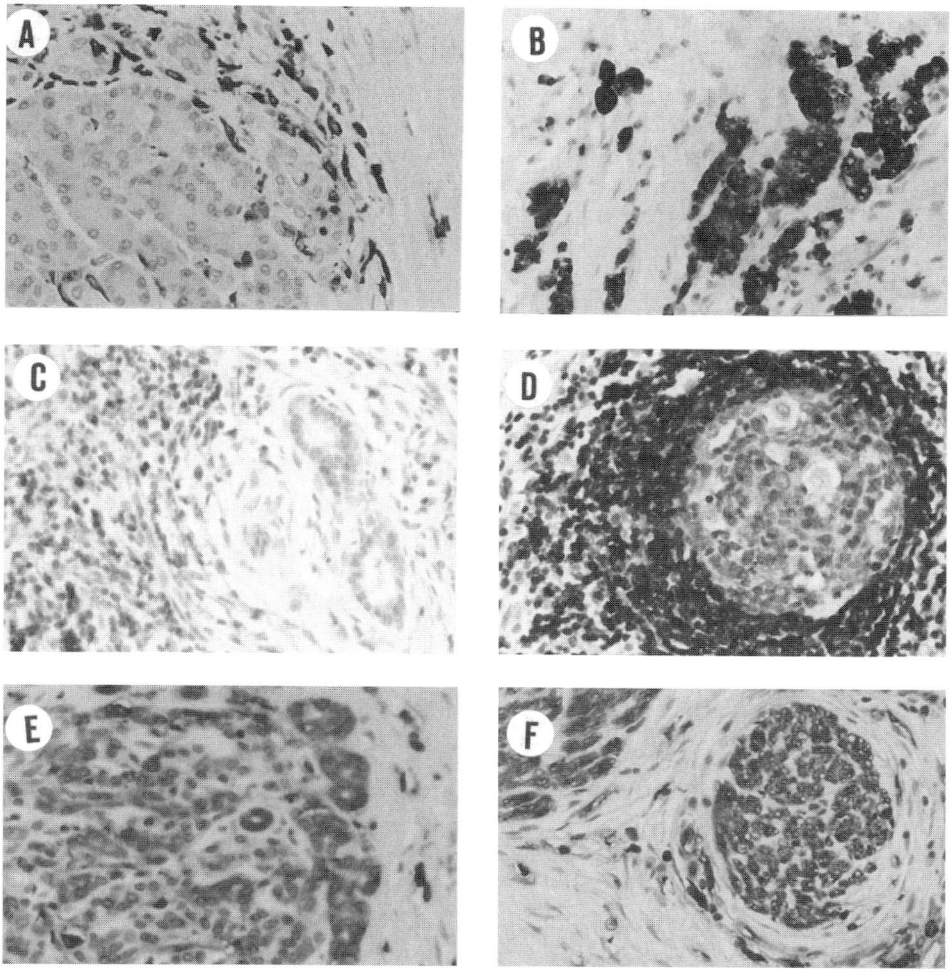

Figure 4.4-1A–F. Immunohistochemical detection of (**A, B**), CD68+ macrophages; (**C**), CD3+ T cells; **D:** CD79+ B-cells and MHC class II (HLA-DR) expression on (**E**) pancreatic centroacinar ducts; and **F:** cross-sectioned nerves and inflammatory cells on tissue sections from patients with CP.

tokines with potent chemoattractant activity for distinct leukocytes, hence termed chemokines, play an important role in upregulating the expression and enhancing the adhesiveness of the integrins. Once a leukocyte has thus become firmly attached to the endothelium it must be guided into the underlying tissue. Together with other chemoattractants (e.g. PAF, C5a, leukotriene B_4) chemokines are involved again in this third step by their ability to selectively attract specific types of leukocytes. Gradients of chemokines have been shown to attract leukocytes *in vitro* and it is assumed that by the ability of chemokines to bind to heparan sulfate in the extracellular matrix such gradients also operate *in vivo* (reviewed in [3, 4]).

General features of chemokines

In the past decade a still growing family of pro-inflammatory cytokines has been identified. The functional characterization of this new superfamily of pro-inflammatory cytokines was initially based on their chemoattractant activity for distinct leukocyte populations, hence these cytokines were collectively termed chemokines [5]. Chemokines are low molecular mass proteins which share 20–70% sequence homology and a common structural motif of four conserved cysteins linked by disulfide bonds. Two main subfamilies are distinguished according to the position of the first two cystein residues. In the α or CXC subfamily these two residues are separated by one amino acid, whereas in the β or CC-chemokines they are adjacent. CXC chemokines include interleukin-8 (IL-8), epithelial neutrophil-activating peptide (ENA 78), melanoma growth-stimulating activity (GRO α, β, and γ), interferon-γ inducible protein (IP-10), and monokine induced by interferon gamma (MIG). Representative members of the CC-chemokines are the monocyte chemotactic proteins (MCP) 1, 2, and 3, macrophage inflammatory protein (MIP)-1 a and b, the chemokine "regulated upon activation normal T cell-expressed and secreted" (RANTES), eotaxin, eotaxin-2 and I-309. However, these are but a few examples, since today over 40 chemokines are known and due to large scale cDNA sequencing programs this family can be expected to grow even more in the future (reviewed in [3, 5, 6]).

The difference between the two major chemokine families is not only a structural but also a functional one: with the exception of IP-10 and MIG, which act specifically on lymphocytes, most CXC-chemokines are capable of attracting and activating neutrophils, whereas CC-chemokines are preferentially chemotactic for mononuclear cell types such as macrophages/monocytes, eosinophils and different lymphocyte subsets and do not seem to considerably affect neutrophil chemotaxis. Besides the CC and CXC families of chemokines, a C(X3)C chemokine family also exists (with so far only one member, i.e. fractalkine) and a C family of chemokines (with so far lymphotactin as its only member).

Cellular sources of chemokines are highly diverse and include inflammatory cells themselves as well as epithelial and endothelial cells, fibroblasts, glial cells and smooth muscle cells. Hence, it may not be too surprising that chemokine expression has been detected during inflammation in most organs. As a general rule chemokines are not stored intracellularly; rather their production is stimulated by a variety of agents, including bacterial products (LPS) and the pro-inflammatory cytokines TNF-α and interleukin-1. One can assume that the different chemokines also interact in a complex manner with each other. Although the nuclear factor NF–K_B has been identified as one of the possible transcription factors involved, on a molecular basis there is still little information available on the induction and regulation mechanisms operative in chemokine gene expression.

The effects of chemokines on leukocytes are mediated by heptahelical transmembrane receptors coupled to GTP-binding proteins. Receptor activation leads to a cascade of intracellular signaling pathways resulting in the release of calcium and a reorganization of the cytoskeleton. So far, five human CXC-chemokine receptors (CXCR1–CXCR5) and nine human CC-chemokine receptors (CCR1–CCR9) have been identified which bind chemokines of the respective families. Most receptors recognize more than one chemokine, and several chemokines bind to more than one receptor, indicating that redundancy and versatility are characteristic of the chemokine system. Whereas some chemokine receptors are widely expressed on a variety of leukocyte populations, others are restricted to certain cell types. Apart from selective expression of receptors, additional specificity and control in response to chemokines may also be conferred by complex up- and downregulation mechanisms that may depend on the presence of other inflammatory mediators and on the activation status of cells (reviewed in [3–6]). Of particular interest is the recent finding that certain chemokine receptors mark subsets of T cells associated with distinct functional phenotypes [7]. Furthermore, chemokine receptors have been shown to play important roles in the pathophysiology of HIV infection [8].

Differential expression of chemokines in normal pancreata and affected pancreatic lobuli from patients with chronic pancreatitis

The central role of chemokines in the early recruitment of inflammatory cells recently prompted us to monitor local expression of distinct chemokine genes in pancreatic lobuli from patients with chronic pancreatitis showing distinct grades of histologic alterations, and from normal pancreatic tissues. Considering the large number of chemokines already identified, we decided to restrict our analysis to five representative members of the CXC- and CC-chemokine families: IL-8 and ENA-78 are two potent CXC-chemokines which are known as major neutrophil attractants [9, 10] and are therefore good indicators for early stages of active inflammation. While ENA-78 is typically expressed by epithelial cells, as evidenced in inflammatory bowel disease (IBD) [11], one of the main sources of IL-8 are inflammatory cells, including neutrophils and monocytes [9, 12]. In IBD, IL-8 expression has indeed been found to be related to the histological grade of active inflammation [12]. In contrast to IL-8 and ENA-78, the third CXC-chemokine analyzed, MIG, mainly acts on activated T cells, as these cells selectively express the specific receptor CXCR3 [13]. The CC-chemokine MCP-1 has been described as major monocyte chemoattractant [14], but also attracts activated T cells [15]. Reports on the potential fibrogenic properties of MCP-1 [16] make this chemokine a particular interesting choice for analysis in chronic pancreatitis. The other CC-chemokine I-309 is less well characterized than MCP-1. Similar to MCP-1, monocytes are an important source of I-309 production [17]. The finding that CCR8, i.e. the only receptor described so far for I-309, is preferentially expressed on functionally differentiated Th2 T cells, i.e. on T cells that support the generation of vigorous humoral immune responses and which may antagonize the functions of Th1 T cells that support potent cellular immune responses, recently rekindled interest in the possible function of this chemokine in regulating inflammatory processes [18, 19].

One of the most striking results obtained in our recent analysis of chemokine gene expression in chronic pancreatitis was the finding that cells of the exocrine pancreatic tissue, and not the inflammatory infiltrate, are the main sources of chemokine production in chronic pancreatitis (Figs. 4.4-2, 4.4-3, 4.4-4). Thus, it is likely that by producing these potent inflammatory mediators the pancreatic parenchyma itself plays an active role in the pathogenesis of this disease. However, as little is known about induction and regulation mechanisms operative in chemokine gene expression, we can only speculate about possible stimuli which might trigger chemokine expression in epithelial cells of the exocrine pancreatic tissue. Possibly, production of chemokines by the parenchyma is not one of the initiating factors but rather an epiphenomenon of the ongoing inflammatory process which, however, may lead to an exacerbating inflammatory response. The expression of MHC class II molecules by cells of the centroacinar ducts (Fig. 4.4-1) might indicate that pro-inflammatory mediators such as TNF-α and IFN-γ, secreted by activated in-

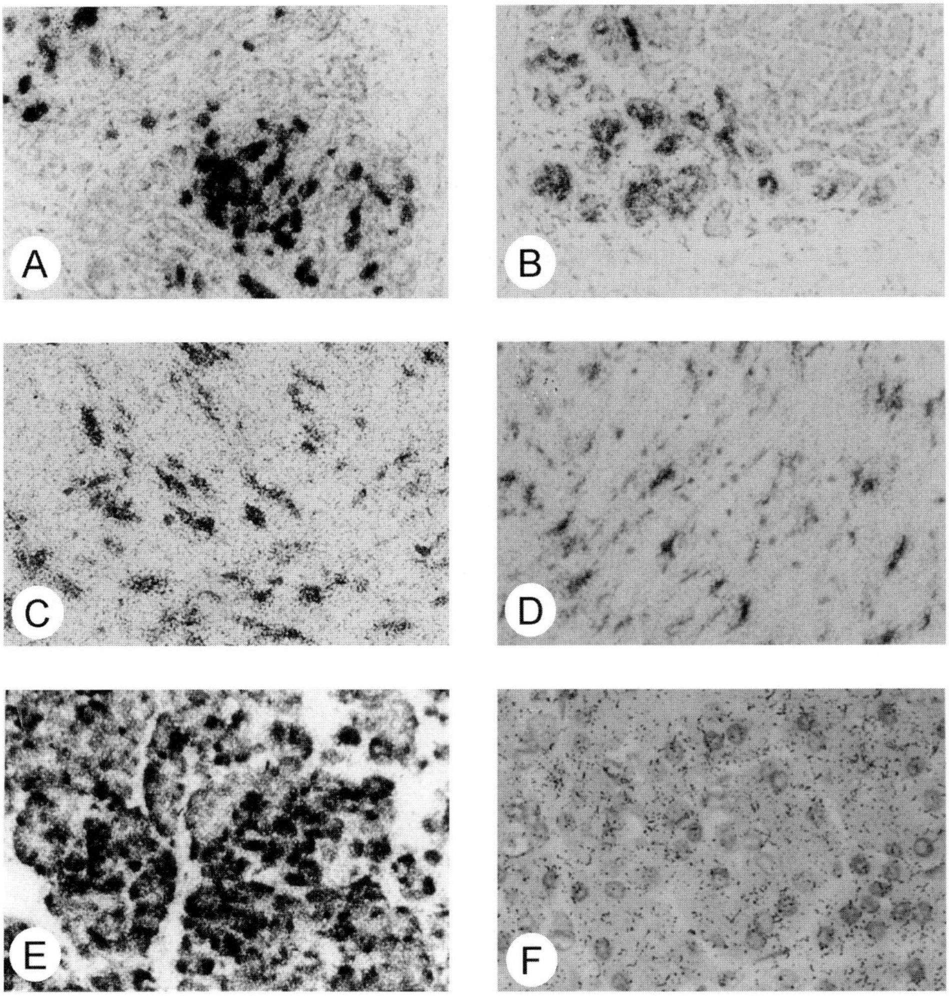

Figure 4.4-2A–F. Representative expression patterns of CC-chemokines in pancreatic tissue sections of (**A–D**) patients with CP and (**E, F**) of a multiorgan donor as a normal control hybridized with antisense probes for (**A, C, E**) I-309 and (**B, D**) MCP-1 or (**F**) hybridized with a sense probe as a negative control. Affected pancreatic lobules are depicted in (**A, B**) with distinct expression patterns of (**A**) I-309 and (**B**) MCP-1 in parenchymal cells. Fibroblasts and occasional inflammatory cells expressing I-309, and MCP-1, are shown in (**C**) and (**D**), respectively. (Adapted from Saurer et al. Gastroenterology 118: 356–367; 2000, with permission).

flammatory cells present in the vicinity of remaining parenchyma, could possibly trigger chemokine gene expression. Although complex interactions and mutual influences between infiltrate and parenchyma are likely, expression of chemokines by pancreatic parenchyma and inflammatory infiltrates is not tightly linked, since in advanced stages of disease activity the extent of CC-chemokine expression in pancreatic parenchyma is decreased (Figs. 4.4-2, 4.4-4) whereas chemokine expressing inflammatory cells are increasingly present in stage 3 of disease activity (Fig. 4.4-4). However, it has also to be taken into account that the observed decline in chemokine expression in pancreatic parenchyma in

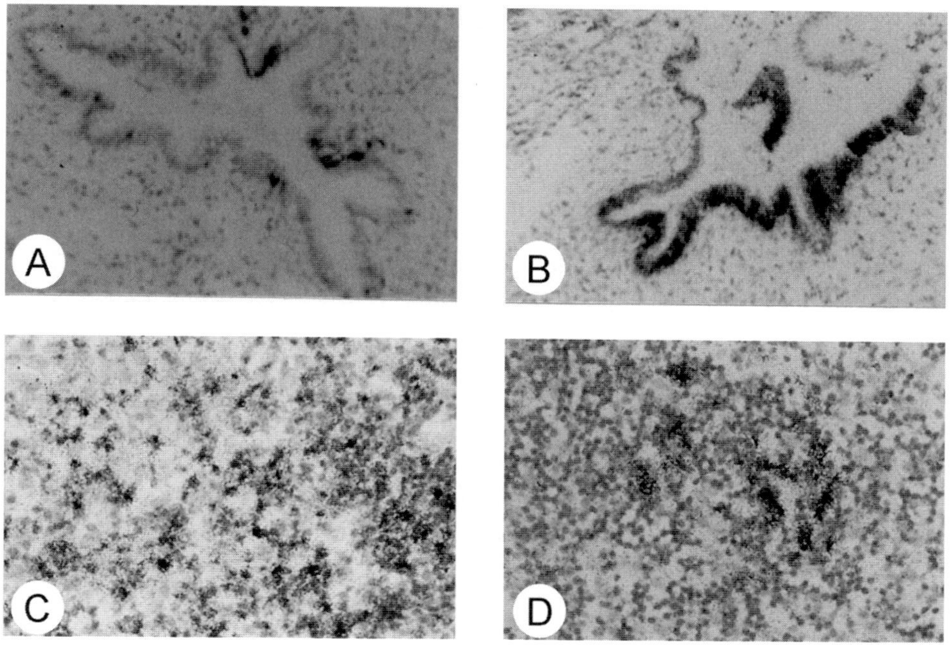

Figure 4.4-3A–D. Representative expression patterns of CXC-chemokines in pancreatic tissue sections of patients with CP hybridized with radioactively labeled antisense probes for specific detection of (**A, C**) IL-8; (**B**) ENA-78, and (**D**) MIG. Affected pancreatic lobules are depicted in (**A, B**) with expression of (**A**) IL-8 and (**B**) ENA-78 by pancreatic duct cells. Inflammatory cells expressing IL-8, and MIG, respectively, are shown in (**C**) and (**D**). (Adapted from Saurer et al. Gastroenterology 118: 356–367; 2000, with permission).

stage 3 of disease activity reflects in part the increasing loss of parenchyma in advanced disease stages. Cellular sources of the CC- chemokines MCP-1 and I-309 in patients with CP are, besides epithelial cells of ducts and centroacinar ducts, also fibroblasts (Fig. 4.4-2), macrophages and to a lesser extent T cells (Table 4.4-1). The great variation in the frequency of chemokine expressing infiltrating cells isolated from tissue samples of different patients (Table 4.4-1) reflects the situation observed for the tissue sections, where the frequency of positive signals varies considerably from one patient to another.

The striking expression pattern observed for MCP-1 at the border of residual pancreatic lobules in transition to fibrous tissue, as well as expression of this chemokine by fibroblasts (Fig. 4.4-2), further suggests a possible role for this chemokine in tissue turnover and fibrogenesis. Increased production of MCP-1 has been described during active hepatic fibrogenesis [20]. More direct evidence for an involvement of MCP-1 in increased extracellular matrix deposition has been provided by a study [36] that reports stimulation of rat lung fibroblast gene collagen expression via endogenous upregulation of transforming growth factor(TGF-)β by MCP-1. TGF-β is known as a cytokine which not only exerts immunomodulatory functions but has also been characterized as a potent fibrogenic mediator by promoting the proliferation of fibroblasts and the production of connective tissue [17]. An upregulated expression of TGF-β in mononuclear and ductal epithelial cells has indeed been observed on tissue sections from patients with chronic

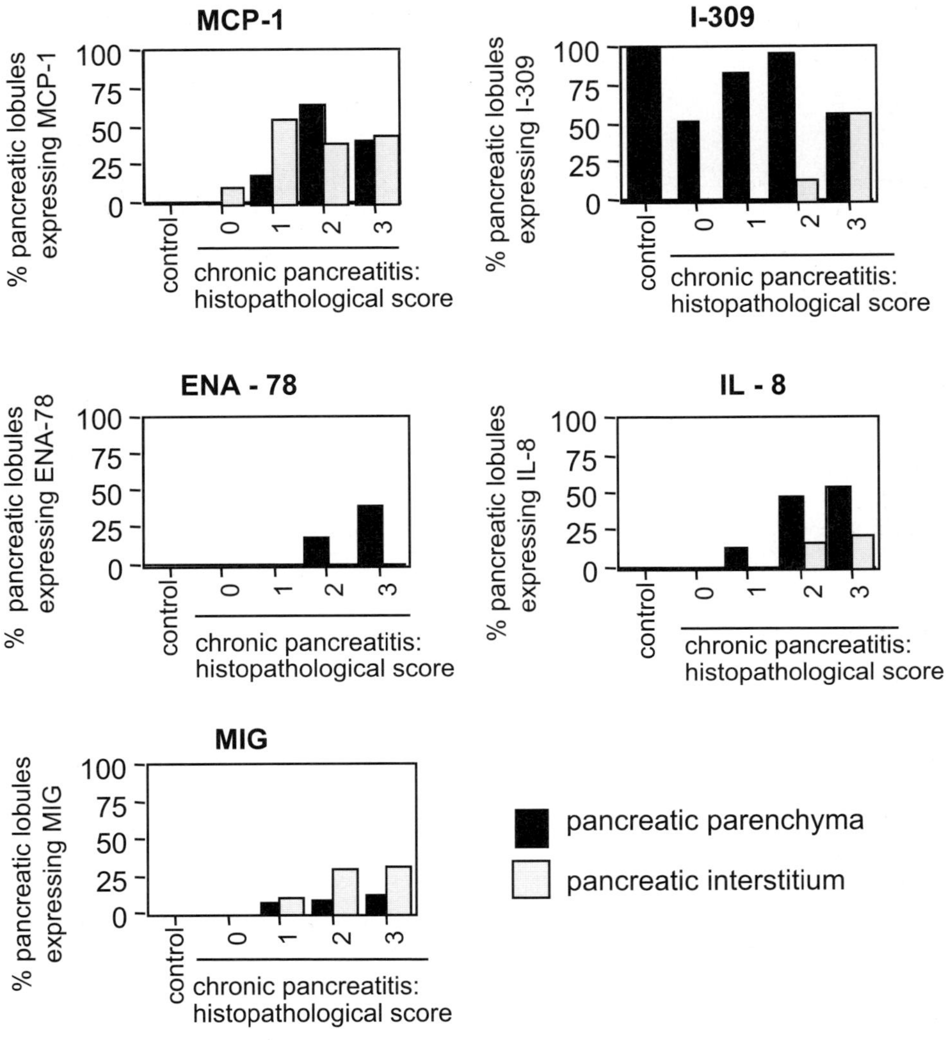

Figure 4.4-4. Chemokine gene expression in pancreatic parenchyma (black bars) and pancreatic interstitium (shaded bars) in normal pancreatic tissues (control) and in tissue samples from patients with chronic pancreatitis. Relative frequency of pancreatic lobules of a distinct grade of histopathologic alteration (scored 0–3) with ≥10 cells expressing detectable amounts of the chemokine mRNA.

pancreatitis [21, 22]. Moreover, in mice TGF-β has been shown to promote development of fibrosis after repeated courses of acute pancreatitis [23]. Due to the multifarious properties of this cytokine, however, it is difficult to determine the precise role of TGF-β in the pathogenesis of chronic pancreatitis. Hence, TGF-β is likely to be involved in the fibrogenetic processes occurring in chronic pancreatitis and thus contributes to the loss of functional exocrine pancreatic tissue. Such fibrosis-promoting effects may also be beneficial, preventing the spreading of the inflammatory reaction. In addition, TGF-β could possibly act by downregulating activated immune cells [24].

Table 4.4-1. Frequency of tissue specimens with distinct cell types expressing the respective chemokine genes in patients with chronic pancreatitis.

Source[1]	ENA-78	IL-8	Chemokine MIG	MCP-1	I-309
Ducts	22	39	0	9	30
Centroacinar cells	35	43	9	43	48
Endothelium	13	0	0	26	0
Cellular infiltrates	13	35	48	57	78
Fibroblasts	0	0	0	39	17
Nerves	0	0	0	17	0
TOTAL[2]	**35**	**57**	**48**	**91**	**87**

Note: Results are expressed as percentage; n = 23.

[1] Cellular sources of chemokine mRNA expression were determined on corresponding H&E-stained sections.

[2] Total: frequency (in percent) of tissue specimens with cells expressing chemokine mRNA at levels detectable by *in situ* hybridization.

(Data from Saurer et al., Gastroenterology 118: 356–367; 2000; reproduced with permission)

At first sight, the expression patterns of I-309 and MCP-I mRNA are comparable in chronic pancreatitis (Fig. 4.4-2, Table 4.4-2) and these two CC-chemokines are expressed simultaneously on tissue. In most tissue sections, it has yet to be determined whether they also mediate – at least in part – overlapping functions. Unlike for MCP-1, studies on possible roles for I-309 are very limited. I-309 has been reported to modulate dexamethasone-induced apoptosis in T-cell lymphomas [37]. Since we observed a surprisingly abundant expression of I-309 in normal pancreatic tissue, I-309 may mediate immunoregulatory functions, thus, preventing excessive stimulation of inflammatory cells, including T cells (see below).

In tissue sections from patients with chronic pancreatitis the CXC-chemokines ENA-78 and IL-8 are often expressed within the same tissue sections. As in IBD [11], epithelial cells appear to be the main contributors of ENA-78 in chronic pancreatitis, but in con-

Table 4.4-2. Frequency of chemokine mRNA-expressing cells in respective cell subsets.

Chemokine	CD14 (%)	CD3 (%)
ENA-78	N.D.	N.D.
IL-8	28.3 (SD ± 16.6)	0
MIG	0	2.6 (SD ± 1)
MCP-1	8.5 (SD ± 6.9)	6.5 (SD ± 3.3)
I-309	11.1 (SD ± 5.1)	8.4 (SD ± 2.3)

Note: The indicated cell populations isolated from patients with CP (n = 4) were sorted on a FACSvantage for subsequent *in situ* hybridization. The percentage of cells expressing chemokine mRNA was determined by counting positive cells in the corresponding cell population. N.D. = not determined.

(Data from Saurer et al., Gastroenterology 118: 356–367; 2000; reproduced with permission) trast to IBD, where IL-8 producing cells are predominantly neutrophils [12], in chronic pancreatitis macrophages significantly contribute to production of this chemokine (Table 4.4-1). Furthermore, in our study epithelial cells of the ducts and centroacinar ducts are additional important cellular sources for IL-8. These cells were also recognized as the main producers in chronic pancreatitis of ENA-78. The CXC-chemokine MIG, which acts preferentially on Th1 T cells [7, 13], is expressed only on a low frequency of isolated T cells. This is in agreement with the observation made on tissue sections from patients with CP where generally only small numbers of MIG mRNA expressing cells are present within inflammatory clusters.

Involvement of T cells in the pathogenesis of chronic pancreatitis

As shown in Figure 4.4-1 T cells are regularly found in affected, but not in normal pancreatic tissues in variable numbers. We previously determined the relative frequency of the pancreas infiltrating CD4, and CD8 T-cell subsets by flow cytometry. Although considerable variation in the CD4:CD8 ratio was found in the T-cell population isolated from pancreatic tissue samples of different patients, there was a tendency to lower CD4:CD8 T-cell ratio in the pancreas infiltrating cells than in the peripheral blood, thus indicating a preferential expansion and/or recruitment of CD8 T cells [25] and confirming work by other groups that determined the distribution of T cells in chronic pancreatitis by immunostainings [1, 26, 27]. CD4 and CD8 T lymphocytes differ not only in their cell surface markers but also in the nature of the antigenic peptides they recognize. Whereas CD4 T cells recognize their antigen when presented by MHC class II antigens (HLA-DR, DP, or DQ in humans), CD8 T cells recognize their antigen on MHC class I molecules (HLA-A, -B, -C in humans). Antigens presented by MHC class I molecules are derived from endogenous proteins synthesized by the cell (e.g. self-proteins and virus-derived antigens). Hence, CD8 T cells preferentially recognize virus-infected cells or altered cells that present an altered pattern of self peptides on their MHC class I molecules. MHC class II molecules are expressed only on a restricted number of cell types and present antigens to CD4 T cells that are derived from exogenous proteins and which had been proteolytically processed upon endocytosis of the intact protein. Functions exerted by T cells after antigen-specific activation are highly diverse even within the same phenotypic T-cell subset. Hence, CD4 T cells are often further divided, according to their functional properties, into cell subsets supporting the generation of a potent cell-mediated immune reaction such as delayed-type hypersensitivity reaction or cell-mediated cytotoxicity reactions (T helper 1 cells, Th1 cells), or into CD4 cells that support a humoral immune response (T helper 2 cells, Th2 cells) and regulatory CD4 T cells (T helper 3 cells, T regulatory 1 cells) that down-regulate a local immune response [10, 11].

Based on the mere presence of infiltrating CD4 and CD8 T cells only limited information can be obtained regarding the possible functions exerted by these cells *in situ,* since activated and resting T cells cannot be distinguished based on the amount if CD4 or CD8 cell surface expression and at the site of inflammation only a minor portion of T cells is activated in an antigen-specific way. One possible way to overcome these limitations is to perform *in situ* hybridizations on tissue sections for detecting mRNA of genes specifically associated with particular effector T-cell functions. In particular, detection of transcripts of the perforin gene has been successfully used to localize activated cytotoxic T cells in tissue sections [28]. Using this approach we were able to demonstrate that in fact

Table 4.4-3. Frequency of cell subsets and perforin mRNA expressing cells in distinct cell subsets isolated from affected pancreatic tissues from patients with chronic pancreatitis.

Cell Subset	Frequency of distinct pancreas infiltrating cell subsets (in % ± SEM)	Frequency of perforin mRNA positive cells in given cell subset (in % ± SEM)
CD4 T cells	30.9 ± 4.1	0.97 ± 0.2
CD8 T cells	26.1 ± 4.3	11.9 ± 2.5
CD56 cells	8.1 ± 3.3	18.0 ± 5.2

in patients with active stages of chronic pancreatitis a considerable fraction of the infiltrating MHC class I restricted CD8 T cells represent activated perforin mRNA (and perforin protein) expressing cells (Table 4.4-3 and [25]). The preferential localization of these activated cytotoxic cells in proximity to remaining parenchyma provided circumstantial evidence for a direct contribution of cytotoxic T cells (and possibly also CD56 positive NK cells) in the destruction of the parenchymal cells.

Intriguingly, this excessive activation of cytotoxic cells and the greatly reduced expression of the I-309 chemokine in chronic pancreatitis may be not completely independent, but may be directly linked. Recent studies on human T-cell clones revealed the preferential expression of the chemokine receptor CCR8 on Th2 T cells, i.e. on the functional T-cell subsets that supports the generation of a potent humoral immune response, and thus down-regulates the activity of Th1 T cells which in turn support the differentiation of CD8 T cells into potent killer T cells. Hence, based on the reported preferential expression of CCR8 on Th2 T cells, it is tempting to speculate that I-309 produced by acinar cells in normal pancreata may act together with other cytokines such as TGF-β or interleukin-10 as a regulatory chemokine that prevents an excessive cell-mediated cytotoxic immune response through the selective recruitment of T cells with an opposing functional phenotype. In normal pancreatic tissues, secretion of I-309 may be limited and most of I-309 may be stored within the acinar cells. Upon injury of the I-309 producing cells, I-309 may be released, leading to the preferential early recruitment of Th2 T cells that initially are able to counteract the generation of potent cell-mediated cytotoxic reactions. However, if acinar cells fail to produce enough I-309 an excessive differentiation of CD8 T cells *in situ* might occur that due to the cytolytic activity of these effector T cells may again lead to a further reduction in the number of I-309 secreting cells in a given pancreatic lobule, thus accelerating the process of fibrotic destruction. Support for this concept of a locally deregulated immune response leading to destruction of pancreatic parenchyma stems from two animal models of spontaneous onset of a chronic pancreatitis-like disease. Vallance and co-workers observed a gradual T-cell infiltration and destruction of the exocrine pancreas in MHC class II deficient mice. These mice lack CD4 T cells (and hence also regulatory CD4 T cells) due to the absence of positive selection of this T-cell subset in the thymus, thus possibly leading to an uncontrolled activation of (auto-)reactive CD8 T cells in the pancreas [29]. Intriguingly, in this mouse model, disease can be induced in immunodeficient recipients of CD8 T cells from these MHC class II deficient mice, thus providing evidence for a CD8 T cell-mediated process leading to pancreatic tissue destruction in the absence of an immunoregulatory network [29]. The other mouse strain that shows spontaneous signs of pancreatic fibrosis is the CTLA-4 deficient mouse [30]. CTLA-4 was initially described as a co-stimulatory molecule expressed on T cells. More recent work with CTLA-4 deficient mice, however, clearly indicated that CTLA-4 is instrumental in down-regulating ongoing T-cell reactions. Hence, it can be concluded that in the absence of CTLA-4 these mice show an excessive activation of pancreas infiltrating T cells that eventually leads to T cell-mediated destruction of the parenchymal cells in the pancreas. A disease exacerbating role has also been ascribed to (mainly) CD4 T cells in a cerulein-induced model of acute pancreatitis in mice [31].

In conclusion, recent work provided compelling evidence for an active involvement of the adaptive immune system in the pathogenesis of chronic pancreatitis. Although major questions still remain open, such as the nature of the (auto-)antigen(s) recognized by infiltrating CD4 and CD8 T cells or whether in recurrent episodes of acute pancreatitis the T-cell clones with identical antigen specificity become reactivated, these new findings will clearly lead to novel concepts of the pathogenesis of chronic pancreatitis. It is hoped that these new concepts will further lead to a careful (re-)evaluation of other animal models, in particular those with an altered immune regulation, for signs of histopathological alterations in the pancreas which might reveal new clues to the possible early steps in the pathogenesis of chronic pancreatitis. The dramatic increase in our understanding of the etiopathogenesis of inflammatory bowel diseases due to the (serendipitous) generations of animal models with specific defects in the immunoregulatory pathways [32] illustrates the potential of combined assessment of animal models and tissue samples from patients with the respective disorders for the elucidation of the etiopathogenesis of complex disorders.

References

1. Jalleh RP, Gilbertson JA, Williamson RC, Slater SD, Foster CS. Expression of major histocompatibility antigens in human chronic pancreatitis. Gut 1993; 34(10): 1452–7.
2. Springer TA. Traffic signals for lymphocyte recirculation and leukocyte emigration: the multistep paradigm. Cell 1994; 76: 301–14.
3. Luster AD. Chemokines-chemotactic cytokines that mediate inflammation. N Engl J Med 1998; 338(7): 436–45.
4. Baggiolini M, Dewald B, Moser B. Human chemokines: an update. Annu Rev Immunol 1997; 15: 675–705.
5. Oppenheim JJ, Zachariae COC, Mukaida N, Matsushima K. Properties of the novel proinflammatory supergene "intercrine" cytokine family. Annu Rev Immunol 1991; 9: 617–48.
6. Rollins BJ. Chemokines. Blood 1997; 90(3): 909–28.
7. Sallusto F, Lanzavecchia A, Mackay CR. Chemokines and chemokine receptors in T-cell priming and Th1/Th2-mediated responses. Immunol Today 1998; 19(12): 568–74.
8. Bates P. Chemokine receptors and HIV-1: an attractive pair? Cell 1996; 86(1): 1–3.
9. Baggiolini M, Dewald B, Walz A. Interleukin-8 and related chemotactic cytokines. In: Gallin JI, Goldstein M, Snyderman R, eds. Inflammation: basic principles and clinical correlates. 2nd ed. New York: Raven Press, 1992.
10. Walz A, Burgener R, Car B, Baggiolini M, Kunkel SL, Strieter RM. Structure and neutrophil-activating properties of a novel inflammatory peptide (ENA-78) with homology to Interleukin 8. J Exp Med 1991; 174: 1355–62.
11. Z'Graggen K, Walz A, Mazzucchelli L, Strieter RM, Mueller C. The C-X-C chemokine ENA-78 is preferentially expressed in intestinal epithelium in inflammatory bowel disease. Gastroenterology 1997; 113(3): 808–16.
12. Mazzucchelli L, Hauser C, Zgraggen K et al. Expression of interleukin-8 gene in inflammatory bowel disease is related to the histological grade of active inflammation. Am J Pathol 1994; 144(5): 997–1007.

13. Loetscher M, Gerber B, Loetscher P et al. Chemokine receptor specific for IP10 and mig: structure, function, and expression in activated T-lymphocytes (see comments). J Exp Med 1996; 184(3): 963–9.
14. Uguccioni M, D'Apuzzo M, Loetscher M, Dewald B, Baggiolini M. Actions of the chemotactic cytokines MCP-1, MCP-2, MCP-3, RANTES, MIP-1alpha and MIP-1beta on human monocytes. Eur J Immunol 1995; 25: 64–8.
15. Loetscher P, Seitz M, Clark-Lewis I, Baggiolini M, Moser B. Monocyte chemotactic proteins MCP-1, MCP-2, and MCP-3 are major attractants for human CD4+ and CD8+ T lymphocytes. FASEB J 1994; 8: 1055–60.
16. Denholm EM. Continuous secretion of monocyte chemotactic factors and fibroblast growth factors by alveolar macrophages following a single exposure to bleomycin in vitro. Am J Pathol 1992; 141(4): 965–71.
17. Selvan RS, Zhou LJ, Krangel MS. Regulation of I-309 gene expression in human monocytes by endogenous interleukin-1. Eur J Immunol 1997; 27(3): 687–94.
18. D'Ambrosio D, Iellem A, Bonecchi R et al. Selective up-regulation of chemokine receptors CCR4 and CCR8 upon activation of polarized human type 2 Th cells. J Immunol 1998; 161(10): 5111–5.
19. Zingoni A, Soto H, Hedrick JA et al. The chemokine receptor CCR8 is preferentially expressed in Th2 but not Th1 cells. J Immunol 1998; 161(2): 547–51.
20. Marra F, De Franco R, Grappone C et al. Increased expression of monocyte chemotactic protein-1 during active hepatic fibrogenesis: correlation with monocyte infiltration. Am J Pathol 1998; 152(2): 423–30.
21. van Laethem JL, Deviere J, Resibois A et al. Localization of transforming growth factor beta 1 and its latent binding protein in human chronic pancreatitis. Gastroenterology 1995; 108(6): 1873–81.
22. Slater SD, Williamson RC, Foster CS. Expression of transforming growth factor-beta 1 in chronic pancreatitis. Digestion 1995; 56(3): 237–41.
23. Van Laethem JL, Robberecht P, Resibois A, Deviere J. Transforming growth factor beta promotes development of fibrosis after repeated courses of acute pancreatitis in mice. Gastroenterology 1996; 110(2): 576–82.
24. Ruscetti F, Varesio L, Ochoa A, Ortaldo J. Pleiotropic effects of transforming growth factor-beta on cells of the immune system. Ann NY Acad Sci 1993; 685: 488–500.
25. Hunger RE, Mueller C, Z'Graggen K, Friess H, Buchler MW. Cytotoxic cells are activated in cellular infiltrates of alcoholic chronic pancreatitis. Gastroenterology 1997; 112(5): 1656–63.
26. Ebert MP, Ademmer K, Muller-Ostermeyer F et al. CD8+ CD103+ T cells analogous to intestinal intraepithelial lymphocytes infiltrate the pancreas in chronic pancreatitis. Am J Gastroenterol 1998; 93(11): 2141–7.
27. Bedossa P, Bacci J, Lemaigre G, Martin E. Lymphocyte subsets and HLA-DR expression in normal pancreas and chronic pancreatitis. Pancreas 1990; 5(4): 415–20.
28. Griffiths GM, Mueller C. Expression of perforin and granzymes in vivo: potential diagnostic markers for activated cytotoxic cells. Immunol Today 1991; 12(11): 415–9.
29. Vallance BA, Hewlett BR, Snider DP, Collins SM. T cell-mediated exocrine pancreatic damage in major histocompatibility complex class II-deficient mice. Gastroenterology 1998; 115(4): 978–87.
30. Waterhouse P, Penninger JM, Timms E et al. Lymphoproliferative disorders with early lethality in mice deficient in CTLA-4. Science 1995; 270: 985–8.
31. Demols A, Le Moine O, Desalle F, Quertinmont E, Van Laethem JL, Deviere J. CD4(+)T Cells Play an Important Role in Acute Experimental Pancreatitis in Mice. Gastroenterology 2000; 118(3): 582–90.
32. Elson CO, Sartor RB, Tennyson GS, Riddell RH. Experimental models of inflammatory bowel disease. Gastroenterology 1995; 109(4): 1344–67.

4.5 The value of p53 mutations in chronic pancreatitis

S. Gansauge

Abstract

In patients suffering from chronic pancreatitis the risk of the development of pancreatic cancer ranges from 4 to 6%. In the present study DNA of 80 tissues of chronic pancreatitis was isolated and SSCP analysis of p53 exons 5–9 was performed. In SSCP-analysis 8 out of 80 cases of chronic pancreatitis showed alterations (2 in exon 5, 4 in exon 6, 2 in exon 7). DNA sequence analysis revealed 1 deletion of 21 amino acids (exon 5), 4 polymorphisms in exon 6 with no change in the amino acid sequence, 1 point mutation in exon 5, and 2 point mutations located in the intron between exon 6 and exon 7. These data show that in some cases of chronic pancreatitis mutations in the p53 gene occur without morphological evidence for pancreatic cancer.

Introduction

Despite improved diagnostic and therapeutic facilities, cancer of the pancreas still has a very poor prognosis [1]. At time of admission to the hospital only one third of the patients are resectable, and even in the group of patients undergoing resection of the tumor, median survival times are seldom longer than two years [2]. Although no specific reasons for the development of pancreatic cancer are known several risk factors, such as alcohol, smoking and nitrosamines are thought to increase the risk for pancreatic cancer development [3–5]. Besides these risk factors several reports provide evidence that chronic pancreatitis itself is associated with an increased risk of pancreatic cancer [6–8]. Analysis of the patients who underwent surgery at our Department for chronic pancreatitis (n = 395) revealed that the frequency of pancreatic cancer in pre-existing chronic pancreatitis was 3.8%, which is significantly higher than that for the normal population [8].

At subcellular and molecular levels chronic pancreatitis and pancreatic carcinoma have been studied extensively (for review see [9]). Although many alterations in mRNA expression were found in chronic pancreatitis as compared to normal pancreatic tissue only a few studies report molecular alterations at the DNA level. Mutations in the p53 gene occur in almost 50% of pancreatic carcinomas [10, 11]. However, only one single observation which investigated 6 cases of chronic pancreatitis for p53 mutations at DNA level exists and in this study no p53 mutations were found in 6 cases of chronic pancreatitis [10]. In pancreatic cancer mutations in the p53 gene seem to be more frequent in advanced tumor stages and seem to be associated with a poorer prognosis than pancreatic tumors bearing wild-type p53 [12].

The aim of the study was to determine whether mutations in the p53 gene occur in chronic pancreatitis providing evidence for a possible screening method for high risk cases of chronic pancreatitis.

Material and methods

Patients

DNA was isolated from 80 tissues of chronic pancreatitis derived from patients undergoing duodenum-preserving pancreatic head resection at the Department of General Surgery from 02/1994 to 08/1995. Immediately following resection the tissue was snap frozen in liquid nitrogen and stored at –80°C until DNA was isolated. The median age was 44 years (range 27–73 years), 64 patients were male, 16 patients were female. No patient died peri- or postoperatively. The diagnosis of chronic pancreatitis was confirmed by a pathologist. DNA was isolated from one random sample. Prior to DNA isolation chronic pancreatitis was assessed by a hematoxylin stain of the tissue block. Only tissue samples which contained more than 80% of chronic pancreatitis areals were included in the analysis.

Detection of p53 mutation

SSCP analysis (single strand conformation polymorphism) was performed as described recently [13]. In brief, PCR (polymerase chain reaction) conditions were as follows: in a total volume of 25 µl, 500 ng of genomic DNA was incubated in 10 mM Tris-HCl (pH 8.3), 2 mM magnesium chloride, 50 mM potassium chloride, 0.01% gelatin, 100 mM dNTPs (deoxy-nucleotid triphosphates), 1 µM of each primer, 5 µCi of α-^{32}P dCTP (deoxy-cytosine triphosphate) and 1 U of Taq polymerase from thermus aquaticus DNA-polymerase (Perkin Elmer, Branchburg, NJ, USA). Amplifications were performed for 35 cycles consisting of 30 s at 94°C, 30s at a range between 50°C and 65°C depending on the primers and 45 s at 72°C. SSCP was performed using MDE gels (long-range gel solution, Boehringer Ingelheim, Heidelberg, Germany) followed by 12 hours exposure to X-ray films. Sequencing was performed using an automated sequencing system (ALF, Pharmacia).

Results

SSCP of exons 5–9 revealed alterations in 8 cases (10%) of the patients investigated (Table 4.5-1). Two cases showed alterations in exon 5, 4 alterations were found in exon 6, and 2 were found in exon 7. All eight alterations were found in different cases.

Table 4.5-1. Alterations in SSCP of DNA from chronic pancreatitis.

	SSCP of p53				
Alteration (n = 80)	**exon 5**	**exon 7**	**exon 6**	**exon 8**	**exon 9**
	2	4	2	0	0

Sequencing of the 8 DNAs which had shown alterations in SSCP analysis of p53 revealed that all cases with alterations in exon 6 showed a CGA → CGG transition at codon 213 without causing a change in amino acid sequence (CGA as well as CGG code for arginine). One case with alterations in exon 5 showed a point mutation GGC → GAC at codon 154 causing an exchange of glycin by asparagin. The other alteration in exon 5 was a frameshift mutation leading to a deletion of 21 nucleotides. The two cases with alter-

Table 4.5-2. Analysis of alterations in p53 by sequencing.

Cases	Exon	Mutation	Type of mutation	Consequence
4	6	CGA → CGG	Point mutation	None, polymorphism
1	5	–	Deletion	Deletion of 21 nucleotides
1	5	GGC → GAC	Point mutation	Glycin → asparagin
2	6–7	G → C	Point mutation	None, polymorphism ?

ations in exon 7 both showed a G → C transversion located in the intron between exon 6 and 7 at position 25 (Table 4.5-2). The polymorphism in exon 6 has also been described in a series of patients with arthrosclerotic lesions [14].

Discussion

The development of pancreatic cancer during chronic pancreatitis is still controversial, in part due to the limited number of cases. In a prospective trial 245 patients with chronic pancreatitis were observed for 10.4 years. Pancreatic carcinoma was diagnosed in seven cases during that period [6]. Löwenfels and coworkers studied a population of 2,015 patients retrospectively. During the observation period of 7.6 years 56 patients developed pancreatic cancer [7]. Molecular analysis on mRNA levels revealed an increased expression of growth factors like TGF-α, aFGF, bFGF as well as the EGF receptor and c-erb B-2 in human pancreatic tissue of chronic pancreatitis [15, 16]. The expression of extracellular matrix molecules and their receptors was also slightly altered in chronic pancreatitis as compared to normal pancreas [17]. These reports suggest a dysregulation of a number of genes resulting in altered mRNA levels in chronic pancreatitis. Some of these changes, especially the overexpression of growth factors and their receptors, might contribute to ductal cell hyperplasia and pseudoductal cell formations. The hypothesis of a sequential development of pancreatic cancer is supported by the observation that in specimens of chronic pancreatitis dysplastic structures are frequently found [18]. A hyperplasia – dysplasia – carcinoma sequence seems to be more likely than an one step process. It is now generally accepted that carcinogenesis is a multistep process [19]. Such a sequence of genetic events was first demonstrated for colon cancer. The accumulation of genetic alterations in both oncogenes and tumor suppressor genes, including activation of the K-ras proto-oncogene and inactivation of the APC, DCC and p53 tumor suppressor genes, is the genetic basis for the adenoma-carcinoma sequence [19]. Mutations in the K-ras gene on chromosome 12p are rare in small adenomas but are found in almost 50% of adenomas bigger than one centimeter in diameter [20], whereas an inactivation of the p53 tumor suppressor gene on chromosome 17p preferentially occurs in large adenomas and in carcinomas, typically at a later stage of the neoplastic process. In the adenoma-carcinoma sequence K-ras mutations always precede p53-inactivation [19, 20]. On the other hand p53 mutations seem to be early genetic events in dysplastic lesions. Patients suffering from colitis ulcerosa develop first p53 mutations and a loss of heterozygocity without evidence of K-ras mutations. Furthermore, p53 mutations have been found in benign or precancerous lesions in other human tissues like hyperplastic prostatic epithelium [21], papillomatous hyperplasia and fibroadenoma of the breast [22], suggesting that p53 mutations can also occur at a very early stage of tumorigenesis in other tissues.

Interestingly we found alterations in the p53 gene in 10% of the cases. Four out of 8 cases showed single base changes at the third position of a codon, not altering the amino acid sequence. The significance of this genetic polymorphism is not clear. However, it is very interesting that in the multitude of reports we only found two studies which described this polymorphism [14, 23]. In 2 cases we found point mutations located in the intron between exon 6 and exon 7, and in 2 cases a mutation either resulted in a loss of 21 nucleotides (exon 5), or caused a change of one amino acid (exon 5). The alterations clearly changed the structure of the p53 protein in terms of alteration of the amino acid sequence. However, we do not know whether these changes also lead to an altered function or a loss of function in the p53 gene product.

These data show that in some cases of chronic pancreatitis, mutations in the p53 gene occur without morphological evidence for pancreatic cancer which could point to precancerous lesions. Since in only two out of 80 cases of the identified mutations the amino acid sequence was altered, we will continue this study to confirm the data presented in a larger series of chronic pancreatitis patients.

References

1. Gudjonsson B. Cancer of the pancreas. 50 years of surgery. Cancer 1987; 60: 2284–303.
2. Beger HG, Büchler MW, Friess H. Surgical results and indications for adjuvant treatment in pancreatic cancer. Chirurg 1994; 65: 246–52.
3. Gold EB, Gordis L, Diener MD, Seltser R, Boitnott JK, Bynum TE, Hutcheon DF. Diet and other risk factors for cancer of the pancreas. Cancer 1985; 55: 460–7.
4. Mack TM, Walker A, Mack W, Bernstein L. Cancer in Hispanics in Los Angeles County. Natl Cancer Inst Monogr 1985; 69: 99–104.
5. Velema JP, Walker AM, Gold EB. Alcohol and pancreatic cancer. Insufficient epidemiologic evidence for a causal relationship. Epidemiol Rev 1986; 8: 28–41.
6. Ammann RW, Akobiantz A, Legardier F, Schueler G. Course and outcome of chronic pancreatitis. Gastroenterology 1984; 86: 820–8.
7. Lowenfels AB, Maisonneuve P, Cavallini G, Ammann RW, Lankisch PG, Andersen JR, DiMagno EP, Andren Sandberg A, Domellof L. Pancreatitis and the risk of pancreatic cancer. International Pancreatitis Study Group. N Engl J Med 1993; 328: 1433–7.
8. Schlosser W, Schoenberg MH, Siech M, Gansauge F, Beger HG. Development of pancreatic cancer in chronic pancreatitis. Z Gastroenterol 1996; 34: 3–8.
9. Gansauge S, Gansauge F, Beger HG. Molecular oncology in pancreatic cancer. J Mol Med 1996; 74: 313–20.
10. Casey G, Yamanaka Y, Friess H, Kobrin MS, Lopez ME, Büchler MW, Beger HG, Korc M. p53 mutations are common in pancreatic cancer and are absent in chronic pancreatitis. Cancer Lett 1993; 69: 151–60.
11. Scarpa A, Capelli P, Mukai K, Zamboni G, Oda T, Iacono C, Hirohashi S. Pancreatic adenocarcinomas frequently show p53 gene mutations. Am J Pathol 1993; 142: 1534–43.
12. Gansauge S, Gansauge F, Negri G, Galle P, Muller J, Poch B, Nussler AK, Beger HG. The role of anti-p53-autoantibodies in pancreatic disorders. Int J Pancreatol 1996; 19: 171–8.
13. Mazars GR, Portier M, Zhang XG, Jourdan M, Bataille R, Theillet C, Klein B. Mutations of the p53 gene in human myeloma cell lines. Oncogene 1992; 7: 1015–8.
14. D'Agostini F, Fronza G, Campomenosi P, Izzotti A, Petrilli GL, Abbondandolo A, De Flora S. Cancer biomarkers in human atherosclerotic lesions: no evidence of p53 involvement. Cancer Epidemiol Biomarkers Prev 1995; 4: 111–5.
15. Barton CM, Hall PA, Hughes CM, Gullick WJ, Lemoine NR. Transforming growth factor alpha and epidermal growth factor in human pancreatic cancer. J Pathol 1991; 163: 111–6.
16. Friess H, Yamanaka Y, Buchler M, Hammer K, Kobrin MS, Beger HG, Korc M. A subgroup of

patients with chronic pancreatitis overexpress the c-erb B-2 protooncogene. Ann Surg 1994; 220: 183–92.
17. Shimoyama S, Gansauge F, Gansauge S, Oohara T, Beger HG. Altered expression of extracellular matrix molecules and their receptors in chronic pancreatitis and adenocarcinoma of the pancreas in comparison to normal pancreas. Int J Pancreatol 1995; 18: 227–34.
18. Cylwik B, Nowak HF, Puchalski Z, Barczyk J. Chronic pancreatitis as a predisposing factor in the development of pancreatic cancer. Histological and histochemical studies. Zentralbl Allg Pathol 1985; 130: 217–24.
19. Vogelstein B, Fearon ER, Hamilton SR, Kern SE, Preisinger AC, Leppert M, Nakamura Y, White R, Smits AM, Bos JL. Genetic alterations during colorectal-tumor development. N Engl J Med 1988; 319: 525–32.
20. Bos JL, Fearon ER, Hamilton SR, Verlaan de Vries M, van Boom JH, van der Eb AJ, Vogelstein B. Prevalence of ras gene mutations in human colorectal cancers. Nature 1987; 327: 293–7.
21. Kallakury BV, Jennings TA, Ross JS, Breese K, Figge HL, Fisher HA, Figge J. Alteration of the p53 locus in benign hyperplastic prostatic epithelium associated with high-grade prostatic adenocarcinoma. Diagn Mol Pathol 1994; 3: 227–32.
22. Millikan R, Hulka B, Thor A, Zhang Y, Edgerton S, Zhang X, Pei H, He M, Wold L, Melton LJ et al. p53 mutations in benign breast tissue. J Clin Oncol 1995; 13: 2293–300.
23. Karameris AM, Worthy E, Gorgoulis VG, Quezado M, Anastassiades OT. p53 gene alterations in special types of breast carcinoma: a molecular and immunohistochemical study in archival material. J Pathol 1995; 176: 361–72.

4.6 Neuroimmune cross-talk: What can we learn from inflammatory disorders?

A. Roggo, H. Friess, E. Weihe

Introduction

Traditionally, the nervous and immune systems have been assumed to function largely independently of each other. Interdisciplinary investigations in the fields of anatomy, molecular biology, neurophysiology and neuro-pharmacology, however, have provided fundamental insights into the complex functional and molecular anatomy of the dialogue between the nervous and immune systems in health and disease, and have provided a basis for novel therapeutic strategies targeted at restoring disturbed neuroimmune interactions [2, 6, 21, 23, 30, 50, 58, 63, 70, 71].

Studies over recent years have revealed that transmitters of the nervous system act on immune cells and messengers of the immune system influence the nervous system. Typical neuronal messengers appear to be synthesized in immune cells, and typical immune cell messengers appear to be produced in neurons. This is a further dimension of interactions between the nervous and immune systems, named neuroimmune interactions. These complex functional interactions are fundamentally important not only for physiological regulation, but also for diverse diseases such as chronic painful inflammations (e.g., arthritis, pancreatitis), degenerative diseases, autoimmune diseases (e.g., multiple sclerosis), and viral infections affecting the nervous system (e.g., neuro-AIDS) [3, 22, 44, 48, 72, 76].

The debate over whether substance P is a nociceptive transmitter has led to a focus on the role of neuropeptides in pain mechanisms [31]. In mammalian species it was originally believed that neuropeptides are the domain of neuronal subpopulations and neuroendocrine cells, but recent evidence suggests that the classical "neuropeptides" have a much wider cellular distribution than previously thought [62, 69, 71]. However, the neuropeptide connection turned out to be very complicated, and its real significance is still debated. A variety of neuropeptides are contained in presumed nociceptive afferents, in spinal interneurons and ascending neurons involved in spinal nociceptive processing and in preganglionic as well as postganglionic sympathetic neurons which are also known to be important in the nociceptive process [12, 19, 26, 29, 34, 57, 63]. Due to characteristic changes of neuropeptide biosynthesis and release in conditions of inflammatory pain [20], it seems reasonable to assume that the synthesis of neuropeptide processing enzymes also may be altered. Furthermore, peripheral and spinal neuropeptide receptor binding is often changed [7, 58]. However, the exact cellular sites of synthesis of the different neuropeptide receptors in the periphery, in the dorsal root ganglionic cells and in the spinal cord are largely unexplored. With the recent cloning of an increasing number of neuropeptide receptor genes it is now possible to determine the sites of synthesis of neuropeptide receptors at the cellular and subcellular levels [31]. Molecular anatomical knowledge of the principles of neuroimmune interactions is meanwhile achieved by applying modern neurobiological, neuroanatomical, immunobiological, and molecular biological methods. Transmitter substances in nerves supplying the immune organs and tissues can be unequivocally identified by immunohistochemistry using transmitter-specific antibodies on both the light and electron microscopic level [23, 24, 67, 69]. The specific spatial relationships of transmitter-identified nerve endings with subtypes of immune cells can be characterized by costaining for neuronal messengers and immune cell markers on identical tissue sections [45, 47].

The regional and cellular localization of neurotransmitter receptors in cells of the immune system can be determined by receptor autoradiography. Furthermore, the immune cell-specific synthesis of receptor proteins can be evaluated and measured on the mRNA level by radioactive and nonradioactive *in situ* hybridization histochemistry, and on the protein level by immunocytochemical localization of the receptor [75]. However, the low abundance of the expression of neurotransmitter receptors in immune cells limits their detectability and localization through immunocytochemical or *in situ* hybridization techniques. In addition, immune cells tend to exhibit nonspecific immunostaining and nonspecific *in situ* hybridization signals. In particular, eosinophilic cells hybridize with many cRNA probes nonspecifically. Therefore, reports of abundant positive immunostaining for neurotransmitter molecules, or hybridization for neurotransmitter mRNAs in immune cells, should be interpreted with caution and have to be reevaluated under *in vivo* conditions [64]. To investigate the pathway-specific origins of transmitter-identified nerve supply to the various immune organs and lymphoid tissues, anterograde and retrograde tracing techniques are combined with immunocytochemistry or *in situ* hybridization [53]. Using this approach, different categories of innervation of the immune organs have been recognized: a) afferent peptidergic sensory nerve fibers projecting to the central nervous system (CNS) via dorsal root or cranial (e.g., vagal) sensory ganglia and b) efferent sympathetic (noradrenergic) and c) parasympathetic (cholinergic) nerve fibers projecting to the peripheral lymphoid tissues. The analysis in immune cells and neurons, experimental neuromanipulation or immune manipulation provides evidence for the functional significance of neuro-immune interactions in health and disease, and reveals underlying cellular and molecular mechanisms [5, 8, 9, 18, 22, 72, 76].

Principles of the neuroimmune dialogue

In the periphery, neuroimmune and immunoneural information exchange require wiring of immune organs, and lymphoid tissues and cells, with different categories of peripheral nerves [72]. The peripheral neuroimmune interactions depend on close spatial relationships of nerve endings with different cells of the immune system (lymphocytes, macrophages, dendritic cells including epidermal Langerhans cells, granulocytes, mast cells), as well as cells of the connective tissue (e.g., fibroblasts), and the terminal vessel structures, especially postcapillary venules. Schwann cells, the glial cells of the peripheral nervous system, also come into play as indirect actors in the complex processes of neuroimmune interactions.

Different messengers of the nervous system (classical neurotransmitters such as noradrenaline and acetylcholine, and neuropeptides such as substance P [SP] and calcitonin gene-related peptide [CGRP]) and their specific receptors on target immune cells, represent in the neuroimmune interactions the "software" by which nerves ("hardware") influence immune cells [39]. These immune cells synthesize cytokines (e.g., interleukins, interferons, tumor necrosis factor [TNF]) acting on cytokine receptors located on the membranes of neurons or on glial cells, to influence neurons directly or indirectly by stimulation of glial-derived messengers [32, 54]. SP and CGRP interact in a complex manner, with CGRP inhibiting the degradation of SP [49], enhancing its pronociceptive and immune-signaling action in the spinal dorsal horn and its proinflammatory and pronociceptive action in the periphery [62]. This is the "software" for immune to neural influences. Furthermore, some researchers believe that neurons themselves may produce cytokines that may act in an autocrine or paracrine fashion, but this view is not supported by our own investigations. Neuropeptides and endocrine messengers may be produced in immune cells to regulate immune cell functions in an autocrine, paracrine, or even intracrine manner [75]. In addition, diverse molecules of the complex families of growth factors and neurotrophins and their receptors are likely to participate directly or indirectly in the interactive neuroimmune "conceit" by being differentially expressed in immune and mast cells, as well as neurons, glial cells, and other types of cells [1].

The "local talk" of the neuroimmune dialogue occurs within the local micro milieu. Different messengers and diverse messenger receptors are directly or indirectly involved in the communication between immune cells and nerve endings. These interactions are characterized by changes in the release of neurotransmitters, which are caused or modulated by changes in local levels of immune mediators (e.g., cytokines, prostaglandins). Released neurotransmitters influence synthesis and release of cytokines from immune cells or support cells [74]. This molecular scenario is complemented by local production of neurotrophins and growth factors acting on pleiotropic receptors localized on heterogeneous immune cell populations, support cells, and neuroglial cells [1, 35, 37]. These factors are crucial for the regulation of the innervation density and spatial connectivity in the lymphoid tissues and in the local neuroimmune territory. Depending on the body region, tissue compartments, and immune organs, the afferent sensory innervation and the efferent sympathetic noradrenergic and/or parasympathetic cholinergic innervation contribute to the interplay in combination or separately [65, 72].

Neuronal chains of the sympathetic and parasympathetic nervous system originating from the CNS are responsible for the "tele-regulation" of the immune system by the CNS. One route of tele-communication from the immune system back to the CNS (immunoendocrine loop) involves cytokines circulating in the bloodstream and entering the brain at sites where there is a reduced blood-brain barrier [6]. Cytokines influence neuroendocrine regulatory centers in the hypothalamus and activate the hypothalamic-pituitary-adrenal (HPA) axis as well as the hypothalamo-sympatho-adrenomedullary axis. In addition to this immunoendocrine loop, immune signaling to the CNS appears to follow a direct immunoneural loop along primary afferents [15, 72].

Peripheral terminals of primary afferent neurons function as "immunoceptors" [25]. This perception of immune signals by primary viscerosensory neurons of the vagal nerve, or by primary somato- or viscerosensory neurons of the dorsal root ganglia (spinal ganglia), is transferred to second-order neurons in the brain stem (vagal nerve) and the spinal cord (primary spinal afferents) [25, 72]. From there, the immune signaling is propagated via further neuronal chains to higher brain centers, particularly to the hypothalamus. It is assumed that the immune activation of these neural pathways also results in an activation of the hypothalamic-pituitary-adrenal (HPA) axis and of the hypothalamo-sympatho-adrenomedullary axis. The long sensory loops that serve the tele-communication from the immune system to the CNS may also be used antidromically as communication pathways from the CNS to the immune system [70, 72]. Primary sensory neurons have a functional duality, perceiving and propagating signals to the CNS, but also exerting local effector functions in the periphery. This prompts the theory that impulses from the brain activate terminals of primary afferents in the CNS and thus activate primary afferents antidromically, which could result in the peripheral release of immuno-modulatory neuropeptides (e.g., CGRP and SP) from sensory terminals in close spatial relationship with immune cells. This may cause priming, exacerbation, or suppression of immune reactions in the periphery, and could explain influences of the psyche on allergic reactions such as asthma.

Furthermore, it can be anticipated that the net signaling generated in immune cells and adjacent support cells is perceived by local endings of sensory, sympathetic, or parasympathetic terminals directly or indirectly (e.g., by Schwann cells) and translated into short- or long-term changes of the gene expression in the respective neuronal cell bodies. Neurons altered in metabolism in this way feed back into local immune target milieu at their peripheral terminal, providing the basis for protracted neuroimmune dialogues and neuroimmune homeostasis. However, as an argument for antidromic activation of sensory efferent functions from the CNS, the possibility has to be proposed that efferent sympathetic or parasympathetic neurons may be influenced antidromically, with the potential of antidromic signaling to the CNS along efferent pathways.

Also within the CNS, there is evidence of mutual intercommunication between nerve endings and resident immunocompetent microglial cells of the CNS, the macrophages of the brain. This interaction will be primarily of a "local talk" type, but also involves long-loop neuronal networks between different brain areas [32, 36, 60]. Microglial cells synthesize cytokines on one side that can modify neurotransmission in the CNS. Neuronal activity on the other side regulates microglial function and cytokine production. Apparently, neuronal IFN-7 receptors are crucially involved. Neuro-mast cell interactions in the brain may be much more important than currently believed, and could represent a causal link in CNS inflammatory and autoimmune disease. Astrocytes are also regarded as sources or targets of cytokines. They express cytokine receptors and neurotransmitter receptors for both classical transmitters and neuropeptide messengers. Microglial and astroglial cells can express neurotrophins and growth factors and are likely to interact with neurons and lymphocytes patrolling the CNS [1]. Endothelial cells express cytokine receptors and possibly also cytokines. Brain endothelial cells could be activated by circulating cytokines to produce cytokines, which when released abluminally influence juxtaendothelial astrocytes, microglial cells, and possibly neurons [72]. Thus, brain endothelial cells may function as transducers of circulating immune signals to the brain parenchyma. The peripheral application of cytokine-inducing LPS or cytokines results in an activation of cytokine synthesis in brain resident cells [4, 11, 54], most likely microglial cells and/or perivascular macrophages. In the course of viral infections (e.g., influenza) or endotoxemia, cytokines produced in the periphery are likely to influence cytokine production in the CNS through an endocrine or neural transmission mechanism, resulting in alteration of neuronal functions as well as sickness behavior. This may be independent of induction of fever.

Molecular anatomy of immune organ innervation

The sympathetic, sensory, and parasympathetic innervation of primary and secondary lymphoid organs differs qualitatively, quantitatively, proportionally, and with respect to neuropeptide content. The innervation is delivered along blood vessels from which fibers branch off to form close spatial relationships with different subsets of immune cells [39, 72].

Knowledge of the specific innervation of the bone marrow is sparse [23, 72]. The presence of vascular and nonvascular fibers staining for CGRP and SP indicates that they are of primary sensory origin. Tyrosine hydroxylase-positive and neuropeptide Y (NPY)-positive fibers mark the sympathetic innervation. Thus, neuroimmune interactions at this level of the bone marrow are conceivable, especially influences of bone marrow innervation on the differentiation and mobilization of hematopoietic cells.

In the mammalian thymus the presence of sensory CGRP/SP innervation and sympathetic noradrenergic NPY innervation is suggested. This is based on double labeling experiments for neuropeptides and markers of the peripheral sympathetic innervation, such as tyrosine hydroxylase (TH) or the vesicular monoamine transporter isoform 2 (VMAT2) [74, 45, 68]. The thymic vasoactive intestinal polypeptide (VIP) innervation has been considered to be cholinergic parasympathetic, although direct evidence of thymic innervation by fibers costaining for VIP and unequivocal markers of cholinergic innervation was absent. In fact, investigations with the recently established highly sensitive marker of peripheral and central cholinergic innervation VAChT, the vesicular acetylcholine transporter, provide no evidence for the presence of cholinergic innervation in the mammalian thymus [56]. The neuropeptidergic and catecholaminergic innervation of the thymus is concentrated in the capsule, in the interlobular septa, in paravascular spaces, and in the corticomedullary boundary zone. SP and CGRP fibers frequently branch off from the perivascular space to run into the surrounding parenchyma. TH/VMAT2-positive noradrenergic fibers are more restricted to the perivascular plexus. Paravascular mast cells and macrophages, but not T cells, are the main targets of sensory and sympathetic thymic innervation [45]. A few fibers containing opioid peptides are also encountered. Some cells of the thymus express neuropeptides (e.g., encephalin, tachykinins, CGRP) or chromogranin A; however, their cellular identities and functions are not yet clearly understood.

Lymph nodes of different body regions receive sensory and sympathetic nerves that accompany blood vessels and lymphatic vessels, and branch off from paravascular spaces to enter the parenchyma [24, 72]. CGRP/SP staining marks the sensory innervation and TH/NPY/VMAT2 staining delineates the sympathetic innervation. VIP, a cotransmitter candidate of acetylcholine innervation, is contained in a low number of nerves, which are most likely of sensory origin as shown by staining of nerve fibers for the cholinergic parasympathetic marker. The presence of VIP innervation was taken as indirect evidence for cholinergic innervation of lymph nodes because VIP is a typical neuropeptide cotransmitter in postganglionic parasympathetic cholinergic neurons. However, the coexistence of VIP and a reliable marker of peripheral cholinergic innervation has not yet been shown. Investigations with VAChT, the novel marker of cholinergic innervation, showed that cholinergic innervation is absent from lymph nodes. Sensory CGRP/SP fibers running independent of the vasculature are more frequent than nonvascular sympathetic TH/NPY/VMAT2 fibers. The presence of SP-containing innervation in conjunction with selective expression of the SP (NK-1) receptor gene in endothelial cells and paravascular macrophages, and perhaps mast cells, suggests that tachykinin-mediated immunomodulation in lymph nodes involves endothelial cells, mast cells, and macrophages but not T cells [75]. In contrast to *in vitro* data providing evidence for NK-1 receptors in T cells, our *in vivo* studies indicate absence or very low abundance of NK-1 receptors in T or B cells. The cellular identity of NPY, VIP, and pituitary adenylate cyclase-activating polypeptide (PACAP) receptors [79] in lymph nodes under *in vivo* conditions is unclear. It remains to be elucidated to what extent the ample evidence of pleiotropic neuropeptide receptor expression in immune cell lines is matched by the *in vivo* situation, when immune cells are naturally exposed to pleiotropic paracrine control mechanisms of their activity by other cell types. Retrograde tracing, combined with immunocytochemistry for opioid peptides, demonstrates a proenkephalin-derived enkephalinergic component of the sympathetic innervation to cervical lymph nodes, originating from the superior cervical ganglion that is segregated from the sympathetic NPY innervation [53]. This is further evidence of a pathway- and transmitter-specific modulation of immune functions in lymph nodes.

In the spleen the sympathetic innervation predominates [23, 72]. Sensory CGRP/SP nerves are rare and cholinergic innervation is absent. The majority of splenic sympathetic fibers costoring noradrenalin and NPY are associated with the vasculature. Some varicose fibers, however, branch off and supply the juxtavascular lymphoid parenchyma with synapse-like target relationships to lymphocytes and close spatial relationships to macrophages. Interleukin-6 secretion is inhibited by electrical stimulation of spleen slices, an effect that is blocked by the opioid antagonist naloxone [59], which indicates the possibility that opioids locally released from immunocytes may control IL-6 secretion in a paracrine manner because murine splenic innervation lacks an opioid component. This inducible opioid expression in splenic immunocytes could be relevant in endotoxic shock. Further cytokines modulate splenic blood flow [52]. The superantigen- and LPS-induced cytokine expression in murine spleen, however, appears to be altered by chemical sympathectomy. This is a further indication that the splenic innervation has functional significance during the immune response. The sympathetic/NPYergic reinnervation of splenic transplants depends on the age of the donor spleen and on the age of the host [78].

Finally, virtually all mucosal tissues are endowed with a defense line of immunocytes, the mucosal-associated lymphoid tissue (MALT). Independent of the location, the innervation of the various MALT systems (e.g., gut-associated lymphoid tissue as Peyer's patches) is predictably similar [46, 47, 65, 72]. The occurrence of nerve fibers is restricted to the outer margins of the lymphoid follicles, while germinal centers (B-cell areas) are regularly spared from innervation. This pattern is similar to that observed in lymph follicles of spleen, tonsils, and lymph nodes. As a rule, sensory fibers containing CGRP/SP, sympathetic noradrenergic NPY fibers, and cholinergic VIP fibers are associated with MALT. This pattern is relatively independent of species and also applies to human palatine tonsils [66]. All three categories of innervation form close spatial relationships with mast cells, macrophages, and plasma cells and with the outer border of lymphoid follicles bearing T cells. Neuro-immunocyte and neuro-mast cell contacts are frequently encountered at sites distant from lymphoid follicles. In the skin, cholinergic/VIPergic neuro-mast cell contacts are less frequent than in visceral mucosal tissues and restricted to sweat gland and paravascular microterritories. In the skin, sensory peptidergic and sympathetic neuro-mast cell contacts prevail. The sensory peptidergic (CGRP) innervation of dendritic epidermal Langerhans cells seems to play a role in the modulation of antigen presentation by Langerhans cells to T cells [33]. This may be of relevance in cutaneous immunological reactions and in neurogenic inflammation [28].

Significance of neuroimmune interactions for underlying diseases

A variety of clinical and experimental observations support the belief that the chemoanatomical substrate for a neuroimmune dialogue is found not only in lymphoid tissue such as thymus, lymph nodes, and spleen. It might also be assumed that a loss of neuroimmune homeostasis may be the common denominator in causing diseases. In fact, neuroimmune dysregulation could even be a crucial pathophysiological principle in a variety of chronifying diseases.

In chronic (alcoholic) pancreatitis, the reason for the generation and continuation of chronic pain and inflammation remains somewhat unclear. A key function has been ascribed to proinflammatory and pronociceptive peptides of the tachykinin (TK) family. Meanwhile, a selective increase in the density of tachykinin receptors in the bowels of patients suffering from Crohn's disease and ulcerative colitis provides evidence that the tachykinin substance P can be involved in painful chronic inflammatory disease of the gastrointestinal system [40, 41, 42, 43]. In addition, light-microscopic immunohistochemical studies have characterized peptide staining patterns in nerves supplying the normal human pancreas and have evaluated changes in peptidergic pancreatic innervation in patients suffering from painful chronic (alcoholic) pancreatitis. Contrary to the more simplistic view in the past that SP and CGRP are of sensory origin, VIP/PHI/PHM of postganglionic parasympathetic origin, and NPY of postganglionic sympathetic origin [13, 62], present results in conjunction with accumulating data in the literature indicate a far more mixed pattern of peptide phenotypes in the main divisions of the pancreatic innervation than previously believed. Nevertheless, SP and particularly CGRP may still be regarded as being mainly sensory, although there may exist a thus-far neglected component of intrinsic SP innervation [62]. The most striking and probably the most pathophysiologically important change is the "lighting up" of close interrelations between peptidergic neuronal elements and inflammatory cells in chronic pancreatitis. Interestingly, mainly the SP/CGRP and the VIP/PHI components form frequent and close contacts with immune cells, while the NPY fibers are much more rarely seen to branch off from blood vessels to intermingle with infiltrated immune cells. SP and CGRP interact in a complex manner, with CGRP inhibiting the degradation of SP [49], enhancing its pronociceptive and immune-signaling action in the spinal dorsal horn and its proinflammatory and pronociceptive action in the periphery [62]. Interestingly, VIP too is involved in some qualities of nociceptive transmission [62]. The fact that SP is mitogenic for fibroblasts could indicate that it is involved in the fibrotic process [14]. Further, there is the intriguing possibility of reciprocal functional interrelation between neuropeptides, immune cells, cytokines, and nerve growth factor. The possible importance of such a constellation in sustaining pain and inflammation has been suggested [38, 62].

Also interesting is the phenomenon that the sensory nervous system responds to peripheral inflammation with an upregulation of the expression of its key neuropeptide transmitters, SP and CGRP [51, 73]. The peripheral release of these transmitters in the inflamed tissue is enhanced and causes increased synthesis and local release of the cytokines IL-1 and TNF-α [70]. These cytokines enhance the release of sensory neuropeptides. Endothelial cells, and possibly macrophages, react with upregulation of the expression of the NK-1 receptor, on which SP exerts its main effects. Endothelial NK-1 receptors may further facilitate the immigration of leukocytes by upregulating the expression of the cell adhesion molecule ICAM. Taken together, these factors enhance inflammatory processes

[75] by entering into a vicious circle. This may be a key mechanism in triggering and sustaining chronification of inflammatory pain, as is commonly observed in conditions such as rheumatoid arthritis and chronic interstitial cystitis, in chronic inflammatory bowel diseases such as sustained appendicitis, Crohn's disease, ulcerative colitis, and anal fissures, as well as in chronic pancreatitis [10, 17, 27, 61].

Peripheral inflammation also causes reactions in the CNS. In the spinal cord, genes encoding the precursors of endogenous opioids, prodynorphin and proenkephalin, are upregulated. This is probably a consequence of an increased spinal release of SP, CGRP, and glutamate from nociceptor terminals in the dorsal horn of primary afferents projecting from the inflamed tissue into the spinal cord [51, 68]. The spinal upregulation of opioid is seen as a mechanism of endogenous pain suppression. The spinal upregulation of NK-1 receptors is regarded as a mechanism to enhance spinal nociceptive neurotransmission, resulting in increased pain [55]. Most interestingly, NK receptors even seem to be expressed on primary afferents themselves, implying autoactivation of immunoceptor signaling by SP. The net effect of pain sensation results from the balance between pain-enhancing and pain-suppressing messengers and receptors along the ascending nociceptive and the descending inhibitory pain pathways. From inflamed tissues, both "immune signals" and nociceptive ("pain") signals are transmitted to the spinal cord, probably by an identical population of small-diameter (C, A-8) afferents. Therefore, for these primary afferents the term "immunonociceptors" might be introduced [75]. This terminology underlines the increasing knowledge of the involvement of neuroimmune interactions in inflammatory pain [61, 72]. In addition, there is mounting evidence that neuroimmune mechanisms within the CNS may be crucially involved in the pathogenesis of chronic neuropathic pain [71, 72]. Consequently, it is an attractive strategy to treat inflammatory, and possibly neuropathic, pain by reestablishing the neuroimmune balance in the "local talk" and "tele talk" of the neuroimmune dialogue.

Therapeutic strategy targets

At multiple intersections, the peripheral and central nervous system and the immune system are directly or indirectly connected to each other and to the endocrine system. Neuroimmune endocrine networks are characterized by anatomical, cellular, and molecular heterogeneity and complexity with tissue, organ-, and cell-specific patterns. As outlined, the bidirectional communication between the nervous and immune systems occurs in short and long loops ("local talk" and "tele talk"). These neuroimmune dialogues are short-term with acute release of messengers and long-term with sustained changes in messenger and messenger receptor gene expression.

The neuroimmune dysregulation underlies a plethora of inflammatory, degenerative, autoimmune, and allergic diseases and also many diseases caused by environmental factors. The neuroimmune connection in pain is obvious. Therefore, the main goal of a neuroimmune-oriented therapeutic strategy is the interruption of a disease-furthering vicious circle. This can be achieved by blocking signals of the nervous system that evoke and sustain pathophysiological immune reactions Thus, presynaptic inhibition of the release of proinflammatory and pronociceptive neuropeptides by opioids acting on peripheral opioid receptors on nociceptor endings may be one way to interrupt the circle under inflammatory pain conditions. Blocking peripheral postsynaptic NK receptors on endothelial cells or macrophages should attenuate the neural stimulus for immune cell immigration and increased cytokine production. Alternatively, the synthesis or release of proinflammatory/pronociceptive cytokines should be blocked, or the released molecules should be neutralized, immunopharmacologically or by antagonists. The combination of the two approaches may be even more efficient in disrupting the assumed vicious circle of neuroimmune dysregulation. In fact, therapeutic trials with TNF-α antibodies reduced inflammation and pain in rheumatoid arthritis and in Crohn's disease. Corticosteroids not only are anti-inflammatory but also regulate the expression of sensory neuropeptides believed to be crucial in the neurogenic inflammatory process [73]. In addition, immunosuppressive therapy with diverse cytokines for the treatment of oncological diseases, in transplantation medicine, or in multiple sclerosis could cause short- and long-term side effects in the nervous system. It will be of paramount importance to recognize the underlying neuroimmune mechanisms of the therapy-induced behavioral effects that are very disturbing for patients. A better understanding of the complex cellular and molecular mechanisms of neuroimmune interactions in health and disease opens far-reaching possibilities for innovative therapies, for long-term disease prevention, and for avoiding unpleasant side effects in ongoing and future pharmacotherapies.

References

1. Acheson A, Lindsay RM. Diverse roles of neurotrophic factors in health and disease. Seminars in the Neurosciences 1994; 6: 333–41.
2. Ader R, Cohen N. Psychoneuroimmunology: conditioning and stress. Annu Rev Psychol 1993; 44: 53–85.
3. Akaike A, Weihe E, Schäfer MKH, Fu ZF, Zheng YM, Vogel W, Schmidt H, Koprowski H, Dietzschold B. Effect of neurotropic virus infection on neuronal and inducible nitric oxide synthase activity in rat brain. Neurovirology 1995; 1: 118–25.
4. Bartholomew SA, Hoffman SA. Effects of peripheral cytokine injections on multiple unit activity in the anterior hypothalamic area of the mouse. Brain Behav Immun 1993; 7: 301–16.
5. Behar O, Ovadia H, Polakiewicz RD, Rosen H. Lipopolysaccharide induces proenkephalin gene expression in rat lymph nodes and adrenal glands. Endocrinology 1994; 134: 475–81.
6. Besedovsky HO, del Rey A. Immuno-neuro-endocrine interactions: facts and hypotheses. Endocrine Reviews 1996; 17: 64–102.
7. Besse D, Weil-Fugazza J, Lombard MC, Butler SH, Besson J. Monoarthritis induces complex changes in /a, 6 and /c opioid binding sites in the superficial dorsal horn of the rat spinal cord. Europ J Pharmacol 1992; 223: 123–31.
8. Bette M, Schäfer MKH, van Rooijen N, Weihe E, Fleischer B. Distribution and kinetics of superantigen-induced cytokine gene expression in mouse spleen. J Exp Med 1993; 178: 1531–40.
9. Bode L, Zimmermann W, Ferszt R, Steinbach F, Ludwig H. Borna disease virus genome transcribed and expressed in psychiatric patients. Nat Med 1995; 1: 232–6.
10. Büchler MW, Weihe E, Friess H, Malfertheiner P, Bockman E, Müller S, Nohr D, Beger HG. Changes in peptidergic innervation in chronic pancreatitis. Pancreas 1992; 7: 183–92.
11. Buttini M, Boddeke H. Peripheral lipopolysaccharide stimulation induces interleukin-β messenger RNA in rat brain microglial cells. Neurosci 1995; 65: 523–30.
12. Coderre TJ, Chan AK, Helms C, Basbaum AI, Levine JD. Increasing sympathetic nerve terminal-dependent plasma extravasation correlates with decreased arthritic joint injury in rats. Neuroscience 1991; 40: 185–9.
13. Dalsgaard CJ. The sensory system. In: Bjorklund A, Hokfelt T, Owman C, eds. Handbook of Chemical Neuroanatomy, Vol 6: The peripheral nervous system. Amsterdam–New York–Oxford: Elsevier, 1988: 599–636.
14. Dalsgaard CJ, Hultgardh-Nilsson A, Haegerstrand A, Nilsson J. Neuropeptides as growth factors. Possible roles in human diseases. Regul Peptides 1989; 25: 1–9.

15. Dantzer R. How do cytokines say hello to the brain? Neural versus humoral mediation. Eur Cytokine Netw 1994; 5: 271–3.
16. da Cunha A, Rausch D, Eiden LE. An early increase in somatostatin mRNA expression in the frontal cortex of monkeys infected with simian immunodeficiency virus. Proc Natl Acad Sci 1995; 92: 1371–5.
17. Di Sebastiano P, Fink T, Weihe E, Friess H, Beger HG, Büchler MW. Changes of protein gene product 9.5 (PGP 9.5) immunoreactive nerves in inflamed appendix. Dig Dis Sci 1995; 40: 366–72.
18. Dietzschold B, Schwäble W, Schäfer MKH, Hooper C, Zheng YM, Petry F, Ṣheng H, Fink T, Loos M, Koprowski H, Weihe E. Expression of C1q, a subcomponent of the rat complement system, is dramatically enhanced in brains of rats with Borna disease or experimental allergic encephalomyelitis. J Neurol Sci 1995; 130: 11–6.
19. Donnerer J, Amann R, Lembeck F. Neurogenic and non-neurogenic inflammation in the rat paw following chemical sympathectomy. Neuroscience 1991; 45: 761–5.
20. Dubner R, Ruda MA. Activity-dependent neuronal plasticity following tissue injury and inflammation. Trends Neurosci 1992; 15: 96–103.
21. Duggan AW, Weihe E. Central transmission of impulses in nociceptors: events in the superficial dorsal horn. In: Basbaum AI, Besson J, eds. Towards a New Pharmacotherapy of Pain. Chichester: John Wiley & Sons Ltd., 1991: 35–67.
22. Eiden LE, Rausch DM, Da Cunha A, Murray EA, Heyes M, Sharer L, Nohr D, Weihe E. AIDS and the central nervous system. Examining pathobiology and testing therapeutic strategies in the SIV-infected rhesus monkey. Ann NY Acad Sci 1993; 693: 229–44.
23. Felten SY, Felten DL. Neural-immune interactions. Prog Brain Res 1994; 100: 157–62.
24. Fink T, Weihe E. Multiple neuropeptides in nerves supplying mammalian lymph nodes: messenger candidates for sensory and autonomic neuroimmunomodulation? Neurosci Lett 1988; 90: 39–44.
25. Fleshner M, Goehler LE, Hermann J, Relton JK, Maier SF, Watkins LR. Interleukin-1 beta induced corticosterone elevation and hypothalamic NE depletion is vagally mediated. Brain Res Bull 1995; 37: 605–10.
26. Freidin M, Kessler JA. Cytokine regulation of substance Pt expression in sympathetic neurons. Proc Natl Acad Sci 1991; 88: 3200–3.
27. Frieling T, Strohmeyer G. Neuroimmune interactions in the gastrointestinal tract. Z Gastroenterol 1995; 33: 219–24.
28. Gillardon F, Moll I, Michel S, Benrath J, Weihe E, Zimmermann M. Calcitonin gene-related peptide and nitric oxide are involved in ultraviolet radiation-induced immuno-suppression. Eur J Pharmacol 1995; 293: 395–400.
29. Gibbins IL. Vasoconstrictor, vasodilator and pilomotor pathways in sympathetic ganglia of guinea-pigs. Neuroscience 1992; 47: 657–72.
30. Handwerker HO. What peripheral mechanisms contribute to nociceptive transmission and hyperalgesia? In: Basbaum AI, Besson J, eds. Towards a New Pharmacotherapy of Pain. Chichester: John Wiley & Sons Ltd., 1991: 5–19.
31. Hökfelt T. Neuropeptides in perspective: The last ten years. Neuron 1991; 7: 867–79.
32. Hopkins SJ, Rothwell NJ. Cytokines and the nervous system. I: Expression and recognition. Trends Neurosci 1995; 18: 83–8.
33. Hosoi J, Murphy GF, Egan CL, Lerner EA, Grabbe S, Asahina A et al. Regulation of Langerhans cell function by nerves containing calcitonin gene-related peptide. Nature 1993; 363: 159–63.
34. Jänig W, Schmidt RF. Reflex Sympathetic Dystrophy: Pathophysiological Mechanisms and Clinical Implications. Weinheim: VCH, 1992: 306.
35. Jonakait GM. Neural-immune interactions in sympathetic ganglia. Trends Neurosci 1993; 16: 419–23.
36. Kreutzberg GW. Microglia, the first line of defence in brain pathologies. Arzneimittelforschung 1995; 45: 357–60.

37. Leon A, Buriani A, Dal TR, Fabris M, Romanello S, Aloe L, Levi-Montalcini R. Mast cells synthesize, store, and release nerve growth factor. Proc Natl Acad Sci USA 1994; 91: 3739–43.
38. Lindsay RM, Harmar AJ. Nerve growth factor regulates expression of neuropeptide genes in adult sensory neurons. Nature 1989; 337: 362–4.
39. Madden KS, Felten DL. Experimental basis for neural-immune interactions. Physiol Rev 1995; 75: 77–106.
40. Malfertheiner P, Büchler MW, Stanescu A, Ditschuneit H. Pancreatic morphology and function in relationship to pain in chronic pancreatitis. Int J Pancreatol 1987; 1: 59–66.
41. Mantyh CR, Gates TS, Zimmerman RP, Welton ML, Passaro Jr EP, Vigna SR, Maggio JE, Kruger L, Mantyh PW. Receptor binding sites for substance P, but not substance K or neuromedin K, are expressed in high concentrations by arterioles, venules, and lymph nodules in surgical specimens obtained from patients with ulcerative colitis and Crohn's disease. Proc Natl Acad Sci USA 1988; 85: 3235–9.
42. Mantyh PW, Catton MD, Boehmer CG, Welton ML, Passaro EP, Maggio JE, Vigna SR. Receptors for sensory neuropeptides in human inflammatory diseases: implications for the effector role of sensory neurons. Peptides 1989; 10: 627–45.
43. Mantyh PW, Mantyh CR, Gates T, Vigna SR, Maggio JE. Receptor binding sites for substance P and substance K in the canine gastrointestinal tract and their possible role in inflammatory bowel disease. Neuroscience 1988; 25: 817–37.
44. McGeer PL, Rogers J, McGeer EG. Neuroimmune mechanisms in Alzheimer disease pathogenesis. Alzheimer Dis Assoc Disord 1994; 8: 149–58.
45. Müller S, Weihe E. Interrelation of peptidergic innervation with mast cells and ED1-positive cells in rat thymus. Brain Behav Immun 1991; 5: 55–72.
46. Nohr D, Buob A, Gärtner K, Weihe E. Changes in pulmonary calcitonin gene-related peptide and protein gene-product 9.5 innervation in mycoplasma pulmonis-infected rats. Cell Tiss Res 1996; 283: 215–9.
47. Nohr D, Weihe E. The neuroimmune link in the bronchus-associated lymphoid tissue (BALT) of cat and rat: peptides and neural markers. Brain Behav Immun 1991; 5: 84–101.
48. Nottet HS, Gendelman HE. Unraveling the neuroimmune mechanisms for the HIV-1-associated cognitive/motor complex. Immunol Today 1995; 16: 441–8.
49. Nyberg F, Legrevos P, Terenius L. Modulation of endopeptidase activity by calcitonin gene-related peptide: a mechanism affecting substance P action? Biochimie 1988; 70: 65–8.
50. Ottaway CA, Husband AJ. The influence of neuroendocrine pathways on lymphocyte migration. Immunol Today 1994; 15: 511–7.
51. Persson S, Schäfer MKH, Nohr D, Ekström G, Post C, Nyberg F, Weihe E. Spinal prodynorphin gene expression in collagen-induced arthritis: influence of the glucocorticosteroid budesonide. Neuroscience 1994; 63: 313–26.
52. Rogausch H, Del RA, Kabiersch A, Besedovsky HO. Interleukin-1 increases splenic blood flow by affecting the sympathetic vasoconstrictor tonus. Am J Physiol 1995; 268: 902–8.
53. Romeo HE, Fink T, Yanaihara N, Weihe E. Distribution and relative proportions of neuropeptide Y- and proenkephalin-containing noradrenergic neurones in rat superior cervical ganglion: separate projections to submaxillary lymph nodes. Peptides 1994; 15: 1479–87.
54. Rothwell NJ, Hopkins SJ. Cytokines and the nervous system II: Actions and mechanisms of action. Trends Neurosci 1995; 18: 130–6.
55. Schäfer MKH, Nohr D, Krause JE, Weihe E. Inflammation-induced upregulation of NK1 receptor mRNA in dorsal horn neurons. Neuroreport 1993; 4: 1007–10.
56. Schäfer MKH, Weihe E, Varoqui H, Eiden LE, Erickson JD. Distribution of the vesicular acetylcholine transporter (VAChT) in the central and peripheral nervous systems of the rat. J Mol Neurosci 1994; 5: 1–26.
57. Schalling M, Franco CA, Hemsen A, Dagerlind A, Seroogy K, Persson H, Hökfelt T, Lundberg JM. Neuropeptide Y and catecholamine synthesizing enzymes and their mRNAs in rat sympathetic neurons and adrenal glands: Studies on expression, synthesis and axonal transport after

pharmacological and experimental manipulations using hybridization techniques and radioimmuno-assay. Neuroscience 1991; 41: 753–66.
58. Stein C, Gramsch C, Herz A. Intrinsic mechanisms of antinociception in inflammation: local opioid receptors and beta-endorphin. J Neurosci 1990; 10: 1292–8.
59. Straub RH, Herrmann M, Berkmiller G, Frauenholz T, Lang B, Scholmerich J, Falk W. Neuronal regulation of interleukin 6 secretion in murine spleen: adrenergic and opioidergic control. J Neurochem 1997; 68: 1633–9.
60. Travis J. Glia: The brain's other cells. Science 1994; 266: 970–2.
61. Watkins LR, Maier SF, Goehler LE. Immune activation: the role of pro-inflammatory cytokines in inflammation, illness responses and pathological pain states. Pain 1995; 63: 289–302.
62. Weihe E. Neuropeptides in primary sensory neurons. In: Zenker W, Neuhuber W, eds. The Primary Afferent Neuron – A Survey of Recent Morpho-Functional Aspects. New York: Plenum, 1990: 127–59.
63. Weihe E. Neurochemical anatomy of the mammalian spinal cord: functional implications. Annals Anatomy 1992; 174: 89–118.
64. Weihe E, Bette M, Fink T, Romeo HE, Schäfer MKH. Molecular Anatomical Basis of Interactions Between Nervous and Immune Systems in Health and Disease. In: Schedlowski M, Tewes U, eds. Psychoneuroimmunology, An Interdisciplinary Introduction. New York, Boston, Dordrecht, London, Moscow: Kluwer Academic/ Plenum Publishers, 1999: 167–85.
65. Weihe E, Hartschuh W. Multiple peptides in cutaneous nerves: regulators under physiological conditions and a pathogenetic role in skin disease? Semin Dermatol 1988; 7: 284–300.
66. Weihe E, Krekel J. The neuroimmune connection in human tonsils. Brain Behav Immun 1991; 5: 41–54.
67. Weihe E, Müller S, Fink T, Zentel HJ. Tachykinins, calcitonin gene-related peptide and neuropeptide Y in nerves of the mammalian thymus: interactions with mast cells in autonomic and sensory neuroimmunomodulation? Neurosci Lett 1989; 100: 77–82.
68. Weihe E, Millan MJ, Höllt V, Nohr D, Herz A. Induction of the gene encoding pro-dynorphin by experimentally induced arthritis enhances staining for dynorphin in the spinal cord of the rat. Neuroscience 1989; 31: 77–95.
69. Weihe E, Müller S, Büchler MW, Friess H, Nohr D. The tachykinin neuroimmune connection in inflammatory pain. In: Leeman SE, Krause JE, Lembeck F, eds. Substance P and Related Peptides: Cellular and Molecular Physiology. New York: New York Academy of Sciences, 1991: 283–95.
70. Weihe E, Nohr D. A neuroimmune sensory-sympathetic link in the pathophysiology and chronic pain cycle of reflex sympathetic dystrophy (RSD)? In: Janig W, Schmidt RF, eds. Reflex Sympathetic Dystrophy: Pathophysiological Mechanisms and Clinical Implications. Weinheim: VCH, 1992: 281–301.
71. Weihe E, Nohr D, Michel S, Müller S, Zentel H, Fink T, Krekel J. Molecular anatomy of the neuro-immune connection. Intern J Neuroscience 1991; 59: 1–23.
72. Weihe E, Nohr D, Müller S, Büchler MW, Friess H, Zentel HJ. The tachykinin neuroimmune connection in inflammatory pain. Ann NY Acad Sci 1991; 632: 283–95.
73. Weihe E, Nohr D, Schäfer MKH, Persson S, Ekström G, Källström J, Nyberg F, Post C. CGRP gene expression in collagen-induced arthritis. Can J Physiol Pharmacol 1995; 73: 1015–19.
74. Weihe E, Schäfer MKH, Erickson JD, Eiden LE. Localization of vesicular monoamine transporter isoforms (VMAT1 and VMAT2) to endocrine cells and neurons in rat. J Mol Neuroscience 1994; 5: 149–64.
75. Weihe E, Schäfer MKH, Nohr D, Persson S. Expression of neuropeptides, neuropeptide receptors and neuropeptide processing enzymes in spinal neurons and peripheral non-neural cells and plasticity in models of inflammatory pain. In: Hökfelt T, Schmidt RF, Schaible HG, eds. Neuropeptides, Nociception and Pain. Weinheim: Chapman & Hall, 1994: 43–69.
76. Wekerle H. T-cell autoimmunity in the central nervous system. Intervirology 1993; 35: 95–100.
77. Wetmore L, Green JJ, Gartner JG, Sanders V, Nance DM. The effects of kainic acid-induced lesions in the lateral septal area on cell-mediated immune function. Brain Behav Immun 1994; 8: 341–54.

78. Westermann J, Michel S, Lopez-Kostka S, Bode U, Rothkotter HJ, Bette M, Weihe E, Straub RH, Pabst R. Regeneration of implanted splenic tissue in the rat: re-innervation is host age-dependent and necessary for tissue development. J Neuroimmunol 1998; 88: 67–76.
79. Yada T, Sakurada M, Ishihara H, Nakata M, Shioda S, Yaekura K, Hamakawa N, Yanagida K, Kikuchi M, Oka Y. Pituitary adenylate cyclase-activating polypeptide (PACAP) is an islet substance serving as an intra-islet amplifier of glucose-induced insulin secretion in rats. J Physiol 1997; 505: 319–28.

5 Diagnosis of chronic pancreatitis: Function tests

5.1 Serological tests to diagnose chronic pancreatitis

A. C. C. Wagner

Introduction

Clearly, if a diagnosis of chronic pancreatitis (CP) is entertained, serological tests do not immediately come to the clinician's mind as the most appropriate procedure to either establish or exclude such a diagnosis. Instead, one more likely would consider imaging or functional studies, all of which are to be discussed in separate chapters of this book. Indeed, it is generally accepted textbook knowledge that *"routine blood tests are usually not helpful for the diagnosis of chronic pancreatitis"*[1].

This indicates that blood tests as a whole, let alone serological tests, will only be helpful to establish a diagnosis of chronic pancreatitis under certain, rare circumstances. Since the title of this chapter specifically refers to serological tests, it is important to consider the definition of serology. Serology generally refers to the study of serum for its antibody content, i.e. to blood tests to detect the presence of antibodies. Thus, in essence, I should discuss in this chapter blood tests detecting the presence of antibodies that may be helpful to establish a diagnosis of chronic pancreatitis.

In order to add a little more substance to the subject, I have, however, allowed myself to extend the definitions given by the title. For the purpose of this chapter, therefore, serology means any test that simply requires that a blood sample be collected. Diagnosis includes tests that, firstly, can help strengthen a suspected diagnosis of CP, secondly, that can be used to establish chronic pancreatitis as a cause of maldigestion and steatorrhea and, most importantly, thirdly, that can help determine the etiology of CP of unknown origin (idiopathic chronic pancreatitis).

Thus, I will briefly discuss the value of serum digestive enzyme determination in the context of chronic pancreatitis. Closing in on serology, I will then discuss the usefulness of blood tests to detect infections as a cause of chronic pancreatitis. Finally, I will discuss chronic pancreatitis related to autoimmune diseases and their diagnosis through blood tests. Particular emphasis will be put on recent evidence of primary autoimmune chronic pancreatitis as entity.

Function tests, stool tests and the like that may include blood sample collection together with application of traceable substances such as the pancreolauryl test are, however, not the subject of this chapter.

Serum digestive enzyme levels to diagnose chronic pancreatitis

When considering the diagnosis of *acute* pancreatitis, serum digestive enzyme levels such as serum amylase and lipase are very useful tests. Unfortunately, there is little evidence that these tests are as beneficial for the diagnosis of *chronic* pancreatitis. If pancreatic insufficiency is present, these enzymes are usually low but diagnosis is mostly self-evident and does not require serum digestive enzyme determination. Sensitivity of serum amylase and lipase levels for CP is accordingly low, between 30 and 45% [2]. Thus, in contrast to acute pancreatitis, serum amylase and lipase levels offer little help for assessment of chronic pancreatitis.

Another digestive enzyme, pancreatic elastase, can be quite helpful to detect pancreatic malfunction, if measured in the stool. However, in contrast to fecal elastase but similar to serum amylase and lipase, serum elastase measurements do not reliably detect chronic pancreatitis nor even insufficiency [3].

The one digestive enzyme whose serum level may be useful under certain circumstances is trypsin, since among digestive enzymes, serum trypsin is the best indicator of pancreatic disease as the cause of steatorrhea, at least in children with cystic fibrosis [4]. However, 50% of patients with chronic pancreatitis have normal serum trypsin levels [5]. Thus, serum trypsin levels may help to define chronic pancreatitis as the cause of maldigestion and steatorrhea but are not useful to diagnose chronic pancreatitis w/o insufficiency.

Taken together, clearly there is not much to be gained by these tests for the diagnosis of chronic pancreatitis.

Blood tests to establish the etiology of chronic pancreatitis

Chronic pancreatitis can develop due to a number of causes as indicated in Table 5.1-1. Most of these cannot, however, be diagnosed through blood tests. Of these, alcoholism stands out as the by far most common etiology. Of course, there is no blood test to diagnose alcoholism. Allelic diseases can lead to chronic pancreatitis and can be diagnosed from a blood specimen if the underlying defect, as in hereditary pancreatitis, is known. Genetic syndromes related to chronic pancreatitis will, however, be discussed elsewhere in this book in great detail and will therefore not be further referred to. Infections certainly can lead to pancreatitis and of course can often be diagnosed serologically. Diagnosis of autoimmune disease related chronic pancreatitis depends on serological detection of antibodies and will, therefore, be discussed in detail together with new insights about autoimmune pancreatitis as an entity.

Table 5.1-1. Etiology of CP (*italics* indicate usefulness of blood tests for diagnosis).

- Alcoholism
- *Infections*
- Drugs
- *Genetic/hereditary diseases/syndromes*
- Malnutrition (Tropical pancreatitis)
- Hypercalcemia
- Pancreas divisum
- Trauma
- Sarcoidosis (arguably no serological diagnosis)
- Unknown causes
- *Autoimmune disease*

Infectious agents inducing recurrent acute pancreatitis and/or chronic pancreatitis

There is a myriad of infectious agents, including viruses, bacteria, protozoa and helminths, that can reportedly induce pancreatitis [6, 7]. Figure 5.1-1 provides an overview of most of the infectious agents that have been implicated as a cause of pancreatitis.

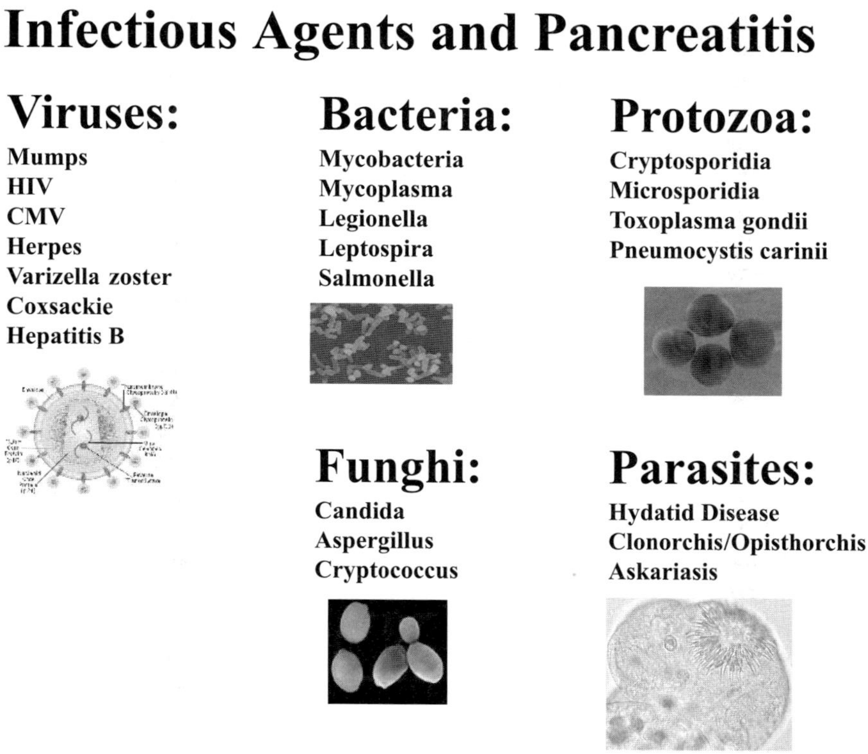

Figure 5.1-1. The figure indicates a comprehensive list of infectious agents reportedly identified in the pancreas. Many of these only cause acute but not chronic pancreatitis, however. Some also represent complications of pancreatitis rather than the cause.

However, most of these induce acute pancreatitis while only a few infectious agents, such as CMV, HIV and parasites, can also lead to chronic pancreatitis. Many agents, such as pneumocystis, aspergillus, toxoplasma, cryptococcus and varicella, have not been reported as a cause of chronic pancreatitis at all. Pancreatic infection with bacteria and candida ssp mainly occurs as a complication, i.e. infected necrosis or pseudocysts, rather than the cause of chronic pancreatitis. Correspondingly, as evidenced by a Medline search, most papers about pancreatitis due to infections deal with acute rather than chronic pancreatitis.

Figure 5.1-2 indicates those infectious agents that have been established as a cause of chronic pancreatitis with reasonable certainty and also compares the numbers of Medline reports relating to individual infectious agents as a cause of either acute or chronic pancreatitis.

Infectious Agents and *Chronic* Pancreatitis

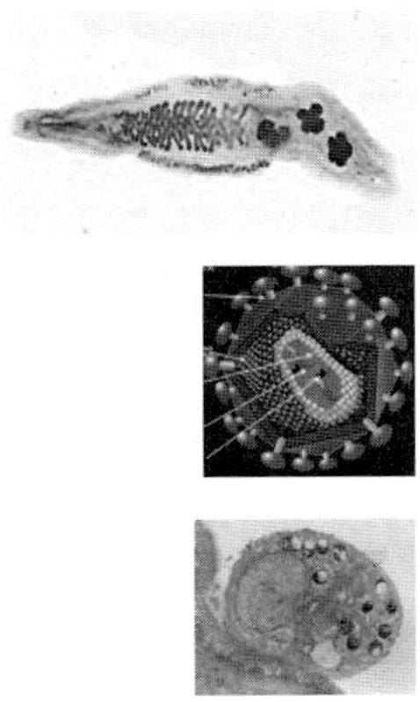

	Ref AP-CP
Echinococcus	54 - 8
Clonorchis	3 - 1
Askaris	45 - 3
Coxsackie	39 - 9
CMV	29 - 2
Mumps	39 - 9
HIV	101 - 9
Microsporidia	5 - 3
Cryptosporidia	28 - 9

Figure 5.1-2. Indicated are infectious agents that have been established as a cause of chronic pancreatitis with reasonable certainty. The columns on the right (Ref AP-CP) indicate the respective numbers of Medline papers dealing with these agents and either acute pancreatitis (AP) or chronic pancreatitis (CP).

Although many of these infections can be diagnosed serologically, under most circumstances, definitive diagnosis of infections as the cause of pancreatitis also requires histological or cultural proof. Worms will mostly be diagnosed through imaging as well. Often, biopsy will be required to make the diagnosis.

In conclusion, the diagnosis of infectious CP will mainly not be made serologically, but serology can provide circumstantial evidence. Other helpful tests may include IgE levels, eosinophil counts (parasitic and helminthic infections), lymphocyte differentiation (HIV) and PCR (viral diseases).

Autoimmune disease and chronic pancreatitis

Many autoimmune diseases such as rheumatoid arthritis (RA), systemic lupus erythematosus (SLE), primary sclerosing cholangitis (PSC), inflammatory bowel disease (IBD) and sarcoidosis have been reported in patients with chronic pancreatitis (Table 5.1-2).

Table 5.1-2. Autoimmune diseases and chronic pancreatitis.

		Serological test
PSC	Association possible but rare (8)	NO
IBD	Association possible but rare (9)	NO
Sarcoidosis	Association possible but quite rare (10)	Arguably NO
RA	Mainly secondary due to gold or sulindac therapy	YES
SLE	Association possible but quite rare (11)	YES
PBC	Association possible but rare (12;13)	YES
SS	Association well established (12;14-19)	YES

Serological tests are available only for a few of these diseases and a causal relationship between the autoimmune disorder and concurrent CP cannot always be established (Table 5.1-2).

Generally, autoimmune disease will more often lead to *acute* rather than *chronic* pancreatitis. In many cases of patients with autoimmune disorders presenting with chronic pancreatitis, it is not clear whether CP is indeed caused by the autoimmune disease rather than alcoholism or drug treatment. Thus, in a study of PSC patients, 7% were found to have mild pancreatic duct changes suggestive of chronic pancreatitis [8] but in 6 of these, alcoholic CP could not be excluded. Thus, CP may occur in PSC patients but is rare, and there is no serological test to diagnose PSC. Of course, IBD patients can have pancreatitis which is also mostly acute rather than chronic and most often related to either gallstone disease or drug treatment [9]. Thus, CP primarily due to IBD does occur but is rare and there is no serological diagnosis of IBD. Sarcoidosis can involve the pancreas in up to 1% of all cases, mostly in the form of a pancreatic mass. Only 2 cases of chronic pancreatitis due to sarcoidosis have been reported however [10]. Whether or not sarcoidosis can be diagnosed serologically (ACE-levels, hyperglobulinemia) is debatable. Often, CP may develop due to treatment of autoimmune disease such as gold- or sulindac-induced CP in patients with RA. SLE can cause acute pancreatitis and probably also chronic pancreatitis in rare cases but there is really only one case report so far [11].

Chronic pancreatitis and Sjögren syndrome (SS)

The single autoimmune disorder most clearly related to chronic pancreatitis is the Sjögren syndrome. It has been reported that up to 27% of patients with SS may have pancreatic ductal changes on ERCP [12]. Up to 54% of SS patients also have antibodies against a pancreatic ductal cell antigen [14. 19]. This antigen has been characterized as a 60 kDa protein on western analysis [16] and identified as carboanhydrase II (CA-II) [15]. Interestingly, in that study it was also shown that mice immunized with CA-II developed sialadenitis. This indicates that CA II antibodies may pathogenetically be relevant for the development of SS. In addition, anti-CA II antibodies (ACAII) can reportedly also be found in some patients with SLE or autoimmune cholangitis as well as PBC. This has been interpreted as supportive evidence for the existence of autoimmune overlap syndromes, sometimes referred to as autoimmune exocrinopathy or dry-gland syndrome [20].

Taken together, it seems reasonable to assume that SS as well as other autoimmune diseases such as PBC or overlap syndromes can lead to chronic pancreatitis. Serology is clearly helpful to diagnose those entities. Thus, in patients with truly idiopathic chronic pancreatitis, an autoimmune disorder should be entertained as a possible diagnosis. For example, in a patient with idiopathic chronic pancreatitis who also complains about dry eye or dry mouth, evaluation for autoimmune disease such as SS seems appropriate. Tests that may be helpful include quantitative IgG and IgM levels, antinuclear-, anti-Ro and anti-La antibodies.

Primary autoimmune chronic pancreatitis as entity

Already in the 60s, cases of chronic pancreatitis presenting with fever, relatively little pain, hypergammaglobulinemia and lymphocytic infiltration were presented and classified as "primary inflammatory pancreatitis" [21]. Only in the 90s, however, was the concept of autoimmune chronic pancreatitis developed when patients with idiopathic chronic pancreatitis, hypergammaglobulinemeia and response to steroid therapy in the absence of any features of Sjögren's disease were reported [22, 23]. This concept was further supported in a study of 362 ERPs performed in one center [24]. Of these, 161 were diagnosed with chronic pancreatitis. Four of these presented with unusual features of a diffusely narrowed pancreatic duct together with hypergammaglobulinemia. One patient had SS while the other three did not show any features of concomitant collagenous disease. Thus, 1.86% of CP patients were diagnosed to have autoimmune chronic pancreatitis. Interestingly, two of these tested positive for the anti-CA II antibody. In a very recent study analyzing data from 313 patients with chronic pancreatitis from one center, 24 patients received a diagnosis of autoimmune chronic pancreatitis [25]. Six of these had concomitant autoimmune disease (SS, PSC, RA, but no case of PBC) leaving 11 with primary autoimmune chronic pancreatitis. These patients were tested for a variety of autoantibodies such as antinuclear antibodies (ANA), anti-lactoferrin antibodies (ALF) and anti-CA II antibodies (ACAII). It has been suggested that all patients with autoimmune chronic pancreatitis, either primary or associated with other collagenous diseases, have either ANA, ALF, ACAII or some combination of these. Most of these patients also had hypergammaglobulinemia while patients with alcohol-induced CP generally had no autoantibodies.

However, neither antibody (ANA, ACAII, ALF) was specific since none was found in all patients and antibody patterns did not differ between patients with underlying autoimmune disease (RA, PSC, SS) and those considered to have primary autoimmune chronic pancreatitis. These antibodies can also be found in other diseases w/o chronic pancreatitis. Thus, ALF, together with antibodies against proteinase 3, myeloperoxidase, bactericidal/permeability-increasing protein, human leukocyte elastase, cathepsin G, belongs to the group of anti-neutrophil cytoplasmic antibodies (ANCA) and can, for example, be found in patients with ulcerative colitis, ankylosing spondylitis or PSC. ACAII, in addition to patients with autoimmune chronic pancreatitis, may also be present in sera from patients with SLE and SS. It is also noteworthy that two thirds of SS patients *without* chronic pancreatitis have ACAII while only 30% of patients with SS *and* chronic pancreatitis are ACAII positive [14].

It has further been reported that many patients with ACAII also have antibodies reacting with anti-carboanhydrase I [14, 26]. Inhibition of ACAI and ACAII activity through mutual absorption revealed that the two antibodies occur independently in these patients. This has been interpreted to mean that antibodies in patients' sera may have been raised against another CA-isoform and that these antibodies crossreact with CAI and II [20]. In the study from Italy [26], 26% of a total 74 patients with CP tested positive for ACAII, 27% for ACAI and 16% for both antibodies. In this study ACAI and ACAII levels could not differentiate between patients with and without alcohol intake.

Thus, although evidence supports the concept of autoimmune pancreatitis, several questions remain unanswered:

- It is unclear whether ACAI and ACAII will indeed be helpful to differentiate between alcoholic and autoimmune pancreatitis.
- The true incidence of autoimmune pancreatitis is unknown.
- It is not clear whether autoimmune pancreatitis truly occurs as a primary rather than a secondary condition.

In conclusion, the paradigm that "routine blood tests are usually not helpful for the diagnosis of chronic pancreatitis" [1] still holds true. However, there is evidence that chronic pancreatitis can develop due to autoimmune phenomena and that in select cases of idiopathic chronic pancreatitis, serological tests may help to strengthen a suspicion of autoimmune chronic pancreatitis. Helpful tests may include quantitative IgG and (IgM?) levels, ANA and, if available, possibly ACAI, ACAII and ALF. Serology may also help to identify infectious causes of CP while serum tryspsin levels may help in the differential diagnosis of maldigestion.

References

1. Owyang C, Levitt MD. Chronic pancreatitis. In: Yamada T, Alpers DH, Owyang C, Powell DW, Silverstein FE, eds. Textbook of Gastroenterology. Philadelphia: J. B. Lippincott, 1997: 2091–2112.
2. Moller-Petersen J, Pedersen JO, Pedersen NT, Andersen BN. Serum cathodic trypsin-like immunoreactivity, pancreatic lipase, and pancreatic isoamylase as diagnostic tests of chronic pancreatitis or pancreatic steatorrhea. Scand J Gastroenterol 1988; 23(3): 287–96.
3. Benini L, Caliari S, Vaona B, Brocco G, Micciolo R, Rizzotti P et al. Variations in time of serum pancreatic enzyme levels in chronic pancreatitis and clinical course of the disease. Int J Pancreatol 1991; 8(4): 279–87.
4. Cleghorn G, Benjamin L, Corey M, Forstner G, Dati F, Durie P. Serum immunoreactive pancreatic lipase and cationic trypsinogen for the assessment of exocrine pancreatic function in older patients with cystic fibrosis. Pediatrics 1986; 77(3): 301–6.
5. Andriulli A, Masoero G, Felder M, Vantini I, Petrillo M, Cavallini G et al. Circulating trypsin-like immunoreactivity in chronic pancreatitis. Dig Dis Sci 1981; 26(6): 532–7.
6. Parenti DM, Steinberg W, Kang P. Infectious causes of acute pancreatitis. Pancreas 1996; 13(4): 356–71.
7. Robbins EG, Stollman NH, Bierman P, Grauer L, Barkin JS. Pancreatic fungal infections: a case report and review of the literature. Pancreas 1996; 12(3): 308–12.
8. Schimanski U, Stiehl A, Stremmel W, Theilmann L. Low prevalence of alterations in the pancreatic duct system in patients with primary sclerosing cholangitis. Endoscopy 1996; 28(4): 346–9.
9. Barthet M, Hastier P, Bernard JP, Bordes G, Frederick J, Allio S et al. Chronic pancreatitis and inflammatory bowel disease: true or coincidental association? [see comments]. Am J Gastroenterol 1999; 94(8): 2141–8.
10. Siavelis HA, Herrmann ME, Aranha GV, Garcia G, Eubanks T, Reyes CV. Sarcoidosis and the pancreas. Surgery 1999; 125(4): 456–61.
11. Borum M, Steinberg W, Steer M, Freedman S, White P. Chronic pancreatitis: a complication of systemic lupus erythematosus [see comments]. Gastroenterology 1993; 104(2): 613–5.
12. Nishimori I, Morita M, Kino J, Onodera M, Nakazawa Y, Okazaki K et al. Pancreatic involvement in patients with Sjögren's syndrome and primary biliary cirrhosis. Int J Pancreatol 1995; 17(1): 47–54.
13. Hastier P, Buckley MJ, Le Gall P, Bellon S, Dumas R, Delmont J. First report of association of chronic pancreatitis, primary biliary cirrhosis, and systemic sclerosis. Dig Dis Sci 1998; 43(11): 2426–8.
14. Kino-Ohsaki J, Nishimori I, Morita M, Okazaki K, Yamamoto Y, Onishi S et al. Serum antibodies to carbonic anhydrase I and II in patients with idiopathic chronic pancreatitis and Sjögren's syndrome. Gastroenterology 1996; 110(5): 1579–86.
15. Nishimori I, Bratanova T, Toshkov I, Caffrey T, Mogaki M, Shibata Y et al. Induction of experimental autoimmune sialoadenitis by immunization of PL/J mice with carbonic anhydrase II. J Immunol 1995; 154(9): 4865–73.
16. Nishimori I, Yamamoto Y, Okazaki K, Morita M, Onodera M, Kino J et al. Identification of autoantibodies to a pancreatic antigen in patients with idiopathic chronic pancreatitis and Sjögren's syndrome. Pancreas 1994; 9(3): 374–81.
17. Onodera M, Okazaki K, Morita M, Nishimori I, Yamamoto Y. Immune complex specific for the

pancreatic duct antigen in patients with idiopathic chronic pancreatitis and Sjögren's syndrome. Autoimmunity 1994; 19(1): 23–9.
18. Nishimori I, Okazaki K, Yamamoto Y, Morita M, Tamura S, Yamamoto Y. Specific cellular immune responses to pancreatic antigen in chronic pancreatitis and Sjögren's syndrome. J Clin Immunol 1993; 13(4): 265–71.
19. Nishimori I, Okazaki K, Yamamoto Y, Morita M, Tamura S, Yamamoto Y. Sensitization against pancreatic antigen in Sjögren's syndrome and chronic pancreatitis. Preliminary communication. Digestion 1992; 51(2): 71–4.
20. Nishimori I, Fujikawa Adachi K, Onishi S, Hollingsworth MA. Carbonic anhydrase in human pancreas: hypotheses for the pathophysiological roles of CA isozymes. Ann NY Acad Sci 1999; 880: 5–16.
21. Sarles H, Sarles JC, Camatte R, Muratore R, Gaini M, Guien C et al. Observations on 205 confirmed cases of acute pancreatitis, recurring pancreatitis, and chronic pancreatitis. Gut 1965; 6(6): 545–59.
22. Yoshida K, Toki F, Takeuchi T, Watanabe S, Shiratori K, Hayashi N. Chronic pancreatitis caused by an autoimmune abnormality. Proposal of the concept of autoimmune pancreatitis. Dig Dis Sci 1995; 40(7): 1561–8.
23. Horiuchi A, Kaneko T, Yamamura N, Nagata A, Nakamura T, Akamatsu T et al. Autoimmune chronic pancreatitis simulating pancreatic lymphoma. Am J Gastroenterol 1996; 91(12): 2607–9.
24. Ito T, Nakano I, Koyanagi S, Miyahara T, Migita Y, Ogoshi K et al. Autoimmune pancreatitis as a new clinical entity. Three cases of autoimmune pancreatitis with effective steroid therapy. Dig Dis Sci 1997; 42(7): 1458–68.
25. Okazaki K, Uchida K, Ohana M, Nakase H, Uose S, Inai M et al. Autoimmune-related pancreatitis is associated with autoantibodies and a Th1/Th2-type cellular immune response [see comments]. Gastroenterology 2000; 118(3): 573–81.
26. Frulloni L, Bovo P, Brunelli S, Vaona B, Di F, V, Nishimori I et al. Elevated serum levels of antibodies to carbonic anhydrase I and II in patients with chronic pancreatitis [In Process Citation]. Pancreas 2000; 20(4): 382–8.

5.2 Noninvasive pancreatic function tests

J. E. Domínguez-Muñoz

Introduction

Because histology is not available for the diagnosis of chronic pancreatitis, detection of the disease is based on the demonstration of the morphological and/or functional changes that develop during the course of the disease. In clinical routine, ductal changes observed by endoscopic retrograde pancreatography or magnetic resonance pancreatography, and parenchymal changes detected by ultrasound, endoscopic ultrasound, computed tomography or magnetic resonance, are the bases for the diagnosis of chronic pancreatitis. Functional evaluation of the pancreas is important to confirm the diagnosis in some controversial cases, to detect pancreatic insufficiency and to follow up the disease.

Direct pancreatic function tests requiring duodenal intubation are without any doubt the gold standard in the evaluation of exocrine pancreatic function. However, these tests are invasive, cumbersome, time-consuming and expensive and thus performed only in some selected medical centers. Indirect pancreatic function tests are easily applicable to the clinical routine and therefore widely used. Among these are oral tests that evaluate the digestive ability of the exocrine pancreas and fecal tests that measure the activity or concentration of pancreatic enzymes in feces. The sensitivity and specificity of these indirect tests are variable and lower than those of the direct tests. Since the information obtained by different indirect tests is different, it is of most importance to select the test to be performed in each clinical situation.

The present chapter tries to bring up to date the clinical utility and diagnostic efficacy of the indirect pancreatic function tests as well as to discuss how these tests can be optimized in order to obtain as much clinical information as possible.

What information are we looking for?

Pancreatic function tests can be used to diagnose chronic pancreatitis in patients with clinical suspicion of the disease but normal imaging. With this aim, only the secretin-caerulein test can be useful since noninvasive pancreatic function tests are unable to detect any abnormality in these patients. In the opposite site, the diagnosis of pancreatic insufficiency with steatorrhea and the indication or control of the efficacy of enzyme substitution therapy requires a test able to detect fat maldigestion. It is easy to understand that in these two clinical situations the test to be used should have a very different sensitivity, the highest in the former case, the lowest in the latter (Fig. 5.2-1). Between both situations, other tests with an intermediate sensitivity are indicated. Among these clinical situations are the screening for chronic pancreatitis in patients with compatible clinical picture and the long-term follow-up of patients with known chronic pancreatitis (Fig.5.2-1).

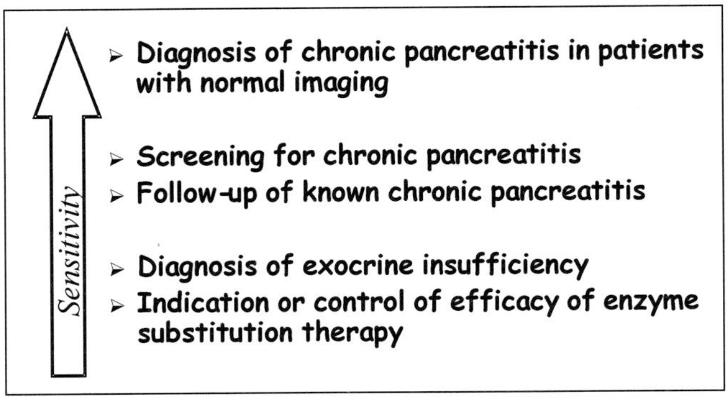

Figure 5.2-1. Indications of functional evaluation of the exocrine pancreas in chronic pancreatitis and the relationship with the required sensitivity of the test to be used.

Which noninvasive tests are available?

From a methodological point of view, tubeless pancreatic function tests can be classified as oral tests and fecal tests. In oral tests a substrate is orally administered together with a test meal. This substrate is hydrolyzed by pancreatic enzymes within the duodenum; the released metabolites are absorbed from the gut and then can be measured in either serum, urine or breath. Oral tests allow therefore an indirect evaluation of the exocrine pancreatic function (indirect test). Among them are the pancreolauryl test, the PABA test and different breath tests mainly using ^{13}C-labelled substrates.

Pancreatic enzyme concentration (elastase) or activity (chymotrypsin) can be measured in feces. These two fecal tests can be considered direct tests, since the amount of pancreatic enzymes secreted by the pancreas are directly measured. Enzymes are deactivated and diluted or concentrated in a variable degree during the intestinal passage, which must be taken into account for an adequate interpretation of the test results. Exocrine pancreatic function can also be measured indirectly in feces by means of the fecal fat quantification. The amount of fat eliminated within the feces reflects indirectly the fat digestion and therefore the pancreatic lipase secretion.

Fecal tests

Fecal fat quantification

Fecal fat quantification by the classical Van de Kamer test is the gold standard for the diagnosis of steatorrhea. Despite that, this test has several and important disadvantages that limit its clinical applicability. Patients must keep on a standard diet containing 80 to 100 g of fat daily during 5 consecutive days. This is an important handicap since the majority of patients with chronic pancreatitis are alcoholics and thus with a limited compliance. Furthermore, patients should collect the whole amount of feces produced over the last 3 days of diet. Again this is not easy to comply with for alcoholic patients.

Not only patient compliance is a limitation for the fecal fat quantification but mainly the handling of stool samples in the lab. Stool samples collected over 3 days must be first homogenized and then processed following a manual method that takes two days and makes this test unpleasant and cumbersome. A new methodology based on near infrared analysis (NIRA) has greatly simplified the quantification of fat in stool and thus can make feasible the wide application of this test in clinical routine [1]. Nevertheless, the difficulties associated with patient compliance remain the same.

Fecal chymotrypsin activity

Quantification of fecal chymotrypsin is a simple test and easy to apply to the clinical routine. This test is based on the enzymatic quantification of the chymotrypsin activity in an isolated small stool sample. Because of that, fecal chymotrypsin has been widely introduced in clinical chemistry labs as an exocrine pancreatic function test. Chymotrypsin is however variably inactivated during the intestinal passage in such a way that fecal chymotrypsin activity does not accurately reflect pancreatic secretion of the enzyme. In addition, dilution of the enzyme in patients with diarrhea of any etiology will also decrease the fecal activity of the enzyme.

Because of that and in order to keep an adequate specificity of the test, a low cut-off (3 U/g of stool) is generally accepted to define a test as abnormal. Patients with fecal chymotrypsin activity less than 3 U/g of stool are thus considered as suffering from exocrine pancreatic insufficiency, but the sensitivity obtained with the test is too low to recommend it for clinical practice. In fact, the test is not able to detect a single case of mild changes of chronic pancreatitis as evidenced by endoscopic retrograde pancreatography (ERP), and only slightly more than half of the patients with moderate or severe changes of the disease [2]. Similar results are obtained when the secretin-caerulein test is used as gold standard [3].

Last but not least, orally administered exogenous pancreatic enzymes as a treatment of exocrine pancreatic insufficiency interact with the determination of chymotrypsin in stool [4] and thus this therapy should be interrupted for at least the 48 hours preceding the stool sample collection. This is not always easy to accomplish for patients with exocrine pancreatic insufficiency.

In conclusion and after taking into consideration all aspects above mentioned, fecal chymotrypsin quantification should not longer be considered as adequate for evaluating exocrine pancreatic function in clinical routine.

Fecal elastase concentration

Compared to chymotrypsin, pancreatic elastase is highly stable along the GI transit and the fecal concentrations of this enzyme significantly correlate with the amount of enzyme secreted by the exocrine pancreas [4]. Furthermore, since the methodology used to quantify this enzyme is based on human specific monoclonal antibodies, the oral enzyme substitution therapy does not interfere with the test [4]. Therefore, interruption of this therapy previous to stool collection is not needed, which is an important advantage of the test.

Although the fecal elastase quantification is not sensitive enough to detect patients with mild changes of chronic pancreatitis, its sensitivity in cases of moderate to severe changes of the disease is very high, reaching values close to 100% [2]. Similar sensitivity values are obtained when the secretin-caerulein test is used as gold standard [3, 5]. The specificity of the fecal elastase is also high, only limited by dilution in cases of watery diarrhea [3].

In summary, fecal elastase based on the use of human specific monoclonal antibodies is a very adequate test for the diagnosis of exocrine pancreatic dysfunction in the context of chronic pancreatitis. Since this test is easy to apply to the clinical routine, it may be used as first-step test for the study of patients with clinically suspected chronic pancreatic disease and for the follow-up of patients with known chronic pancreatitis.

Oral tests

Oral pancreatic function tests are based on the administration of a substrate together with a standardized test meal. The substrate is hydrolyzed into the intestinal lumen by specific pancreatic enzymes and the resulting products are absorbed from the gut and can be measured either in serum or in urine or even in expired air (breath tests) after renal or respiratory elimination respectively.

Several extrapancreatic factors are known to limit the accuracy of oral pancreatic function tests [6], mainly those interfering with a normal digestion (slow gastric emptying rate, decreased bile acid secretion) and intestinal absorption (intestinal diseases) as well as those affecting the elimination of the digestion products (renal insufficiency). Variability in gastric emptying rate can be to some extent avoided by intravenous administration of metoclopramide just after ingestion of the test meal [6, 7]. Moreover, the potential negative role of renal disturbances is avoided by the quantification of the digestion products in serum instead of urine [6, 7].

Serum pancreolauryl test

Among oral pancreatic function tests, the serum pancreolauryl test is the most widely used to evaluate exocrine pancreatic function and to grade the functional impairment of the gland [7, 8]. In this test, fluorescein dilaurate is administered orally together with a standardized breakfast. A pancreas-specific cholesterol ester hydrolase acts on this compound and water-soluble fluorescein is released, absorbed from the gut and then measured in serum (Fig. 5.2-2).

The advantage of this test is that it is easily applicable to the clinical routine and can be used not only for supporting the diagnosis of chronic pancreatitis but also for the follow-up of patients with this disease [9]. The limiting factors of oral tests described above and a limited sensitivity for the early diagnosis of chronic pancreatitis are the major disadvantages of the test.

In patients suffering from mild chronic pancreatitis, the pancreas is able to respond normally to a physiological stimulus, i.e. meal. Indirect pancreatic function tests are thus unable to detect any abnormality in these patients [9]. The initial pancreatic response to the intravenous administration of supraphysiological doses of secretin and CCK is also frequently normal in these patients, but decreases if the stimulus is maintained [10]. In the same way, the pancreas affected by chronic pancreatitis can normally respond to the test meal given after an overnight fast in the context of the pancreolauryl test and the re-

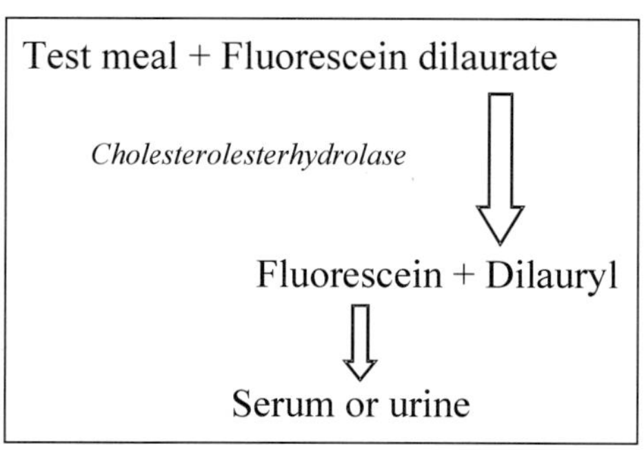

Figure 5.2-2. Basis of the pancreolauryl test.

sult of the test can thus be normal. Intravenous administration of secretin just before ingestion of the test meal increases significantly the sensitivity of the test by inducing a washout of the pancreatic enzymes stored overnight [8]. Thus the test meal given immediately thereafter requires new enzyme synthesis for digestion. This new synthesis is likely impaired in chronic pancreatitis, as supported by our data [8]. In fact, patients with mild changes of chronic pancreatitis in the endoscopic retrograde pancreatography and some with moderate and even severe changes of the disease are able to digest normally the test meal given after an overnight fast if secretin is not previously administered. Thus serum levels of fluorescein attained in these cases are normal. If a previous washout of pancreatic enzymes is performed by intravenous administration of secretin, the test result turns to abnormal in the majority of patients [8]. This maneuver leads thus to a significant increase in the proportion of patients with chronic pancreatitis with abnormal pancreolauryl test result. Moreover, intravenous injection of secretin influences neither the test result in healthy subjects or patients with any extrapancreatic gastrointestinal disorders nor the time curve of the test and, therefore, does not influence the specificity of the test and the optimal sampling time (Fig. 5.2-3).

Calculation of serum fluorescein concentration in the pancreolauryl test has been routinely performed by multiplying the extinction of each sample by a standard calibration factor [6, 7, 11]. This standard calibration factor was calculated in our laboratory by adding different amounts of fluorescein to a serum pool (obtaining final fluorescein concentrations from 0 to 10 mg/L) and thus drawing a standard curve. By linear regression analysis we obtained a calibration factor of 20.83 [6]. The extinction of serum at 492 nm shows however a significant intraindividual day to day variation as well as interindividual variation depending on the characteristics of serum (e.g. concentration of lipids) and conditions of the analysis (e.g. centrifugation, room temperature). Furthermore, the use of a standard curve including a wide range of fluorescein concentrations does not assure the highest accuracy of the method at the range of 4.0–4.5 mg/L fluorescein, which is critical to define a test result as abnormal. We confirmed these facts and showed that the use of the same standard factor for all patients influences the accuracy of the pancreolauryl test [8]. This limitation is overcome by applying a specimen-specific calibration factor for each subject at each day. The fluorescein concentration of the calibration serum obtained was 4.0 mg/L, thus assuring the highest accuracy of the test at that level.

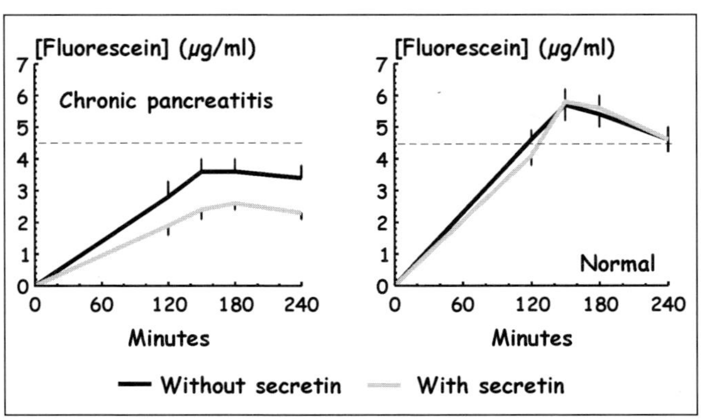

Figure 5.2-3. Curves of serum fluorescein concentrations (mean ± SEM) in the pancreolauryl test in patients with chronic pancreatitis (left) and patients with digestive extrapancreatic diseases (right) according to the administration (gray line) or not (black line) of secretin before the ingestion of the test meal. Modified from reference [8].

The urine PLT has been reported to have an overall accuracy of around 70% for the detection of pancreatic dysfunction in patients with chronic pancreatitis [12–16]. This accuracy was further improved up to 84% by the determination of fluorescein in serum [17] and the introduction of some test modifications [6, 7]. The sensitivity of the PLT in patients with mild morphological changes of chronic pancreatitis was however still as low as 52% [7]. This sensitivity can be increased in about 30% by applying all test modifications described above (from 46% to 75% in patients with mild chronic pancreatitis and from 71% to 100% in those with moderate disease) [8]. Therefore, applying all modifications described above, the sensitivity of the serum pancreolauryl test can be significantly increased to figures close to 100% in patients with moderate and severe chronic pancreatitis and to values as high as 75% in patients with mild disease [8].

In summary, and based on the experience accumulated over many years, we have developed a tubeless pancreatic function test that provides a high sensitivity for chronic pancreatitis, close to that obtained by means of the invasive secretin-CCK test and higher than any other indirect test [8]. This high sensitivity is however reached at the cost of introducing some invasive maneuvers (i.e. intravenous injection of secretin and metoclopramide and collection of blood samples). Potential side effects of metoclopramide and secretin present very rarely after a single dose. In our experience, transient mouth dryness is observed occasionally after metoclopramide administration. A few patients suffer from nausea after secretin, which can be prevented by the slow injection of the drug (over 2–3 minutes). The specificity of the pancreolauryl test is not affected by the modifications used. False-positive results can be obtained in patients with other pancreatic diseases (e.g. pancreatic cancer) and gastrointestinal extrapancreatic diseases leading to maldigestion of the fluorescein-dilaurate (e.g. partial gastric resection with Billroth II anastomosis, obstructive jaundice) or to malabsorption of the released fluorescein (e.g. sprue) [7, 18].

Breath tests

Several substrates, mainly ^{13}C-marked, are being used to evaluate exocrine pancreatic function by means of breath tests. In these tests, the marked substrate is given orally together with a test meal. After intraduodenal hydrolysis of the substrate by specific pancreatic enzymes, ^{13}C-marked metabolites are released, absorbed from the gut and metabolized within the liver. As a consequence of the hepatic metabolism $^{13}CO_2$ is released and thereafter eliminated with the expired air (Fig. 5.2-4). The amount of $^{13}CO_2$ expired, which indirectly reflects the exocrine pancreatic function, can be measured by means of mass spectrometry or infrared analysis.

Most substrates used in breath tests, among them the mixed ^{13}C-triglyceride, the cholesteryl ^{13}C-octanoate, the ^{13}C-hiolein and the ^{13}C-triolein, are hydrolyzed by the pancre-

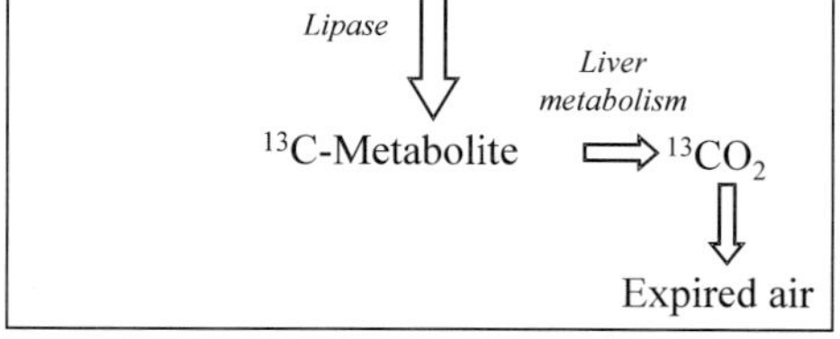

Figure 5.2-4. Basis of the breath pancreatic function tests.

atic lipases. In this way pancreatic function breath tests should be seen as fat digestion tests and thus be considered as an alternative to fecal fat quantification. For the diagnosis of steatorrhea, pancreatic function breath tests have a sensitivity ranging from 80% to 92% and a specificity ranging from 81% to 96% [19–22]. These figures are logically lower when also milder degrees of exocrine pancreatic dysfunction are considered [23].

Nevertheless, no exocrine pancreatic breath test has been optimized up to now and therefore previously reported data have to be considered with caution. In the near future, breath tests should be a real alternative to fecal fat quantification for the diagnosis of steatorrhea in clinical practice. Furthermore, since breath tests are simple and easily applicable to the clinical routine, pancreatic enzymes substitution therapy in patients with steatorrhea could be individualized and monitored for follow-up.

Summary

- Compared with the direct intubation tests, noninvasive pancreatic function tests are simple and applicable to the clinical routine.
- Among fecal pancreatic function tests, elastase is significantly superior to chymotrypsin determination. In fact, fecal chymotrypsin no longer plays a role in the diagnostic approach to chronic pancreatitis in clinical routine.
- Fecal elastase is easy to apply to the clinical routine and is very adequate to be used as first step test for the study of patients with clinically suspected chronic pancreatic disease and for the follow-up of patients with known chronic pancreatitis.
- The optimized serum pancreolauryl test is the most sensitive noninvasive test for the detection of exocrine pancreatic dysfunction. Without the modifications described above the diagnostic accuracy of the test is low and it cannot be recommended for clinical practice.
- Noninvasive tests are useful for the screening of chronic pancreatitis in patients with clinical suspicion of the disease and for the follow-up of known chronic pancreatitis. In both cases, the test to be used should have a high sensitivity.
- Diagnosis of exocrine pancreatic insufficiency is easily done by means of noninvasive tests. Steatorrhea can be diagnosed by any pancreatic function test, since a high diagnostic sensitivity is not required, but fecal fat quantification is still considered the gold standard.
- The efficacy of enzyme substitution therapy can be objectively controlled only by fecal fat quantification. Breath tests can be a simple alternative to fecal fat quantification, easily applicable to clinical routine.

References

1. Ventrucci M, Cipolla A, Di Stefano M, Ubalducci GM, Middonno M, Ligabue A, Roda E. Determination of fecal fat concentration by near infrared spectrometry for screening of pancreatic steatorrhea. Int J Pancreatol 1998; 23: 17–23.
2. Domínguez-Muñoz JE, Hyeronimus C, Sauerbruch T, Malfertheiner P. Fecal elastase test: Evaluation of a new noninvasive pancreatic function test. Am J Gastroenterol 1995; 90: 1834–7.
3. Lankisch PG, Schmidt I, Konig H, Lehnick D, Knollmann R, Lohr M, Liebe S. Fecal elastase 1: not helpful in diagnosing chronic pancreatitis associated to mild to moderate exocrine pancreatic insufficiency. Gut 1998; 42: 551–4.
4. Stein J, Jung M, Sziegoleit A, Zeuzem S, Caspary F, Lembcke B. Immunoreactive elastase 1: Clinical evaluation of a new noninvasive test of pancreatic function. Clin Chem 1996; 42: 222–6.

5. Löser C, Möllgaard A, Fölsch UR. Faecal elastase 1: A novel, highly sensitive and specific tubeless pancreatic function test. Gut 1996; 39: 580–6.
6. Malfertheiner P, Büchler MW, Müller A, Ditschuneit H. Fluorescein dilaurate serum test: A rapid tubeless pancreatic function test. Pancreas 1987; 2: 53–60.
7. Domínguez-Muñoz JE, Pieramico O, Büchler MW, Malfertheiner P. Clinical utility of the serum pancreolauryl test in diagnosing and staging of chronic pancreatitis. Am J Gastroenterol 1993; 88: 1237–41.
8. Domínguez-Muñoz JE, Malfertheiner P. Optimized serum pancreolauryl test for differentiating patients with and without chronic pancreatitis. Clin Chem 1998; 44: 869–75.
9. Malfertheiner P, Domínguez-Muñoz JE, Büchler MW. Diagnosis and staging of chronic pancreatitis. In: Beger HG, Büchler MW, Malfertheiner P, eds. Standards in pancreatic surgery. Berlin–Heidelberg: Springer-Verlag, 1993: 297–313.
10. Gullo L. Value and clinical role of intubation tests in chronic pancreatitis. In: Beger HG, Büchler MW, Ditschuneit H, Malfertheiner P, eds. Chronic pancreatitis. Berlin–Heidelberg: Springer-Verlag, 1990: 287–90.
11. Domínguez-Muñoz JE, Manes G, Pieramico O, Büchler MW, Malfertheiner P. Effect of ductal and parenchymal changes on exocrine function in chronic pancreatitis. Pancreas 1995; 10: 31–5.
12. Malfertheiner P, Peter M, Junge U, Ditschuneit H. Indirect pancreatic function test pancreolauryl: Its value in diagnosis of chronic pancreatitis. Klin Wochenschr 1983; 61: 193–8.
13. Ammann RW, Bühler H, Pei P. Comparative diagnostic accuracy of four tubeless pancreatic function tests in chronic pancreatitis. Scand J Gastroenterol 1982; 17: 997–1002.
14. Lankisch PG. Exocrine pancreatic function test. Gut 1982; 23: 777–98.
15. Barry RE, Barry R, Ene MK, Parker G. Fluorescein dilaurate-tubeless test for pancreatic exocrine failure. Lancet 1982; 2: 742–4.
16. Boyd JS, Cumming JGR, Cushieri A, Wood RAB, Worsmley KG. Prospective comparison of the fluorescein dilaurate test with the secretin-cholecystokinin test for pancreatic exocrine function. J Clin Pathol 1982; 35: 1240–3.
17. Lankisch PG, Brauneis J, Otto J, Goke B. Pancreolauryl and PABA tests. Are serum tests more practicable alternatives to urine tests in the diagnosis of exocrine pancreatic insufficiency? Gastroenterology 1986; 80: 350–4.
18. Malfertheiner P, Büchler MW, Müller A et al. Influence of extrapancreatic digestive disorders on the indirect pancreatic function test with fluorescein dilaurate. Clin Physiol Biochem 1985; 3: 166–73.
19. Dominguez-Muñoz JE, Leodolter A, Malfertheiner P. Accuracy of the 13C-mixed triglyceride breath test for the diagnosis of exocrine pancreatic insufficiency. Gut 1997 (suppl).
20. Löser C, Brauer C, Aygen S, Hennemann O, Fölsch UR. Comparative clinical evaluation of the 13C-mixed triglyceride breath test as an indirect pancreatic function test. Scand J Gastroenterol 1998; 33: 327–34.
21. Lembcke B, Braden B, Caspary WF. Exocrine pancreatic insufficiency: accuracy and clinical value of the uniformly labelled 13C-Hiolein breath test. Gut 1996; 39: 668–74.
22. Vantrappen GR, Rutgeerts PJ, Ghoos YF, Hiele MI. Mixed triglyceride breath test: a noninvasive test of pancreatic lipase activity in the duodenum. Gastroenterology 1989; 96: 1126–34.
23. Ventrucci M, Cipolla A, Ubalducci, Roda A, Roda E. 13C-labelled cholesteryl octanoate breath test for assessing pancreatic exocrine insufficiency. Gut 1998; 42: 81–7.

5.3 How to make use of pancreatic function tests and do we need them?

P. Layer, J. Keller

Introduction

An ideal pancreatic exocrine function test should be specific for pancreatic insufficiency and exclude other causes of maldigestion. It should be sensitive enough to detect early stages of impaired pancreatic exocrine function and define the level of insufficiency even in the absence of overt malabsorption, be noninvasive, inexpensive, easily performed, reproducible and able to monitor pancreatic function during the course of pancreatic disease. Moreover, lack of interference from exogenous pancreatic supplements would be desirable. Unfortunately, such an ideal test does not exist and all available ones have several disadvantages: The more sensitive, invasive tests are not only unpleasant for the patient, but also expensive and hardly standardized among different laboratories. On the other hand, it is virtually impossible to diagnose mild to moderate pancreatic insufficiency by noninvasive tests. Sensitivity and specificity of these tests are only satisfactory in cases of severe pancreatic insufficiency after loss of 90–95% of the secretory capacity of the pancreas (Fig. 5.3-1). However, such patients usually suffer from steatorrhea [1] which can be diagnosed visually with considerable accuracy, though not in mild to moderate cases [2]. Moreover, in a patient with known chronic pancreatitis who develops steatorrhea enzyme supplementation without further diagnostic measures might be justified. This renders the question, whether routine performance of pancreatic function tests makes sense at all.

Methodology, advantages and disadvantages of the available pancreatic function tests and why we still need them are discussed below.

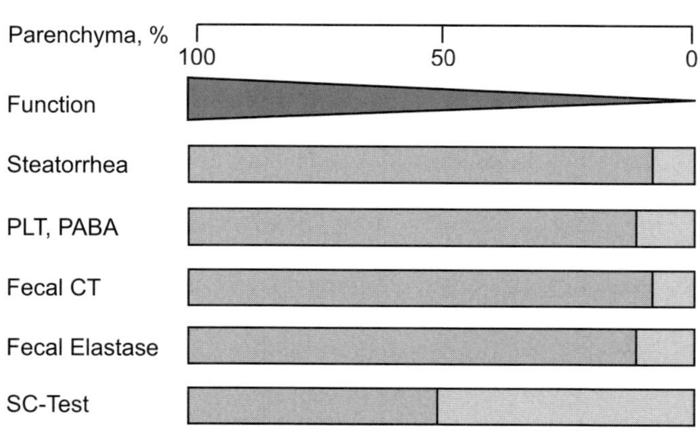

Figure 5.3-1. Sensitivity of pancreatic function tests in progressive pancreatic exocrine insufficiency.

Pathophysiologic background

Maldigestion of macronutrients caused by low intraluminal enzymatic activities may result from disturbances of enzyme synthesis or secretion or from intraluminal inactivation. In chronic pancreatitis, the most common cause of pancreatic exocrine insufficiency, these mechanisms interact: Enzyme synthesis and consequently enzyme output decreases by 60–90% within the first 5–10 years of alcoholic chronic pancreatitis [3] with an earlier decrease in lipase synthesis and secretion compared with other enzymes. This significant decrease in enzyme output is still associated with normal fecal fat excretion (compensated pancreatic insufficiency). The critical threshold of less than 5–10% of normal lipase activity leading to overt steatorrhea (decompensated pancreatic insufficiency) is usually reached after about 15 years [4]. In addition residual intraluminal enzymes are partly destroyed by increased intraluminal acidity due to loss of bicarbonate secretion and by proteolytic destruction during small intestinal transit [5, 6]. Again, lipase is most sensitive to acidic and proteolytic inactivation and this explains the pivotal clinical importance of lipid maldigestion (often associated with malabsortion of the lipid soluble vitamins A, D, E and K) which is more severe and occurs several years prior to clinical malabsorption of protein or starch.

While chronic pancreatitis leads to disturbances of enzyme synthesis and secretion as well as to intraluminal inactivation, other diseases such as cancer of the head of the pancreas or periampullary tumors may obstruct the main pancreatic duct and impair secretion of pancreatic juice despite normal synthetic capacity. In celiac sprue, on the other hand, decreased release of CCK by the diseased intestinal mucosa reduces pancreatic secretory response to nutrients, despite normal secretory capacity and absence of obstruction [7, 8]. Zollinger-Ellison-syndrome patients may suffer from maldigestion due to intraluminal inactivation of especially lipase caused by duodenal hyperacidity [5] and gastrointestinal surgery, e.g. gastrectomy may induce malabsorption due to impaired coordination between secretory and motor functions.

The available pancreatic function tests reflect the impairment of pancreatic enzyme secretion on different levels: Direct tests measure the secretory capacity of the pancreas during exogenous or endogenous stimulation and collection of duodenal juice via tubes or estimate fecal excretion of pancreatic enzymes. Indirect tests assess pancreatic function by measurement of a digestive function or malfunction.

Direct pancreatic function tests

Secretin-cerulein test (SC test)

Direct measurement of pancreatic enzyme and bicarbonate output in response to a defined hormonal stimulus (CCK or an analogue such as cerulein, alone or in combination with secretin) is considered the gold standard for determining pancreatic exocrine function. Sensitivity and specificity of this test both exceed 90% [1, 5, 7, 9, 10] and it is the only means of reliably diagnosing mild to moderate pancreatic insufficiency. However, the test is invasive, costly and not standardized among different centers. It requires placement of a double lumen naso-duodenal tube for constant elimination of gastric juice and complete and fractionated collection of duodenal juice on ice during intravenous infusion of secretin and cerulein. Incomplete collection of intestinal juice can be compensated for by constant duodenal perfusion of a dilution marker, but this requires a triple lumen tube and further complicates the performance of the test. The protocol performed in our laboratory [11] includes:

1. positioning of a double lumen naso-duodenal tube with fluoroscopic control,
2. complete aspiration and elimination of gastric juice,
3. complete collection of duodenal juice in 10 min intervals for 30 min during a basal period, for 60 min during intravenous application of 1 CU/kg secretin and for a further 60 min during intravenous infusion of 1 CU/kg secretin and 75 ng/kg cerulein (doses are chosen to achieve maximal stimulation of pancreatic secretion),
4. subsequent measurement of volume, bicarbonate, trypsin, chymotrypsin, lipase and amylase outputs.

Lundh test

The Lundh test [12–14] also includes intestinal intubation and direct measurement of enzyme output in duodenal juice, however, it uses a different stimulus. Instead of exogenous stimulation, pancreatic exocrine secretion is stimulated by a test meal which requires release of regulatory mediators from the intestinal mucosa. As a consequence, this test is less specific than the SC test and may render false-positive results in intestinal diseases such as celiac sprue.

Fecal tests

Fecal output of individual enzymes correlates with duodenal enzyme output [15], though all pancreatic enzymes are inactivated during intestinal transit. The degree of inactivation varies among different enzymes, however [6]. As stated above, pancreatic lipase is most susceptible to various inactivating mechanisms and almost completely lost during small intestinal transit following a carbohydrate meal. By contrast, pancreatic amylase is relatively stable within the small intestinal lumen so that about 60% of duodenal amylase activity is delivered to the colon. Proteases show intermediary inactivation rates of about 50%. Within the large intestine further destruction of pancreatic enzymes due to bacterial metabolism may take place [16].

Nevertheless, fecal excretion of certain pancreatic enzymes is used routinely as a test of pancreatic exocrine function:

Fecal *chymotrypsin* activity can be measured by a commercially available photometric test kit [17]. When performed on three consecutive days, this test reliably detects patients with severe pancreatic exocrine insufficiency (decompensated pancreatic insufficiency), but sensitivity and specificity are inadequate in mild to moderate cases (compensated pancreatic insufficiency) [18–20]. In addition, the test does not differentiate between porcine and human chymotrypsin, so that pancreatin preparations need to be discontinued at least 5 days in advance.This disadvantage is in part compensated for by the ability to monitor patients' compliance in severe pancreatic insufficiency refractory to enzyme treatment. Patients who still suffer from steatorrhea although they take the advised amount of pancreatin supplements will have high fecal chymotrypsin activities; others who fail to take (all) the medication will have low chymotrypsin activities.

Fecal *elastase-1* excretion can be measured by an ELISA test using an antibody highly specific for the human enzyme. Therefore, pancreatin supplements do not interfere with this pancreatic function test and need not be discontinued. Measurement of fecal elastase-1 excretion appears to be more sensitive and specific than fecal chymotrypsin

[21–23]; however, there are numerous false-positive results in patients with intestinal diseases and mild to moderate stages of pancreatic exocrine insufficiency cannot be diagnosed reliably [24, 25].

ELISA tests for measurement of fecal *amylase* and *lipase* [26] excretion are being developed, but have so far not been introduced into routine clinical procedures.

Pancreatic enzyme serum levels

Even in healthy humans, small amounts of pancreatic enzymes are released from the pancreas into the circulation and are detectable as low serum levels of lipase, amylase, trypsin(ogen) and chymotrypsin(ogen). Theoretically, in chronic pancreatitis, progressive destruction of the organ should be reflected by decreasing serum levels of pancreatic enzymes. However, because of their low accuracy, serum tests are not useful as routine procedures [27, 28].

Indirect tests

Indirect pancreatic function tests assess pancreatic function or malfunction by measurement of a physiological or synthetic substrate or its metabolic product that needs to be enzymatically cleaved before absorption and/or excretion, e.g. in urine or breath.

Stool weight and quantitative fecal fat excretion

Measurement of stool weight on three consecutive days during ingestion of a normal, balanced diet is a rather crude test, but may suggest pancreatic insufficiency if stool weight exceeds 200 g/d. Measurement of quantitative fecal fat excretion is the "gold standard" test for malabsorption, though it is an insensitive and nonspecific pancreatic function test because steatorrhea only occurs after loss of more than 90% of exocrine function [1]. In addition, other causes of malabsorption, e.g. celiac sprue or Crohn's disease, may also induce abnormal fecal fat excretion of more than 7 g/day or more than 5 g/100 g. In chronic pancreatitis, however, steatorrhea is usually more severe (fecal fat concentration usually > 10 g/100 g stool) [29] compared with mild to moderate steatorrhea in intestinal diseases.

Fluorescein dilaurate test (pancreolauryl test)

Orally administered fluorescein dilaurate cannot be absorbed unless it is cleaved by the pancreatic cholesterol esterase. Enzymatic cleavage leads to liberation of lauric acid and fluorescein. Free fluorescein is water soluble and readily absorbed by the small intestine, partially glucoronidated in the liver and excreted in the urine, predominantly as fluorescein diglucoronide. In pancreatic insufficient patients, lack of cholesterol esterase prevents (complete) cleavage of fluorescein dilaurate and, consequently, absorption of free fluorescein.

The commercially available pancreolauryl test is based on the above described test principle and includes ingestion of a standard breakfast together with 0.5 mmol of fluorescein dilaurate. Urine is collected completely for 10 hours postprandially and allows measurement of fluorescein excretion. In order to enhance diuresis, 1 L unsweetened tea is administered during the first three hours postprandially. After a wash-out period of at least 24 hours, the protocol is repeated using equimolar amounts of free fluorescein instead of fluorescein dilaurate as substrate. This repetition serves as a control for individual differences in intestinal absorption, conjugation and urinary excretion of free fluorescein.

The results are expressed as the ratio of fluorescein excreted on the test and the control day in percent. A ratio of less than 20% is abnormal, 20–30% is equivocal and more than 30% is considered normal.

Recently, a serum test was developed which eliminates the need for urine collection and can be performed on one day only. However, additional application of secretin and metoclopramide increases costs considerably and superior sensitivity and specificity of the serum compared with the urine test still need to be established [30, 31].

Again, both tests, the serum as well as the urine test, diagnose severe pancreatic exocrine insufficiency reliably, but are not capable of detecting mild to moderate impairment of pancreatic function [19]. False-positive results occur in patients with biliary diseases, chronic inflammatory bowel disease or other malassimilation syndromes and following extensive gastrointestinal surgery, e.g. gastrectomy [32–34]. In the latter patients, intraluminal lack of pancreatic enzymes is caused predominantly by postprandial asynchrony of secretory and motor functions and subsequent reduced release of stimulatory mediators, but not by reduced secretory capacity of the pancreas. Nevertheless, the pancreolauryl test may be a useful tool to estimate the degree of nutrient assimilation in such patients and to monitor the effect of enzyme therapy.

Breath tests

The common, noninvasive and easy to handle H2 breath test has been employed for measurement of pancreatic function [35, 36] based on the principle that starch which is not digested due to pancreatic exocrine insufficiency is delivered to the colon and metabolized by the colonic flora leading to an increase in H2 exhalation. However, there are numerous possibilities of false-positive (e.g. bacterial overgrowth) and negative (e.g. insufficient H2 production by colonic bacteria) results, so that the H2 breath test is an inaccurate tool for measurement of pancreatic function [36].

During the recent years, breath tests using ^{13}C-labeled substrates have been developed for measurement of pancreatic function. In these tests, duodenal lipolysis as the rate-limiting step of lipid absorption is reflected by the ratio of breath $^{13}CO_2/^{12}CO_2$ over time. Available substrates include 1,3 distearyl-2[^{13}C]-octanoate, uniformly labeled Hiolein® (mixture of long chain triglycerides) and cholesteryl-^{13}C-octanoate [37–40]. These tests are noninvasive and rather comfortable. However, expensive substrates and lack of superior sensitivity and specificity compared with other noninvasive techniques have prevented routine clinical use so far. One potential advantage of these kinetic tests might be the ability to detect not only a decrease in overall lipolysis but also a shift to more distal intestinal sites.

Concluding considerations

How to use pancreatic function tests

As stated above, all pancreatic function tests available have several disadvantages which may question clinical usefulness. In particular, diagnosis of mild pancreatic insufficiency is virtually impossible using indirect or noninvasive tests (Fig. 5.3-1). The accurracy of fecal elastase-1 measurements, a function test which is currently favored by many clinicians due to its noninvasiveness and convenience, is low in mild pancreatic insufficiency. In addition, false-positive results may occur due to dilution of feces in diarrheal states. Hence, pancreatic insufficiency tends to be substantially underdiagnosed in the early course of chronic pancreatitis and overdiagnosed in the differential diagnosis of patients with diarrhea and steatorrhea of uncertain origin [41].

These considerations support the use of the invasive SC test despite its costs and patient discomfort in selected cases. This test allows a reliable diagnosis of even mild to moderate pancreatic insufficiency. Although few patients develop steatorrhea in this state, decreased pancreatic enzyme output may still be clinically significant for several reasons [42, 43] (compare below).

Is functional impairment reflected by morphological findings?

In most patients, clinically overt steatorrhea is a late event in the course of chronic pancreatitis, which is the most common cause of pancreatic exocrine insufficiency [4]. Up to one third of patients with chronic alcoholic pancreatitis, however, have no or little pain at the onset of the disease. Instead, pancreatic insufficiency may be the first or leading symptom and should be confirmed by pancreatic function tests. In addition, in chronic pancreatitis, morphological changes and functional impairment do not always develop in parallel. Thus, about 15% of patients have severe pancreatic exocrine insufficiency and no or only mild morphological signs of chronic pancreatitis, or vice versa [44, 45]. In other words, normal morphological findings do not exclude pancreatic exocrine insufficiency as the cause of malabsorption, so that pancreatic function tests are needed.

Is detection of mild pancreatic insufficiency clinically relevant?

Under physiological circumstances, up to 80% of nutrients, in particular lipids, are absorbed proximal to the Ligament of Treitz [42, 46, 47]. Rapid and effective absorption is achieved by a complex interplay between gastric and small intestinal motility, on the one hand, and secretion of pancreatic and biliary juice, on the other hand. Postprandially, only small portions of nutrients (2–3 kcal/min) are delivered from the stomach in a regulated fashion, mixed thoroughly with pancreatic and biliary secretions and brought into contact with the absorptive epithelium by segmenting contractions of the small intestine. In mild to moderate pancreatic insufficiency enzymatic activity may be sufficient to achieve digestion and absorption of normal amounts of nutrients, but the site of main digestion is shifted to more distal segments of the small intestine. In response to increased nutrient exposure, release of distal intestinal (mostly inhibitory) mediators is enhanced [42]. This, in turn, causes regulatory disturbances of motor and secretory functions which can be corrected by enzyme treatment [42, 43]. Therefore, in the therapy of pain, the response to enzyme treatment even in the absence of steatorrhea [48] may be explained by restoration of regulatory disturbances. However, there are no controlled studies available so far demonstrating clinical benefit of enzyme treatment in this patient subgroup. Hence, it is conceivable but unproven that diagnosis and supplementation therapy of mild exocrine pancreatic insufficiency is of clinical relevance in a subset of patients.

Taken together, pancreatic function tests are needed whenever we consider it important for the assessment, management and guidance of a patient to clarify one or more of the following aspects:

- Is a specific symptom or sign caused by pancreatic insufficiency (due to chronic pancreatitis or other causes)?
- Has pancreatic insufficiency developed in the course of chronic pancreatitis?
- Does a patient require enzyme treatment?

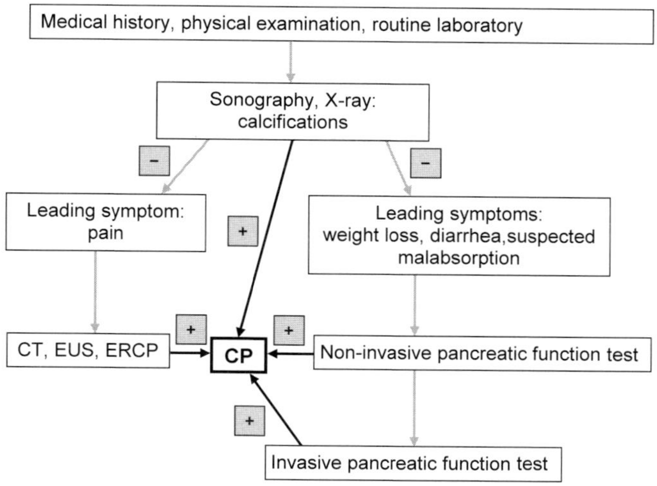

Figure 5.3-2. Diagnostic algorithm in chronic pancreatitis.

Pancreatic function tests are particularly important for the diagnostic algorithm in patients with chronic pancreatitis who present with weight loss, diarrhea and features of malabsorption as leading symptoms (Fig. 5.3-2) [49]. If the main diagnostic goal consists in confirmation of chronic pancreatitis, noninvasive tests of secretory function such as fecal chymotrypsin and elastase-1 are the tests of first choice. If the main goal is to verify maldigestion (which need not be due to loss of pancreatic secretory capacity) or optimize enzyme treatment, indirect tests such as the pancreolauryl test may be preferred. In specific cases in which noninvasive, direct or indirect tests are negative or equivocal and diagnosis or exclusion of pancreatic exocrine insufficiency appears relevant, the invasive SC test should be considered (Fig. 5.3-3).

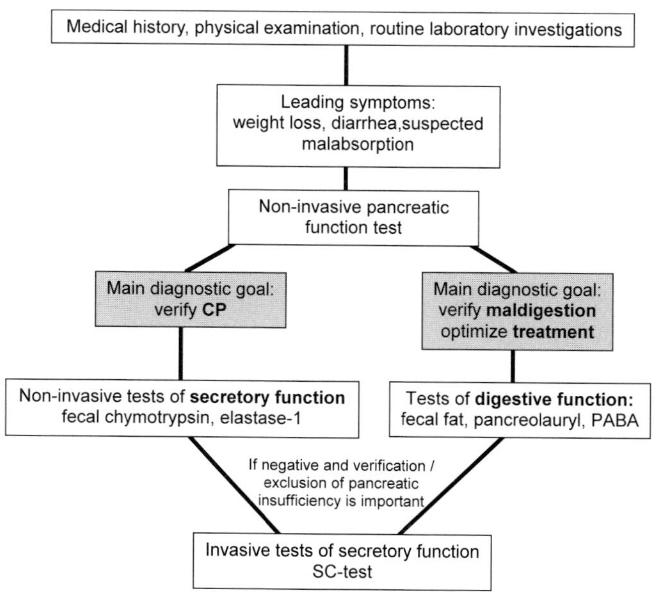

Figure 5.3-3. Differential use of pancreatic function tests.

Acknowledgements

Own studies cited in this article were supported by the German Research Foundation (DFG, grants La 483/5-3).

References

1. DiMagno EP, Go VL, Summerskill WH. Relations between pancreatic enzyme outputs and malabsorption in severe pancreatic insufficiency. N Engl J Med 1973; 288: 813–5.
2. Lankisch PG, Droge M, Hofses S, Konig H, Lembcke B. Steatorrhoea: you cannot trust your eyes when it comes to diagnosis [letter] [see comments]. Lancet 1996; 347: 1620–1.
3. DiMagno EP, Malagelada JR, Go VL. Relationship between alcoholism and pancreatic insufficiency. Ann NY Acad Sci 1975; 252: 200–7.
4. Layer P, Yamamoto H, Kalthoff L, Clain JE, Bakken LJ, DiMagno EP. The different courses of early- and late-onset idiopathic and alcoholic chronic pancreatitis. Gastroenterology 1994; 107: 1481–7.
5. DiMagno EP, Malagelada JR, Go VL, Moertel CG. Fate of orally ingested enzymes in pancreatic insufficiency. Comparison of two dosage schedules. N Engl J Med 1977; 296: 1318–22.
6. Layer P, Go VL, DiMagno EP. Fate of pancreatic enzymes during small intestinal aboral transit in humans. Am J Physiol 1986; 251: 475–80.
7. DiMagno EP, Go WL, Summerskill WH. Impaired cholecystokinin-pancreozymin secretion, intraluminal dilution, and maldigestion of fat in sprue. Gastroenterology 1972; 63: 25–32.
8. Maton PN, Selden AC, Fitzpatrick ML, Chadwick VS. Defective gallbladder emptying and cholecystokinin release in celiac disease. Reversal by gluten-free diet. Gastroenterology 1985; 88: 391–6.
9. Lankisch PG, Schmidt I. Exocrine pancreatic function tests, 1999: is the best we have good enough? [editorial]. Scand J Gastroenterol 1999; 34: 945–7.
10. Wormsley KG. Tests of pancreatic secretion. Clin Gastroenterol 1978; 7: 529–44.
11. Rosien U, Holtmann G, Layer P. Funktionsdiagnostik von Sekretion, Absorption und Motilität. In: Layer P, Rosien U, Goebell H, eds. Praktische Gastroenterologie, 1st ed. München, Wien, Baltimore: Urban & Schwarzenberg, 1996: 74–5.
12. Ihse I, Lilja P, Evander A, Skude G. Time-related enzyme concentrations in duodenal aspirates after ingestion of a test meal. Scand J Gastroenterol 1977; 12: 629–35.
13. Moeller DD, Dunn GD, Klotz AP. Comparison of the pancreozymin-secretin test and the Lundh test meal. Am J Dig Dis 1972; 17: 799–805.
14. James O. The Lundh test. Gut 1973; 14: 582–91.
15. Katschinski M, Schirra J, Bross A, Goke B, Arnold R. Duodenal secretion and fecal excretion of pancreatic elastase-1 in healthy humans and patients with chronic pancreatitis. Pancreas 1997; 15: 191–200.
16. Macfarlane GT, Cummings JH, Macfarlane S, Gibson GR. Influence of retention time on degradation of pancreatic enzymes by human colonic bacteria grown in a 3-stage continuous culture system. J Appl Bacteriol 1989; 67: 520–7.
17. Kaspar P, Moller G, Wahlefeld A. New photometric assay for chymotrypsin in stool. Clin Chem 1984; 30: 1753–7.
18. Bonin A, Roy CC, Lasalle R, Weber A, Morin CL. Fecal chymotrypsin: a reliable index of exocrine pancreatic function in children. J Pediatr 1973; 83: 594–600.
19. Lankisch PG, Schreiber A, Otto J. Pancreolauryl test. Evaluation of a tubeless pancreatic function test in comparison with other indirect and direct tests for exocrine pancreatic function. Dig Dis Sci 1983; 28: 490–3.
20. Ammann RW, Akovbiantz A, Hacki W, Largiader F, Schmid M. Diagnostic value of the fecal chymotrypsin test in pancreatic insufficiency, particularly chronic pancreatitis: correlation with the pancreozymin-secretin test, fecal fat excretion and final clinical diagnosis. Digestion 1981; 21: 281–9.

21. Domínguez-Muñoz JE, Hieronymus C, Sauerbruch T, Malfertheiner P. Fecal elastase test: evaluation of a new noninvasive pancreatic function test. Am J Gastroenterol 1995; 90: 1834–7.
22. Glasbrenner B, Schon A, Klatt S, Beckh K, Adler G. Clinical evaluation of the faecal elastase test in the diagnosis and staging of chronic pancreatitis. Eur J Gastroenterol Hepatol 1996; 8: 1117–20.
23. Loser C, Mollgaard A, Folsch UR. Faecal elastase 1: a novel, highly sensitive, and specific tubeless pancreatic function test [see comments]. Gut 1996; 39: 580–6.
24. Lankisch PG, Schmidt I, Konig H et al. Faecal elastase 1: not helpful in diagnosing chronic pancreatitis associated with mild to moderate exocrine pancreatic insufficiency [see comments]. Gut 1998; 42: 551–4.
25. Lankisch PG, Schmidt I. Fecal elastase 1 is not the indirect pancreatic function test we have been waiting for [letter; comment]. Dig Dis Sci 2000; 45: 166–7.
26. Muench R, Ammann RW. Fecal immunoreactive lipase: a new tubeless pancreatic function test. Scand J Gastroenterol 1992; 27: 289–94.
27. Jacobson DG, Curington C, Connery K, Toskes PP. Trypsin-like immunoreactivity as a test for pancreatic insufficiency. N Engl J Med 1984; 310: 1307–9.
28. Ammann RW, Buhler H, Pei P. Comparative diagnostic accuracy of four tubeless pancreatic function tests in chronic pancreatitis. Scand J Gastroenterol 1982; 17: 997–1002.
29. Bo-Linn GW, Fordtran JS. Fecal fat concentration in patients with steatorrhea. Gastroenterology 1984; 87: 319–22.
30. Lock G, Kadow R, Messmann H, Zirngibl H, Scholmerich J, Holstege A. Modified serum pancreolauryl test in chronic pancreatitis: evaluation in comparison to endoscopic retrograde pancreatography. Hepatogastroenterology 1997; 44: 1110–6.
31. Malfertheiner P, Büchler MW, Muller A, Ditschuneit H. Fluorescein dilaurate serum test: a rapid tubeless pancreatic function test. Pancreas 1987; 2: 53–60.
32. Malfertheiner P, Büchler MW, Muller A, Ditschuneit H. Influence of extrapancreatic digestive disorders on the indirect pancreatic function test with fluorescein dilaurate. Clin Physiol Biochem 1985; 3: 166–73.
33. Kay G, Hine P, Braganza J. The pancreolauryl test. A method of assessing the combined functional efficacy of pancreatic esterase and bile salts in vivo? Digestion 1982; 24: 241–5.
34. Heptner G, Domschke S, Domschke W. Exocrine pancreatic function after gastrectomy. Specificity of indirect tests. Gastroenterology 1989; 97: 147–53.
35. Ladas SD, Giorgiotis K, Raptis SA. Complex carbohydrate malabsorption in exocrine pancreatic insufficiency. Gut 1993; 34: 984–7.
36. Patel VP, Jain NK, Agarwal N, GeeVarghese PJ, Pitchumoni CS. Comparison of bentiromide test and rice flour breath hydrogen test in the detection of exocrine pancreatic insufficiency. Pancreas 1986; 1: 172–5.
37. Loser C, Brauer C, Aygen S, Hennemann O, Folsch UR. Comparative clinical evaluation of the ^{13}C-mixed triglyceride breath test as an indirect pancreatic function test [see comments]. Scand J Gastroenterol 1998; 33: 327–34.
38. Lembcke B, Braden B, Caspary WF. Exocrine pancreatic insufficiency: accuracy and clinical value of the uniformly labelled ^{13}C-Hiolein breath test. Gut 1996; 39: 668–74.
39. Lembcke B. Current role of breath tests in gastroenterology. Z Gastroenterol 1996; 34, Suppl. 4: 46–53.
40. Wutzke KD, Radke M, Breuel K, Gurk S, Lafrenz JD, Heine WE. Triglyceride oxidation in cystic fibrosis: a comparison between different ^{13}C-labeled tracer substances. J Pediatr Gastroenterol Nutr 1999; 29: 148–54.
41. Layer P, Rünzi MGV. Diagnosis of chronic pancreatitis. In: Howard J, Idezuki Y, Ihse I, Prinz R, eds. Surgical diseases of the pancreas, 3rd ed. Baltimore: Williams & Wilkins, 1998: 329–33.
42. Layer P, von der O, Holst JJ et al. Altered postprandial motility in chronic pancreatitis: role of malabsorption. Gastroenterology 1997; 112: 1624–34.
43. Layer P, Keller J. Pancreatic enzymes: secretion and luminal nutrient digestion in health and disease. J Clin Gastroenterol 1999; 28: 3–10.

44. Malfertheiner P, Büchler MW, Stanescu A, Ditschuneit H. Exocrine pancreatic function in correlation to ductal and parenchymal morphology in chronic pancreatitis. Hepatogastroenterology 1986; 33: 110–4.
45. Lankisch PG, Seidensticker F, Otto J et al. Secretin-pancreozymin test (SPT) and endoscopic retrograde cholangiopancreatography (ERCP): both are necessary for diagnosing or excluding chronic pancreatitis. Pancreas 1996; 12: 149–52.
46. Keller J, Runzi M, Goebell H, Layer P. Duodenal and ileal nutrient deliveries regulate human intestinal motor and pancreatic responses to a meal. Am J Physiol 1997; 272: 632–7.
47. Holtmann G, Kelly DG, Sternby B, DiMagno EP. Survival of human pancreatic enzymes during small bowel transit: effect of nutrients, bile acids, and enzymes. Am J Physiol 1997; 273: 553–8.
48. Slaff J, Jacobson D, Tillman CR, Curington C, Toskes P. Protease-specific suppression of pancreatic exocrine secretion. Gastroenterology 1984; 87: 44–52.
49. Lankisch PG, Layer P. Chronische Pankreatitis: Update Diagnostik und Therapie 2000. Deutsches Ärzteblatt 2000; 97: A2169.

6 Chronic pancreatitis: Diagnostic imaging

6.1 Ultrasound in chronic pancreatitis

A. Lügering, M. M. Lerch

Introduction

In different parts of the world the usage of abdominal ultrasound varies considerably. In most Anglo-Saxon countries ultrasound studies are performed by technicians and the ultrasound films they generate are read and evaluated by radiologists. In many European countries clinicians, including surgeons and internists, are trained to perform ultrasound studies on their own patients in real time and they evaluate them as part of the patients' clinical assessment and without further involvement of a radiologist. Under both of these approaches abdominal ultrasound has been found to be a cost-effective and reproducible imaging technique. Its advantages are the absence of radiation, the option to perform the study in real time and at the patient's bedside, and the possibility to perform sonographic interventions. Its disadvantages are the requirement for a high level of training and experience on the part of the person who performs the study and the varying image quality.

An ultrasound image of the pancreas was first reported in 1969. In the last 30 years many technical improvements have contributed to much better imaging of this rather inaccessible organ. Despite these advances in imaging quality and image resolution, the accuracy of conventional ultrasound has improved little over the past 10 years. Provided that interference from body fat and bowel gas is limited an ultrasound of the pancreas can contribute significantly to the accurate diagnosis of pancreatic disease and can often spare the patient much more invasive procedures.

Under physiological conditions the pancreas is located in the upper retroperitoneum and consists of three anatomical parts (head, body, and tail) which can be sonographically identified ventral of the splenic vein. The examination is usually carried out in a supine position with a minimum of two longitudinal and two transverse projections, but flexible techniques are necessary to avoid artefacts caused by neighbouring structures, e.g. the stomach or transverse colon. An additional view through the splenic window can occasionally reveal processes that are located in the tail of the pancreas. If the organ is covered by mobile structures like the stomach it can be helpful to change the patient's position, to apply pressure to the applicator and compress hollow structures, or to use the liver or spleen as an acoustic window. In some cases it may be necessary to fill the stomach with fluid (300 ml fruit juice or water) to replace gas overlying the pancreas. Under optimal circumstances the pancreas can be evaluated in up to 90% by an experienced investigator [1]. On routine examination multiple forms and positions of the organ can be differentiated, and the ventro-dorsal diameters of the head, the body and the tail should be measured. Another important characteristic of the pancreas is its main duct whose visualization is a marker for image quality. The normal duct should be measurable in 90% of the examinations, and typical alterations such as strictures, dilatations, and intraductal stones are valuable diagnostic features in patients with chronic pancreatitis [2]. The echogenicity of the pancreas is slightly more intense than that of normal liver tissue and is age-dependent – which means a more dense parenchyma is found in older patients due to pancreatic lipomatosis. Echogenicity can also increase in diabetic or adipose patients. Additional age-dependent changes are atrophy and fibrosis, which must be differentiated from early alterations in chronic pancreatitis. Another important characteristic during ultrasound examination is the pain or discomfort the patient reports during palpation of the organ. Malformation of the organ (Pancreas divisum, Pancreas anulare) can only occasionally be identified by pancreatic ultrasound.

Use of ultrasound in chronic pancreatitis

Chronic pancreatitis is an inflammatory process in which irreversible and progressive structural changes occur. Its pathophysiology and histopathology are discussed elsewhere in this volume. In contrast to acute pancreatitis where changes often resolve after an acute attack the alterations in chronic pancreatitis are usually progressive and permanent. In most patients with chronic pancreatitis (75%) the underlying etiology is alcohol abuse but other causes such as obstructive, traumatic, and metabolic factors exist and can usually not be differentiated by pancreatic ultrasound [3]. Recently a number of genetic factors have been identified and the hereditary variety of pancreatitis they cause appears to be much more common than previously assumed. Patients in which no cause of chronic pancreatitis can be identified are referred to as suffering from chronic idiopathic pancreatitis.

Initial alterations of the parenchyma that can be detected by ultrasound consist in a diffuse enhancement of the echogenicity, a discrete dilatation of the main pancreatic duct (> 3 mm) or the formation of cysts (< 10 mm), all of which can involve either distinct parts of the organ or the entire pancreas. The size and contour are usually not altered at this early stage. The main diagnostic problem in early chronic pancreatitis is the fact that there are considerable differences between morphological and functional alterations. Initial lesions can only be diagnosed with difficulty and are often not detectable at all, whereas advanced stages can be more easily identified. The latter include an enlarged or atrophied organ with an irregular contour that appears indiscernible from the surrounding tissue and the fibrosis of the organ that results in a reduced flexibility and mobility during examination. The inhomogeneous parenchyma often contains large (> 10mm) cystic alterations. If calcium deposits are detected either within the pancreatic duct or in the parenchyma this sign is usually regarded as pathognomonic for chronic pancreatitis regardless of the underlying etiology. If calcifications involve the pancreatic duct they often impair the flow of pancreatic juice and lead to a dilatation of the duct (Fig. 6.1-1). In addition, focal strictures of the duct are common, but complete obstruction of the duct should always prompt a search for pancreatic neoplasm. The dilatation of the bile duct caused by an inflammatory mass in the head of the pancreas is a frequently observed extrapancreatic feature of chronic pancreatitis. It is also quite common in a rare subform of pancreatitis that involves the pancreatic tissue surrounding the duodenum, which is referred to as "groove pancreatitis" ("Rinnenpankreatitis") and is very hard to diagnose by either ultrasound or CT because most of the pancreas itself appears normal. Other more common extrapancreatic complications of chronic pancreatitis are a thrombosis of the retropancreatic splenic vein that can most easily be detected by Color-Flow-Mapping (CFM) ultrasound, a constriction of the duodenum or stomach, and most often pseudocyst formation. Some of the early and late features of chronic pancreatitis are summarized

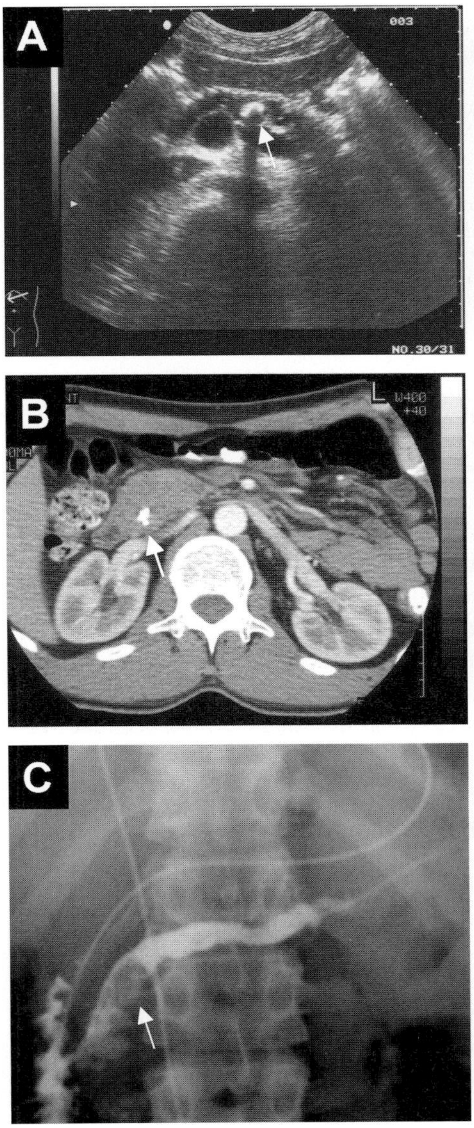

Figure 6.1-1A–C. Intraductal pancreatic stones. All images in this figure were taken from the same patient with hereditary chronic pancreatitis. Arrows in each panel indicate the pancreatic stones. Panel **A** shows the patient's abdominal ultrasound on which intraductal calcifications can be clearly identified. Panel **B** shows the corresponding CT scan with an unequivocal calcification in the head of the pancreas. In panel **C** an endoscopically inserted drainage catheter was used to fill the pancreatic duct with contrast agent and allow for the resolution and removal of the intraductal stone by lithotrypsy.

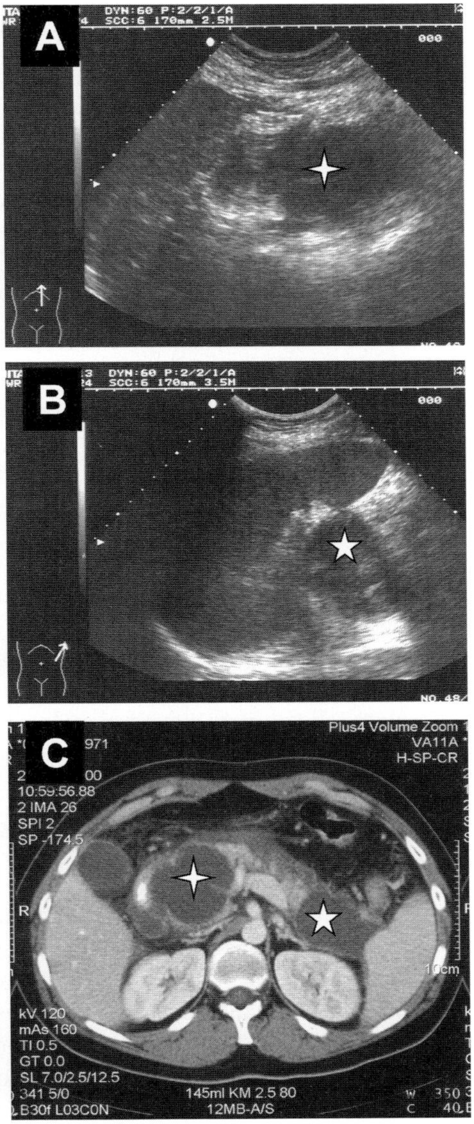

Figure 6.1-2A–C. Cystic lesions of the pancreas. All image studies shown were performed on the same patient. In the panel **A** ultrasound study of the pancreas is shown in a longitudinal plane and a large cystic lesion is clearly identifiable (asterisk) in the head of the pancreas. In panel **B** a second cystic lesion (asterisk) is shown in the tail of the pancreas using an acoustic window through the spleen. Panel **C** represents both cysts as seen on the patient's CT scan and indicated with their respective asterisks.

Table 6.1-1. Ultrasound characteristics in chronic pancreatitis.

Early alterations	• Echogenic foci within the pancreatic parenchyma • Cysts < 10 mm • Discrete irregularities/enlargement of the main duct
Late alterations	• Calculi in the duct • Large cysts > 10 mm • Irregular anatomical contour • Duct obstruction/duct dilatation, major irregularities of the ductal wall
Complications	• Dilatation of the common bile duct • From pancreatic pseudocysts: – obstruction – bleeding – infection • Thrombosis of the portal vein • Neoplasm • Inflammatory pseudotumor

in Table 6.1-1. Pseudocysts that are larger than 1 cm are generally detectable by ultrasound. Often they show a homogeneous and echo-free fluid content that can become echogenic when the cyst is infected. Other important complications of pseudocyst formation are a compression of the intestine, the common bile duct or the portal vein and bleeding from arterial erosion. Cystic lesions greater than 5 cm in diameter therefore require close follow-up or interventional treatment to reduce the risk of subsequent complications (Fig. 6.1-2).

Diagnostic value of ultrasound in chronic pancreatitis

As mentioned before, the diagnostic value of an ultrasound examination is highly dependent on the experience of the investigator. Various studies that evaluated the overall sensitivity and specificity of ultrasound in chronic pancreatitis have resulted in sensitivities ranging from 52% [4] to 82% [5]. Some of these variations are probably related to differences in the study design and the different inclusion criteria for patients. Especially minimal-change pancreatitis and early chronic pancreatitis remain a highly controversial issue and are difficult to diagnose with any confidence or precision. In contrast, when typical alterations are detected ultrasound is a remarkably good diagnostic tool and the specificity of the method can reach over 90% [6, 7]. The most frequently identified pathological findings are inhomogeneous parenchymal texture (50–92%) with an irregular anatomical contour (23–60%), dilatation of the main pancreatic duct (20–77%), and a diffuse or partial hypertrophy of the pancreas (12–57%, [2]). Coexisting gallstones are also routinely detectable. A distinction between chronic pancreatitis and recurrent acute pancreatitis by means of ultrasound is often not possible. Pancreatic cancer arising in a chronically inflamed pancreas is notoriously difficult to diagnose by any imaging technique and this drawback is particularly true for abdominal ultrasound. As a consequence regions of a poorly echogenic mass with almost no internal echoes remain a major problem in differentiating lesions due to chronic pancreatitis, necrosis, and neoplasm. Another problem is a massively dilated pancreatic duct which can arise from an intraductal tumor that occasionally cannot be differentiated from cystic or pseudocystic lesions. These

Table 6.1-2. Alterations in chronic pancreatitis as detectable by conventional US.

Routinely detectable	Sometimes detectable	Rarely detectable
• Cystic lesions • Pancreatic masses • Coexisting gallstones	• Calcifications • Duct stones • Neoplasm • Morphological alterations of the pancreatic main duct	• Anatomic abnormalities

main local complications of chronic pancreatitis occur with an incidence of between 5 and 32% [8]. Ultrasound routinely detects them with a sensitivity of up to 94% [9]. The most commonly detectable characteristics of chronic pancreatitis are summarized in Table 6.1-2.

Some more recent studies have tried to improve the diagnostic accuracy of pancreatic ultrasound by secretin-stimulation in order to dilate the pancreatic duct. Most authors today agree that this functional test adds little if anything to the diagnostic accuracy in most patients [10].

Comparison of computed tomography (CT) and ultrasound in chronic pancreatitis

The second most common noninvasive pancreas imaging technique is computed tomography (CT). CT is a well standardized and highly reproducible imaging technique and its diagnostic accuracy appears to be less investigator-dependent than that of ultrasound. Additionally, CT can better differentiate between benign and malignant pancreatic lesions. Its disadvantages compared to ultrasound are the facts that CT is not a bedside technique because CT scanners are still very immobile machines, and CT studies involve high levels of radiation. The main advantage of CT in the diagnosis of chronic pancreatitis is its superiority in detecting typical signs of the disease such as pancreatic calcifications, peripancreatic fascial thickening, and small intrapancreatic pseudocysts, which can be more easily differentiated from neighbouring structures [11]. In addition, the tail of the pancreas, which is generally the most difficult part to visualize on ultrasound examination, can be much more easily evaluated by CT. Acute pancreatitis can also be better differentiated when intravenous contrast agents are used because non-perfused necrotic areas can be distinguished from vital pancreatic parenchyma. In contrast to its superior diagnostic value in assessing the complications and late changes of pancreatitis, CT is a less sensitive imaging technique for the early stages of the disease.

Many studies in the 1980s focused on the comparison of CT and ultrasound in diagnosing chronic pancreatitis and evaluated their diagnostic accuracy [12–14]. While several reports found that CT is the more accurate imaging technique, others reported an almost equal accuracy for both techniques. Wherever the two imaging techniques gave different results Hessel et al. [15] found CT to give the correct diagnosis in 85%, and other investigators have confirmed these results. Hollerbach et al. [16] have demonstrated in a more recent study that a false negative result occurred in only 14% of ultrasound examinations when study conditions were adequate and concluded that further investigations by CT in patients with a negative ultrasound is only necessary when clinical data strongly suggest chronic pancreatitis.

Table 6.1-3. Sensitivity of different imaging methods in diagnosing chronic pancreatitis.

	Ultrasound	CT	ERCP
Foley et al., 1980 [13]	0.40	0.90	0.68
Lackner et al., 1980 [23]	0.70	0.84	n. d.
Hessel et al., 1982 [15]	0.69	0.87	n. d.
Swobodnik et al., 1983 [4]	0.52	0.74	0.93
Gebel et al., 1985 [5]	0.82	n. d.	0.56

n. d. = not determined

Mayer et al. [9] compared the diagnostic value of CT and ultrasound and showed that intra- or extrapancreatic pseudocysts are the most common local complications of chronic pancreatitis. They demonstrated that CT is only marginally superior in detecting cystic lesions and concluded that these alterations should be regularly re-evaluated by ultrasound. Some of the studies comparing CT and ultrasound in chronic pancreatitis are summarized in Table 6.1-3.

Pancreatic cancer in chronic pancreatitis – relevance of conventional ultrasound

The relative risk to develop pancreatic cancer for a patient with chronic pancreatitis is still a matter of debate. Recent studies estimate a relative risk of more than 50 in comparison to the normal population [17] but other authors have calculated that risk as being between 4- and 16-fold. On the other hand, the development of chronic pancreatitis caused by a duct-obstructing and slow-growing tumor has also been reported. Chronic pancreatitis and pancreatic carcinoma share many clinical features such as weight loss, anorexia, obstructive jaundice, upper abdominal pain, steatorrhoea, and diabetes mellitus [18]. The main diagnostic problem for conventional ultrasound is the differentiation of malignant processes from the surrounding alterations caused by the chronic inflammation. Multiple studies suggest that ERCP is probably the most sensitive technique to identify a malignant process in the pancreas, although even the specificity of ERCP is not higher than 85% [19]. Studies that have focused on the value of ultrasound in detecting a neoplasm in the chronically inflamed pancreatitis have demonstrated a reasonably good diagnostic value of this method and found it, surprisingly, to be comparable to CT [20]. Nevertheless, endoscopic ultrasound and a CT- or ultrasound-guided needle biopsy are often necessary. Whether biopsy of the pancreas is still required where a distinction between chronic pancreatitis and pancreatic cancer cannot be achieved by imaging techniques or, alternatively, open laparotomy should be the procedure of choice will be discussed elsewhere in this volume. The extent of a pancreatic mass and its possible infiltration into the surrounding structures can be evaluated much better by CT than by ultrasound. An enlargement of the peripancreatic and periaortic lymph nodes is usually impossible to detect by abdominal ultrasound. Because even an array of diagnostic tests including ultrasound, CT and needle biopsy of serum tumor markers often cannot distinguish between malignant and benign pancreatic lesion some authors have suggested early resection as the procedure of choice [21]. The main advantages and disadvantages of CT and ultrasound are summarized in Table 6.1-4.

Table 6.1-4. Advantages and disadvantages of US and CT diagnosis.

	Ultrasound	Computered tomography
Advantage	• Real-time technique • Bedside examination • No risk from radiation • Noninvasive	• Highly reproducible • Good anatomic view • Measurable densities • Contrast enhancement • No interference from surrounding structures other than metal
Disadvantage	• Highly dependent on investigator • Interference from surrounding structures • Poorly standardized	• Time-consuming • Radiation exposure • Not a bedside technique

Conclusions

Conventional abdominal ultrasound is a specific diagnostic tool in patients with chronic pancreatitis when typical morphologic signs such as parenchymal (Fig. 6.1-3) or intraductal calcifications are present. It is also a very sensitive diagnostic tool to detect early lesions in chronic pancreatitis such as an increase in tissue density and changes in the shape of the organ – albeit at the price of a very low specificity. Tumors of the pancreas can be

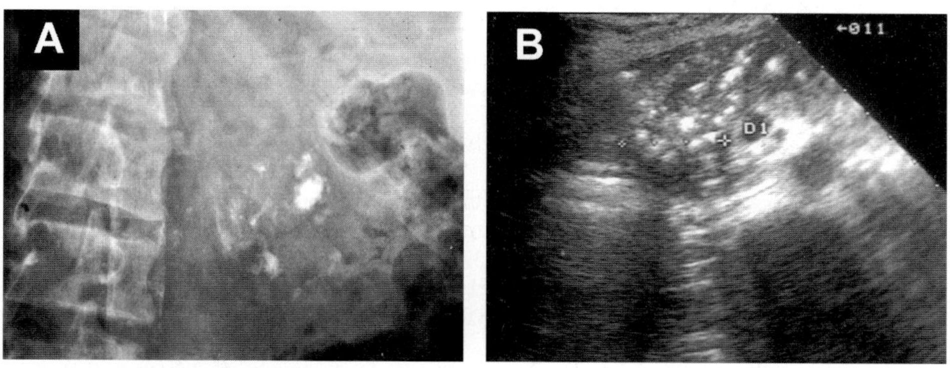

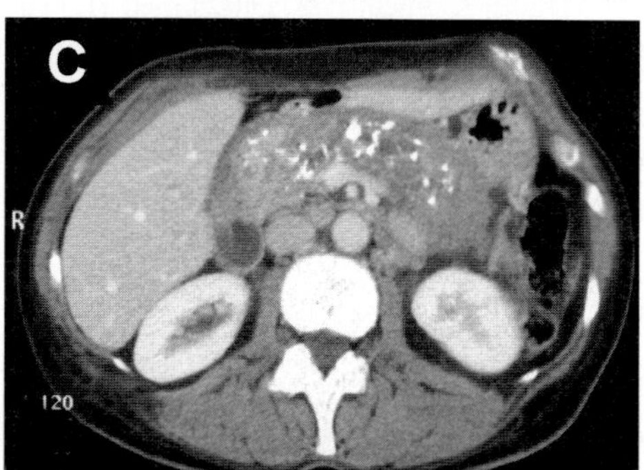

Figure 6.1-3A–C. Calcifications of the pancreatic parenchyma. Calcifications in the head and body of the pancreas are shown on plain X-ray film (panel **A**), on abdominal ultrasound (panel **B**), and on a CT scan (panel **C**). While ultrasound is clearly more sensitive than plain film to detect pancreatic calcifications, its sensitivity in comparison to CT scanning is probably comparable if not better. Each of these techniques, however, is superior to magnetic resonance imaging of the pancreas in the detection of calcifications.

easily detected on ultrasound but distinction between benign and malignant lesions in a chronically inflamed organ is usually not possible and attempts to establish ultrasound as a screening method for pancreatic cancer have failed. Complications of chronic pancreatitis such as pseudocyst formation and dilatation of the common bile duct or main pancreatic duct can be effectively detected by ultrasound and the advantages of ultrasound include the option to repeat equivocal studies without the risks involved in radiation exposure and to perform interventions such as needle biopsy or drainage of fluid collections at the patients' bedside. This is a particular advantage when dealing with critically ill patients in an intensive care setting [22]. At our institution ultrasound is still the first imaging technique for patients with suspected pancreatic disease or chronic pancreatitis. However, this choice of approach is based as much on logistic considerations such as patient scheduling, referral habits, reimbursement practices, and training requirements for young internists and gastroenterologists as it is on the diagnostic advantages of ultrasound. Between 25 and 40% of pathological findings on ultrasound are still being referred to either CT or ERCP for confirmation.

References

1. Simon C, Hoffmann V, Richter GM, Seelos, R, Senninger N, Kauffmann GW. [Hydrosonographie of the pancreas: initial results of a pilot study]. Radiologie 1996; 36: 389–96.
2. Lankisch PG, Staritz M, Freise J. [Reliability of the diagnosis of chronic pancreatitis]. Z Gastroenterol 1990; 28: 253–8.
3. Mergerer K, Baillie J. Chronic pancreatitis. Lancet 1997; 350: 1379–85.
4. Swobodnik W, Meyer W, Brecht-Kraus D, Wechsler JG, Geiger S, Malfertheiner P, Junge U, Ditschuneit H. Ultrasound, computed tomography and endoscopic retrograde cholangiopancreatography in the morphologic diagnosis of pancreatic disease. Klin Wochenschr 1983; 61: 291–6.
5. Gebel M, Stiehl M, Freise J. [Value of sonographic imaging of the pancreatic duct for the diagnosis of chronic pancreatitis and pancreatic cancer compared to ERCP]. Ultraschall Med 1985; 6: 127–30.
6. Bolondi L, Li Bassi S, Gaiani S, Barbara L. Sonography of chronic pancreatitis. Radiol Clin North Am 1989; 27: 815–33.
7. Fiegler W, Claussen C, Hedde JP. [Comparison of computed tomography, automated multisector scanner (Octoson) and conventional ultrasound in pancreatic diseases]. ROFO Fortschr Geb Röntgenstr Nuklearmed 1984; 140: 50–3.
8. Bradley EL, III. Pseudocysts in chronic pancreatitis: development and clinical implications. In: Beger HG, Büchler M, Ditschuneit H, Mafertheimer P, eds. Chronic pancreatitis. Heidelberg: Springer-Verlag, 1990: 260.
9. Mayer D, Malfertheiner P, Kemmer TP, Stanescu A, Kuhn K, Büchler M, Ditschuneit H. [The value of ultrasound and computerized tomography in detection of cystic changes in chronic pancreatitis]. Z Gastroenterol 1992; 30: 709–12.
10. Topazian M. Acute pancreatitis, pancreatic duct obstruction, and the secretin-ultrasound test. J Clin Gastroenterol 1994; 18: 277–9.
11. Luetmer PH, Stephens DH, Ward EM. Chronic pancreatitis: reassessment with current CT. Radiology 1989; 171: 353–7.
12. Brasch RC, Abols IB, Gooding CA, Filly RA. Abdominal disease in children: a comparison of computed tomography and ultrasound. Am J Roentgenol 1980; 134: 153–8.
13. Foley WD, Stewart ET, Lawson TL, Geenan J, Loguidice J, Maher L, Unger GF. Computed tomography, ultrasonography, and endoscopic retrograde cholangiopancreatography in the diagnosis of pancreatic disease: a comparative study. Gastrointest Radiol 1980; 1(5): 29–35.

14. Gmelin E, Weiss HD, Fuchs HD, Reiser M. [A comparison of the diagnostic accuracy of ultrasound, computer tomography and ERPC in chronic pancreatitis and carcinoma of the pancreas]. Fortschr Röntgenstr Nuklearmed 1981; 134: 136–41.
15. Hessel SJ, Siegelman SS, McNeil BJ, Sanders R, Adams DF, Alderson PO, Finberg HJ, Abrams HL. A prospective evaluation of computed tomography and ultrasound of the pancreas. Radiology 1982; 143(1): 29–33.
16. Hollerbach S, Ruser J, Ochs A, Frick E, Scholmerich J. [Current status of abdominal pancreatic ultrasound. A retrospective analysis of 585 pancreatic ultrasound examinations]. Med Klin 1994; 15(89): 7–13.
17. Schlosser W, Schoenberg MH, Rhein E, Siech M, Gansauge F, Beger HG. [Pancreatic carcinoma in chronic pancreatitis with inflammatory tumor of the head of the pancreas]. Z Gastroenterol 1996; 34: 3–8.
18. Carter, DC. Cancer of the head of pancreas or chronic pancreatitis? A diagnostic dilemma. Surgery 1992; 111: 602–3.
19. Menges M, Lerch MM, Zeitz M. The double duct sign in patients with malignant and benign pancreatic lesions. Gastrointest Endosc 2000; 52: 74–7.
20. Gronen G, Dombrowski H, Adler G, Lorenz-Meyer H. [Differential diagnostic evaluation of chronic pancreatitis in relation to pancreatic cancer based on clinical, laboratory, chemical and diagnostic parameters. Studies of 174 patients in 10 years]. Z Gastroenterol 1986; 24: 416–25.
21. Wharton SM, Rahman Z, Johnson CD. Missed curable carcinoma of the pancreas presenting as chronic pancreatitis. Postgrad Med J 1997; 73: 577–9.
22. Lerch MM, Riehl J, Buechsel R, Kierdorf H, Winkeltau G, Matern S. Bedside ultrasound in the decision making for emergency surgery – its role in medical intensive care patients. Am J Emerg Med 1992; 10: 35–8.
23. Lackner K, Frommhold H, Grauthoff H, Modder U, Heuser L, Braun G, Buurman R, Scherer K. [The value of computer tomography and sonography in the investigation of the pancreas]. ROFO Fortschr Geb Rontgenstr Nuklearmed 1980; 132: 509–13.

6.2 ERCP – still needed for diagnosis of chronic pancreatitis or outmoded?

P. Bauerfeind

Abstract

ERCP (endoscopic retrograde cholangiopancreaticography) allows diagnosis of CP (chronic pancreatitis) with a sensitivity and specificity of more than 90%. ERCP findings in CP are well standardized and the method is broadly available. However, up to 10% of the patients with CP and impaired exocrine function may have a normal pancreatogram. ERCP has a complication risk of 1–10%. Alternative imaging methods, such as US (abdominal ultrasound), CT (computed tomography), EUS (endoscopic ultrasound) or MRCP (magnetic resonance cholangiopancreaticography) are slightly less sensitive but without the risk of complications. Broad experience with the new and more sensitive methods (EUS, MRCP) is lacking and they are more likely to be examiner-dependent than ERCP. Thus, ERCP remains the "gold standard" for imaging of CP. In the clinical situation ERCP has limited impact on the management of patients with CP. ERCP should be performed only with a therapeutic intention.

Introduction

Diagnosis of chronic pancreatitis is based on imaging methods, functional tests, patient history and clinical signs. No single method allows unequivocal diagnosis of chronic pancreatitis. Therefore, the combination of all methods is usually applied. Among the imaging methods, ERCP is considered as the one with the highest sensitivity and specificity. The aim of this review is to discuss the strength and the problems of ERCP and to define the role of ERCP in clinical application in patients in whom chronic pancreatitis is suspected.

Strength of ERCP

Imaging of the pancreatic duct system by ERCP shows typical changes depending on the stage of the disease. The changes were described and classified in the "Cambridge Classification" of chronic pancreatitis [1] (Table 6.2-1). This classification is widely accepted and allows comparison of ERCP results for CP among different centers. ERCP is considered to be the most sensitive imaging method, with a sensitivity and specificity of above 90 [2, 3]. Sensitivity of ERCP in most studies was determined in patients with clinically clear diagnosis of chronic pancreatitis and/or impaired exocrine function measured by function tests. The ideal gold standard for diagnosis of CP is not available yet. Histology could be used as the final arbiter in diagnosis of chronic pancreatitis. However, tissue sampling from the pancreas has a complication rate of around 1% [4] and is rarely performed. Since diagnosis of CP is most difficult in mild stages of the disease, controlled trials including different stages of CP comparing ERCP and histology would be necessary.

Table 6.2-1. Cambridge grading of chronic pancreatitis by ERCP.

Grade	Main Duct	Abnormal side branches	Additional features
Normal	Normal	None	
Equivocal	Normal	< 3	
Mild	Normal	3 or more	
Moderate	Abnormal	> 3	
Marked	Abnormal	> 3	One or more of the following signs: • Large cavity (> 10 mm) • Duct obstruction • Filling defects or calculi • Sever duct dilatation or irregularities

However these studies are lacking. Correlation of histology and ERCP findings seemed to be high in the late stages of the disease only [5]; however, this is true for all other diagnostic methods as well. Based on the high sensitivity, ERCP serves as the gold standard to determine the sensitivity of other imaging methods, such as MRCP or EUS.

Besides sensitivity and specificity, ERCP has the advantage of being easily available in most gastroenterology departments all over the world. The technique is well standardized and the images are interpretable by most gastroenterologists and radiologists. The film documents of ERCP also allow the quality of the examination to be assessed. Documentation of ERCP is one main advantage compared to abdominal ultrasound or EUS. Although ultrasound images can be documented on plain film, most examiners agree that only the dynamic examination allows conclusive diagnosis. The only way to re-evaluate an EUS examination is by video documentation, as done in most comparative studies with EUS [6].

In summary, the strength of ERCP in the diagnosis of CP is based on its wide distribution, the standardized classification and the high sensitivity. In addition, ERCP offers the possibility to perform therapeutic procedures such as dilatation and stenting of the duct.

Disadvantages of ERCP

The main disadvantage of ERCP is the risk of complications. In diagnostic ERCP (i.e. without papillotomy) the complication rate is around 1.5% and the mortality rate is 0.2% [7]. If papillotomy is performed the complication rate increases to 5–10% and the risk of mortality is around 0.5% [7–10]. However, papillotomy is rarely necessary for diagnostic ERCP, depending on the experience of the examiner. The complication rate for ERCP also depends largely on the experience of the examiner: a minimum of 150 examinations per year and per examiner are necessary to ensure best quality [11]. However, even in large centers this minimum number of examinations per year is not guaranteed. The most frequent adverse event of ERCP is acute pancreatitis. According to anecdotical reports, the risk of acute pancreatitis after ERCP seemed to be lower in patients with chronic pancreatitis. However, controlled trials to prove the observation are missing. In two recent studies, complication rates in patients with and without a history of pancreatitis were similar [8, 10]. From our clinical experience it seems that in cases of severe CP with large dilatation of the duct system the risk of acute pancreatitis induced by ERCP is low. However, in these cases diagnosis is usually possible with non-invasive methods such as abdominal ultrasound or CT scan. In cases of suspected mild CP the rate of adverse events is probably in the same range as found in all other cases of ERCP. In addition, sensitivity of ERCP seems to be lower in mild pancreatitis than in end stage CP [5]. ERCP may be normal in up to 14% of patients with mild or moderate impairment of pancreatic function. On the other hand, ERCP may show mild changes in cases without chronic pancreatitis [12]. Minor changes of the pancreatic duct were found in old patients, patients with HIV or after an episode of acute pancreatitis.

In summary, the main disadvantages of ERCP as a diagnostic tool for CP are the substantial complication risk and its decreased or unknown sensitivity in mild CP.

Comparison of ERCP and other imaging methods

The classical imaging methods for diagnosis of CP are plain abdominal film and CT scan. Both methods allow calcifications of the pancreas to be detected. Sensitivity in detecting calcifications seems slightly higher for CT scan than for plain film. The specificity of this finding is very high, since calcifications in the pancreas are considered to be proof of CP in most classifications [13]. However, calcifications are present only in 30% of patients with CP. In addition, pancreatic calcification does not indicate severity of the disease. US, CT and EUS have the advantage that they allow examination of the duct and of the parenchyma of the pancreas. The diagnostic sensitivity and specificity of US for CP are 60–70% and 80–90%, respectively [14]. CT seems to have a sensitivity of above 90%, compared to ERCP [5]; however, in mild forms of CP the sensitivity is unknown and is most likely inferior to ERCP. Recently endoscopic ultrasound (EUS) evolved as a new method of diagnosing chronic pancreatitis. Although endoscopy is necessary for this method, the risk of complications is negligible compared to ERCP. Diagnosis of chronic pancreatitis by EUS is based on a scoring system which includes structure of the tissue, duct size and form [15]. In a recent paper the interobserver reliability of the method was tested [6]. The rate of agreement among leading EUS specialists was determined as a kappa value of 0.42, which is considered as moderate, certainly not excellent. Even among these highly specialized EUS examiners the rate of CP diagnosed in the same set of patients with suspected CP ranged between 40 and 80%. The advantage of EUS being noninvasive compared to ERCP is counterbalanced by the fact that EUS is even more examiner-dependent than ERCP. In addition, as discussed above, documentation of EUS is more difficult than ERCP. However, EUS is superior to ERCP for ruling out pancreatic masses. This is most likely more important in the clinical situation than its weakness in diagnosing mild forms of CP. Another new and promising technique for diagnosis of chronic pancreatitis is MRI-based cholangiopancreaticography (MRCP). This method allows imaging of the duct system without endoscopy. The results of the first studies show a high sensitivity of 80–90% compared to ERCP [2, 16] and even to histology [2]. Filling of the duct system may be enhanced by stimulation with secretin [17]. In these studies most patients had severe CP; thus, as for most other imaging methods, comparative studies including patients with mild CP are not available yet.

In summary, modern imaging methods such as US, CT, EUS and MRCP have only a slightly lower sensitivity for detecting CP without the risk of complication. However, these methods are more examiner-dependent and broad experience is lacking.

Clinical role of ERCP in diagnosis and management of chronic CP

In the clinical situation of an individual patient the value of a diagnostic test is not determined only by its sensitivity. It is usually more important that a diagnostic result changes the treatment. In CP the consequences of a diagnostic result depend on the symptoms of the patient and the stage of the disease. In the case of clinically severe CP with exocrine insufficiency and clear signs of CP at US, plain film or CT no further diagnostic measures such as ERCP are necessary. In these cases ERCP should only be performed if stenting of the pancreatic duct or the common bile duct is considered. Another good indication for ERCP and duodenoscopy is if a tumor of the papilla is suspected. The most difficult situation occurs in the patient with suspected mild CP who presents only part of the clinical picture. For example, in patients with nonspecific dyspepsia mild pancreatitis may be suspected if all other diagnostic efforts have failed to reveal an explanation. In these patients the complication rate militates against ERCP. It was recently shown that EUS may allow diagnosis of CP in some of these patients [18]. The EUS finding of a mild CP will not substantially change the treatment, but EUS will also rule out a tumor of the pancreas which frequently is a main concern of the patient and the physician. To exclude a pancreatic tumor is also the focus in cases of steatorrhea without other signs of CP. In these cases EUS, CT and MRCP are more appropriate than ERCP. One rare indication for ERCP is in patients with recurring episodes of acute pancreatitis and suspicion of sphincter Oddi dysfunction.

In summary, ERCP is rarely indicated in CP. It should be limited to those cases in which therapeutic measures are intended.

Conclusions

ERCP is still the gold standard of the imaging methods for chronic pancreatitis. Its main advantages are high sensitivity and high negative predictive value, good standardization, wide availability and good documentation. However, ERCP entails a high risk of complications and may change the treatment only in very few patients. Thus, ERCP should only be performed if therapeutic measures such as papillotomy or stenting are planned.

References

1. Axon ATR, Classen M, Cotton PB, Cremer M, Freeny PC, Lees WR. Pancreatography in chronic pancreatitis: international definitions. Gut 1984; 25: 1107–12.
2. Adamek H, Albert J, Breer H, Weitz M, Schilling D, Riemann J. Pancreatic cancer detection with magnetic resonance cholangiopancreatography and endoscopic retrograde cholangiopancreatography: a prospective controlled study. Lancet 2000; 356(9225): 190–3.
3. Caletti G, Brocchi E, Agostini D, Balduzzi A, Bolondi L, Labo G. Sensitivity of endoscopic retrograde pancreatography in chronic pancreatitis. Br J Surg 1982; 69(9): 507–9.
4. Welch T, Sheedy PN, Johnson C, Stephens D. CT-guided biopsy: prospective analysis of 1,000 procedures. Radiology 1989; 171(2): 493–6.
5. Malfertheiner P, Büchler MW. Correlation of imaging and function in chronic pancreatitis. Radiol Clin North Am 1989; 27(1): 51–64.
6. Wallace M, Hawes R, Durkalski V, Chak A, Mallery S, Catalano M et al. The reliability of EUS for the diagnosis of chronic pancreatitis: interobserver agreement among experienced endosonographers. Gastrointest Endosc 2001; 53(3): 294–9.

7. Loperfido S, Angelini G, Benedetti G, Chilovi F, Costan F, Berardinis F et al. Major early complications from diagnostic and therapeutic ERCP: a prospective multicenter study. Gastrointest Endosc 1998; 48(1): 1–10.
8. Freeman M, Nelson D, Sherman S, Haber G, Herman M, Dorsher P et al. Complications of endoscopic biliary sphincterotomy. N Engl J Med 1996; 335(13): 909–18.
9. Masci E, Toti G, Mariani A, Curioni S, Lomazzi A, Dinelli M et al. Complications of diagnostic and therapeutic ERCP: a prospective multicenter study. Am J Gastroenterol 2001; 96(2): 417–23.
10. Mehta S, Pavone E, Barkun J, Bouchard S, Barkun A. Predictors of post-ERCP complications in patients with suspected choledocholithiasis. Endoscopy 1998; 30(5): 457–63.
11. Freeman M. Toward improving outcomes of ERCP. Gastrointest Endosc 1998; 48(1): 96–102.
12. Lankisch P, Seidensticker F, Otto J, Lubbers H, Mahlke R, Stockmann F et al. Secretin-pancreozymin test (SPT) and endoscopic retrograde cholangiopancreatography (ERCP): both are necessary for diagnosing or excluding chronic pancreatitis. Pancreas 1996; 12(2): 149–52.
13. Etemad B, Whitcomb D. Chronic pancreatitis: diagnosis, classification, and new genetic developments. Gastroenterology 2001; 120(3): 682–707.
14. Bolondi L, Li Bassi S, Gaiani S, Barbara L. Sonography of chronic pancreatitis. Radiol Clin North Am 1989; 27(4): 815–33.
15. Sahai A, Zimmermann M, Aabakken L, Tarnasky P, Cunningham J, van Velse A et al. Prospective assessment of the ability of endoscopic ultrasound to diagnose, exclude, or establish the severity of chronic pancreatitis found by endoscopic retrograde cholangiopancreatography. Gastrointest Endosc 1998; 48(1): 18–25.
16. Sica G, Braver J, Cooney M, Miller F, Chai J, Adams D. Comparison of endoscopic retrograde cholangiopancreatography with MR cholangiopancreatography in patients with pancreatitis. Radiology 1999; 210(3): 605–10.
17. Manfredi R, Costamagna G, Brizi M, Maresca G, Vecchioli A, Colagrande C et al. Severe chronic pancreatitis versus suspected pancreatic disease: dynamic MR cholangiopancreatography after secretin stimulation. Radiology 2000; 214(3): 849–55.
18. Sahai A, Mishra G, Penman I, Williams D, Wallace M, Hadzijahic N et al. EUS to detect evidence of pancreatic disease in patients with persistent or nonspecific dyspepsia. Gastrointest Endosc 2000; 52(2): 153–9.

6.3 Endosonography in chronic pancreatitis: New developments

T. M. Gress

Since its introduction in the early 1980s endoscopic ultrasonography (EUS) has revolutionized the imaging of the pancreas. It has become a standard in the detection and assessment of small pancreatic lesions and accurate in the preoperative staging of pancreatic carcinoma when compared with other techniques such as abdominal ultrasound (US), endoscopic retrograde cholangiopancreaticography (ERCP), computed tomography (CT) and nuclear magnetic resonance tomography (MRI) [15]. The major advantages of EUS over standard transabdominal US imaging being the possibility to place the US-transducer close to the pancreas. In standard EUS imaging of the pancreas the transducer located at the tip of a side viewing duodenoscope is forwarded into the third portion of the duodenum and then slowly withdrawn to allow a transduodenal and transgastric visualization of the pancreas. The close proximity to the organ of interest and the absence of intervening structures such as fat, bowel and gas allows to use high frequency transducers (5–20 Mhz) for a higher spatial resolution. In contrast to ERCP, EUS evaluates both, the parenchyma and the ducts at a low risk. Furthermore it allows to perform interventional approaches and fine-needle-aspiration cytologies only penetrating the gastric or duodenal wall, thus decreasing the risk of complications.

The standard EUS instruments for imaging the pancreas are radial scanning echoendoscopes using a mechanical transducer which is housed at the tip of a side-viewing duodenoscope and is rotated within its plastic casing by a motor located in the handle of the endoscope. Three hundred sixty degree images are generated in a plane perpendicular to the long axis of the instrument. This type of instrument is widely used for routine imaging of the pancreas and represents the standard for diagnostic imaging to date. In recent years electronic linear array echoendoscopes have been introduced which acquire 2-dimensional images by using multiple tiny transducers configured in a line or arc at the tip of the instrument. Images are formed by electronic mixing of signals from combinations of these transducers. The image plane is parallel to the long axis of the endoscope, resulting in a completely different orientation than that produced by radial scanning instruments. The major advantage of this system is the capability of imaging a needle passed through the working channel to direct fine-needle aspiration (FNA) or interventional approaches. Doppler imaging is also available only with the electronic array instruments [17]. One of the newest developments in instrumentation is endosonographic imaging with miniprobes or catheter probes that can be passed through the accessory channel of a standard endoscope. They provide excellent, high-resolution images of the bile duct and pancreatic duct because of generally higher sonographic frequencies of up to 30 Mhz [4]. The use of these probes for intraductal ultrasound (IDUS) of the pancreas is being increasingly tested in clinical studies, but its role in the routine diagnostic workup of the pancreas has not been established to date [8, 10].

Once the role of radial EUS for imaging of pancreatic tumors was established it soon became obvious that EUS would be useful in assessing chronic pancreatitis as well. Many studies have shown that both parenchymal and ductal criteria are indicative of chronic pancreatitis [5, 16, 19]. Parenchymal changes include hyperechoic foci (calcifications), hyperechoic strands (fibrosis), accentuation of lobular pattern (fibrosis), cysts, shadowing calcifications and the gland size. Ductal changes comprise dilatation of the main pancreatic duct (MPD) or side branches, irregularity of the MPD, hyperechoic duct margins and stones (Fig. 6.3-1). Calcifications and the presence of pancreatic stones are generally judged to have the highest predictive values for the diagnosis of chronic pancreatitis [5, 16, 18, 19]. However, there is consensus that the total number of criteria in a given patient is more predictive than any individual criterion [5, 16]. In general the presence of 3 or more criteria is sufficient to allow the diagnosis of chronic pancreatitis e.g. at 80% sensitivity, 86% specificity, 84% accuracy and high interobserver agreement (92%), always relative to data obtained by ERCP, secretin test (ST), pure pancreatic juice analysis (PPJ) and clinical data [5, 16, 19].

In recent years a number of clinical studies have focused on the evaluation of the role of EUS in diagnosing severity and early forms of chronic pancreatitis. Sahai and col-

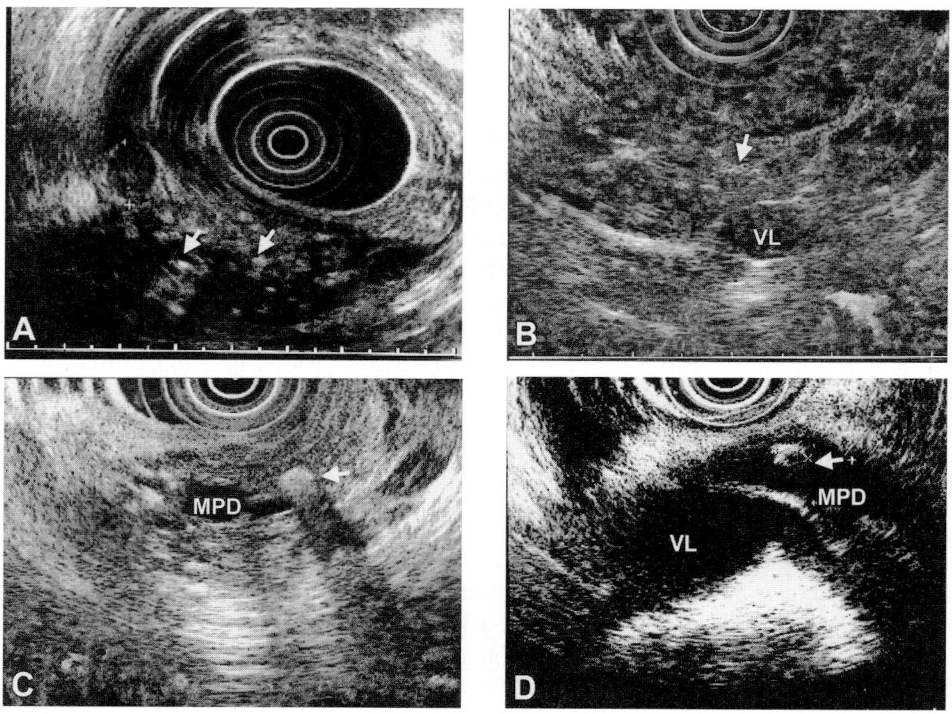

Figure 6.3-1A–D. EUS images of various regions of the pancreas showing signs of chronic pancreatitis obtained with an Olympus GF-UM20 radial scanning echoendoscope. All images were obtained from patients with alcoholic chronic pancreatitis. **A:** Hyperechoic foci in the head of the pancreas (arrow). **B:** Hyperechoic septa (arrow) and an accentuated lobular pattern in the region of the pancreatic head/body. **C:** Dilatation and caliber irregularity of the main pancreatic duct and a shadowing calcification in the parenchyma (arrow). **D:** Dilated main pancreatic duct with an intraductal stone (arrow).
VL = vena lienalis, MPD = main pancreatic duct

leagues (1998) studied the correlation of EUS criteria to the severity of chronic pancreatitis found by ERCP and classified according to the Cambridge classification [1]. In this study the presence of more than 6 EUS criteria allowed to diagnose moderate and/or severe (Cambridge III and/or IV) chronic pancreatitis with a positive predictive value (PPV) larger than 85%. The presence of less than 3 criteria excludes Cambridge III/IV chronic pancreatitis with a negative predictive value (NPV) of more than 85%. However, EUS could not reliably exclude less severe disease and the NPV never reached values of more than 50%. Similar results were obtained by Catalano and colleagues who compared the agreement between EUS criteria and ERCP and/or secretin test (ST) [5]. Severity of chronic pancreatitis was empirically classified as mild (1–2 criteria), moderate (3–5 criteria) and severe (> 5 criteria) based on the total number of criteria present in a given patient. There was good agreement between the presence of abnormal ERCP findings (Cambridge II–IV) and moderate (92%) and severe (100%) chronic pancreatitis by EUS, as well as between the absence of ERCP findings and the absence of EUS criteria (100%). Similar results were obtained for the secretin test, which showed 100% agreement between normal pancreas by EUS and normal ST test as well as between severe chronic pancreatitis by EUS and abnormal ST test. Only 50% agreement was found between moderate chronic pancreatitis by EUS and abnormal ST test values. In contrast, mild chronic pancreatitis in the presence of 1–2 EUS criteria showed only poor agreement with abnormal findings by ERCP (17%) and ST test (13%). Furthermore, there was only a poor agreement between the severity of chronic pancreatitis judged by EUS and ERCP. Similar results have been obtained in two recent studies which have only been published in abstract form [7, 21]. Both studies show that in general EUS is useful in diagnosing advanced, but not early or mild chronic pancreatitis. The significance of mild changes noted by EUS, e.g. the presence of 1–2 criteria, is not known to date. These mild EUS changes could be diagnostic of early forms of chronic pancreatitis that cannot be assessed by the conventional diagnostic tools, e.g. ERCP, CT, ST or PPJ. Long-term follow-up of patients with the diagnosis of mild chronic pancreatitis by EUS will be required to determine the validity of EUS in diagnosing early changes of chronic pancreatitis.

A number of new developments have been made possible by the introduction of linear array electronic echoendoscopes with the possibility of performing fine-needle aspiration (FNA) cytology and interventional approaches. EUS FNA cytology of a pancreatic mass or cyst is an elegant approach allowing performance of a biopsy only penetrating the duodenal or gastric wall, thus reducing the potential risk of complications such as perforation, bleeding and tumor spreading (Fig. 6.3-2). To date no large prospective studies are available evaluating the aspect of tumor spreading after EUS FNA as compared to standard US- or CT-guided transabdominal FNA. In recent studies EUS FNA was shown to have a sensitivity of 65–90%, a specificity of 85–100%, a PPV of 99–100% and a NPV of 3% in the diagnosis of pancreatic tumors [2].

In the same way it has been shown that EUS-guided transgastric or transduodenal drainage of pancreatic pseudocysts, in particular those not bulging the GI wall and thus not accessible to standard endoscopic drainage, is safe and feasible and reduces the risk of complications by visualizing intervening structures, e.g. gastric varices or bowel [9, 13]. These studies indicate that EUS-guided drainage should be preferred when endoscopic therapy is considered for patients with large pseudocysts.

EUS-guided celiac plexus neurolysis using alcohol has been reported as a safe and effective palliative technique for improving pain control in patients with pancreatic cancer

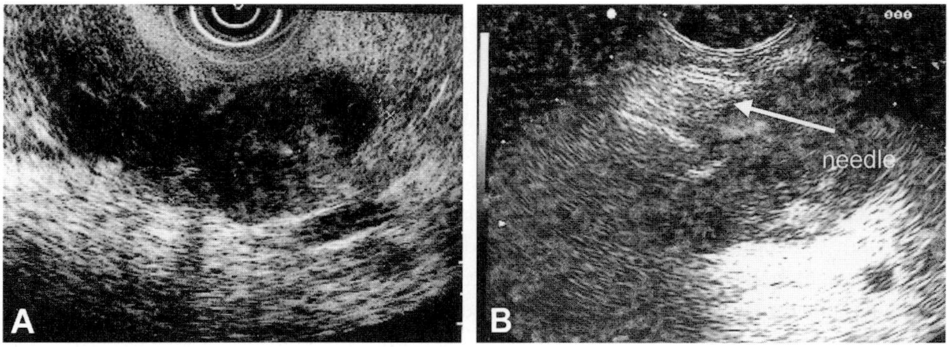

Figure 6.3-2A, B. EUS image of a large tumor in the head of the pancreas visualized first with a radial (**A**) and then with a linear array echoendoscope (**B**) to perform fine-needle-aspiration cytology. The image shown in B was obtained with a Pentax-Hitachi FG 32-UA linear array echoendoscope. The arrow indicates the position of the needle.

which could even be performed on an outpatient basis due to the presence of only minor complications [20]. The same technique using bupivacaine in combination with triamcinolone was recently applied by Gress and coworkers in a randomized trial comparing CT-guided and EUS-guided celiac neurolysis in patients with chronic pancreatitis pain [12]. 50% of the patients in the EUS group as compared to 25% of the CT group reported transient pain relief. Furthermore, pain relief was more pronounced and persistent in the EUS group, which was speculated to be due to the possibility to more accurately locate the celiac trunk and to insert the needle closer to the celiac trunk. However, the pain relief was not persistent (only 30% after 24 weeks) and the method has the risk of infectious complications. The same authors reported the occurrence of a peripancreatic abscess 5 days post EUS-guided celiac plexus block [11]. Thus, though these results are promising, further improvements are necessary to allow this technique to play a significant role in the management of these patients.

A further new development is the use of EUS imaging with secretin stimulation for evaluating the obstructive pathology of chronic pancreatitis [6]. Marked (> 1 mm diameter increase) and sustained (> 15 min) dilatation of the main pancreatic duct after secretin stimulation (1 IU/kg) correlated well with the obstructive pathology and the response to endoscopic therapy, e.g. in patients with pancreas divisum. In the same way as for transabdominal US, contrast agents are being tested for use with EUS. Hirooka and coworkers, for example, reported the use of air-filled albumin microspheres (Albunex®) for the differential diagnosis of tumors and cysts in the pancreas. They showed that pancreatic pseudocysts and ductal cell carcinoma did not enhance, whereas mucin-producing neoplasms showed enhancement with this contrast agent during EUS [14]. The use of Levovist®, another ultrasound contrast agent, may help in EUS assessment of the celiac artery and superior mesenteric artery [2]. The use of catheter probes or miniprobes for intraductal ultrasound (IDUS) of the pancreas may have some advantages in diagnosis of small pancreatic tumors and in the differential diagnosis of localized stenosis of the MPD [8, 10]. However, the experience with IDUS reported to date is limited, it has not been systematically compared to other imaging modalities such as ERCP, MRCP or spiral CT, and a number of technical aspects have to be addressed prior to allowing widespread use and application of this technique [4]. IDUS probes are fragile and expensive and thus are of limited durability, in particular when used with side-viewing duodenoscopes to cannulate the MPD, e.g. with the help of an elevator. It may be necessary to perform papillotomy in some patients for intubation of the MPD and it is not always possible to advance the probe all the way to the tail of the pancreas, in particular in the absence of MPD dilatation. Furthermore, in contrast to standard radial EUS, the technique has the risk of complications such as acute pancreatitis, which has been reported to be 0.4% in preliminary studies [8].

To summarize, EUS should be added to the standard diagnostic armamentarium available to diagnose chronic pancreatitis as it has been proven to be accurate and safe for this application. PPV and NPV of the method depend on the number of EUS criteria in a given patient rather than on the presence of any individual criterion. Under these conditions high interobserver agreement in the diagnosis of chronic pancreatitis is achieved in the hands of experienced investigators. Although EUS can reliably diagnose or exclude moderate to severe chronic pancreatitis it is less reliable for the diagnosis of mild chronic pancreatitis. No consensus has been reached on whether mild changes identified by EUS are indicative of early changes in chronic pancreatitis. This should be one of the major topics of future studies and should include the long-term follow-up of patients with mild EUS changes. The introduction of linear array electronic EUS has allowed the development of interventional approaches. EUS-FNA and EUS-guided transgastric/transduodenal drainage of pancreatic pseudocysts have the potential to become standard techniques, in the same way as secretin-stimulated EUS. Newer developments such as EUS-guided celiac plexus neurolysis, intraductal ultrasound and contrast-enhanced EUS are still experimental and await evaluation in large clinical trials.

Acknowledgements

I would like to thank Dr. A. Römpp, Dr. M. P. Lutz and Dr. M. Reinshagen for their assistance in collecting suitable EUS images of patients with chronic pancreatitis.

References

1. Axon ATR, Classen M, Cotton PB, Cremer M, Freeny PC, Lees WR. Pancreatography in chronic pancreatitis: international definitions. Gut 1984; 25: 1107–12.
2. Bhutani MS, Hoffman BJ, Van Velse A et al. Contrast-enhanced endoscopic ultrasonography with galactose microparticles: SHU508A (Levovist). Endoscopy 1997; 29: 635–9.
3. Bhutani MS. Interventional endoscopic ultrasonography: state of the art at the new millenium. Endoscopy 2000; 32: 62–71.
4. Canto MIF. Endosonographic imaging with catheter probes. Techn Gastrointest Endosc 2000; 2: 110–20.
5. Catalano MF, Lahoti S, Geenen JE, Hogan WJ. Prospective evaluation of endoscopic ultrasonography, endoscopic retrograde pancreatography, and secretin test in the diagnosis of chronic pancreatitis. Gastrointest Endosc 1998; 48: 11–7.
6. Catalano MF, Lahoti S, Alcocer E, Geenen JE, Hogan W. Dynamic imaging of the pancreas using real-time endoscopic ultrasonography with secretin stimulation. Gastrointest Endosc 1998; 48: 580–7.
7. Catalano MF, Sial SH, Maher WE, Greenen JE, Hogan WJ. Prospective evaluation of endoscopic ultrasonography and endoscopic retrograde cholangiopancreatography in the diagnosis of chronic pancreatitis in an adolescent population. Gastrointest Endosc 2000; 51 (Part 2): AB133.

8. Furukawa T, Oohashi K, Yamao K et al. Intraductal ultrasonography of the pancreas: development and clinical potential. Endoscopy 1997; 29: 561–9.
9. Giovanni M, Bernardi D, Seitz JF. Cystogastrostomy entirely performed under endosonography guidance for pancreatic pseudocyst: results in 6 patients. Gastrointest Endosc 1998; 48: 200–3.
10. Gress F, Chen YK, Sherman S et al. Experience with catheter-based ultrasound probe in the bile duct and pancreas. Endoscopy 1995; 27: 178–84.
11. Gress F, Ciaccia D, Kiel J et al. Endoscopic ultrasound (EUS) guided celiac plexus block (CB) for management of pain due to chronic pancreatitis (CP): A large single center experience. Gastrointest Endosc 1997; 45: 594A.
12. Gress F, Schmitt C, Sherman S, Ikenberry S, Lehman G. A prospective randomized comparison of endoscopic ultrasound- and computed tomography-guided celiac plexus block for managing chronic pancreatitis pain. Am J Gastroenterol 1999; 94: 900–5.
13. Grimm HA, Doniec MJ, Kuemmel K, Henne-Bruns DH. Prospective evaluation of endosonography (EUS) in therapeutic approach to pancreatic pseudocysts (PPC). Endoscopy 2000; 32: A39.
14. HirookaY, Goto H, Ito A et al. Contrast-enhanced endoscopic ultrasonography in pancreatic diseases: A preliminary study. Am J Gastroenterol 1998; 93: 632–5.
15. Kassem AM, Rösch T. Endosonographic imaging in pancreatic disease. Techn Gastrointest Endosc 2000; 2: 94–100.
16. Sahai A, Zimmermann M, Aabakken L et al. Prospective evaluation of the ability of endoscopic ultrasound to diagnose, exclude, or establish the severity of chronic pancreatitis found by endoscopic retrograde cholangiopancreatography. Gastrointest Endosc 1998; 48: 18–25.
17. Shaw S, Kimmey MB. General principles of endoscopic ultrasonographic imaging. Techn. Gastrointest Endosc 2000; 2: 50–5.
18. Wallace MB, Hawes RH, Durkaski VL et al. Towards consensus in the EUS diagnosis of chronic pancreatitis. Interobserver agreement among expert endosonographers. Gastrointest Endosc 2000; 51 (Part 2): AB173.
19. Wiersema MJ, Hawes RH, Lehman GA, Kochman ML, Sherman S, Kopecky KK. Prospective evaluation of endoscopic ultrasonography and endoscopic retrograde cholangiopancreatography in patients with chronic abdominal pain of suspected pancreatic origin. Endoscopy 1993; 25: 555–64.
20. Wiersema MJ, Wiersema LM. Endosonography-guided celiac plexus neurolysis. Gastrointest Endosc 1996; 44: 656–62.
21. Zuccaro G, Conwell DL, Vargo JJ et al.The role of endoscopic ultrasound (EUS) in the diagnosis of early and advanced chronic pancreatitis (CP). Gastroenterol 2000; 118: A674.

6.4 Role of EUS in the diagnosis of chronic pancreatitis: Mayo Clinic experience

J. Clain

Human endoscopic ultrasound (EUS) using a prototype instrument consisting of an endoscope with an ultrasound probe incorporated into its distal tip was first performed at the Mayo Clinic more than two decades ago. Initial studies were reported in dogs [1], and subsequently in humans [2]. Human EUS was recognized to be feasible when we reported our results in 22 human subjects. In one of these subjects, gross changes of pancreatitis were noted in a patient with a pancreatic pseudocyst, and although subtle changes of chronic pancreatitis were not appreciated, this appears to be the first description of chronic pancreatitis visualized with an echoendoscope.

The subsequent development of EUS and the ability of the instrument to visualize the entire pancreas both from the duodenum (including the uncinate, head, periampullary area) and from the stomach (body and tail) led to the concept that this was a technique which could potentially be used for the diagnosis of chronic pancreatitis. The proximity of the high frequency ultrasound probe to the pancreas from both the duodenum and the stomach and the absence of intervening air permits high spatial resolution, and thus detailed views of pancreatic parenchymal and ductal structure not possible with transabdominal ultrasound or computed tomography. Combining information available from transabdominal imaging and endoscopic retrograde pancreatography (ERP), criteria were developed describing abnormalities in both parenchyma and duct anatomy, which were felt to be characteristic of chronic pancreatitis (see Table 6.4-1) [3].

In this initial description, 20 normal volunteers and 69 patients suspected to have chronic pancreatitis (CP) were assessed for these features using either the Olympus EUM 20 or EUM 30 instrument, which incorporates a mechanical transducer in the endoscope tip. (It is important to emphasize that all reported studies assessing EUS for the diagnosis of CP have used a mechanical transducer. The pancreas, as viewed with the currently available electronic array instruments, does not yield the same information with regard to the subtle parenchymal changes because the electronic probe produces a "smoothing out" of the image.)

In this report [3], all patients (but not controls) were submitted to ERP, and some patients had analysis of pure pancreatic juice. This is one of the few studies that have as-

Table 6.4-1. Endoscopic ultrasound: ductular and parenchymal features of chronic pancreatitis.

Ductular	Parenchymal
Narrowing	Gland size
Dilatation	Areas of reduced echogenicity
Irregular contour	Echogenic foci
Increased wall echogenicity	Cysts
Calculi	Accentuation of the lobular pattern
Side branch dilatation	

sessed endoscopic ultrasound interpretation in an objective manner. Interobserver error was assessed and correlation was good. A receiver operating characteristic curve was constructed for sensitivity versus specificity. When three of the criteria described in Table 6.4-1 were present, it provided the best compromise of sensitivity and specificity for the diagnosis of chronic pancreatitis. The correlation with ERP was assessed, and EUS was shown to be a sensitive test for the diagnosis of chronic pancreatitis using the "gold standard" provided, but was only 79% specific, i.e., abnormalities seen at EUS were not borne out by ERP. This difference in findings cannot be adequately resolved since a "gold standard" diagnosis is not available. Thus, it is possible that EUS may be a good test for early chronic pancreatitis even before the changes are apparent at ERP, or it may be that parenchymal abnormalities interpreted as chronic pancreatitis may in fact be a normal variant. Unfortunately, histology is not obtainable in subjects with early pancreatitis, and long-term follow-up to determine whether these patients ultimately develop progressive changes of chronic pancreatitis is not available.

For this reason, it appears that for lack of a reliable gold standard in the diagnosis of early chronic pancreatitis, the task of examining the value of the EUS is fraught with difficulty. Two recent studies published in 1998 attest to these difficulties. In one study [4], 126 patients with abdominal pain suspected to have pancreatitis were evaluated with EUS and ERP. In a second study [5], 80 consecutive patients with recurrent acute pancreatitis underwent ERP and a secretin test as well as endoscopic ultrasound. In both studies, the results were predictable. Thus, the diagnosis of chronic pancreatitis correlated well when disease was moderate or severe on the one hand or absent on the other. However, EUS was often abnormal when the gold standard test (ERP or function test or both) was negative. In both studies, a major shortcoming was the lack of follow-up, so that abnormal EUS examination in patients with normal ERP or function tests could not definitively be attributed to a false-positive EUS or a false-negative ERP/function test. Since there is no reliable gold standard for the diagnosis of chronic pancreatitis on the horizon, long-term follow-up is the only way to resolve the issue.

Mayo Clinic experience

We have used EUS and pancreatic function testing to address the question of whether EUS can detect early or severe pancreatitis [6]. Firstly, we devised a simple "through-the-endoscope" direct pancreatic function test. Secretin, 1 clinical unit/kilogram, was administered intravenously. With the endoscope in the postbulbar duodenum, a catheter was placed through the biopsy channel and positioned near the papilla, and 25 cc of duodenal juice was collected under ice over a period of 10 minutes. Lipolytic activity concentration was subsequently measured.

A validation test was performed for the through-the-endoscope secretin test in 10 patients, who were also submitted to a standard pancreatic function test employing duodenal intubation. The correlation between our standard pancreatic function test and the through-the-scope secretin test is demonstrated in Figure 6.4-1.

Ninety-two patients were prospectively evaluated with EUS and "through-the-scope" pancreatic function testing.

(a) Control group of 43 patients (26 females) with a mean age of 57 years (32–84 years). Criteria for a normal pancreas included findings at surgery, a normal CCK test, a normal CT, and uneventful clinical follow-up (not all patients underwent all tests).

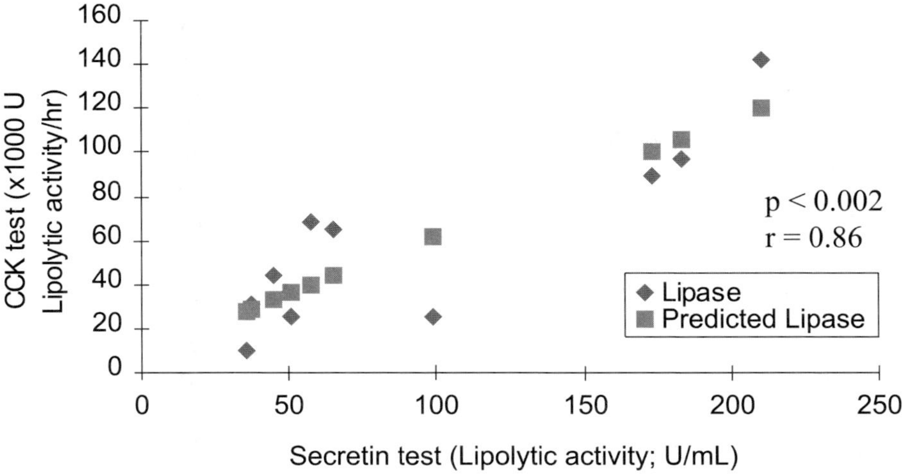

Figure 6.4-1. Comparison of EUS with pancreatic function in chronic pancreatitis. Validation: Comparison between CCK and secretin tests.

(b) Forty-one patients with definite chronic pancreatitis (23 females) with a mean age of 55 (31–75 years) were examined. Criteria for diagnosis included histology (n = 17), abnormal CCK test (n = 7), calcification (n = 8), and an abnormal CT and/or ERCP (n = 29).

(c) Eight patients with "early" chronic pancreatitis were identified (2 females) with a mean age of 52 years (39–62 years). Criteria for diagnosis were normal imaging studies exclusive of EUS, a pain syndrome consistent with pain of pancreatic origin (n = 6), or recurrent episodes of pancreatitis (n = 2).

The results showed that the through-the-endoscope test of lipolytic activity in the duodenum segregated control patients from those with early chronic pancreatitis and pa-

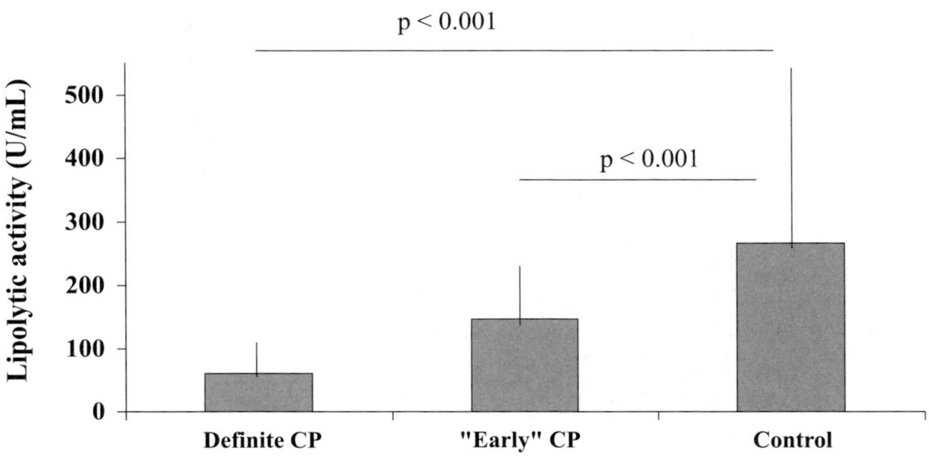

Figure 6.4-2. Comparison of secretin test results among normal and chronic pancreatitis groups.

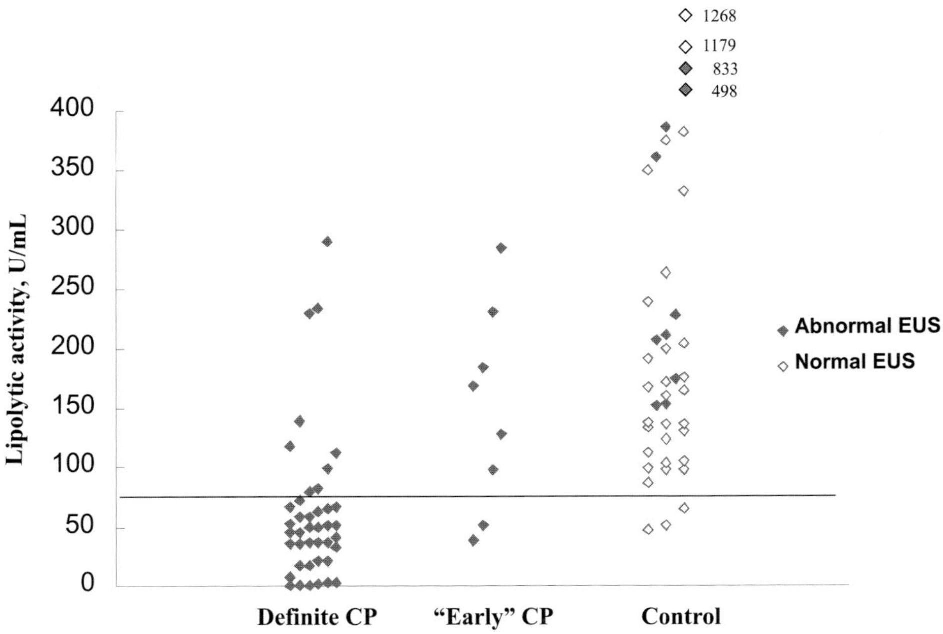

Figure 6.4-3. Comparison between EUS and secretin test in chronic pancreatitis.

tients with definite chronic pancreatitis. Although these differences were significant, there was considerable overlap (Figure 6.4-2).

When EUS was performed, the diagnosis of chronic pancreatitis was made when one or more features described in Table 6.4-1 were identified. Using these criteria, all patients with definite chronic pancreatitis and early chronic pancreatitis had abnormal EUS findings. However, in the control subjects, 23% of patients who were felt to have a normal pancreas had an abnormal EUS, confirming the lack of specificity of this examination. These results are shown in Figure 6.4-3.

We concluded that there is a role for EUS in the diagnosis of chronic pancreatitis, provided the following points are taken into account:

1. A normal EUS rules out the diagnosis of chronic pancreatitis with a high negative predictive value.
2. The diagnosis of chronic pancreatitis by EUS without other imaging or functional criteria had a 23% false-positive rate in our experience.
3. An abnormal EUS alone cannot be relied upon for the diagnosis of early chronic pancreatitis.
4. Additional functional and structural tests (possibly the newly devised through-the-endoscope secretin test could be refined and incorporated) are required in order to make a diagnosis.

Age-related changes in normal subjects

As described above, from our experience and that of others, it is apparent that while EUS may be the most sensitive test of early chronic pancreatitis, false-positive results fre-

Table 6.4-2. Age-related changes in normal subjects (Rajan E, Clain JE, Norton ID, Wiersema MJ. Preliminary data, 2000).

	Greater than 60 yrs.	40–60 yrs.	Less than 40 yrs.
1 abnormality	7/29	1/18	No data
Greater than 1 abnormality	3/29	0/18	No data

quently occur. In part, the abnormalities, which simulate those of chronic pancreatitis, appear to be age-related.

To date, there has been no rigorous appraisal of this phenomenon reported. At present, we are conducting a study in control subjects to document abnormal parenchymal and ductular features described in Table 6.4-1 in three age groups as shown.

Preliminary data (which at this point has not been blindly reviewed) is shown in Table 6.4-2.

Computer-assisted interpretation of EUS images; differentiation of inflammatory mass from pancreatic cancer

Differentiation of focal pancreatitis from pancreatic cancer may be difficult, and no current imaging modality is wholly satisfactory for this purpose. Needle biopsy of the mass can be performed, but a negative result is not reassuring that malignancy is absent. At most institutions, 3–6% of pancreaticoduodenectomies performed for presumed cancer yield benign disease. EUS is the most sensitive test for the identification of small pancreatic masses, but the echosonographic features of the mass cannot definitively differentiate pancreatitis from cancer.

EUS is a subjective technique, and interpretation of subtle differences is difficult. We thus employed a self-teaching “neuronet” or “artificial intelligence” program. These programs have previously been developed to interpret electrocardiograms and more recently applied to the interpretation of benign from malignant breast lesions [7].

We set out to investigate the potential role of a "neuronet" in differentiating inflammatory from neoplastic pancreatic masses. Patients identified from the Pancreas Clinic database were selected provided they had undergone an EUS and a surgically obtained histologic diagnosis was available.

EUS images from archived film were scanned from 14 patients with focal pancreatitis and 21 patients with pancreatic cancer. The computer analyzed the data by examining the rows of pixels and expressed gray scale pattern by mathematical formulation. The computer then determined the gray scale characteristics that discriminated malignancy from pancreatitis.

When the computer sensitivity was set at 100% for the diagnosis of cancer, the sensitivity of blinded interpretation and interpretation during the EUS examination (with all clinical data available) was 73% and 89% respectively. Diagnostic accuracy was 80%, 83%, and 85% from computer (when set to optimal sensitivity and specificity), blinded interpretation and interpretation at EUS examination respectively. We thus have demonstrated that this technology, if further refined, may play a role in the interpretation of EUS images when focal pancreatitis versus pancreatic neoplasm is an issue, and this may be a further situation where EUS may be useful in the realm of the diagnosis of chronic pancreatitis [8].

Utility of EUS in the endoscopic drainage of pancreatic pseudocysts

Endoscopic drainage of pancreatic pseudocysts has gained wide acceptance. There is little information available addressing the role of EUS for selecting appropriate candidates and detecting the optimal drainage site.

We performed EUS in 16 patients with 17 pseudocysts and in 1 patient with organizing pancreatic necrosis [9]. There were 11 males, median age 45 years (34–75 years). The cause of the pseudocysts was chronic pancreatitis in 9 and acute pancreatitis in 8. Pain was the presenting symptom in all patients. The median pseudocyst size was 8 cm (5–12 cm).

Three of 17 patients did not have endoscopic drainage performed based upon the EUS findings. One patient had extensive gastric collaterals, a second patient lacked apposition between the gastric wall and the pseudocyst, and a third patient had a spontaneous reduction in the size of the pseudocyst that was recognized at EUS.

Drainage was successful in 13 of 14 patients. In one patient the cyst could not be punctured. In all cases the optimal puncture site, as assessed by EUS, was marked with a biopsy forceps. A puncture site was later obtained by using a needle knife, introduction of a wire into the cyst, balloon dilatation, and subsequently multiple stents were placed through the fistula so formed. In two patients the entire procedure was performed using a therapeutic echoendoscope. Pseudocysts resolved in 13 of 14 patients. In one patient surgery was required for a septic complication, probably due to inadequate drainage of the pseudocyst during our initial learning experience.

We concluded that EUS altered management in a significant proportion of patients and that EUS was felt to be useful for selecting an optimal and safe drainage site.

Summary

1. We consider that EUS is a useful tool in conjunction with other diagnostic modalities for the diagnosis of chronic pancreatitis. Problems related to the specificity of subtle changes of chronic pancreatitis versus normal changes of aging remain a problem area.
2. Computer-assisted interpretation of EUS images for the differentiation of patients with pancreatic neoplasms versus focal pancreatitis shows promise.
3. EUS is a useful technique in selecting appropriate patients for endoscopic drainage and for localizing the optimal site of drainage.

References

1. DiMagno EP, Buxton JL, Regan PT et al. The ultrasonic endoscope. Lancet 1980; i: 629–31.
2. DiMagno EP, Regan PT, Clain JE et al. Human endoscopic ultrasonography. Gastroenterology 1982; 83: 824–9.
3. Wiersema MJ, Hawes RH, Lehman GA et al. Prospective evaluation of endoscopic ultrasonography and endoscopic retrograde cholangiopancreatography in patients with chronic abdominal pain of suspected pancreatic origin. Endoscopy 1993; 25: 555–64.
4. Sahai AV, Zimmermann M, Aabakken L et al. A prospective assessment of the ability of endoscopic ultrasound to diagnose, exclude, or establish the severity of chronic pancreatitis found by endoscopic retrograde pancreatography. Gastrointest Endosc 1998; 48: 18–25.
5. Catalano MF, Lahoti S, Geenen JE, Hogan WJ. Prospective evaluation of endoscopic ultrasonography, endoscopic retrograde pancreatography and secretin test in the diagnosis of chronic pancreatitis. Gastrointest Endosc 1998; 48: 11–7.

6. Raimondo M, Clain JE, Wang KK, DiMagno EP. Can EUS detect early or severe chronic pancreatitis (CP)? Comparison of endoscopic ultrasonography with pancreatic function. Gastroenterology 1998; 114: A492.
7. Zheng Y, Greenleaf JF, Gisvold JJ. Reduction of breast biopsies with a modified self-organizing map. IEEE Trans Neural Net 1997; 8: 1386–96.
8. Norton ID, Zheng Y, Wiersema MJ et al. Computer analysis of endoscopic ultrasound images to differentiate between pancreatic malignancy and pancreatitis. Accepted for publication in Gastrointest Endosc 2001.
9. Norton ID, Clain JE, DiMagno EP et al. Endoscopic management of pancreatic pseudocyst by EUS localization of puncture site and balloon dilatation of fistulae. Gastrointest Endosc 1998; 47: AB139.

6.5 Computed tomography and magnetic resonance pancreatography in chronic pancreatitis

P. C. Freeny

Endoscopic retrograde cholangiopancreatography (ERCP) has long been considered to be the "gold standard" for the imaging diagnosis of chronic pancreatitis [4]. More recently, however, computed tomography (CT) and magnetic resonance cholangiopancreatography (MRCP) have been shown to be highly accurate methods for depiction of the major imaging findings of chronic pancreatitis, namely main pancreatic duct dilatation, stenosis, or irregularity, pancreatic duct calculi, parenchymal atrophy, bile duct stenosis or obstruction, and pseudocysts [2–5, 9, 12, 13]. While routine axial MR imaging can depict many of these changes, it has received little attention in the literature [11]. This is most likely owing to the fact that calculi are not readily demonstrated by MR, the examination is more costly and complex than CT, in the absence of any contraindication to intravenous contrast administration, MR does not appear to offer any significant advantage over CT. However, MRCP now can be considered to be highly competitive with ERCP for depiction of main pancreatic duct changes.

Imaging diagnosis of chronic pancreatitis

The most widely used classification of the imaging findings of chronic pancreatitis was developed at the Cambridge meeting in 1983 [1, 10]. The Cambridge classification (Table 6.5-1) categorizes the imaging findings (ERCP, CT) of chronic pancreatitis into mild, moderate and severe changes.

Computed tomography

The CT findings of chronic pancreatitis consist of a broad spectrum of changes which include alterations in size and shape of the gland, changes in parenchymal attenuation, pancreatic duct calculi and dilatation, bile duct dilatation, fluid collections, and gastrointestinal tract or vascular involvement (portal venous obstruction, arterial pseudoaneurysms). Luetmer and co-workers reported a false-negative rate of only 7% (4 of 56 patients) in CT detection of the imaging findings of chronic pancreatitis [5]. However, the spectrum of the clinical and/or functional severity of the disease in their patients was not reported. This is important because, in mild chronic pancreatitis, the CT findings often are normal.

The advantages of CT include wide availability, short examination time (< 2 min), and minimal invasiveness (radiation and injection of intravenous contrast comprise its minimally invasive techniques). It has a high sensitivity for detection of ductal calculi and accurately depicts the pancreatic vasculature, pancreatic parenchyma, and peripancreatic structures, easily detecting complications, involvement, or abnormalities in these areas (Fig. 6.5-1A).

The disadvantages of CT include inability to diagnose pancreatic duct-fluid collection/pseudocyst communication, which may influence the type of treatment, and fre-

Table 6.5-1. Cambridge Classification of pancreatic morphology in chronic pancreatitis.

Changes	ERCP	CT and US
Normal	• No abnormal LSB	• Normal gland size, shape • Homogeneous parenchyma
Equivocal	• MPD normal	• ONE of the following: – < 3 abnormal LSB – MPD 2–4 mm – gland enlarged < 2 × normal Heterogeneous parenchyma
Mild	• MPD normal	• Two or more signs for diagnosis: – > 3 abnormal LSB – MPD 2–4 mm – Slight gland enlargement – Heterogeneous parenchyma
Moderate	• MPD changes • LSB changes	• Small cysts < 10 mm • MPD irregularity • Focal acute pancreatitis • Increased echogenicity of MPD walls • Gland contour irregularity
Severe Any of the above changes plus one or more of the following: Cyst > 10 mm • Intraductal filling defects • Calculi • MPD obstruction, stricture • Severe MPD irregularity • Contiguous organ invasion		

MPD = main pancreatic duct; LSB = lateral side branch ducts
Focal change: less than one-third of gland involved

quent lack of depiction of subtle pancreatic duct irregularity, stenosis, or lateral side branch abnormalities (Fig. 6.5-1B).

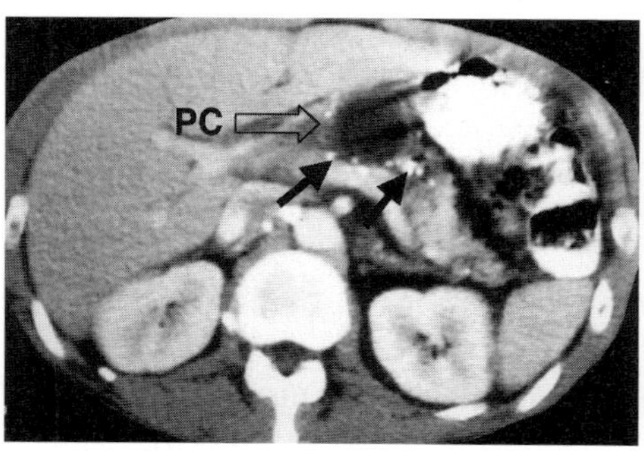

Figure 6.5-1A. Helical CT of patient with chronic pancreatitis shows small ductal calcifications (arrows) within a dilated pancreatic duct and a pseudocyst (open arrow).

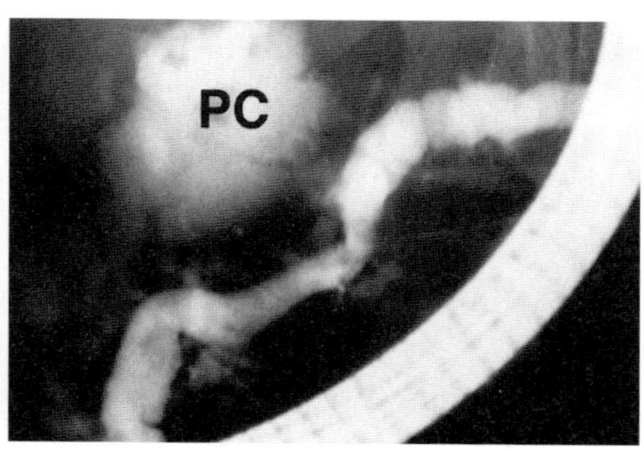

Figure 6.5-1B. ERCP confirms pancreatic duct dilatation and demonstrated communication between the pseudocyst (PC) and the main duct.

MR cholangiopancreatography (MRCP)

MRCP with 3-D rendering of main pancreatic duct anatomy has been used successfully in patients with chronic pancreatitis. In one series of patients with chronic pancreatitis, MRCP and ERCP agreed in 83–92% of cases of pancreatic duct dilatation, 70–92% of cases of ductal narrowing, and 92–100% of cases of intraductal filling defects [14]. More recently, Manfredi and co-workers have used secretin stimulation of the pancreas during MRCP and have shown a significant improvement in detection of pancreatic duct stenosis, intraductal filling defects (calculi), and visualization of the lateral side branches, the latter of which is critical for detection of Cambridge mild to moderate disease [9].

The advantages of MRCP include a short examination time (< 10 min) and lack of invasive techniques. It can accurately display the anatomy of the pancreatic and common bile duct without contrast medium administration (Fig. 6.5-2A). The disadvantages include the lack of widespread availability of MR scanners and difficulty in obtaining high detail images except on current generation state-of-the-art scanners. Similar to CT, MR accurately depicts pancreatic fluid collections/pseudocysts, but cannot establish if there is communication with the pancreatic duct (Fig. 6.5-2B).

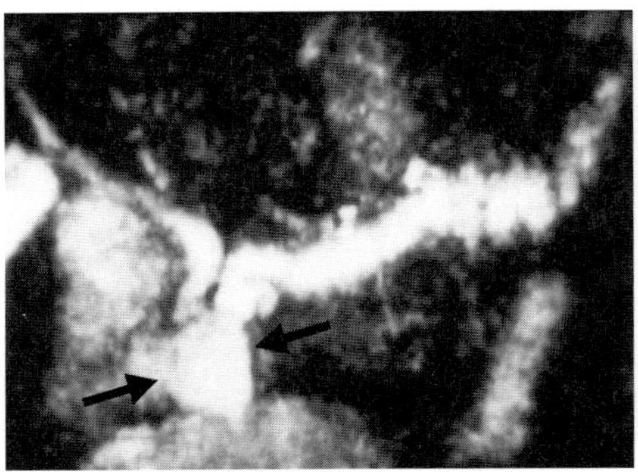

Figure 6.5-2A. MRCP of patient with chronic pancreatitis shows dilatation of the main pancreatic duct and lateral sidebranches. A small pseudocyst (arrows) is seen to communicate with the main duct. The common bile duct is mildly dilated.

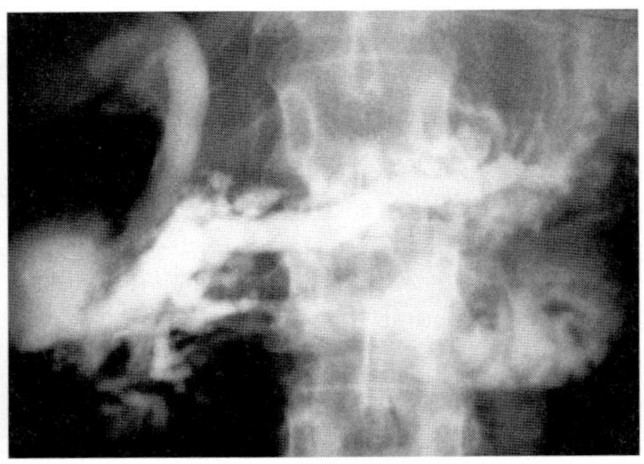

Figure 6.5-2B. ERCP confirms main pancreatic duct and lateral side branch changes of chronic pancreatitis. However, the small pseudocyst in the head of the pancreas shown on the MRCP does not fill during opacification of the main duct. The common bile duct is mildly dilated.

Correlation of imaging and clinical severity of chronic pancreatitis

In a recent study, we have compared the severity of the imaging findings depicted by ERCP and CT (Cambridge classification) with the clinical severity of the disease (pancreatic exocrine and endocrine function, severity of pain syndrome, associated biliary duct obstruction) in 100 patients with chronic pancreatitis (unpublished data). In our series, CT and ERCP up-staged 71% of patients with mild disease and 91% of patients with moderate disease, while it down-staged 14% of patients with mild and 5% of patients with severe disease. There was positive correlation between imaging and clinical severity of the disease in only 10% of patients with mild to moderate disease, but in 95% in patients with severe disease.

Published reports comparing imaging and function can be summarized by saying that in mild or early chronic pancreatitis, the most accurate diagnosis and assessment of the patient is achieved by the use of both function tests and imaging modalities, primarily CT and ERCP [6–8]. In more severe disease, imaging is most efficacious when used to detect complications of chronic pancreatitis or to define main pancreatic ductal anatomy. Imaging also may be used to select the most appropriate therapy for the patient and particularly to identify patients who may benefit from surgery.

Conclusions

MRCP should be considered as the initial imaging test in patients with suspected chronic pancreatitis. It can accurately detect chronic pancreatitis by depicting changes in the main pancreatic duct and lateral side branches. If MRCP is unsuccessful, or if additional information is required, such as a question of pancreatic duct-fluid collection/pseudocyst communication, ERCP can then be performed.

CT is believed to be the single best imaging test for detection of pancreatic duct calculi and for detection of complications of chronic pancreatitis, particularly fluid collections or pseudocysts, involvement of the vascular system, biliary duct, or gastrointestinal tract.

References

1. Axon ATR. Endoscopic retrograde cholangiopancreatography in chronic pancreatitis. The Cambridge classification. Radiologic Clinics of North Am 1989; 27: 39–50.
2. Barish M, Soto J, Ferrucci J. Magnetic resonance pancreatography. Endoscopy 1997; 29: 487–95.
3. Freeny PC. Radiologic imaging of chronic pancreatitis. In: Malfertheiner P, Domínguez-Muñoz J, Schulz U, Lippert H, eds. Diagnostic Procedures in Pancreatic Disease. Berlin: Springer-Verlag, 1997: 203–14.
4. Freeny PC, Lawson TL. Radiology of the Pancreas. New York: Springer-Verlag, 1982.
5. Luetmer PH, Stephens DH, Ward EM. Chronic pancreatitis: reassessment with current CT. Radiology 1989; 171: 353–7.
6. Malfertheiner P. Combined functional and morphological diagnostic approach in chronic pancreatitis. In: Malfertheiner P, Ditschuneit H, eds. Diagnostic Procedures in Pancreatic Disease. Berlin: Springer-Verlag, 1986: 262–7.
7. Malfertheiner P, Büchler MW. Correlation of imaging and function in chronic pancreatitis. Radiologic Clinics of North Am 1989; 27: 51–64.
8. Malfertheiner P, Büchler MW, Stanescu A et al. Correlation of morphological lesions, functional changes, and clinical stages in chronic pancreatitis. In: Malfertheiner P, Ditschuneit H, eds. Diagnostic Procedures in Pancreatic Disease. Berlin: Springer-Verlag, 1986: 268–73.
9. Manfredi R, Costamagna G, Brizi MG et al. Severe chronic pancreatitis versus suspected pancreatic disease: dynamic MR cholangiopancreatography after secretin stimulation. Radiology 2000; 214(3): 849–55.
10. Sarner M, Cotton PB. Definitions of acute and chronic pancreatitis. Clin Gastroenterol 1984; 13: 865–70.
11. Semelka RC, Shoenut JP, Kroeker MA, Micflikier AB. Chronic pancreatitis: MR imaging features before and after administration of gadopentetate dimeglumine. J Magn Reson Imaging 1993; 3(1): 79–82.

12. Soto JA, Barish MA, Yucel EK et al. Pancreatic duct: MR cholangiopancreatography with a three-dimensional fast spin-echo technique. Radiology 1995; 196: 459–64.
13. Takehara Y. MR pancreatography: technique and applications. Top Magn Reson Imaging 1996; 8(5): 290–301.
14. Takehara Y, Ichijo K, Tooyama N et al. Breath-hold MR cholangiopancreatography with a long echo-train fast spin-echo sequence and a surface coil in chronic pancreatitis. Radiology 1994; 192: 19–21.

6.6 Integrated radiology for surgical resection in chronic pancreatitis

J. P. Neoptolemos, P. Ghaneh, R. Sutton, M. Hartley, M. Hughes, C. J. Garvey, M. Lombard, H. Smart, I. Gilmore

Introduction

Chronic pancreatitis represents an increasing medical and surgical challenge. The incidence of chronic pancreatitis is around 1–10 per 100,000 population per year in Europe [1]. There is a steady rise in incidence, linked to increasing alcohol consumption. In advanced chronic pancreatitis surgery has a major role to play. Chronic pancreatitis is a complex medical, surgical and social disease that must be fully understood in order to optimize treatment. Radiological imaging is mandatory for correct diagnosis, patient selection for surgery and choosing the surgical procedure that is most appropriate for any particular patient.

Indications for surgery

Until recently there were two main classical indications for surgery: chronic debilitating pain and the surgical complications of chronic pancreatitis itself [2]. The surgical complications include pancreatic pseudocyst, biliary obstruction, duodenal obstruction, pancreatic ascites, pancreatic fistula, hepatic portal venous compression or occlusion, left-sided (sinistral) portal hypertension with gastric varices and hemorrhage, and pseudoaneurysm.

During the past decade it has been recognized that there is an approximate 10-fold increased incidence of pancreatic ductal adenocarcinoma in non-genetically linked (sporadic) forms of chronic pancreatitis and a 40- to 70-fold risk in hereditary pancreatitis [3–6]. Given the dramatic reduction in mortality from pancreatic resectional surgery over a similar period [6–16], there is increasing use of pancreatic resection for discrete lesions of uncertain etiology (fear of cancer) in patients with a background of chronic pancreatitis (as well as those without such a history on presentation). In patients from families with hereditary pancreatitis, prophylactic pancreatectomy may also be indicated in certain circumstances [17].

Traditional surgical procedures

The continuing controversy for resection centers on both the usefulness of surgery for chronic pain and inter-linked with this question, the optimum means of surgical intervention. Patients with a dilated main pancreatic duct (MPD) classically were and are treated by a side-to-side ("longitudinal") pancreatojejunostomy. The success rates in terms of controlling pain long-term from different series were highly variable, suggesting different selection approaches [18–22]. Recently this surgical procedure has been challenged by the increasing use of endoscopic procedures, notably stenting, but also with variable results [23, 24].

In the past there have been advocates of total pancreatectomy but with post-operative mortality rates of around 10% and a late mortality of some 20%, there was an increasing tendency towards more conservative procedures [12, 13, 15, 25]. Notably there was extensive use of left-sided (incorrectly labelled "distal") pancreatectomy, in part due to a perception that this procedure was an "easier" operation with apparently fewer complications than total pancreatectomy. The results of left-sided pancreatectomy for controlling the pain of chronic pancreatitis long-term have been disappointing in some but not all series [8, 26, 27]. The right-sided pancreatectomy (Kausch-Whipple pancreatoduodenectomy) was and is still reserved for cases with dominant disease of the head of the pancreas, often complicated by obstruction of the intrapancreatic main bile duct (MBD), duodenal obstruction and hepatic portal vein/superior mesenteric vein (HPV/SMV) compression.

Changing surgical philosophy

While individual success stories of surgery for pain in chronic pancreatitis have been dramatic the less than successful overall results prompted important changes in surgical philosophy. The key elements of this change have been the following:

1. There has been a great improvement in surgical results from resectional procedures of the pancreas, both for pancreatic cancer and for chronic pancreatitis [6–16].
2. Several hypotheses to explain the causes of pain in chronic pancreatitis have been refined and developed [28–31].
3. There has been empirical validation of the notion that limited resection of the dominant focus of disease may help to break the vicious cycle of pain, increasing analgesia and addiction to opiates (often being compounded by an alcohol addiction tendency) [7, 8].
4. In addition there has been a move in pancreatic resection towards preserving adjacent anatomy, the gastric antrum, the pylorus, the duodenum, the intrapancreatic main bile duct and the spleen [7, 10, 12, 13, 15].

The mortality from surgical resection has been reduced from 20–30% in the past 15 years or so to 5–6% or less and in the case of chronic pancreatitis to around 1–3% or less, at least in specialist centers [6–16, 25–27, 32].

Three theories have emerged to explain the pain in chronic pancreatitis and *pari passu*, the evolution of surgical concepts:

1. There is the notion that pain is due to increased pressure in the MPD [28]. The implication is that relief of ductal hypertension by pancreatojejunostomy or endoscopic stenting will relieve the pain [29] and may even slow down the rate of progression of at least mild disease [20]. This particularly applies to cases in which the MPD is dilated to say > 6–10 mm in diameter ("large duct" disease). In the situation in which the MPD is < 6 mm ("small duct" disease) there may still be ductal hypertension because extensive parenchymal fibrosis prevents duct dilatation. In this case improved drainage by resecting strictures present within the head of the gland or removing the tail/body of the gland for left-sided strictures should also relieve pancreatic pain.
2. Chronic pancreatitis may be regarded as a compartment syndrome with an external capsule explaining the increased parenchymal tissue pressure [30, 31] and perhaps also the reduced blood flow through the gland [33]. These aspects of the compartment syndrome may explain the pain of chronic pancreatitis. According to this theory

the success of pancreatojejunostomy and perhaps the Frey procedure, which combines the latter with the additional removal of tissue around the MPD in the head of the gland, is due to the release of compartmental pressure. A recent surgical study, however, failed to show that pain was correlated with parenchymal tissue pressure [34].

3. There is now considerable evidence in favor of the "neuronal-inflammatory mediator" theory as the principle cause of pain in chronic pancreatitis [35–37]. During the progression of chronic pancreatitis there is an incremental loss of pancreatic acini and normal stroma, increasing fibrosis and loss of architecture, whilst intra-pancreatic nerves are preserved. Electron microscopy of such nerves demonstrates destruction of protective nerve sheaths [35]. Moreover there is an increase of inflammatory mediators, largely derived from infiltrating leukocytes, around these nerves that are likely to be responsible for increased signals along the axons of pain-sensitive neurons [36, 37]. Thus, according to this theory, pain relief is best achieved by resecting the most affected and inflammatory active part of the gland. This is elegantly demonstrated by the exceptionally good results obtained by the Beger procedure, which removes the head of the gland in cases of "dominant head" disease or "inflammatory mass of the head of the pancreas" [7].

From a pragmatic viewpoint it is important to consider all three hypotheses as being potential elements of the cause of the pain in chronic pancreatitis in any individual patient. Ignoring one or more of these in undertaking intervention may be a reason for subsequent failure.

The development of more sophisticated forms of surgical, as well as endoscopic and radiological, interventions has been entirely contingent on integrating detailed mapping of the anatomy and pathology by endoscopic and radiological means in each patient with the overall clinical picture.

Standard clinical radiological and endoscopic work-up prior to surgery

Each patient needs detailed assessment combining clinical information, the results of pancreatic function tests and endoscopic and radiological findings. The primary objectives of such investigations are as follows:

- to help confirm the diagnosis of chronic pancreatitis;
- to look for a possible anatomical or pathological cause for the chronic pancreatitis;
- to assess the severity of involvement of the pancreas;
- to determine the involvement of surrounding organs and blood vessels and the presence of other complications, including cancer;
- to plan radiological and endoscopic interventions;
- to assess the patient prior to surgery.

There is a wide range of radiological investigations available that can be applied to the study of patients with chronic pancreatitis. These include the plain abdominal radiograph, ultrasound (US), computed tomography (CT) and magnetic resonance (MR) scanning; dynamic investigations include the secretin-enhanced US or MR tests. Important forms of imaging obtained with the aid of endoscopy are endoscopic retrograde cholangiopancreatography (ERCP) and endoluminal ultrasound (EUS). All of these tests may play a part in the assessment process.

At our institution we proceed routinely with the following investigations:
1. Detailed clinical work-up including history, physical examination and blood investigations.
2. Tubeless pancreatic function tests (pancreato-lauryl test and fecal elastase [38]).
3. Oral glucose tolerance test in patients who are not insulin-dependent.
4. Plain chest and abdominal X-rays.
5. Dual-phase contrast-enhanced computed tomography.
6. Endoscopic retrograde cholangiopancreatography.
7. Endoluminal ultrasound is used in selected cases with an uncertain diagnosis or discrete pancreatic lesions of an uncertain nature.
8. Magnetic resonance cholangiopancreatography (MRCP) is only used if ERCP fails and there is insufficient information from CT and EUS.

Radiological confirmation of the diagnosis

The presence of calcification within the gland is the key to establishing the diagnosis radiologically. This is detected with greatest accuracy using CT (Fig. 6.6-1) scanning but abdominal radiographs (Fig. 6.6-2), ultrasound and MR can also show calcification. MR,

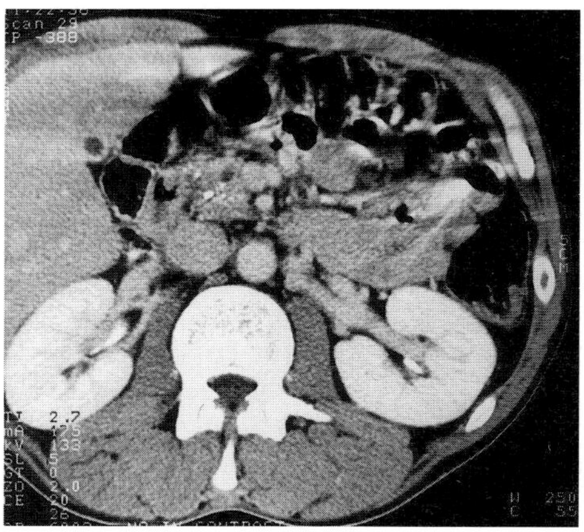

Figure 6.6.-1. CT scan showing specs of calcification within the head of the pancreas and a cross section of a slightly dilated main pancreatic duct. Note that there is only marginal inflammatory enlargement of the head of the pancreas. Operation performed: Beger's procedure.

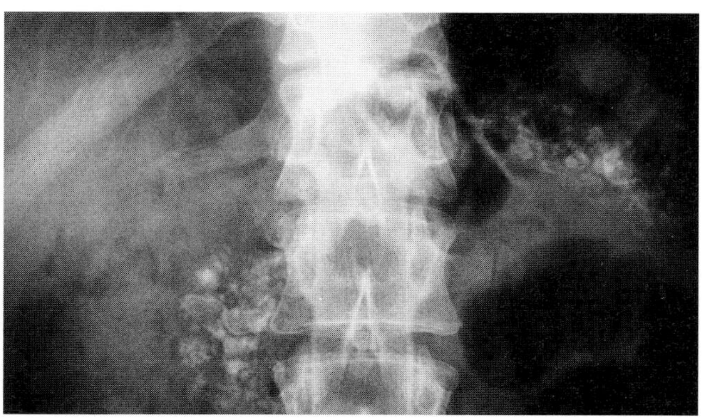

Figure 6.6.-2. Plain abdominal radiograph showing calcification in the whole of the pancreas confirmed by CT. Operation performed: duodenum and spleen-preserving total pancreatectomy.

though useful in assessing other aspects of chronic pancreatitis, is the least dependable at detecting calcification [39–41].

In the absence of calcification, diagnostic features of chronic pancreatitis have been difficult to characterize with imaging techniques. Also there is a poor morphological correlation between symptoms, functional defects and radiology and similarly between imaging and histology [42]. Transabdominal US has a diagnostic sensitivity and specificity of about 70% and then in only about 65% of patients in whom the pancreas can be adequately examined. Conventional CT scanning has the advantage of imaging the pancreas in every case with a sensitivity of 50–90% and a specificity of 50–85% [43]. Dual phase, spiral CT is more sensitive but again, specificity for abnormalities characteristic of chronic pancreatitis is not much improved.

ERCP has traditionally been regarded as the most sensitive (71–90%) and specific test (90–93%) against which other investigations have been compared [44]. ERCP outlines only ductal changes, however, cannot examine the parenchyma, and has the distinct disadvantage of provoking an acute bout of pancreatitis in 5–10% of patients.

Radial array EUS can be used to examine the entire pancreatic gland in most patients without fear of complication and has the advantage of demonstrating both duct and parenchyma in some detail. The normal pancreas has a homogenous "salt and pepper" echo pattern with smooth borders and the main pancreatic duct is a smooth, well-defined structure, tapering from head to tail [45, 46].

In chronic pancreatitis, the organ may appear either enlarged or shrunken. It can have an irregular border and some loss of its homogeneity, with areas of hypo- and hyper-echogenicity. Fine areas of bright speckling may be seen, which are thought to represent calcification. The duct can appear to have brighter walls than usual in mild cases, become irregular in more severe cases and occasionally contain calculi (Fig. 6.6-3). Some of the more subtle changes are not specific and can be seen, for example, in the elderly pancreas.

Lees et al. [45] identified several EUS features that may be present in chronic pancreatitis (Table 6.6-1). Demonstration of three or more of these features was shown to be more than 80% sensitive and specific for chronic pancreatitis in several subsequent studies. Natterman et al. [47] compared EUS findings (Table 6.6-1) with the ERCP fea-

Table 6.6-1. Features of EUS compared to ERCP.

Grade of chronic pancreatitis	**EUS findings** [45]	**ERCP (Cambridge I–III)** [48]
Mild	Increasing heterogeneity of hypo- and hyper-echoic areas in a diffuse pattern. Lobulated or irregular border. No changes in main pancreatic duct.	Minor changes in < 3 side branches
Moderate	As above, but more extensive focal areas of hypo- or hyper-echogenicity. Brighter duct walls, duct dilatation or irregularity.	Changes in > 3 side branches and main duct
Severe	As above, more extensive. Duct dilatation and/or irregularity, with side branches involved. Calcification in parenchyma or duct.	Above plus severe dilatation and irregularity of ducts, cystic change, calcification.
Other	Pseudocyst formation	

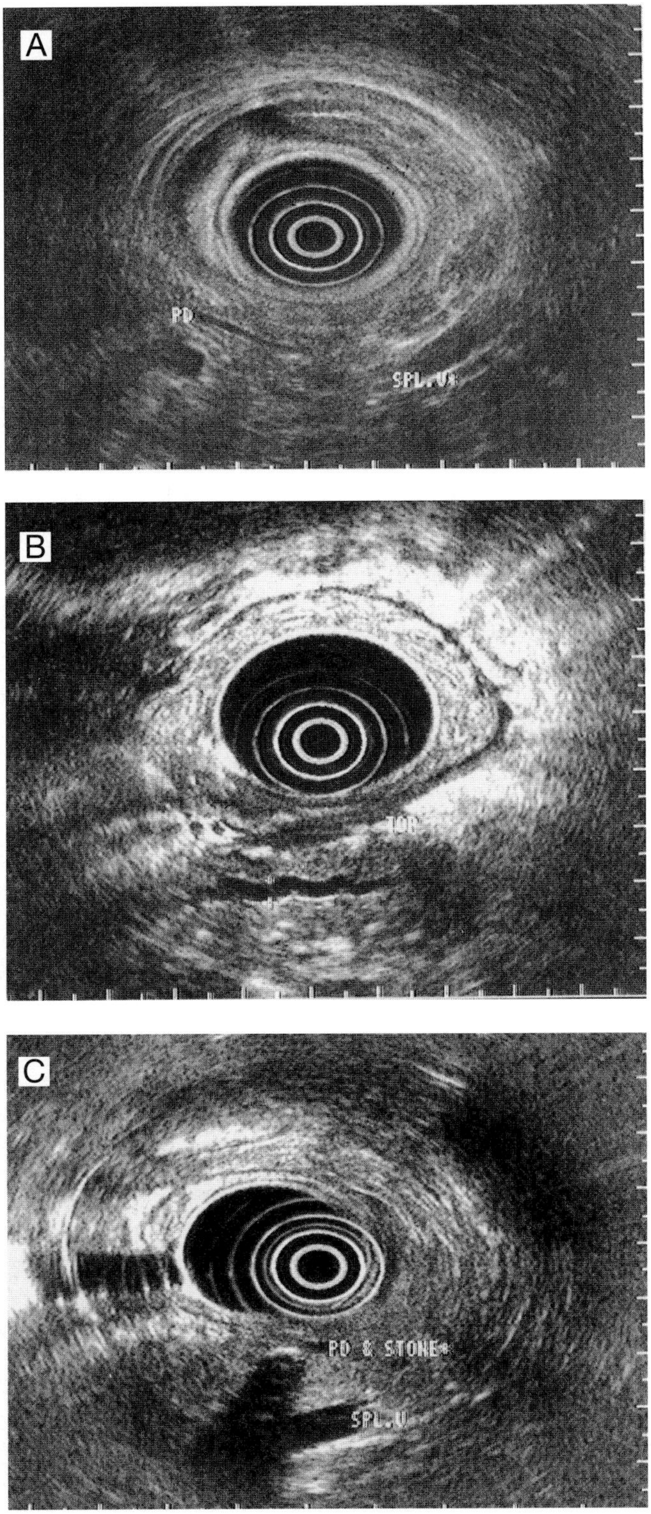

Figure 6.6.-3A–C. Endoluminal ultrasound. **A:** Normal pancreas: the body of the pancreas is shown with a typical granular appearance. There is a normal main pancreatic duct (PD) and the splenic vein is also seen (SPL.V.). **B:** Chronic pancreatitis: the body of the pancreas is shown with lobulated irregular borders, hyperechoic flecks and an irregular dilated main pancreatic duct. **C:** Chronic pancreatitis: there is a stone lying within the main pancreatic duct (PD); the splenic vein (SPL.V.) lies posteriorly.

tures defined by the Cambridge Classification [48]. The study comprised 94 patients with chronic pancreatitis "or status post acute edematous pancreatitis" and 20 "controls" with a normal ERP. There was an excellent correlation of EUS with ERCP, respectively: for Group I, 7 vs 8 (88%); Group II, 16 vs 16 (100%); and Group III, 27 vs 27 (100%). EUS changes were also identified in 63% of the remaining patients in whom ERCP was interpreted as normal whilst EUS was entirely normal in the "controls". Other studies have also indicated that EUS is at least as sensitive as ERCP or tests of pancreatic function in chronic pancreatitis and probably more so in early disease [45, 49–52].

The importance of ERCP, however, also lies in providing detailed information on the state of the MBD and MPD for surgical planning [44].

Radiologically determined causes of chronic pancreatitis

Important obstructive causes of chronic pancreatitis include strictures associated with pancreas divisum and small tumors. In pancreas divisum there may be a stricture of the duct of Santorini (rarely the duct of Wirsung) as it drains into the duodenum (minor papilla) or a partial pancreas divisum in which there is a tenuous connection between the ducts of Santorini and Wirsung and a duct of Santorini that stops short of the duodenal lumen [53]. Cannulation of the minor papilla is difficult at ERCP and other forms of imaging are often required to establish the diagnosis of chronic pancreatitis such as MRCP [54, 55]. The use of secretin to stimulate pancreatic secretion will often cause abnormal and prolonged dilatation of the MPD in the body and tail. Detection of abnormal duct dilatation after intravenous injection of secretin allows the presence of a stricture of the minor papilla to be inferred. This technique was originally described using ultrasound [56] but more recently with MR [57].

Severity of gland involvement

CT is particularly helpful in demonstrating the site of dominant lesions such as an inflammatory mass in the head of the pancreas, the extent of parenchymal calcification (Fig. 6.6-4), MPD (Fig. 6.6-5) and/or MBD (Fig. 6.6-6) dilatation and the presence of pseudocysts (Fig. 6.6-7) [42, 43]. Intraductal calculi may sometimes be seen on CT

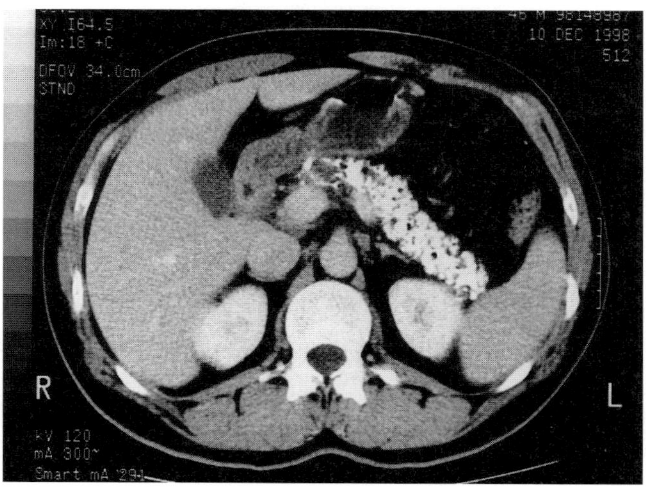

Figure 6.6.-4. CT scan demonstrating calcification in the whole of the pancreas. Operation performed: total pancreatectomy.

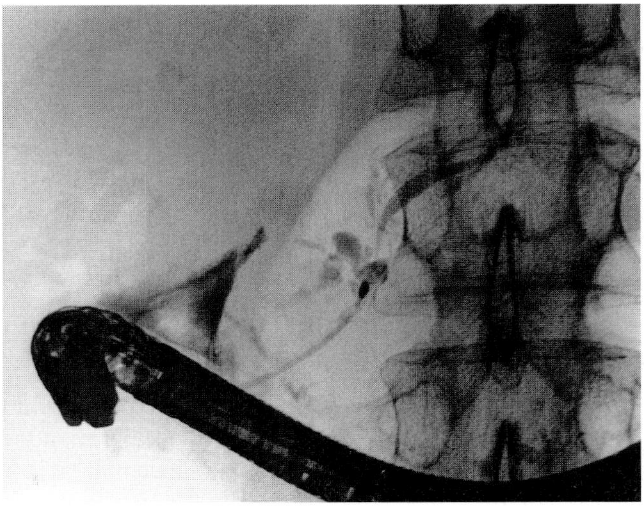

Figure 6.6.-5. Endoscopic retrograde pancreatography showing a stricture of the main pancreatic duct in the head of the pancreas, but without proximal main pancreatic duct dilatation. On CT, the pancreas appeared to be "normal". Operation performed: Beger's operation.

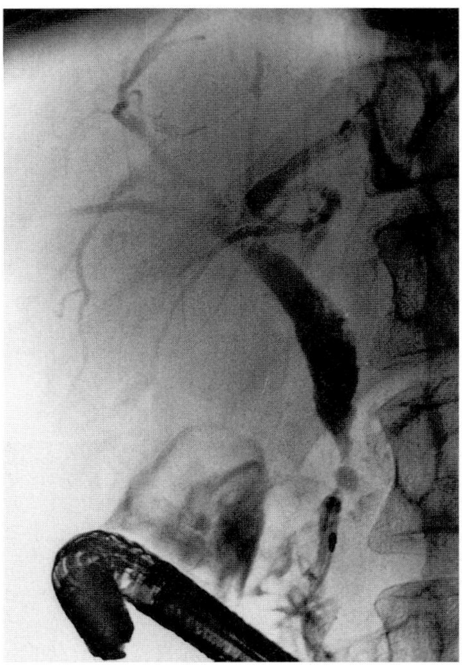

Figure 6.6.-6. Endoscopic retrograde cholangiography showing a stricture of the main bile duct in the head of the pancreas. On CT, the pancreas appeared to be "normal". Operation performed: Beger's operation.

but this feature, along with pancreatic duct strictures, is best established by ERCP or MRCP. Sometimes the gland may appear normal or atrophic, yet ERCP will clearly show features of chronic pancreatitis subsequently confirmed by histology of the resected specimen.

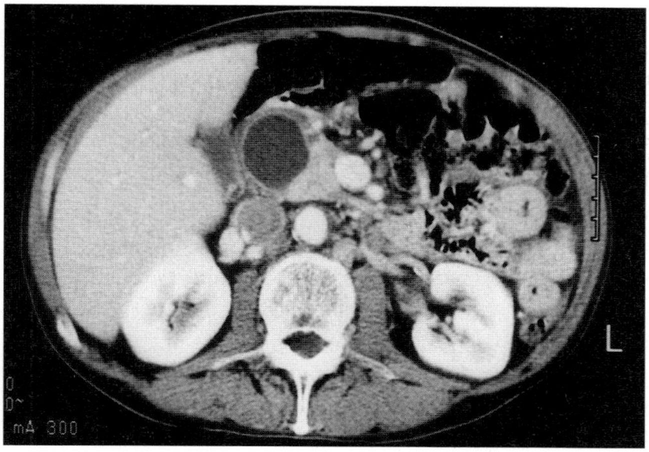

Figure 6.6.-7. CT scan showing a pseudocyst in the head of the pancreas. Endoscopic retrograde cholangiopancreatography showed strictures with proximal dilatation of both the main bile and pancreatic ducts. Operation performed: Beger's operation.

Associated complications of chronic pancreatitis

Important associated complications of chronic pancreatitis amenable to surgical intervention include [2, 41]:

- Pancreatic duct strictures.
- Pseudocysts.
- Main bile duct obstruction.
- Duodenal obstruction.
- Pancreatic ascites.
- Cancer. The incidence of cancer arising in chronic pancreatitis is higher than in the general population [3–6]. Alternatively a small tumor may cause secondary obstructive chronic pancreatitis in an otherwise non-inflamed gland. Cystic tumors may be difficult to differentiate from pancreatic pseudocysts, especially in the presence of calcification [58].
- Venous thrombosis, usually involving the splenic vein, and compression or occlusion of the superior mesenteric and hepatic portal veins. The incidence of splenic vein thrombosis in the published literature varies from 3–10% [59, 60]. Our experience of over 100 patients suggests a much higher incidence, closer to 30%.
- Varices and portal hypertension secondary to venous thrombosis.
- Pseudoaneurysm, particularly of the gastroduodenal and splenic arteries [61].
- Haemosuccus pancreaticus.

Conventional CT scanners will usually suffice to assess the presence of pseudocysts but spiral (helical) CT is normally required to detect more complex complications, particularly those affecting the vascular system. The detection of duodenal obstruction may not be so easy on CT but should be identified during ERCP. A barium meal X-ray examination remains an excellent investigation for this complication. ERCP will often reveal clear compression of the intrapancreatic MBD not so easily detected by CT. Extrapancreatic MBD compression seen on ERCP may be shown by CT to be due to a large pseudocyst.

ERCP is essential for demonstrating a communication between the MPD and a pseudocyst or identifying MPD or pseudocyst disruption in pancreatic ascites [62].

Because of the many changes that may occur in the gland as a consequence of chronic pancreatitis, it can be extremely difficult to detect the presence of a cancer pre-operatively by any imaging modality [41, 44, 45, 63]. Much work is currently taking place trying to identify changes that will allow cancer to be detected by CT or MR but, so far, there is no conclusive appearance. EUS cannot reliably differentiate focal pancreatitis from carcinoma, nor determine whether a tumor has developed in the presence of severe chronic pancreatitis [64]. The presence of lymphadenopathy detected by EUS in such cases has also been shown to be not specific for either. Linear array echo-endoscopy provides the possibility of biopsy either of pancreatic tissue or lymph nodes. In the presence of chronic pancreatitis, however, concerns regarding sampling error in the context of negative histology are likely to limit its role.

Thus it remains unclear which imaging modality offers the best chance of detecting cancer. Because of this difficulty, we along with many other surgeons will remove a suspect mass in a patient with known chronic pancreatitis and leave it to the pathologist to establish the final diagnosis.

Calcification in the wall of a cystadenocarcinoma may be difficult to distinguish from a pseudocyst in chronic pancreatitis [58]. The absence of a long history of chronic pain may not be especially helpful. A normal MPD on ERCP should point to neoplasia being the more likely cause but is only really helpful in lesions of the tail of the gland.

Gastric varices from portal hypertension and bleeding from the ampulla of Vater due to haemosuccus pancreaticus may be seen during endoscopy. Selective angiography (arteriography and/or phlebography) may be necessary to demonstrate the site of a pancreato-vascular fistula. ERCP may also demonstrate the presence and site of a pancreato-venous fistula.

Planning of endoscopic and radiological interventions

The main endoscopic interventions using ERCP include the following:

- Drainage of accessible chronic pancreatic pseudocysts into the stomach or duodenum. The use of EUS is important to plan a route free of major intervening vessels if a trans-gastric or trans-duodenal route is chosen.
- Placement of endoscopic stents through MPD strictures and across a leaking MPD associated with pancreatic ascites.
- Placement of endoscopic stents through a strictured minor papilla in pancreas divisum.
- Relief of biliary obstruction secondary to bile duct compression.

The principle radiological interventions are performed using image guidance, primarily CT or US; these are:

- Embolization of bleeding pseudoaneurysm of the gastroduodenal or splenic arteries.
- Percutaneous pancreatic duct puncture to facilitate pancreatic duct stent insertion when ERCP is impossible.
- Percutaneous transhepatic insertion of vascular stent into compressed HPV/SMV.
- Occasionally, assisting in the placement of a percutaneous jejunal feeding tube in patients with gastric outlet obstruction due to duodenal loop compression.

As for surgical interventions, detailed mapping of the anatomy and pathology is required before choosing the type of intervention and the most appropriate route.

Pre-operative assessment

A combination of contrast-enhanced CT scanning and either ERCP or MRCP will usually provide the surgeon with all the information required to allow surgery to proceed. The information required includes:

1. The area of maximal involvement of the pancreatic gland.
2. The location and number of pancreatic duct strictures to enable a decision to be made about the optimum procedure (partial resection and/or pancreatojejunostomy, or total pancreatectomy).
3. The location, size and appearance of any pseudocysts and their relation to adjacent organs, particularly spleen, colon, kidney and major vessels
4. The state of the local arterial supply. Dynamic spiral CT with reformatting can show the arterial anatomy with a high degree of accuracy. This can allow important vascular anomalies to be detected pre-operatively and the patency and degree of encasement of arteries can usually be established.
5. The patency of the important veins, including the splenic, superior mesenteric and hepatic portal veins and the inferior vena cava. When venous occlusion is present, CT can reveal the presence of major venous collaterals, which can be helpful in planning the surgical approach.

Modern-day operations for chronic pancreatitis

The detailed work-up of the patient described in the previous section will enable the patient to be selected for one of the following procedures. It is of course vital that the patient is well motivated and in relevant cases has demonstrated a strong desire to escape from opiate and alcohol addiction.

Beger's operation (duodenum-preserving resection of the head of the pancreas)

This operation is principally undertaken for an inflammatory mass in the head of the pancreas. This is associated with a single stricture in the MPD in around 40% and is often complicated by obstruction to the duodenum (5–10%), intrapancreatic MBD obstruction (50%) and HPV/SMV compression (18%) [7,65]. The operation will relieve the obstruction of all these structures. Unlike lateral pancreatojejunostomy, the Beger procedure will improve spleno-portal venous blood flow in cases in which segmental portal hypertension has been demonstrated [66]. There is almost invariably stricturing of the MPD within the head of the pancreas. The extent of resection must encompass these MPD strictures to ensure unimpeded flow of pancreatic juice. Moreover an inflammatory mass in the head of the pancreas may be accompanied by more proximal (left-sided) MPD stricturing associated with a dilated MPD. In this case it is essential to include a pancreatojejunostomy across any strictures to ensure adequate drainage of the proximal MPD [65].

The Beger procedure is particularly challenging and needs to be properly understood before the operation can be safely performed independently. Preservation of an adequate rim of pancreatic tissue around the "C" of the duodenum and at least part of the intrapancreatic bile duct as well as preservation of the posterior inferior pancreatoduodenal artery is necessary to maintain an adequate blood supply.

The Frey operation [67] may be considered a modification of the Beger operation, or alternatively an extended variant of the pancreatojejunostomy. A rather small randomized study by Izbicki et al. suggested that these two procedures produced a similar outcome [68] but can be criticized on the basis of no predetermined end-point in setting power calculations. Indeed it would be rather naïve to consider these two operations as being in any way equivalent. Interestingly the same group concluded in another trial that adding a "longitudinal" pancreatojejunostomy to the Beger procedure made little difference to outcome [69], which is a reasonable conclusion provided left-sided strictures are dealt with.

In cases of chronic pancreatitis with small duct disease affecting the whole pancreas and with at least some exocrine and endocrine function but without dominant head disease, the Beger operation also appears to be quite effective, at least in our hands (unpublished data).

Alternatively Izbicki et al. [70] claim good results by an operation which involves cutting a longitudinal "V" shaped gutter along the length of a narrow main pancreatic duct. A Roux-en-Y anastomosis to the parenchyma alongside the MPD is then performed. The rationale for this operation is based on the "compartment syndrome" theory [30, 31].

Pylorus-preserving partial pancreatoduodenectomy (PPPD) and the Kausch-Whipple (KW) operations

Although there is now extensive experience with the Beger operation this is not universally accepted and both the PPPD and KW procedures are still commonly used for dominant head disease [9–11, 14, 32]. This is despite the fact that a randomized study has suggested that the Beger operation is superior to the PPPD procedure [71] and that unlike the PPPD, the Beger operation is not especially prone to delayed gastric emptying [72]. Indeed there is still some preference for the KW rather than the PPPD procedure because of greater frequency of delayed gastric emptying with PPPD, albeit based on retrospective non-randomized data [14].

Pancreatic cancer is found unexpectedly in 5–10% of cases being operated upon for chronic pancreatitis, an issue that favors the routine use of the PPPD and KW. Alternatively it is suggested that pre-operative Tru-Cut frozen biopsies from the head of the pancreas should be performed routinely prior to any Beger operation. It is not clear how successful this proposal is, given the problems of sampling and diagnostic error in such a scenario. Developments in molecular diagnosis may prove to be of particular value in the near future [17].

Left pancreatic resection (spleen-preserving)

The presence of strictures in the body and/or tail of the pancreas with relatively normal parenchyma in the remainder of the pancreas warrants a left pancreatectomy. Ideally the spleen should be preserved; the technique described by Warshaw [73] of preserving the spleen on the vasa brevia enables this to be achieved in virtually all cases. The long-term results of this procedure have been variable dependent upon the appropriateness of patient selection, as well as the accuracy of long-term follow-up [8, 26, 27].

Total pancreatectomy (spleen-preserving and/or duodenum-preserving)

There are three main indications for this procedure.

1. Complete loss of endocrine and exocrine function with severe pain.
2. Recurrence of a severe chronic pancreatic pain following a previous partial resection (either a right- or left-sided resection).

3. Prophylaxis against pancreatic cancer in hereditary pancreatitis (rare) or familial pancreatic cancer (even more rare) in highly selected individuals. Ideally there should be no endocrine or exocrine function. The involvement of a unit that is highly experienced in this area, which will include a clinical genetics input, is mandatory [17].

Preservation of either the duodenum [15] or the spleen [12] with total pancreatectomy has been described. We prefer to do both in the same operation, preserving a splenic blood supply via the vasa brevia. We would not support the use of total pancreatectomy as an initial procedure in patients with sporadic chronic pancreatitis who are not insulin-dependent.

Lateral pancreatojejunostomy

The indication for this drainage procedure is a dilated MPD with minimal parenchymal disease. Typically there is a small area of focal disease in the head of the gland close to the distal part of the MPD near its insertion into the ampulla of Vater. This may be associated with a solitary stone in the head of the gland in idiopathic chronic pancreatitis, which in the case of senile pancreatitis may not be calcified. Rarely there may be a distal stricture in the duct of Santorini in a patient with pancreas divisum. In these former cases there is a modest success rate with endoscopic stenting [74] and therefore it should be attempted, with surgery being reserved for technical failures or recurrence following stent removal. If there is gross disease in the head of the gland, the Beger procedure is the operation of choice.

Procedures for pancreatic pseudocyst

It is essential that pseudocysts are not confused with cystic tumors – both may demonstrate wall calcification [42]. With limited wall thickness, an absence of varices and clear bulging of the pseudocyst into the stomach or duodenum, drainage can be undertaken safely with endoscopic internal drainage. In the absence of these features or if there is recurrence, large pseudocysts should be drained internally by a Roux-en-Y procedure [75–77]. Small pseudocysts in the tail of the gland or in the head of the pancreas associated with MPD strictures should be included in the resectional procedure [77].

Procedures for pancreatic ascites

This is invariably associated with an intra-peritoneal leak of pancreatic juice either from a disruption of the MPD itself or a communicating pseudocyst. The pathological picture may be quite complex, often involving downstream stricturing of the MPD [62]. A clear anatomical and pathological radiological map is required to optimize the choice of therapeutic procedures, which include endoscopic stenting (with octreotide), internal Roux-en-Y stenting and partial pancreatic resection.

Procedures for hemorrhage

The most common cause is bleeding from gastric (usually fundal) varices associated with HPV/SMV stenosis or splenic vein thrombosis [2]. Stenosis of the HPV/SMV may best be treated by percutaneous transhepatic stenting. Recurrent or massive gastric bleeding warrants gastric vascular isolation and sometimes sub-total gastrectomy. Rare causes of hemorrhage are leaking pseudoaneurysm and haemosuccus pancreaticus (due to a ruptured pseudoaneurysm or venous-pancreatic duct fistula). Embolization should be tried initially following selective angiography, with surgery being reserved for failure.

Reasons for surgical failure

The outcome from surgery may prove to be disappointing for any one of a number of reasons.

1. The initial diagnosis of pain from chronic pancreatitis was incorrect. The patient may have a clinical picture of abdominal pain and chronic pancreatitis but may have had another cause for abdominal pain (such as a peptic ulcer) or not have had chronic pancreatitis at all.
2. The patient may have had an associated cancer (cystic or solid) that was not recognized at the initial operation [78]. The tumor may have arisen in pre-existing chronic pancreatitis or actually have been the cause of an obstructive chronic pancreatitis.
3. The incorrect technical procedure was performed [78]. Common examples include the following. (a) The performance of a pancreatojejunostomy when in fact a Beger operation was required because of major disease in the head of the gland. (b) A left pancreatectomy in a gland that is equally affected throughout or with predominant disease in the head of the gland. (c) Any resectional or drainage procedure which fails to ensure adequate MPD drainage of the remaining pancreas.
4. Complications of the surgical procedure itself. Although these are relatively uncommon they may include the following. (a) MBD stricture following a Beger's, PPPD or KW procedure. (b) Duodenal obstruction following a Beger's procedure. (c) Anastomotic ulceration following a PPPD (duodeno-jejunal) or KW (gastro-jejunal) operation. (d) Dumping associated with the partial gastrectomy of the KW operation.
5. Progression of the chronic pancreatitis in the remaining pancreas following a drainage or partial resection procedure.
6. Failure to optimize medical measures, notably pancreatic enzyme supplementation and glucose homeostasis, and to pursue a healthy diet and generally good life-style.
7. Failure of the patient to be psychologically and socially rehabilitated resulting in a return to opiate addiction and/or alcohol addiction, social and professional disruption and extreme loss of self-esteem.

From the above it should be readily apparent that the management of patients with severe chronic pancreatitis is a major multi-disciplinary commitment both before and after any major surgery.

Outcome from surgery

The operative mortality from surgery of the pancreas for chronic pancreatitis is now widely reported to be in the region of 1–3% or even less and with a morbidity of 20–40% [6–16, 18–22, 77]. The immediate results of surgery for chronic pancreatitis in the past 46 months at our own institution are shown in Table 6.6-2. Many of the patients suffer from malnutrition and other extreme consequences of pancreatic organ failure. Often these features are superimposed upon the debilitating effects of long-term alcohol and opiate abuse. These factors need to be taken into account in selecting patients for surgery. Nevertheless with appropriate patient selection 80–90% of patients may be rendered completely or largely pain-free and a significant proportion socially and professionally rehabilitated [7–11, 13–16, 18–22].

Table 6.6-2. Operations performed for chronic pancreatitis at the Royal Liverpool University Hospital from 1.10.96 to 1.8.2000

Procedure	Number	Deaths
Beger's Operation	34	0
Pylorus-preserving PD	10	0
Kausch-Whipple	6	0
Total pancreatectomy	12	2
Left pancreatectomy	6	0
Pseudocyst Roux-en-Y	11	0
Biliary bypass	2	0
Total	**81**	**2***

* 2.5% of all cases and 2.9% of resections

Conclusions

There is no absolute relationship between the morphological appearances of the pancreas and the severity of pain [42]. Moreover the pathological consequences of chronic pancreatitis can be quite complex, requiring a sophisticated algorithm for the optimum treatment. Therefore the synthesis of clinical, radiological and endoscopic information is an absolute requirement for management.

One of the most fascinating observations in recent years is the wide discrepancy in the types of procedure performed in major centers. For example there is a high relative incidence of inflammatory mass of the head of the pancreas reported by Ulm [7, 65]. In contrast the Verona group [6] report a continuing rise over the past 28 years in drainage procedures for chronic pancreatitis, such that resection is now performed in only 13% of all operations. In contrast our experience in both the Birmingham and the Liverpool regions evinces hardly any cases of main pancreatic duct dilatation and relatively few cases with a dominant inflammatory mass in the head of the pancreas; small duct disease with severe fibrosis and parenchymal calcification is a much more typical presentation. Whether these differences simply reflect different referral patterns or whether there is a genuine difference in disease manifestation requires investigation.

Radiology, including imaging obtained by endoscopy, plays an important part in the management of patients with chronic pancreatitis. Close liaison between the pancreatic surgical team and the radiological and endoscopic teams is essential at all stages of management. This includes diagnosis, detection of complications, the planning and performance of radiological, endoscopic and surgical interventions and long-term follow-up.

References

1. Worning H. Alcoholic chronic pancreatitis. In: Beger HG, Warshaw AL, Büchler MW, Carr-Locke DL, Neoptolemos JP, Russell C, Sarr MG, eds. The Pancreas. Oxford: Blackwell Science, 1998: 672–82.
2. Russell R. Indications for surgery. In: Beger HG, Warshaw AL, Büchler MW, Carr-Locke DL, Neoptolemos JP, Russell C, Sarr MG, eds. The Pancreas. Oxford: Blackwell Science, 1998: 815–23.
3. Lowenfels A, Maisonneuve P, Cavallini G, Amman, Lankisch P, Andersen J, DiMagno E, Andrén-Sandberg A, Domellöf L. Pancreatitis and the risk of pancreatic cancer. N Eng J Med 1993; 328: 1433–7.

4. Lowenfels A, Maisonneuve P, DiMagno E, Elitsur Y, Gates LK, Perrault J, Whitcomb DC: Hereditary pancreatitis and the risk of pancreatic cancer. J Natl Cancer Inst. 1997; 89: 442–6.
5. Finch M, Howes N, Ellis I, Mountford R, Sutton R, Raraty M, Neoptolemos JP. Hereditary pancreatitis and familial pancreatic cancer. Digestion 1997; 58: 564–9.
6. Falconi M, Valerio A, Caldiron E, Salvia R, Sartori N, Talamini G, Bassi C, Pederzoli P. Changes in pancreatic resection for chronic pancreatitis over 28 years in a single institution. Br J Surg 2000; 87: 428–33.
7. Beger HG, Schlosser W, Friess HM, Büchler MW. Duodenum-preserving head resection in chronic pancreatitis changes the natural course of the disease: a single-center 26-year experience. Ann Surg 1999; 230: 512–9.
8. Schöenberg MH, Schlosser W, Ruck W, Beger HG. Distal pancreatectomy in chronic pancreatitis. Dig Surg 1999; 16:130–6.
9. Stapleton GN, Williamson RC. Proximal pancreatoduodenectomy for chronic pancreatitis. Br J Surg 1996; 83:1433–40.
10. Martin RF, Rossi RL, Leslie KA. Long-term results of pylorus-preserving pancreatoduodenectomy for chronic pancreatitis. Arch Surg 1996; 131: 247–52.
11. Sakorafas GH, Farnell MB, Nagorney DM, Sarr MG, Rowland CM. Pancreatoduodenectomy for chronic pancreatitis: long-term results in 105 patients. Arch Surg 2000; 135: 517–23.
12. White SA, Sutton CD, Weymss-Holden S, Berry DP, Pollard C, Rees Y, Dennison AR. The feasibility of spleen-preserving pancreatectomy for end-stage chronic pancreatitis. Am J Surg 2000; 179: 294–7.
13. Fleming WR, Williamson RCN. Role of total pancreatectomy in the treatment of patients with end-stage chronic pancreatitis. Br J Surg 1995; 82: 1409–12.
14. Jimenez RE, Fernandez-del Castillo C, Rattner DW, Chang Y, Warshaw AL. Outcome of pancreaticoduodenectomy with pylorus preservation or with antrectomy in the treatment of chronic pancreatitis. Ann Surg 2000; 231: 293–300.
15. Linehan IP, Lambert MA, Brown DC, Kurtz AB, Cotton PB, Russell RC. Total pancreatectomy for chronic pancreatitis. Gut 1988; 29: 358–65.
16. Evans JD, Wilson P, Carver C, Bramhall SR, Buckels JAC, Mayer AD, McMaster P, Neoptolemos JP. Outcome of surgery for chronic pancreatitis. British Journal of Surgery 1997; 84: 624–9.
17. Howes N, Greenhalf W, Neoptolemos JP. Screening for early pancreatic ductal adenocarcinoma in hereditary pancreatitis. Medical Clinics of North America 2000; 84: 719–38.
18. Bradley EL III. Long-term results of pancreato-jejunostomy in patients with chronic pancreatitis. Am J Surg 1987; 153: 207–13.
19. Lucas CE, McIntosh B, Paley D, Ledgerwood AM, Vlahos A. Surgical decompression of ductal obstruction in patients with chronic pancreatitis. Surgery 1999; 126: 790–5.
20. Nealon WH, Thompson JC. Progressive loss of pancreatic function in chronic pancreatitis is delayed by main pancreatic duct decompression. A longitudinal prospective analysis of the modified Puestow procedure. Ann Surg 1993; 217: 458–66.
21. Adams DB, Ford MC, Anderson MC. Outcome after lateral pancreaticojejunostomy for chronic pancreatitis. Ann Surg 1994; 219: 481–7.
22. Prinz RA. Pancreatic duct drainage. In: Beger HG, Warshaw AL, Büchler MW, Carr-Locke DL, Neoptolemos JP, Russell C, Sarr MG, eds. The Pancreas. Oxford: Blackwell Science, 1998: 829–36.
23. Somogyi L, Forsmark CE. Pancreatic duct stenting in benign pancreatic disease. Semin Gastrointest Dis 1998; 9: 73–9.
24. Binmoeller KF, Soehendra N. Endoscopic treatment. Part 5 Chronic Pancreatitis. In: Beger HG, Warshaw AL, Büchler MW, Carr-Locke DL, Neoptolemos JP, Russell C, Sarr MG, eds. The Pancreas. Oxford: Blackwell Science, 1998: 794–807.
25. Russell R. Surgical failures-total pancreatectomy. Part 5 Chronic Pancreatitis. In: Beger HG, Warshaw AL, Büchler MW, Carr-Locke DL, Neoptolemos JP, Russell C, Sarr MG, eds. The Pancreas. Oxford: Blackwell Science, 1998: 877–85.
26. Govil S, Imrie CW. Value of splenic preservation during distal pancreatectomy for chronic pancreatitis. Br J Surg 1999; 86: 895–8.

27. Brancatisano RP, Williamson RCN. Distal pancreatectomy with or without splenectomy. Part 5 Chronic Pancreatitis. In: Beger HG, Warshaw AL, Büchler MW, Carr-Locke DL, Neoptolemos JP, Russell C, Sarr MG, eds. The Pancreas. Oxford: Blackwell Science, 1998: 855–62.
28. Okazaki K, Yamamoto Y, Kagiyama S, Tamura S, Sakamoto Y, Nakazawa Y, Morita M, Yamamoto Y. Pressure of papillary sphincter zone and pancreatic main duct in patients with chronic pancreatitis in the early stage. Scand J Gastroenterol 1988; 23: 501–7.
29. Renou C, Grandval P, Ville E, Laugier R. Endoscopic treatment of the main pancreatic duct – correlations among manometry, and clinical follow-up. Int J Pancreatol. 2000; 27: 143–9.
30. Ebbehoj N, Borly L, Bulow J, Rasmussen SG, Madsen P, Matzen P, Owre A. Pancreatic tissue fluid pressure in chronic pancreatitis. Relation to pain, morphology, and function. Scand J Gastroenterol 1990; 25: 1046–51.
31. Jalleh RP, Aslam M, Williamson RCN. Pancreatic tissue and ductal pressures in chronic pancreatitis. Br J Surg 1991; 78: 1235–7.
32. Martin RF, Rossi RL. Pancreatoduodenectomy with or without pylorus preservation. Part 5 Chronic Pancreatitis. In: Beger HG, Warshaw AL, Büchler MW, Carr-Locke DL, Neoptolemos JP, Russell C, Sarr MG, eds. The Pancreas. Oxford: Blackwell Science, 1998: 863–9.
33. Schilling MK, Redaelli C, Reber PU, Friess H, Signer C, Stoupis C, Büchler MW. Microcirculation in chronic alcoholic pancreatitis: a laser Doppler flow study. Pancreas 1999; 19: 21–5.
34. Manes G, Büchler MW, Pieramico O, Di Sebastiano P, Malfertheiner P. Is increased pancreatic pressure related to pain in chronic pancreatitis? Int J Pancreatol 1994; 15: 113–7.
35. Bockman DE, Büchler MW, Malfertheiner P, Beger HG. Analysis of nerves in chronic pancreatitis. Gastroenterology 1988; 94: 1459–69.
36. Di Sebastiano P, Fink T, Weihe E, Friess H, Innocenti P, Beger HG, Büchler MW. Immune cell infiltration and growth-associated protein 43 expression correlate with pain in chronic pancreatitis. Gastroenterology 1997; 112: 1648–55.
37. Friess H, Zhu ZW, di Mola FF, Kulli C, Graber HU, Andren-Sandberg A, Zimmermann A, Korc M, Reinshagen M, Büchler MW. Nerve growth factor and its high-affinity receptor in chronic pancreatitis. Ann Surg 1999; 230: 615–24.
38. Loser C, Mollgaard A, Fölsch UR. Faecal elastase 1: a novel, highly sensitive, and specific tubeless pancreatic function test. Gut 1996; 39: 580–6.
39. Manes G, Kahl S et al. Chronic pancreatitis: diagnosis and staging. Ann Ital Chir 2000 Jan–Feb; 71: 22–32.
40. Homma T. Criteria for pancreatic disease diagnosis in Japan: diagnostic criteria for chronic pancreatitis. Pancreas 1998; 16: 250–4.
41. Freeny PC. Radiology. Part 5 Chronic Pancreatitis. In: Beger HG, Warshaw AL, Büchler MW, Carr-Locke DL, Neoptolemos JP, Russell C, Sarr MG. eds. The Pancreas. Oxford: Blackwell Science, 1998: 728–39.
42. Malfertheiner P, Büchler MW, Stanescu A, Ditschuneit H. Pancreatic morphology and function in relationship to pain in chronic pancreatitis. Int J Pancreatol 1987; 2: 59–66.
43. Balthazar EJ. Computed tomography of the pancreas. In: Beger HG, Warshaw AL, Büchler MW, Carr-Locke DL, Neoptolemos JP, Russell C, Sarr MG, eds. The Pancreas. Oxford: Blackwell Science, 1998: 205–30.
44. Parsons WG, Carr-Locke DL. In: Beger HG, Warshaw AL, Büchler MW, Carr-Locke DL, Neoptolemos JP, Russell C, Sarr MG, eds. The Pancreas. Oxford: Blackwell Science, 1998: 230–46.
45. Lees WR. Endoscopic ultrasonography of chronic pancreatitis and pancreatic pseudocysts. Scandinavian Journal of Gastroenterology – Supplement 1986; 123: 123–9.
46. Sahai AV, Zimmermann M, Aabakken L, Tarnasky PR, Cunningham JT, van Velse A, Hawes RH, Hoffman BJ. Prospective assessment of the ability of endoscopic ultrasound to diagnose, exclude, or establish the severity of chronic pancreatitis found by endoscopic retrograde cholangiopancreatography. Gastrointest Endosc 1998; 48: 18–25.
47. Natterman C, Goldschmidt AJ, Dancygier H. Endosonography in chronic pancreatitis – a comparison between endoscopic retrograde pancreatography and endoscopic ultrasonography. Endoscopy 1993; 25: 565–70.

48. Sarner M, Cotton PB. Classification of pancreatitis. Gut 1984; 25: 756–9.
49. Catalano MF, Lahoti S, Alcocer E, Geenen JE, Hogan WJ. Dynamic imaging of the pancreas using real-time endoscopic ultrasonography with secretin stimulation. Gastrointestinal Endoscopy 1998; 48: 580–7.
50. Wiersema MJ, Hawes RH, Lehman GA, Kochman ML, Sherman S, Kopecky KK. Prospective evaluation of endoscopic ultrasonography and endoscopic retrograde cholangiopancreatography in patients with chronic abdominal pain of suspected pancreatic origin. Endoscopy 1993; 25: 555–64.
51. Wiersema MJ, Wiersema LM. Endosonography of the pancreas: normal variation versus changes of early chronic pancreatitis. Gastrointestinal Endoscopy Clinics of North America 1995; 5: 487–96.
52. Zuccaro G, Jr, Sivak MV, Jr. Endoscopic ultrasonography in the diagnosis of chronic pancreatitis. Endoscopy 1992; 24(Suppl 1): 347–9.
53. Lindstrom E, Ihse I. Pancreatic disease caused by pancreas divisum. Eur J Surg 1994; 160: 385–7.
54. Fulcher AS, Turner MA. Magnetic resonance pancreatography. Crit Rev Diagn Imaging 1999; 40: 285–322.
55. Coakley FV, Schwartz LH. Magnetic resonance cholangiopancreatography. J Magn Reson Imaging 1999; 9: 157–62.
56. Glaser J. Clinical perspectives of a sonographic secretin test. Z Gastroenterol 1997; 35: 579–83.
57. Matos C et al. Secretin-enhanced MR pancreatography. Semin Ultrasound CT MR 1999; 20: 340–51.
58. Le Borgne J, de Calan L, Partensky C. Cystadenomas and cystadenocarcinomas of the pancreas: a multiinstitutional retrospective study of 398 cases. French Surgical Association. Ann Surg 1999; 230: 152–61.
59. Sakorafas GH, Tsiotou AG. Splenic vein thrombosis complicating chronic pancreatitis. Scand J Gastroenterol 1999; 34: 1171–7.
60. Seiler CA, Friess H, Büchler MW. Thrombosis of the portal and splenic vein. Part 5 Chronic Pancreatitis. In: Beger HG, Warshaw AL, Büchler MW, Carr-Locke DL, Neoptolemos JP, Russell C, Sarr MG, eds. The Pancreas. Oxford: Blackwell Science, 1998: 761–5.
61. LiPuma JP et al. Splenic artery pseudoaneurysm associated with chronic pancreatitis. Amer J Roentgenology 1997; 169: 259.
62. Neoptolemos JP, Winslet M. Pancreatic ascites. In: Beger H, Büchler MW. Ditschuneit H, Malfertheiner P, eds. Chronic Pancreatitis. Berlin: Springer-Verlag, 1990: 268–79.
63. Johnson PT. Pancreatic cancer v. chronic pancreatitis: dynamic MR imaging. Radiology 1999; 212: 213.
64. Barthet M, Portal I, Boujaoude J, Bernard JP, Sahel J. Endoscopic ultrasonographic diagnosis of pancreatic cancer complicating chronic pancreatitis. Endoscopy 1996; 28: 487–91.
65. Beger HG, Kunz R, Schoenberg MH. Duodenum preserving resection of the pancreatic head – a standard procedure for chronic pancreatitis. Part 5 Chronic Pancreatitis. In: Beger HG, Warshaw AL, Büchler MW, Carr-Locke DL, Neoptolemos JP, Russell C, Sarr MG, eds. The Pancreas. Oxford: Blackwell Science, 1998: 870–6.
66. Bloechle C, Busch C, Tesch C, Nicolas V, Binmoeller KF, Soehendra N, Izbicki JR. Prospective randomized study of drainage and resection on non-occlusive segmental portal hypertension in chronic pancreatitis. Br J Surg 1997; 84: 477–82.
67. Frey CF, Amikura K. Local resection of the head of the pancreas combined with longitudinal pancreaticojejunostomy in the management of patients with chronic pancreatitis. Ann Surg 1994; 220: 492–504.
68. Izbicki JR, Bloechle C, Knoefel WT, Kuechler T, Binmoeller KF, Broelsch CE. Duodenum-preserving resection of the head of the pancreas in chronic pancreatitis. A prospective, randomized trial. Ann Surg 1995; 221: 350–8.
69. Izbicki JR, Bloechle C, Broering DC, Knoefel WT, Kuechler T, Broelsch CE. Extended drainage versus resection in surgery for chronic pancreatitis: a prospective randomized trial comparing

the longitudinal pancreaticojejunostomy combined with local pancreatic head excision with the pylorus-preserving pancreatoduodenectomy. Ann Surg 1998; 228: 771–9.
70. Izbicki JR, Bloechle C, Broering DC, Kuechler T, Broelsch CE. Longitudinal V-shaped excision of the ventral pancreas for small duct disease in severe chronic pancreatitis: prospective evaluation of a new surgical procedure. Ann Surg 1998; 227: 213–9.
71. Büchler MW, Friess H, Muller MW, Wheatley AM, Beger HG. Randomized trial of duodenum-preserving pancreatic head resection versus pylorus-preserving Whipple in chronic pancreatitis. Am J Surg 1995; 169: 65–9.
72. Muller MW, Friess H, Beger HG, Kleeff J, Lauterburg B, Glasbrenner B, Riepl RL, Büchler MW. Gastric emptying following pylorus-preserving Whipple and duodenum-preserving pancreatic head resection in patients with chronic pancreatitis. Am J Surg. 1997; 173: 257–63.
73. Warshaw AL. Conservation of the spleen with distal pancreatectomy. Arch Surg 1988; 123: 550–3.
74. Boerma D, Huibregtse K, Gulik TM, Rauws EAJ, Obertop H, Gouma DJ. Long-term outcome of endoscopic stent placement for chronic pancreatitis associated with pancreas divisum. Endoscopy 2000: 32: 452–6.
75. Boerma D, Obertop H, Gouma DJ. Pancreatic pseudocysts in chronic pancreatitis. Surgical or interventional drainage? Ann Chir Ital 2000; 71: 43–50.
76. Pitchumoni CS, Agarwal N. Pancreatic pseudocysts. When and how should drainage be performed? Gastroenterol Clin Nor Amer 1999; 28: 615–39.
77. Yeo C, Cameron JL. Surgical treatment of pseudocysts. Part 5 Chronic Pancreatitis. In: Beger HG, Warshaw AL, Büchler MW, Carr-Locke DL, Neoptolemos JP, Russell C, Sarr MG, eds. The Pancreas. Oxford: Blackwell Science, 1998: 845–53.
78. Rattner DW, Fernandez-del Castillo C, Warshaw AL. Pitfalls of distal pancreatectomy for relief of pain in chronic pancreatitis. Am J Surg 1996; 171: 142–5.

7 Chronic pancreatitis: An attempt to classify

7.1 Classification of liver cirrhosis

J. Reichen

The liver and pancreas have many things in common, not the least of which is the stellate cell or myofibroblast as the originator of the wound healing reaction. The classification of liver diseases could be done on the level of etiology, anatomy or functional reserve. The latter is our prime research focus and will also be the main topic of this overview.

Etiology

When one looks at the etiologies of chronic liver disease leading to cirrhosis it is immediately apparent that there are many commonalities but also major discrepancies (Table 7.1-1).

Table 7.1-1. Classification of chronic liver diseases based on etiology.

- Toxic (drugs, alcohol, bile salts)
- Infectious
- Autoimmune diseases
- Obstructive
- Inborn errors of metabolism (hemochromatosis, α_1-antitrypsin deficiency, Wilson's disease)

Among the toxins listed in Table 7.1-1, I would like to draw particular attention to alcohol as the cause of a substantial number of both chronic pancreatic and chronic liver disease. The central role of endotoxin and the following activation of a cytokine cascade beginning with tumor necrosis factor α (TNF-α) has now been well worked out to explain alcoholic hepatitis [1]. Similar experiments are carried out by pancreatic pathophysiologists and understanding of this cascade may open new therapeutic avenues.

The second class of toxins of major interest to both hepatologists and pancreatologists are the bile salts. Taurocholate has long been used to induce pancreatitis [2]. Serum bile salt levels are elevated in both chronic liver and chronic pancreatic disease, in particular when there is cholestasis. Bile salts are an early signal for hepatocyte apoptosis in the liver by a novel, caspase-independent pathway [3]. Hepatocyte death increases TGF-β, the major fibrogenic signal in the liver; thus, bile salts may also be indirectly involved in hepatic fibrosis [3]. The role of cholestasis in hepatic fibrosis is underlined by a recent report on its reversibility in man [4] as we have previously described in animal models [5].

While pancreatologists might feel that autoimmune disorders are an irrelevant part of patients with pancreatic disease, I would like to point out that the major cholestatic autoimmune diseases – primary biliary cirrhosis and primary sclerosing cholangitis – often exhibit pancreatic involvement [6, 7]. Pancreatitis can even be the first presenting sign of primary sclerosing cholangitis and – in contrast to the liver disease – might be responsive to steroid treatment [8].

Anatomy

Another way to classify liver disease – in particular that involving the biliary tree – is based on anatomy. In this respect I would like to draw the reader's attention to the classification of biliary cirrhosis proposed by Ludwig (Table 7.1-2) [9]. As discussed in the previous paragraph, a variety of the diseases, in particular the autoimmune ones, can also affect the pancreas.

Cirrhosis	Cholangitis	Examples
Small duct	Granulomatous	PBC, sarcoidosis
	Lymphocytic, pleomorphic	GVHD, chronic rejection, adult ductopenia
	Fibrous, obliterative	PSC, drugs, infantile ductopenia
Large duct		

Table 7.1-2. Classification of biliary cirrhosis [9].

Of major interest to pancreatologists is obviously the large duct disease. Here one should also point out that hepatic fibrosis, often of the biliary type, is frequently seen in alcoholic pancreatitis. Thus, Lesur *et al.* found significant biliary pathology in 69% of patients with alcoholic pancreatitis; 19% had unrecognized alcoholic hepatitis which was predictive of postoperative death [10]. No clinical, biochemical or imaging test was able to predict hepatic lesions. Similar data were recently reported by another group: 75% of patients with alcoholic pancreatitis had increased fibrogenic activity of the liver [11].

Function

Finally, liver diseases can be classified by their functional impairment. The most popular classification is the Child-Pugh classification. It was originally designed to evaluate patients for portosystemic shunt surgery [12] and used five variables, namely serum bilirubin, serum albumin, ascites, encephalopathy and nutritional state. The latter was replaced with the prothrombin time as a more objective parameter by Pugh *et al.* [13] leading to the most frequently used Child-Pugh classification of cirrhotic liver disease (Table 7.1-3). The classification into Child A, B or C has never been unambiguous [14]; replacing this by a numerical score as indicated in the legend to Table 7.1-3 is recommended.

While the Child-Pugh classification was designed to select patients for portosystemic surgery, it is increasingly also used to prognosticate liver disease *per se*. Indeed, it has been shown to reliably predict survival in patients with cirrhosis [15], but the overlap between the different studies can be sizable [14]. One of the challenges of modern hepatobiliary surgery is selection of patients with hepatocellular cancer. For this purpose, besides the Child-Pugh classification, the Okuda score is used most frequently [16]. However, both of

Table 7.1-3. The Child-Pugh [13] classification of cirrhotic liver disease. The classification of A, B or C should be abandoned in favor of a numerical score, assigning 1, 2 or 3 to each criterion and summing this up.

	A = 1	B = 2	C = 3
Albumin (g/l)	> 35	30–35	< 30
Bilirubin (µmol/l)	< 35	35–50	> 50
Prothrombin time (sec prolonged)	1–4	4–6	> 6
Ascites	None	Slight	Moderate
Encephalopathy	None	Grade 1–2	Grade 3–4

these scores are mainly useful to exclude patients from surgery but are unable to really predict functional reserve and thereby tolerance of hepatic resection.

For the purpose of predicting functional reserve the so-called quantitative or dynamic liver function tests have been used. They are based on the hepatic clearance principle [17]. In particular Asian groups have demonstrated that such tests – in particular the ICG clearance or retention – are superior to the Child or Okuda classification[18, 19]. A recent study from Berne demonstrated galactose elimination capacity to predict postoperative morbidity and mortality in hepatic resections not only for hepatocellular cancer but also for metastatic liver disease [20]. For an overview of this topic the reader is referred to a recent review [21].

The inexorable loss of liver function as disease progresses is of major interest. We were able to first demonstrate this in animal models of cirrhosis [22]. In this and other studies function could be correlated with stereologically determined hepatocellular mass [23, 24]. A similar evolution of quantitative liver function can also be observed in patients, in particular in primary biliary cirrhosis [25]. Kawasaki *et al.* demonstrated also in patients that the intact cell hypothesis – lying at the base of these observations – is applicable to man [26].

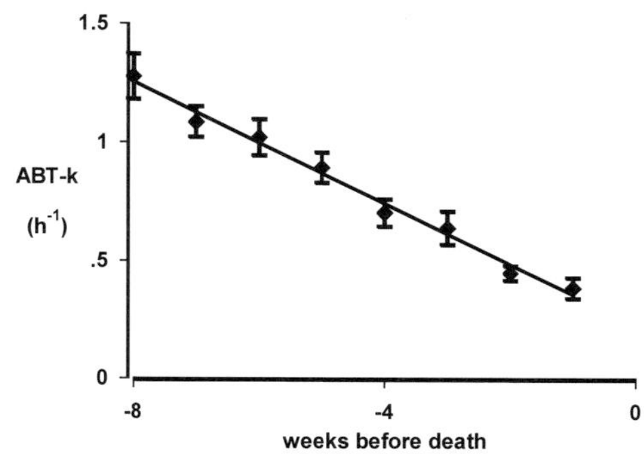

Figure 7.1-1. Decline in microsomal function as measured by the aminopyrine breath test (ABT) in bile duct ligated rats. There is a linear decline in function when calculated backwards from the time of death. Modified from [22] with permission from the publisher.

We believe that this loss of function is related to an exhaustion of the regenerative potential of the liver. Indeed, comparing two models of cirrhosis we were able to show that loss of hepatocyte mass is associated with a lack of nuclear translocation of EGF receptor [27, 28], an early event in initiation of regeneration. In line with this – and extending it to man – Delhaye and colleagues observed a decrease of PCNA expressing cells with increasing Child classification [29].

Acknowledgements

The author acknowledges the support of his research by the Swiss National Foundation for Scientific Research (45349.95 and 63476.00).

References

1. Tilg H, Diehl AM. Mechanisms of disease: Cytokines in alcoholic and nonalcoholic steatohepatitis. N Engl J Med 2000; 343(20): 1467–76.
2. Alvarez C, Nelms C, D'Addio V, Bass BL. The pancreatic duct epithelium in vitro: Bile acid injury and the effect of epidermal growth factor. Surgery 1997; 122(2): 476–83.
3. Jones BA, Gores GJ. Physiology and pathophysiology of apoptosis in epithelial cells of the liver, pancreas, and intestine. Am J Physiol Gastrointest Liver Physiol 1997; 273(6): G1174–88.
4. Hammel P, Couvelard A, O'Toole D, Ratouis A, Sauvanet A, Fléjou JF et al. Regression of liver fibrosis after biliary drainage in patients with chronic pancreatitis and stenosis of the common bile duct. N Engl J Med 2001; 344(6): 418–23.
5. Zimmermann H, Reichen J, Zimmermann A, Sägesser H, Tenisch B, Höflin F. Reversibility of secondary biliary fibrosis by biliodigestive anastomosis in the rat. GE 1992; 103: 579–89.
6. Epstein O, Chapman RWG, Lake-Bakaar G, Foo AY, Rosalki SB, Sherlock S. The pancreas in primary biliary cirrhosis and primary sclerosing cholangitis. GE 1982; 83: 1177–82.
7. Fausa O, Kolmanskog F, Ritland S. The pancreatic ducts in primary biliary cirrhosis and sclerosing cholangitis. Scand J Gastroenterol 1985; 107: 32–5.
8. Kazumori H, Ashizawa N, Moriyama H, Arima N, Hirakawa K, Adachi K et al. Primary sclerosing pancreatitis and cholangitis. Int J Pancreatol 1998; 24(2): 123–7.
9. Ludwig J. New concepts in biliary cirrhosis. Semin Liver Dis 1987; 7: 293–301.
10. Lesur G, Levy P, Flejou JF, Belghiti J, Fekete F, Bernades P. Factors predictive of liver histopathological appearance in chronic alcoholic pancreatitis with common bile duct stenosis and increased serum alkaline phosphatase. Hepatology 1993; 18: 1078–81.
11. Valderrama R, Navarro S, Bruguera M, López JM, Caballería J, Bianchi L et al. Hepatic fibrogenic activity in chronic alcoholic pancreatitis. Pancreas 1999; 19(3): 276–80.
12. Child CG, Turcotte JG. Surgery and portal hypertension. In: Child CG, ed. The liver and portal hypertension. Philadelphia: W. B. Saunders & Co., 1964: 50–1.
13. Pugh RN, Murray-Lyon IM, Dawson JL, Pietroni MC, Williams R. Transection of the esophagus for bleeding esophageal varices. Br J Surg 1973; 60: 646–9.
14. Conn HO. A peek at the Child-Turcotte classification. Hepatology 1981; 1: 673–6.
15. Villeneuve JP, Infante Rivard C, Ampelas M, Pomier-Layrargues G, Huet PM, Marleau D. Prognostic value of the aminopyrine breath test in cirrhotic patients. Hepatology 1986; 6: 928–31.
16. Okuda K, Ohtsuki T, Obata H et al. Natural history of hepatocellular carcinoma and prognosis in relation to treatment. Study of 850 patients. Cancer 1985; 56: 918–28.
17. Reichen J. Assessment of hepatic function with xenobiotics. Semin Liver Dis 1995; 15: 189–201.
18. Matsumata T, Kanematsu T, Yoshida Y, Furuta T, Yanaga K, Sugimachi K. The indocyanine green test enables prediction of postoperative complications after hepatic resection. World J Surg 1987; 11: 678–81.
19. Fan ST, Lai ECS, Lo CM, Ng IOL, Wong J. Hospital mortality of major hepatectomy for hepatocellular carcinoma associated with cirrhosis. Arch Surg 1995; 130(2): 198–203.
20. Redaelli C, Dufour JF, Krähenbühl L, Schilling M, Wagner M, Büchler MW et al. Preoperative Galactose Elimination Capacity predicts Morbidity and Survival after Hepatic Resection. Ann Surg 2001. (in revision.)
21. Zimmermann H, Reichen J. Hepatectomy: Preoperative analysis of hepatic function and postoperative liver failure. Dig Surg 1998; 15(1): 1–11.
22. Gross JB, Reichen J, Zeltner T, Zimmermann A. The evolution of changes in quantitative liver function tests in a rat model of cirrhosis: Correlation with morphometric measurement of hepatocyte mass. Hepatology 1987; 7: 457–63.

23. Reichen J, Arts B, Schafroth U, Zimmermann A, Zeltner TB, Zysset T. Aminopyrine N-demethylation by rats with liver cirrhosis: Evidence for the intact cell hypothesis. A morphometric-functional study. GE 1987; 93: 719–26.
24. Reichen J, Egger B, Ohara N, Zeltner TB, Zysset T, Zimmermann A. Determinants of hepatic functions in liver cirrhosis in the rat: A multivariate analysis. J Clin Invest 1988; 82: 2069–76.
25. Reichen J, Widmer T, Cotting J. Accurate prediction of death by serial determination of the galactose elimination capacity in primary biliary cirrhosis – A comparison with the Mayo model. Hepatology 1991; 14: 504–10.
26. Kawasaki S, Imamura H, Bandai Y, Sanjo K, Idezuki Y. Direct evidence for the intact hepatocyte therory in patients with liver cirrhosis. GE 1992; 102: 1351–5.
27. Oguey D, Marti U, Reichen J. Epidermal growth factor receptor: Its possible implication in the maintenance of hepatocellular mass in biliary cirrhosis in the rat. Eur J Cell Biol 1992; 59: 187–95.
28. Oguey D, Reichen J, Marti U. Differential effect of micronodular and biliary cirrhosis on epidermal growth factor receptor expression in the rat. J Hepatol 1994; 21(6): 997–1005.
29. Delhaye M, Louis H, DeGraef C, Le Moine O, Devière J, Gulbis B et al. Relationship between hepatocyte proliferative activity and liver functional reserve in human cirrhosis. Hepatology 1996; 23: 1003–11.

7.2 The natural history of alcoholic chronic pancreatitis

R. W. Ammann

Abstract

An improved knowledge of the natural history is the indispensable basis for a rational concept in respect of diagnosis, classification, understanding and management of pain in chronic pancreatitis. Unfortunately, data on the natural history of CP are scarce and conflicting. Some relevant observations from our prospective long-term study of a mixed medical-surgical cohort comprising 207 patients with alcoholic CP (mean follow-up 17 years from onset) are summarized. In early-stage CP, episodes of recurrent pancreatitis predominated. Severe persistent pain was typically associated with local complications (mainly postnecrotic cysts in 54%; symptomatic cholestasis in 24%) definitely relieved by a drainage procedure. Lasting pain remission was documented in > 80% of the whole cohort within 10 years from onset in association with marked pancreatic dysfunction. In our experience, relief of "chronic" pain regularly follows selective surgery tailored to the presumptive pain cause or occurs spontaneously in uncomplicated advanced CP (excluding narcotic addiction).

Introduction

Chronic pancreatitis (CP) is characterized clinically by a broad spectrum of variable features depending on many factors such as etiology, stage of the disease process, presence (or absence) of local complications. The large overlap of clinical features in early-stage CP both with pancreatic cancer and recurrent acute pancreatitis is a major diagnostic problem. Particularly, the lack of a standardized definition of "early" CP enhances the controversy on diagnosis, pathogenesis, and treatment of CP in the current literature. An improved knowledge of the natural history of ACP – the "backbone" of the diagnosis in the absence of the gold standard histopathology – could be helpful for resolving these problems. Unfortunately, data on the natural history are scarce and conflicting.

Chronic alcohol abuse is the major etiological factor in CP in industrialized countries, accounting for about 70% of patients [1]. Nevertheless, it has become clear that the development of pancreatitis is not simply due to the amount and type of alcohol consumed. Indeed, only a small proportion of chronic alcoholics (less than 10%) suffer from clinical pancreatitis. A number of individual predisposing factors have been proposed, such as environmental factors, e.g. diet [2, 3], xenobiotics [4], smoking [2, 3, 5] and/or a genetic predisposition, e.g. CF-gene mutations, HLA-antigens, mutations of the trypsinogen gene [2, 6]. This problem is one of the current top research issues but despite a large number of studies, present knowledge is still limited. Interestingly, different risk-cofactors have to be assumed for alcoholic CP and alcoholic liver cirrhosis, since the latter is associated with alcoholic CP in only 2–10% [7, 8].

The diagnosis of CP is readily possible in advanced stages based on pancreatic calcification, steatorrhea and/or diabetes. However, there is no reliable routine method available for early-stage CP because, in contrast to liver biopsy, no comparable diagnostic tool exists for CP. The role of modern imaging techniques, e.g. sonography, endoscopic sonography, ERCP, CT and magnetic resonance pancreatography, for the diagnosis of early-stage CP is debated. Scientific validation of these techniques for detecting minor alterations specific to CP is lacking. Furthermore, a rather large interobserver variation regarding sensitivity and specificity of these methods is observed [9].

Clinically, alcoholic CP (ACP) is a multifaceted disease characterized in most instances chronologically by 2 phases, i) an early stage of recurrent clinical acute pancreatitis and ii) a late stage dominated by steatorrhea, diabetes and pancreatic calcification. Pain is the cardinal (initial) symptom in up to 90% of patients. The typical pain pattern in early-stage ACP corresponds closely to recurrent pancreatitis of other etiology, e.g. biliary pancreatitis with short attacks of variable intensity separated by long asymptomatic periods (months or ≥ one year) [10]. A rather large group of ACP patients experience, mainly in early-stage CP, periods of protracted pain severe enough to warrant surgical intervention (27–67%) [10]. The tactic of surgery (indication) and surgical technique (drainage vs resection) in such situations is debated [11]. Recently, endoscopic procedures and/or lithotripsy for pain relief have been advocated but the value of this new therapeutic option remains to be documented [12]. A major reason for the ongoing controversy regarding the optimal therapy of pain in ACP is the fact that most published series provide insufficient data on the pertinent variables, in particular the clinical pain pattern and its relation to the probable pain cause. Therefore, data from different centers are difficult to compare [10].

In view of the many controversial issues, most experts would probably agree that without an improved knowledge of the natural history, no progress in developing a rational concept of classification of CP and the understanding of the pathomechanisms and management of pain will be achieved. The main purpose of this article is to emphasize some aspects of the natural history of ACP based on the current literature.

Classification of CP

A number of attempts at classification of CP has been made in the past 40 years (see ref [9]) but none of them can identify early-stage CP reliably in comparison with histopathology, the diagnostic gold standard which is rarely available in clinical practice. A clinically based classification system, based on the combination of clinical, functional and morphological criteria, was worked out at the international workshop at Zurich in 1996 [9]. Two categories of ACP are distinguished: a) definite ACP and b) probable ACP (Table 7.2-1). The experts agreed that the final diagnosis should be deferred until the disease has reached the stage of definite ACP. This proposal is not perfect but it eliminates the current confusion due to the many published series comprising a rough mixture of patients with definite CP pooled with ill-defined "CP" such as pancreatic cancer, probable CP etc. Monitoring the long-term course from onset to late-stage ACP, in which a definite diagnosis can be established, is at present a *"conditio sine qua non"* for a rational therapy concept. This goal has not been reached despite > 20 years of clinical research [11]. *Mutatis mutandis*, the terminology may also be applied for non-alcoholic CP.

Table 7.2-1. Diagnostic criteria of alcoholic chronic pancreatitis (ACP) (Classification of Zurich 1996; see ref. [9]).

Note: Clinically 2 forms of ACP are distinguished:

a) Definite ACP and

b) Probable ACP (i.e. initial working diagnosis)

Both forms have the following features in common:

> 1) A typical history of recurrent pancreatitis, except primary painless ACP (which is rare in alcoholics)

> 2) A history of excessive alcohol intake (usually > 80 g/day for some years in males, smaller amounts in females)

a) Definite ACP

One or more of the following criteria establish definite ACP (in addition to the typical history, see above):

- Pancreatic calcification
- Moderate or marked ductal lesions ("Cambridge classification")
- Marked (and persistent) exocrine insufficiency defined as pancreatic steatorrhea, markedly reduced by enzyme supplementation)
- Typical histology of an adequate surgical specimen

b) Probable ACP

This diagnosis is likely based on one or more of the following criteria (in addition to the typical history, see above):

- Mild ductal alterations ("Cambridge classification")
- Recurrent or persistent pseudocysts
- Pathological secretin test
- Endocrine insufficiency i.e. abnormal glucose tolerance test

Etiology is a diagnostic cornerstone in the initial clinical phase characterized usually by acute (recurrent) pancreatitis. It is generally recognized that biliary and alcoholic pancreatitis (in around 80% the 2 major etiological factors) differ in their natural history since biliary in contrast to alcoholic pancreatitis virtually never progresses to CP (Table 7.2-2) [9].

Table 7.2-2. Clinicoetiological categories of recurrent pancreatitis: impact of etiology on course and outcome.

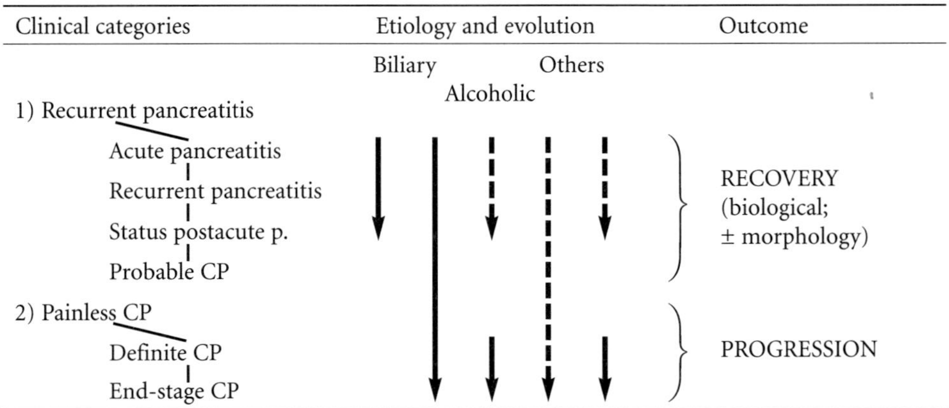

Knowledge of the natural history is of special interest for the following 3 issues:

i) Can the progression of ACP be assessed clinically?
ii) What is the impact of etiology on the course and outcome of CP? and
iii) Is knowledge of the natural history helpful for understanding the pathomechanisms and management of pain? The relevant factors for evaluating the natural history are listed in Table 7.2-3.

Table 7.2-3. The long-term course of CP is defined by:

I Etiology and		
II Clinical Triad		
i) Clinical pattern	}	evolving from onset to end-stage CP
ii) Morphology		
iii) Function		

Can progression of ACP be assessed clinically? or Is exocrine insufficiency a reliable replacement for histopathology?

According to most experts CP is a dynamic evolutive process associated with progressive fibrosis resulting over a period of several years in end-stage disease, i.e. "cirrhosis" of the pancreas. Pancreatic function testing is probably the most reliable routine method for the assessment of progressive glandular atrophy during the evolution of CP. Because of the large secretory capacity, persistent exocrine and endocrine insufficiency develops with a considerable delay during the evolution of CP. The interval between onset of disease and the occurrence of persistent exocrine insufficiency (± calcification) averages 4.8–5.5 years in ACP (see ref. [9]). A close (significant) relationship between fibrosis and pancreatic dysfunction in relation to the duration of ACP from onset has been documented by our group (Fig. 7.2-1 and Fig. 7.2-2) [1]. These studies also have an important impact on the

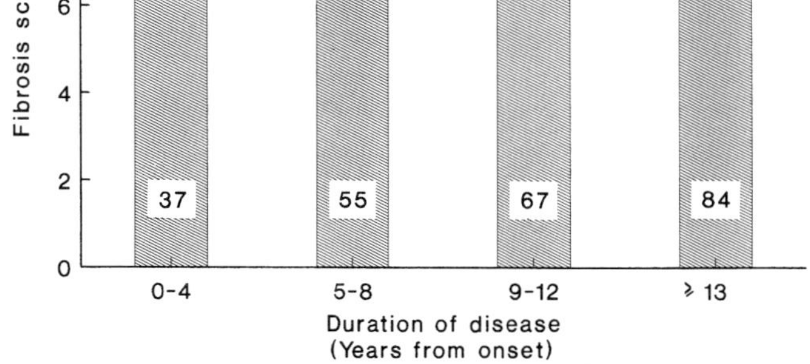

Figure 7.2-1. Evolution of fibrosis (FS; mean ± SEM) in relation to duration of ACP from onset. Numbers in parentheses at the top of the bars are numbers of patients with histology; numbers inside bars are the percentage of patients with calcifications. Figure 7.2-1 reproduced from Ammann *et al.* [1] with kind permission from the publisher.

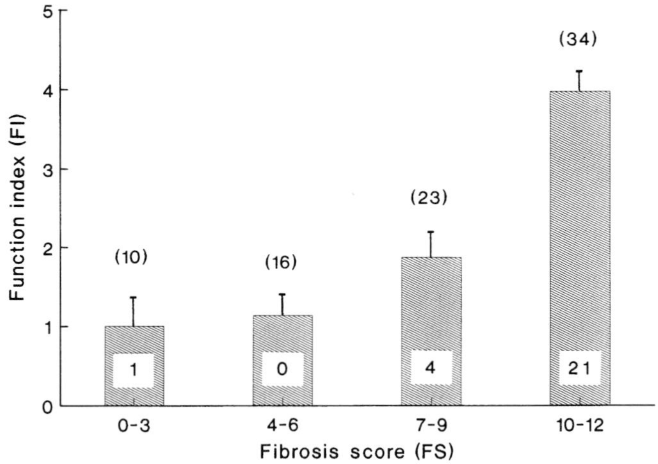

Figure 7.2-2. Relationship between degree of fibrosis and pancreatic dysfunction in ACP (FI; mean ± SEM). Numbers in parentheses at the top are the numbers of patients; numbers inside bars are the numbers of patients with diabetes. The correlation of the two variables (FS and FI) is statistically significant (P = 0.001). Fig. 7.2.-2 reproduced from Ammann *et al.* [1] with kind permission from the publisher.

pathogenetic link between alcoholic acute pancreatitis and ACP, a clinically relevant issue of controversy for the past 40 years [8, 9, 13, 14]. Former studies on the covariation of function and morphology [15] and ERCP [16] respectively in CP are of interest but, in contrast to our study [1], no data were provided of these alterations in relation to the evolution of CP from onset.

Pancreatic function testing has become discredited in recent years and has been abandoned in many Anglo-Saxon centers for the primary reasons that i) the (CCK) secretin test, considered to be the gold standard, is too laborious and invasive and ii) the indirect function tests, e.g. PABA, fecal chymotrypsin test, are not sensitive enough for detection of mild exocrine insufficiency. This line of argument has to be questioned since CP leads to progressive exocrine insufficiency which may be assessed accurately by indirect function tests as shown previously [1, 7,10] (Fig. 7.2-2). It should be noted that staging into early- and late-stage ACP is best based primarily on pancreatic function testing and not on imaging techniques [9] because i) morphologic features such as ductal dilatation do not predict whether or not a patient experiences pain [10] and ii) exocrine insufficiency is the most accurate replacement for histopathology (see above). The new fecal elastase test appears to be more specific (and sensitive) than the fecal chymotrypsin test, primarily because oral enzyme substitution therapy does not affect this test [17]. The impact of exocrine function testing on the pain profile of CP will be discussed below.

The impact of etiology on the natural history of CP

CP can be classified according to the etiology primarily into two main subgroups, alcoholic and non-alcoholic CP (Table 7.2-4). ACP accounts for about 70% of all patients with CP in our series, the rest being etiologically classified as idiopathic (around 24%) or due to rare causes (6%) [7, 10].

Recently, the experts of the Mayo Clinic have shown that idiopathic CP (ICP) comprises, based on the age distribution, 2 subgroups, i) an early-onset and ii) a late-onset ICP. The two subgroups differ in their natural history from each other and from ACP

Table 7.2-4. Etiologic Factors of CP.

I	Alcoholic CP
II	Non-alcoholic CP
	Tropical (nutritional) CP
	Hereditary CP
	Metabolic CP (e.g. hypercalcemia, hypertriglyceridemia)
	Idiopathic CP (ICP)
	> early-onset ("juvenile") type of ICP
	> late-onset ("senile") type of ICP
	"Autoimmune" CP
	CP due to miscellaneous causes, e.g. trauma, postradiation

[18]. These observations corroborate results previously published by our group on "juvenile" (IJCP) and "senile" (ISCP) ICP, first published in 1976 in German (see ref. [19]) and summarized in English [19].

The age distribution of our cohort of ICP is shown in Figure 7.2-3. With the clinical pattern of recurrent pancreatitis starting at a young age, IJCP mimics hereditary CP. However, the former lacks clinical evidence of heredity. Nevertheless a genetic factor seems likely in IJCP. In fact, 16 patients of our group classified as IJCP have been tested recently for trypsinogen gene mutations and 2 of the youngest patients with onset of disease below the age of 10 (Fig. 7.2-3) tested positive (one for R 117H, one for A 16 V) while the rest were negative [20].

Progressive exocrine and endocrine insufficiency are typically observed both in IJCP and ISCP but compared to ACP, pancreatic dysfunction develops with a marked delay in relation to onset of the disease [18, 19]. Furthermore, recurrent episodes of pancreatitis

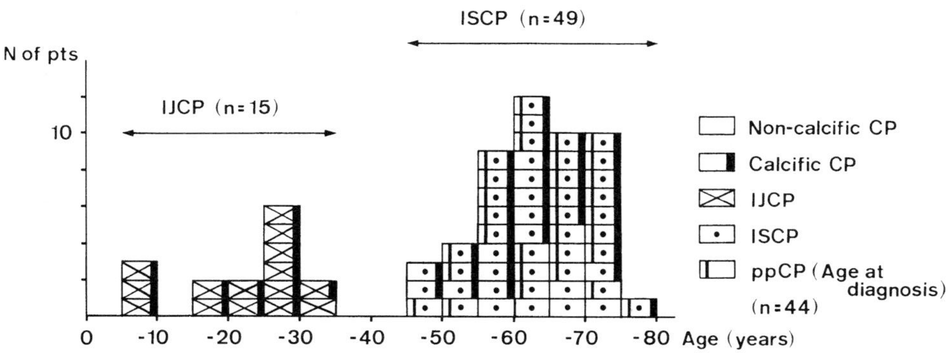

Figure 7.2-3. The bimodal age distribution of patients with idiopathic CP is indicative of two subgroups, an idiopathic juvenile form (IJCP) with a peak age of about 25 years and an idiopathic senile form (ISCP) with a peak around 65 years. *Note:* The two subgroups differ in their natural history from each other and from ACP. Primary painless CP is common in ISCP (about 70%) in contrast to ACP (< 10%) and IJCP (0%). Pancreatic calcification occurs in both subgroups in a high percentage comparable to ACP. Figure 7.2-3 is a modified reproduction from Ammann [19].

occur over a prolonged period of time in IJCP in contrast to ACP and ISCP. The latter exhibits a primary painless course in 50–70% of patients. Differences in natural history between ACP and ICP have to be taken into account and probably explain some disagreement of results, e.g. duration of pain between our ACP and other CP series, the latter including 25–38 % of ICP patients [21].

The relationship between pain and pancreatic (dys-)function in early- and late-stage ACP

In the last 3–4 decades a large amount of conflicting data on pain in CP have been published. This clinically relevant issue has not been resolved mainly because 1) CP (early stage) is not a clinically precisely defined entity, 2) the mechanisms of pain induction in CP are controversial and 3) the long-term evolution of the pain profile from onset to end-stage CP (without and with surgery) is ill-defined.

A distorted pain pattern is often reported in the current literature and in some textbooks as being typical for CP. For instance, it is stated that "ACP is typically associated with chronic truly intractable pain leading to ever-increasing needs of narcotics which can be altered successfully only by surgery in patients who stop alcohol abuse"[21]. This "horror-scenario" is inaccurate and misleading.

The long-term pain profile in ACP has been characterized recently in a large mixed medical-surgical cohort observed prospectively for an average of 17 years [10]. Two typical pain patterns based on frequency, duration and intensity were distinguished (Fig. 7.2-4). Of a total of 207 patients, all started with recurrent attacks of clinical acute pancreatitis (A-type pain), 91 of them (44%) never experienced chronic severe pain (non-surgical series). In 116 patients (56%) with prolonged periods of severe B-type pain, interspersed between attacks of A-type pain, surgical intervention became necessary (surgical series). Some of the latter group experienced postoperative pain recurrences (n = 69). A second operation for B-type pain recurrence became necessary in 39 patients. No second operation was necessary in the remaining 26 patients with recurrence of A-type pain. The 3 main causes of B-type pain (first and second operation; n = 155) were pseudocysts

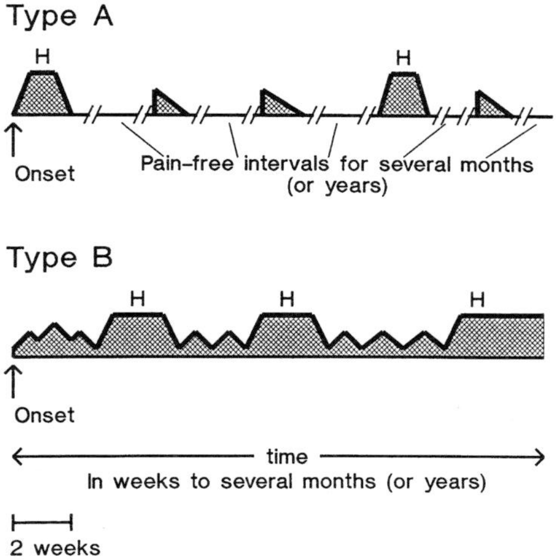

Figure 7.2-4. Two typical pain patterns can be distinguished in ACP according to a clinically based staging system; A-type pain, which corresponds to clinical acute (recurrent) pancreatitis, shows typically short pain attacks lasting less than 7 days and long pain-free intervals of several months (or ≥ 1 year). The intensity of A-type pain may be severe (with need of hospitalization: = H).
B-type pain is characterized by prolonged periods of unremitting pain usually for > 2 months with need of repeated hospitalizations (= H). Figure 7.2-4 reproduced from Ammann *et al.* [10] with kind permission from the publisher.

(n = 84; 54 %), obstructive cholestasis (n = 37; 24%) and presumptive ductal hypertension (n = 21; 14%). Prompt relief of B-type pain was achieved by surgical correction of the complication, usually a drainage procedure. The second operation for B-type recurrence (in about 50% due to cholestasis) became necessary 5.5 to 7 years after the first operation, typically in late-stage ACP.

Pain episodes of A- or B-type pain occurred predominately in early-stage ACP and the duration of the initial phase of pain from onset to pain relief (i.e. no pain for at least 2 years) averaged 5.5 years in both the non-surgical and the surgical series. Interesting and of major clinical relevance is the fact that lasting complete pain remission was documented in late-stage ACP over a period of about 11 years both in the non-surgical (n = 91)and surgical series with one operation (n = 77) and for about 7 years in the subgroup with two surgical interventions [10]. Thus, our observations on lasting pain relief in late-stage ACP differ distinctly from the "horror scenario" of pain [21].

Over 80% of patients got lasting pain relief within 10 years from onset of disease in both the non-surgical and the surgical series (Fig. 7.2-5). The close relationship between pain relief and pancreatic exocrine insufficiency (Fig. 7.2-6) corroborates the "burnout" hypothesis first reported in 1970 by our group and evaluated prospectively since (see ref. [1]). Forty years ago, Gambill *et al.* reported that in the long-term study of the Mayo Clinic about 80% of 48 CP patients treated surgically got partial or complete pain relief for an average of 13.8 years [22]. Forty-one of the 48 patients had a biliary drainage procedure suggesting that pain relief followed biliary surgery. This conclusion was already questioned in the discussion of the paper at the AGA meeting in 1960 [22]. The permanent pain relief observed in our series in over 80% within 10 years is in accordance with Gambill. However, in contrast to the latter experts, pain relief was closely related with marked exocrine insufficiency, an observation confirmed by Girdwood et al. in 1981 [23]. This topic is still controversial and requires further investigations. In 1977 a multicenter study of the problem was started with 2 German centers but unfortunately the trial ended when one center discontinued collaboration in 1982.

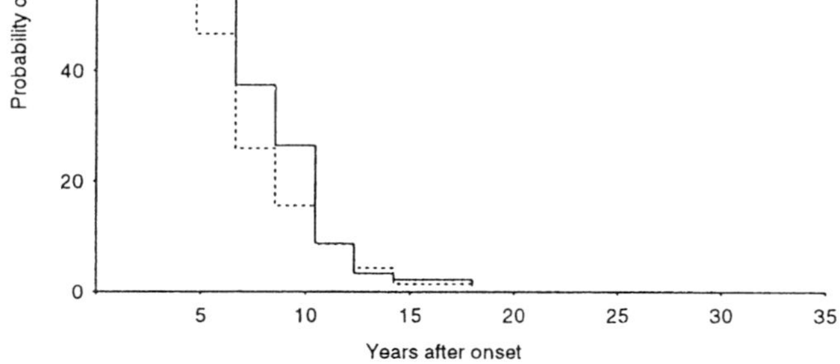

Figure 7.2-5. Probability of remaining free from pain recurrences for non-surgical (—) and surgical (....) patients. *Note:* Both subgroups got lasting pain relief in > 80% within 10 years from onset of ACP (Fig. reproduced from Ammann *et al.* [10] with kind permission from the publisher).

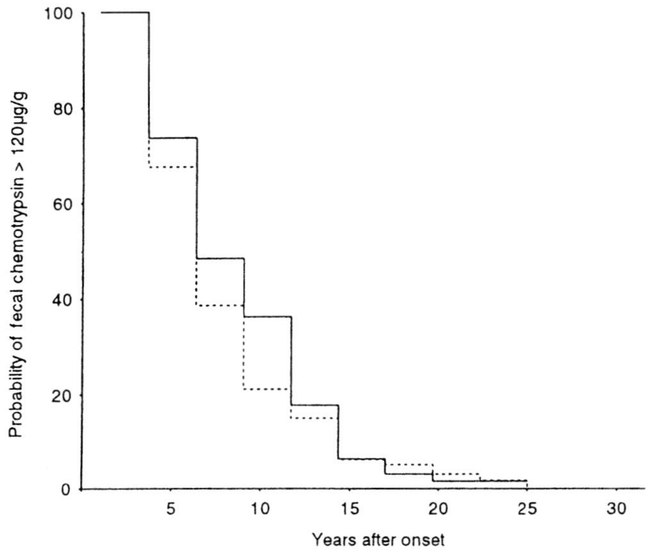

Figure 7.2-6. Probability of remaining free of exocrine insufficiency for non-surgical (—) and surgical (……) patients. A fecal chymotrypsin value < 120 μg/g is indicative of exocrine insufficiency. *Note:* About 80% of patients of both subgroups developed exocrine insufficiency within 10 years from onset of ACP, which, in combination with the data in Figure 7.2-5, is supporting evidence for the "burn-out" thesis of ACP (see text). Figure 7.2-6 reproduced from Ammann et al. [10] with kind permission from the publisher.

The tactic of our center in the management of pain may be summarized as follows:

1. Episodes of clinical acute pancreatitis (A-type pain) are treated conservatively according to the rules for acute pancreatitis (Fig. 7.2-7). This approach is also indicated for postoperative A-type pain episodes.
2. Severe persistent pain (B-type pain) is best managed by surgical correction of the underlying local complication i.e. usually a drainage procedure (Fig. 7.2-8).
3. Prevention of A-type pain recurrence is not a surgical but a medical problem and implies in uncomplicated early-stage ACP primarily alcohol abstinence, which succeeds in preventing A-type pain recurrences in most instances [24]. Lasting pain relief will occur in unreformed alcoholics in uncomplicated late-stage ACP ("burned-out" ACP).

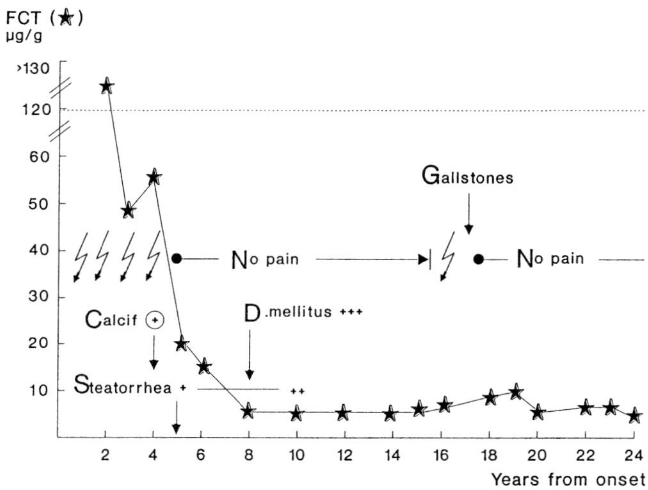

Figure 7.2-7. Typical example of the long-term course of a patient with ACP (non-surgical series) who got lasting pain relief despite continued alcohol abuse following 4 severe episodes of clinical acute pancreatitis in the first 4–5 years from onset. Lasting pain relief was associated with marked exocrine insufficiency, steatorrhea, calcification (and later diabetes), 5 years from onset of ACP.

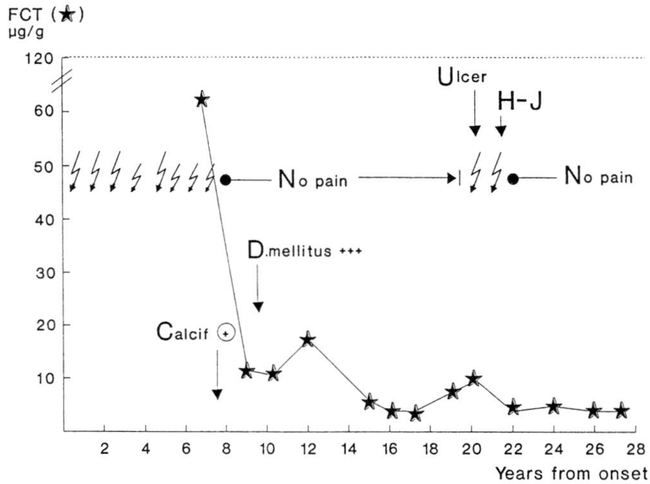

Figure 7.2-8. Typical example of the long-term course of a patient with ACP (surgical series) who suffered initially for about 8 years of recurrent episodes of clinical acute pancreatitis. The patient got pain-free 8 years from onset of ACP (despite continued alcohol abuse) in association with marked exocrine insufficiency, diabetes and calcification. Pain recurred, however, 18 years from onset in association with a peptic ulcer (healed medically) and symptomatic cholestasis. Prompt and lasting pain relief was achieved by a hepaticojejunostomy (H–J) with a postoperative follow-up of 13 years.

Note: these rules cannot be applied to patients with narcotic addiction (i.e. a psychiatric problem) or in ACP with pain of extrapancreatic origin or due to pancreatic cancer (in some CP series in up to 15%) [11].

Impact of alcohol, smoking and additional factors on course and outcome of ACP

There are a number of additional factors which may influence quantity (survival) and quality of life in ACP, in particular chronic alcohol abuse, smoking and narcotic addiction. The average survival of ACP patients 15–20 years from onset is 50% and most of them die at a mean age of 54 years [1, 25]. Mortality is not directly related to ACP and its complications in about 80% of patients [1, 8, 18, 25]; the most common causes of death are heavy smoking (e.g. extrapancreatic malignancy, cardio-vascular or sudden death) and/or alcohol abuse (i.e. severe infections, non-pancreatic surgery, gastrointestinal hemorrhage, suicide or hepatic disease) [7]. As shown recently, alcohol abuse plays an important role after onset of ACP in respect of mortality and invalidity, since both are increased by a factor of about 3 in ACP patients with continued alcohol abuse compared to those with reduced or discontinued alcohol intake [10].

Smoking has been proposed as an additional risk factor in the pathogenesis of CP. The assessment of the relative importance of smoking is difficult, mainly because alcohol abuse and heavy smoking are closely associated in ACP (in 95% in our series). In a controlled prospective study of 100 chronic alcoholics, half of them with pancreatitis, the other half without pancreatic disease, Haber et al. found no statistical difference in the 2 subgroups with regard to smoking [2]. The issue remains highly controversial [4, 59]. On

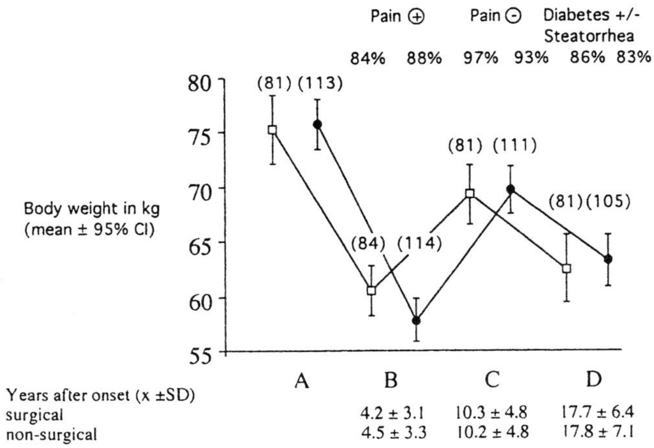

Figure 7.2-9. Changes of body weight from onset (A) to final weight (D; at end of follow-up) in ACP-patients without (□) or with surgery (●). A marked weight loss is observed in both subgroups initially related to pain (A to B). In association with pain relief in late-stage ACP, both subgroups show a distinct gain of weight (B to C) but in association with diabetes and/or steatorrhea, the weight curves turn down in both subgroups (C to D). There was no significant difference in weight between the surgical and non-surgical series at any stage of the disease. Figure 7.2-9 reproduced from Ammann *et al.* [10] with kind permission from the publisher.

the other hand, about 5% of CP patients develop pancreatic cancer about 20 years from onset and smoking plays an important role in this condition [25]. One should, however, note that most ACP patients do not have such a long survival. Furthermore, the rate of pancreatic to extrapancreatic cancer was 3:18 in 173 patients with ACP and 4:7 in 72 patients with non-alcoholic CP [7].

Maintenance or gain of weight is one parameter which reflects quality of life in ACP. It is often postulated that weight gain is a reliable criterion to document pain-relieving surgery. According to our experience, the curve of the body weight in ACP is bimodal, irrespective of surgery, with a first phase of weight loss in early-stage ACP, probably related to pain. A marked weight gain is typically observed in late-stage ACP, followed by a second phase of weight loss in advanced ACP probably due to steatorrhea and/or diabetes (Fig. 7.2-9) [10].

The impact of the ill-defined predisposing factors (environmental and/or genetic) on the long-term course of ACP needs further investigation [20].

Acknowledgement

The work of the Zurich Pancreatitis Study Group was supported by the Amélie Waring Foundation, CH-Zürich (see ref [10]).

References

1. Ammann RW, Heitz PhU, Klöppel G. Course of alcoholic chronic pancreatitis: a prospective clinico-morphological long-term study. Gastroenterology 1996; 111: 224–31.
2. Haber P, Wilson J, Apte M, Korsten M, Pirola R. Individual susceptibility to alcoholic pancreatitis: still an enigma. J Lab Clin Med 1995; 125: 305–12.

3. Levy P, Mathurin P, Roqueplo A, Rueff B, Bernardes P. A multidimensional case-control study of dietary, alcohol and tobacco habits in alcoholic men with chronic pancreatitis. Pancreas 1995; 10: 231–8.
4. Braganza JM. A framework for the aetiogenesis of chronic pancreatitis. Digestion 1998; 59: 1–12.
5. Lin Y, Tamakoshi A, Hayakawa T, Ogawa M, Ohno Y et al. Cigarette smoking as a risk factor for chronic pancreatitis. Pancreas 2000; 21: 109–14.
6. Whitcomb DC, Cohn JA, Ulrich CD. Inherited Diseases of the Pancreas. Med Clin N Am 2000; 84, May issue.
7. Ammann RW, Akovbiantz A, Largiader F, Schueler G. Course and outcome of chronic pancreatitis. Gastroenterology 1984; 86: 820–8.
8. Bank S. Chronic pancreatitis: clinical features and medical management. Am J Gastroenterol 1986; 81: 153–67.
9. Ammann RW and symposium participants. A clinically based classification system for alcoholic chronic pancreatitis: Summary of the International Workshop in Zurich 1996 (Conference report). Pancreas 1997; 14: 215–21.
10. Ammann RW, Muellhaupt B and Zurich Pancreatitis Study Group. The natural history of pain in alcoholic chronic pancreatitis. Gastroenterology 1999; 116: 1132–40.
11. Warshaw AL, Banks PA, Fernandez-del Castillo C. Treatment of pain in chronic pancreatitis. AGA Technical Review. Gastroenterology 1998; 115: 765–76.
12. DiMagno EP. Toward understanding (and management) of painful chronic pancreatitis. Gastroenterology 1999; 116: 1252–7 (editorial).
13. Sarles H, Bernard JP, Gullo L. Pathogenesis of chronic pancreatitis. Gut 1990; 31: 629–32.
14. Whitcomb DC. Hereditary pancreatitis: new insights into acute and chronic pancreatitis. Gut 1999; 45: 317–22.
15. Hayakawa T, Kondo T, Shibata T, Noda A, Suzuki T, Nakano S. Relationship between pancreatic exocrine function and histological changes in chronic pancreatitis. Amer J Gastroenterol 1992; 87: 1170–4.
16. Nagata A, Homma T, Oguchi H, Tamura Y, Hirabayashi H et al. Study of chronic alcoholic pancreatitis by means of serial pancreozymin-secretin tests. Digestion 1986; 33: 135–45.
17. Löser C, Möllgaard A, Fölsch UR. Faecal elatase 1; a novel, highly sensitive, and specific pancreatic function test. Gut 1996; 39: 580–6.
18. Layer P, Yamamoto H, Kalthoff L, Clain JE, Bakken LJ, DiMagno EP. The different courses of early- and late-onset idiopathic and alcoholic chronic pancreatitis. Gastroenterology 1994; 107: 1481–7.
19. Ammann RW. Alcohol- and non-alcohol-induced pancreatitis: clinical aspects. In: Burns GP, Bank S, eds. Disorders of the Pancreas. New York: McGraw-Hill, Inc, 1992: 253–72.
20. Truninger K, Köck J, Wirth HP, Muellhaupt B, Arnold C et al. Trypsinogen gene mutations in patients with chronic or recurrent acute pancreatitis. Pancreas 2001; 22: 18–23.
21. Blackstone MO, Ammann RW. Pain in alcoholic chronic pancreatitis. Gastroenterology 1999; 117: 1026–8 (Letter to editor).
22. Gambill EE, Baggenstoss AH, Priestley JT. Chronic relapsing pancreatitis. Fate of 56 patients first encountered in the years 1939 to 1943 inclusive. Gastroenterology 1960; 39: 404–11.
23. Girdwood AH, Marks IN, Bornman PC, Kottler RE, Cohen M. Does progressive pancreatic insufficiency limit pain in calcific pancreatitis with duct stricture or continued alcohol insult? Clin Gastroenterol 1981; 3: 241–5.
24. Strum WB. Abstinence in alcoholic chronic pancreatitis. Effect on pain and outcome. J Clin Gastroenterol 1995; 20: 37–41.
25. Lowenfels A, Maisonneuve P, Cavallini G, Ammann RW, Lankisch P et al. Prognosis of chronic pancreatitis: an international multicenter study. Am J Gastroenterol 1994; 89: 1467–71.

7.3 Natural history of idiopathic chronic pancreatitis

G. G. Tsiotos

Introduction

In the past, chronic pancreatitis (CP) was considered to be almost exclusively associated with overconsumption of alcohol (alcoholic chronic pancreatitis – ACP). During the past two decades idiopathic chronic pancreatitis (ICP) was recognized as a new entity. This was identified as CP with all its classical features, which was not associated to any alcohol intake. Thus, until very recently, CP was considered to be either ACP in about 70% to 90% of the time, or ICP in the remaining 10–30%. However, this convenient scheme has been challenged based on last decade's findings.

Until the early 1990s, all patients with non-ACP were automatically labeled as having ICP. Within this group however, there have been recognized several other conditions predisposing to or causing CP. Among them, more common and conceptually more important is the cystic fibrosis gene mutation (CFTR mutation – Cystic Fibrosis Transmembrane Regulator gene), which is now recognized in 25–48% of patients who were previously considered as having ICP [1–5]. About 15% of patients with "ICP" are now recognized as suffering from sphincter of Oddi dysfunction – type 1 (SOD-1). Another 5% have autoimmune CP, 1–5% hereditary CP [6], and about 1% pancreas divisum. Thus, from the initial 10–30% of patients with "ICP", there remains only 25–30% of these patients with *true ICP*. Consequently, from the whole group of patients with CP, *only 3–9% are recognized today as truly having ICP.*

In addition to some very crucial terminology problems, which seriously affect the understanding of both ACP and ICP (see later), there have been yet other, even more exciting new epidemiologic findings, which altogether put the understanding of ICP and, for that matter, of CP as a whole into a totally new perspective [23–25]. Based on modern analysis, *it now seems that CP may be just two distinct forms of ICP (early-onset ICP and late-onset ICP), and the expression of one of them (late-onset ICP) depends a lot on environmental factors, such as alcohol intake or, to a lesser extent, smoking.* Thus, a deep and thorough understanding of ICP is of paramount importance for the appropriate, modern understanding of CP.

Terminology

The term "idiopathic chronic pancreatitis" was first introduced in the literature in 1976, when Rudolph Ammann identified a distinct group of older patients with all the clinical, biochemical, and imaging features of CP, with no history of alcohol intake whatsoever; for this subgroup he coined the term "senile chronic pancreatitis" [20]. After the introduction of this revolutionary concept, the pancreatic literature and the understanding of ACP and ICP has been hampered by one very important factor: *the lack of a universally accepted level of daily alcohol intake* above which patients are considered as having ACP. This issue, although seemingly trivial, is in fact crucial. Based on various studies, patients are categorized in the ACP group if they consume more than 80 grams of alcohol daily [7, 8], or more than 50 grams [9], or 2 liters of beer [7], or if they simply have a "history of frequent and high alcohol intake". The implications are obvious: for example a patient whose daily alcohol intake is 60 grams will be included in the ACP group by some authors [9], but in the ICP by others [7, 8]. Similarly, a patient with 1.5 liters of daily beer consumption for several years would be included in the ICP group [7] despite the fact that very few clinicians would deny that this patient has ACP. This proves the inherent inability to draw definitive and reliable conclusions from the literature, as well as to compare the results of the various studies on common grounds, since different kinds of patients may be under the same "label" in different studies.

In summary, today two new factors have emerged in the understanding of ICP. First, genetic factors are increasingly recognized as causes of "ICP", and second, it is very hard to make an absolute distinction between ACP and ICP in the literature and consequently to study them in comparison. With these provisions in mind, this chapter will discuss the natural history of ICP and this will be compared to that of ACP. The natural history will be analyzed based on the presentation (symptoms, signs, demographics), development of pancreatic calcifications, exocrine and endocrine pancreatic insufficiency, development of pancreatic cancer and other complications, and finally survival.

Idiopathic chronic pancreatitis

As previously mentioned, there is a lot of "flexibility" as to the criteria on which patients are included in the ICP or the ACP group. Using the arbitrary level of 80 grams of daily alcohol intake (equivalent to one bottle of wine or six bottles of beer) allows the inclusion of patients with daily intake of i.e. half a bottle of wine or four bottles of beer for many years in the ICP group, although it may be clinically obvious that this is not right [21]. This leads to artificial increase of the subgroup of patients with ICP, due to the inclusion of patients with considerable daily alcohol intake, not enough though to formally include them in the ACP subgroup. Even worse, the observations and conclusions on the different natural histories of ACP and ICP cannot be relied upon. This is a very big problem in the pancreatic literature and there has been unfortunately only one clinical study in which it has been solved and thus its results are considered reliable [9]. This study from the Mayo Clinic, because of its very strict methodological criteria, is considered up to the present time as the only one that describes reliably and accurately the natural history of ICP and ACP and their differences. Because of its importance, it will be presented in detail.

The authors studied 448 patients with CP managed at the Mayo Clinic between 1976 and 1982. Patients with daily alcohol intake higher than 50 grams were considered as having ACP; their number was 249. Obviously, if the level used was 80 grams, the number of patients with ACP would have been lower and the number of patients with ICP would have been much higher. For patients to be included in the ICP group, they had to have *no alcohol intake at all*; their number was 66. Patients with daily alcohol intake lower than 50 grams, those in whom it was uncertain whether they consumed any alcohol, and those who had other known causes of CP (i.e.: hereditary CP, SOD-1, autoimmune CP, pancreas divisum) were excluded from the study altogether; their number was 133, or 30% of the initial group. It is interesting and revealing to note that these 133 totally excluded patients would have comprised two thirds of all patients included in the ICP group based on the criteria of all other studies. Thus, by applying these strict methodology criteria, one can create "clean" subgroups, so their comparison can be reliable. Mean duration of observation was 18.1 years for the ICP subgroup and 14.6 years for the ACP subgroup.

Presentation of ICP and ACP

Analysis of the 66 patients with ICP demonstrated a bimodal age distribution (Fig. 7.3-1A). If these patients are grouped as younger and older than 35 years, then two distinct subgroups clearly emerge: patients with *early-onset ICP* (median age at presentation: 19.2 years) and patients with *late-onset ICP* (median age at presentation: 56.2 years). In ACP median age at presentation was 43.9 years, between, that is, early-onset and late-onset ICP (Fig. 7.3-1B). Sex distribution, although equal in early-onset and late-onset ICP (men: 44% and 56% respectively), was not so in ACP, which was far more frequent among men (72%, $p < 0.001$).

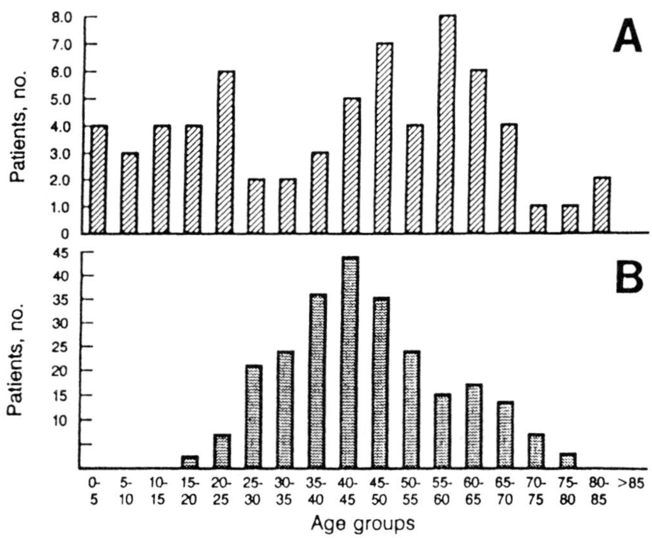

Figure 7.3-1A, B. Age distribution of patients with ICP (**A**) and ACP (**B**). Note the bimodal pattern of age distribution in ICP, which forms the basis for distinction between early-onset ICP and late-onset ICP. Median age at onset of ACP is higher than early-onset ICP, but lower than late-onset ICP. Reprinted from Gastroenterology 1994; 107: 1481–1487.

Development and evolution of abdominal pain

Abdominal pain, as a *presenting* symptom, was much more common in patients with early-onset ICP (96%) compared to late-onset ICP (54%, $p = 0.0005$), or ACP (77%, $p = 0.003$). Again, one can see that ACP "lies between" early-onset and late-onset ICP, a feature that will be observed again repeatedly later. Similarly, severity of pain was higher in early-onset ICP than late-onset ICP ($p = 0.001$), or ACP ($p = 0.04$). Interestingly, both the frequency of pain as a presenting symptom, and its severity prove to be quite similar in late-onset ICP and ACP. Over time, pain was improved in all groups. In early-onset ICP, late-onset ICP, and ACP pain improved or disappeared in 67%, 64% and 77% of patients respectively and became worse only in 8%, 18%, and 7% respectively. The course of pain did not correlate with development of pancreatic calcifications or pancreatic insufficiency.

Development of pancreatic calcifications

Parenchymal and ductal calcifications generally develop later in both early- and late-onset ICP than in ACP (Fig. 7.3-2). Median time for development of calcifications since the onset of symptoms was 24.9 years in early-onset ICP, 19.4 years for late-onset ICP, and only 8.7 years for ACP. Here we can see that ACP behaves as the "worse" form of CP, since calcifications develop a decade earlier than in late-onset ICP, in which in turn they develop five years earlier than early-onset ICP.

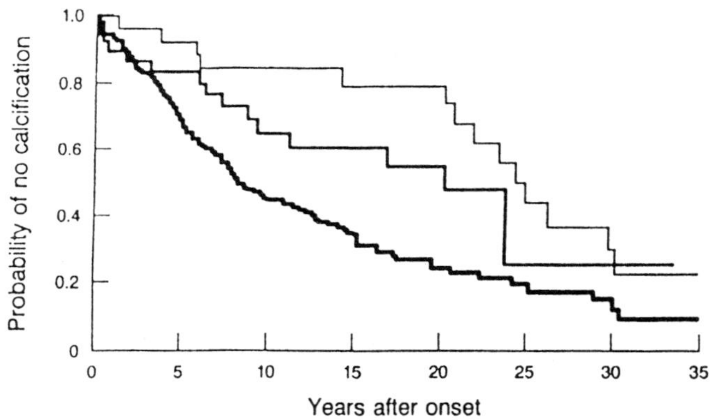

Figure 7.3-2. Probability of remaining free of pancreatic calcifications for patients with early-onset ICP (top curve), late-onset ICP (middle curve), and ACP (lower curve). Reprinted from Gastroenterology 1994; 107: 1481–1487.

Exocrine pancreatic insufficiency

Precisely the same pattern is present here as well (Fig. 7.3-3). Median time for development of exocrine insufficiency since the onset of symptoms was 26.3 years in early-onset ICP, 16.9 years for late-onset ICP, and 13.1 years for ACP. Here ACP proves "worse" than late-onset ICP by four years, which in turn proves "worse" than early-onset ICP by a decade.

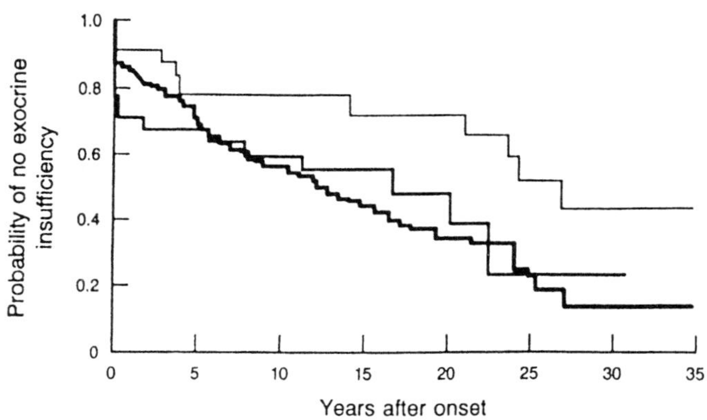

Figure 7.3-3. Probability of remaining free of exocrine insufficiency for patients with early-onset ICP (top curve), late-onset ICP (middle curve), and ACP (lower curve). Reprinted from Gastroenterology 1994; 107: 1481–1487.

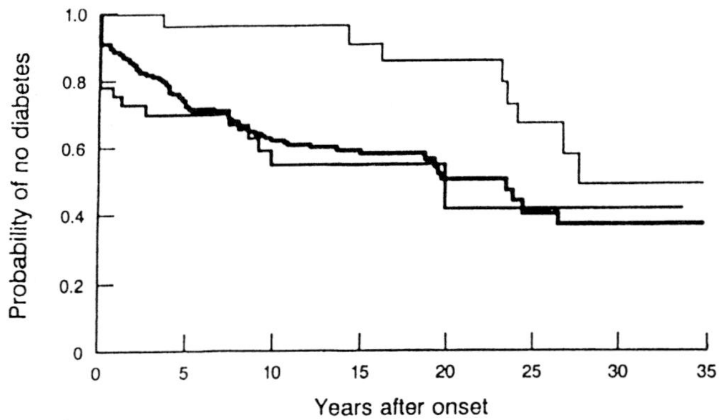

Figure 7.3-4. Probability of remaining free of diabetes mellitus for patients with early-onset ICP (top curve), late-onset ICP (lower curve), and ACP (middle curve). Reprinted from Gastroenterology 1994; 107: 1481–1487.

Endocrine pancreatic insufficiency

Median time for development of diabetes mellitus since the diagnosis of CP was 27.5 years in early-onset ICP, 11.9 years for late-onset ICP, and 19.8 years for ACP (Fig. 7.3-4). Diabetes was never a presenting feature in early-onset ICP, as opposed to late-onset ICP (22% of patients) and ACP (8% of patients).

Other complications – Need for surgery

Complications, such as pancreatic pseudocysts, abscesses or fistulae and jaundice due to an inflammatory pancreatic head mass are more common in ACP. Although such complications occurred in 20% and 27% of patients with early- and late-onset ICP respectively, they were manifested in 43% in patients with ACP. These particular complications required operative treatment in 50–65% of the patients and this was similar among the three groups. Overall however, more patients with early-onset ICP required operative treatment than with late-onset ICP (60% versus 32%). Median time between development of symptoms and need for operative treatment was 21.9 years in early-onset ICP, 20.6 years in late-onset ICP, and 18.8 years in ACP. Incapacitating pain was by far the most common indication for operative treatment, similar in all three groups: 100% in early-onset ICP, 85% in late-onset ICP, and 80% in ACP.

Survival and development of cancer

Overall, survival was longer for patients with ICP (80 years) than for those with ACP (72 years). During the period of observation mortality was 24% in patients with ICP (16 of 66 patients) and 29% in those with ACP (72 of 249 patients). Cause of death in patients with ICP was: pancreatic cancer (13%), nonpancreatic cancer (31%), cardiovascular complications (13%), and complications directly related to CP (13%). Cause of death in patients with ACP was: pancreatic cancer (10%), nonpancreatic cancer (13%), cardiovascular complications (18%), and complications directly related to CP (14%). These observations are similar to those in other studies on the natural history of CP [7, 11, 13, 16].

Development of pancreatic cancer in patients with CP is of particular interest. Empirically, pancreatic cancer was observed to occur more commonly among patients with a history of CP. In addition to the findings presented above, this relation was proved by a large, multicentric epidemiologic study which included more than 1500 patients with CP of all etiologies who were followed for many years and determined the risk of development of pancreatic cancer at 2% per decade [18]. This is of particular importance to pancreatic surgeons and pancreatologists alike when they are faced with patients with a mass in the head of the pancreas in whom absolute differentiation between CP and pancreatic cancer cannot be made based on the usual clinical and imaging criteria. It is then reasonable for such patients to be managed as having pancreatic cancer and submitted to pancreatoduodenectomy, since even if they may not prove to have it at that particular moment they carry a much higher risk of developing it in the near future [19].

Summary

By applying strict criteria (as discussed earlier), two forms of ICP emerge: early-onset ICP and late-onset ICP, with definite and different characteristics. Compared to ACP, ICP (in general) has equal sex distribution and is associated less with pancreatic calcifications, exocrine insufficiency, and other complications. Thus, *ICP presents as a milder form of CP* compared to ACP. Comparing early-onset ICP and late-onset ICP, it seems that the former is associated more often with severe pain, but with less calcifications, exocrine and endocrine insufficiency than the latter. Thus, *early-onset ICP presents as milder than late-onset ICP*. Based on this analysis, the following pattern seems to emerge: *early-onset ICP is milder than late-onset ICP, which in turn is milder than ACP.* At the same time, there seem to be a lot of similarities between late-onset ICP and ACP. Although early-onset ICP seems to be a distinctly unique entity (probably related to certain gene mutation(s), which are clinically expressed at a young age), late-onset ICP and ACP seem to be more similar than different. All the characteristics of ACP are similar to those of late-onset ICP, only they are manifested either a little earlier or a little worse.

Novel concepts

These observations lead to the hypothesis that there may be some (yet unknown) genetic predisposition to the development of late-onset ICP, which can be accelerated or deteriorated by an environmental factor such as alcohol. This would very well explain the widely known fact that only a slim minority of alcoholics develop ACP as opposed to alcoholic liver cirrhosis for example, which is prevalent in the majority of alcoholics. Thus, alcohol may not be the sole cause of ACP, but rather an accelerating factor in a process that may in fact be already set in motion and would otherwise be manifested much later. At the same time there has been evidence of pancreatic histologic changes compatible with early chronic pancreatitis in autopsies of elderly people who died from other causes and with no history of alcohol intake whatsoever [22].

All this evidence led the same Mayo Clinic group [23] to look again into their data, but this time include also those patients with moderate alcohol intake (< 50 grams daily) who were excluded from the first study. If the hypothesis stated previously were correct then this subgroup with moderate alcohol intake would have a form of CP milder than ACP (> 50 grams daily alcohol), but worse than late-onset ICP (no alcohol at all), or, in other words they would have slower progression of disease than ACP, but faster than late-onset ICP. Patients with uncertain alcohol consumption were again excluded. The authors determined whether there were different rates of developing calcification, exocrine or endocrine insufficiency, pain and complications. More importantly, in this study they specifically investigated the hypothesis that an increasing intake of alcohol accelerates the course of CP by separately comparing results among these three groups.

Median age of patients at onset was: 19 years for early-onset ICP, 56 years for late-onset ICP, 53 years for alcohol < 50 g/day, and 44 years for alcohol > 50 g/day. An increasing alcohol intake from zero (late-onset ICP and no alcohol) to less than 50 grams daily to 50 grams or more was associated with earlier inception of disease ($p < 0.001$; Fig. 7.3-5A). The frequency of pain as a presenting symptom increased as alcohol intake increased from zero (late-onset ICP and no alcohol) to < 50 grams daily to > 50 grams ($p = 0.005$; Fig. 7.3-5B). Severity of pain increased similarly ($p = 0.001$; Fig. 7.3-5C). The overall frequency of calcification was significantly associated with alcohol intake. As alcohol intake increased from zero (late-onset ICP and no alcohol) to < 50 grams daily to > 50 grams, more patients developed calcification (37%, 42%, and 59% respectively; $p = 0.004$; Fig. 7.3-5D). However, level of alcohol consumption was not associated to the development of either exocrine or endocrine pancreatic insufficiency. The overall frequency of other complications (i.e.: pseudocysts, abscesses, fistulae, jaundice) was also significantly associated with alcohol intake. As alcohol intake increased from zero (late-onset ICP and no alcohol) to < 50 grams daily to > 50 grams, more patients developed calcification (29%, 39%, and 52% respectively; $p = 0.009$; Fig. 7.5-5E). In addition, sur-

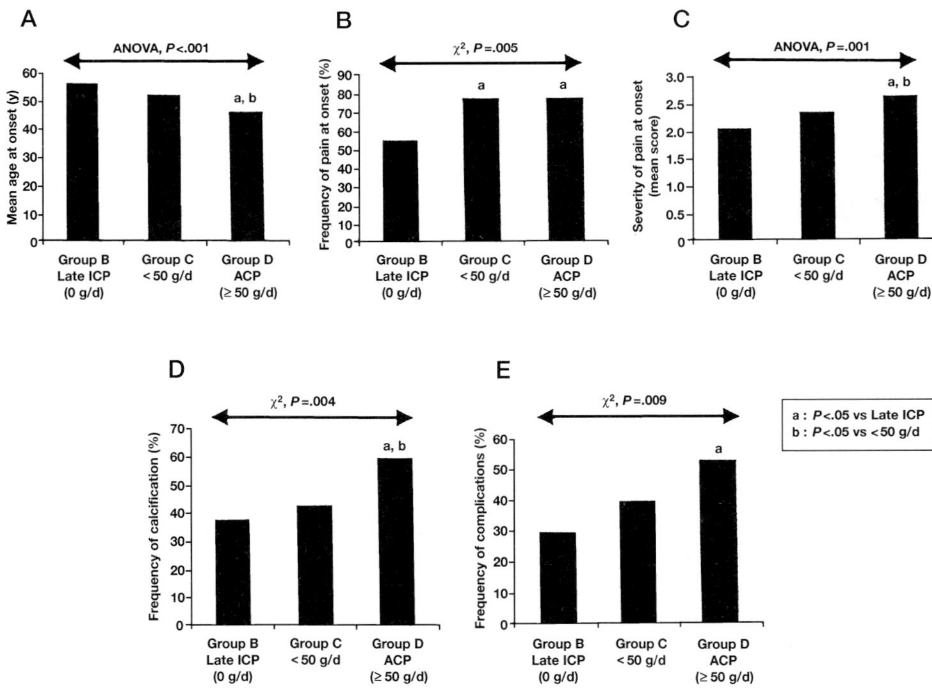

Figure 7.3-5A–E. **A:** Mean age at onset among patients with late onset ICP: group B, no alcohol; group C, less than 50 grams of alcohol daily; and group D, 50 grams or more of alcohol daily (ACP). ANOVA: analysis of variance. **B:** Frequency of pain at onset among groups B, C, and D. **C:** Severity of pain at onset among groups B, C, and D. **D:** Frequency of developing calcifications among groups B, C, and D. **E:** Frequency of developing complications among groups B, C, and D.

vival was significantly associated with the level of alcohol intake; earlier death was associated with larger amounts of alcohol intake. Survival was significantly longer in patients with late-onset ICP and no alcohol intake (81 years) than in those with < 50 grams daily (79 years), in whom it was significantly longer than in those with > 50 grams (72 years) ($p < 0.05$).

This data suggests that there are basically two forms of CP: early-onset ICP and late-onset ICP. The expression of late-onset ICP and no alcohol intake, low alcohol intake, and high alcohol intake differs significantly from early-onset ICP and no alcohol (earlier age at onset and greater proportion of patients with pain). The late-onset ICP forms (with alcohol intake ranging from zero to > 50 grams daily) are more similar than different, suggesting that they may in fact be just different expressions of the same form of CP. Thus, in patients with ACP, increasing alcohol intake accelerates and worsens the expression of the same underlying predisposing condition which is present in late-onset ICP with no alcohol consumption. ACP could then represent just a "modification of the basic expression of CP exemplified by the late-onset ICP group" [23]. Previous observations that smoking affects features of the natural history of CP [25, 26] also lend support to the assumption that environmental factors regulate the expression of this underlying condition predisposing to CP. In conclusion, today it seems that "a common underlying genetic defect(s) exists for the basis of most CP, which is responsible for the expression of the disease in 'late-onset ICP', but the expression of the disease is modified by environmental (alcohol, cigarette smoking) or additional genetic factors" [23].

In the beginning of the 21st century, the understanding of CP has changed dramatically. In addition to the increasing recognition of CFTR as the underlying genetic disorder in the pathogenesis of CP (mainly early-onset ICP), there is now evidence accumulating suggesting that also late-onset ICP and, more excitingly, even ACP may in fact have a genetic cause. In these questions, the study of the human genome will certainly have a lot to offer.

References

1. Cohn JA, Bornstein JD, Jowell PS. Cystic fibrosis mutations and genetic predisposition to idiopathic chronic pancreatitis. Med Clin N America 2000; 84(3): 621–31.
2. Cohn JA, Friedman KJ, Noone PG, Knowles MR, Silverman LM, Jowell PS. Relation between mutations of the cystic fibrosis gene and idiopathic chronic pancreatitis. N Engl J Med 1998; 339(10): 653–8.
3. Durie PR. Pancreatic aspects of cystic fibrosis and other inherited causes of pancreatic dysfunction. Med Clin N America 2000; 84(3): 609–19.
4. Sharer N, Schwartz M, Malone G, Howarth A, Painter J, Super M, Braganza J. Mutations of the cystic fibrosis gene in patients with chronic pancreatitis. N Engl J Med 1998; 339(10): 645–52.
5. Freedman SD. Personal communication. May 2000.
6. Gates LK, Ulrich CD, Whitcomb DC. Hereditary pancreatitis: gene defects and their complications. Surg Clin N America 1999; 79(4): 711–22.
7. Lankisch MR, Imoto M, Layer P, DiMagno EP. The effect of small amounts of alcohol on the clinical course of chronic pancreatitis. Mayo Clin Proc 2001; 76: 242–51.
8. Toskes PP. Alcohol consumption and chronic pancreatitis. Mayo Clin Proc 2001; 76: 241.
9. Imoto M, DiMagno EP. Cigarette smoking increases the risk of pancreatic calcification in late-onset but not early-onset idiopathic chronic pancreatitis. Pancreas 2000; 21: 115–9.
10. Ammann RW, Sulser H. Die senile chronische Pankreatitis: Eine neue nosologische Einheit? Schweiz Med Wochenschr 1976; 106: 429–37.

11. Lankisch PG, Lohr-Happe A, Otto J, Creutzfeldt W. Natural course in chronic pancreatitis. Digestion 1993; 54: 148–55.
12. Ammann RW, Muellhaupt B. The natural history of pain in alcoholic chronic pancreatitis. Gastroenterology 1999; 116: 1132–40.
13. Layer P, Yamamoto H, Kalthoff L, Clain JE, Bakken L, DiMagno EP. The different courses of early- and late-onset idiopathic and alcoholic chronic pancreatitis. Gastroenterology 1994; 107: 1481–7.
14. Layer P, DiMagno EP. Early and late onset in idiopathic and alcoholic chronic pancreatitis: different clinical courses. Surg Clin N Amer 1999; 79(4): 847–60.
15. Ammann RW, Akovbiantz A, Largiader F, Schueler G. Course and outcome of chronic pancreatitis: longitudinal study of a mixed medical-surgical series of 245 patients. Gastroenterology 1984; 86: 820–8.
16. Hayakawa T, Kondo T, Shibata T, Sugimoto Y, Kitagawa M. Chronic alcoholism and evolution of pain and prognosis in chronic pancreatitis. Dig Dis Sci 1989; 34: 33–8.
17. Miyake H, Harada H, Kunichika K, Ochi K, Kimura I. Clinical course and prognosis of chronic pancreatitis. Pancreas 1987; 2: 378–85.
18. Lowenfels AB, Maisonneauve P, Cavallini G, Ammann RW, Lankisch PG, Andersen JR, DiMagno EP, Andren-Sandberg A, Domellof L, and the International Pancreatitis Study Group. Pancreatitis and the risk of pancreatic cancer. N Engl J Med 1993; 328: 1433–7.
19. Tsiotos GG, Sarr MG. Diagnosis of pancreatic cancer. In: Howard JM, Idezuki I, Ihse I, Prinz RA, eds. Surgical Diseases of the Pancreas. Media, PA: Williams & Wilkins, 1998: 497–515.
20. Avram RM, Iancu M. Pancreatic disease in uremia and parathyroid hormone excess. Nephron 1982; 32: 60–2.
21. Cavallini G, Talamini G, Vaona B et al. Effect of alcohol and smoking on pancreatic lithogenesis in the course of chronic pancreatitis. Pancreas 1994; 9: 42–6.

7.4 Imaging and function and their implications for classification

B. Glasbrenner, St. Kahl, A. Leodolter, P. Malfertheiner

Introduction

There are several more or less accepted *definitions of chronic pancreatitis*. Sarner defines chronic pancreatitis as a "continuing inflammatory disease characterized by irreversible morphological changes and typically causing pain and/or permanent impairment of function" [1]. In the absence of histology, diagnosis of chronic pancreatitis is based on clinical features and findings from imaging procedures and/or function tests. In clinical practice, the starting point for diagnostic procedures in most cases is either an acute first-onset pancreatitis or a patient with abdominal pain of unknown etiology. For the large subgroup of patients with alcoholic chronic pancreatitis (ACP), it has recently been suggested that a distinction be drawn between *probable and definite ACP*, and criteria for both categories have been defined [2]. This classification system includes etiological and clinical features as well as imaging and function test results.

Concerning the controversial term of "early chronic pancreatitis", it is increasingly being accepted that the recurrent transformation from autodigestive focal necrosis to perilobular and intralobular fibrosis is a central event in the pathogenesis and/or progression of alcoholic chronic pancreatitis [3]. The clinical implication is that the majority of cases with chronic pancreatitis develop from recurrent acute pancreatitis. At this point, one shortcoming of the *classification systems of Cambridge and Marseille* becomes obvious: they do not sufficiently elucidate the "gray zone" between acute and chronic pancreatitis [4, 5]. Alcoholic chronic pancreatitis often starts with episodes of recurrent acute pancreatitis, and the unanswered question is at which timepoint or by which diagnostic procedures a distinction between alcoholic acute (without progression) or chronic (with progression) pancreatitis becomes possible (Fig. 7.4-1).

An attractive approach would be to have a serum marker that reveals pancreatic fibrosis, but there is none available as yet. Fibrogenesis indicator candidates are not specific for the pancreas, and their upregulation needs to be seen in the context of proinflammatory markers [6, 7]. In the absence of histopathology as the diagnostic gold standard, the differential diagnosis between recurrent acute pancreatitis and chronic pancreatitis at an early stage by means of imaging procedures or function tests remains uncertain, and confirmation needs to await the results from follow-up. This review deals with recent progress and persisting dilemmas in the diagnosis and classification of chronic pancreatitis, with focus on imaging and function.

Imaging procedures

Invasive and noninvasive imaging procedures are the most important diagnostic tools for the primary diagnosis of chronic pancreatitis. *Transabdominal ultrasonography* is the noninvasive and well-tolerated modality of first choice in a patient with history and

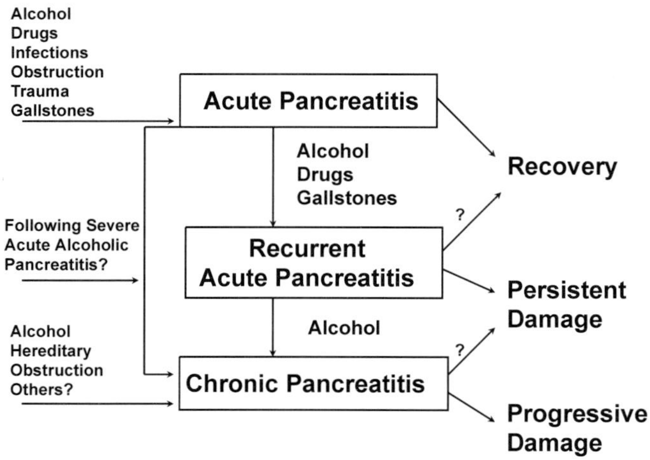

Figure 7.4-1. Interrelationship between etiology and different inflammatory pancreatic diseases. The major diagnostic problem is the differentiation between alcoholic recurrent acute and chronic pancreatitis at an early stage, which is presently only soluble by follow-up.

symptoms suggestive of pancreatic disease. The diagnostic accuracy depends of course on the visualization of the organ and the investigator's experience. It is well known that the predominant role of transabdominal ultrasound is also coupled to aspects like costs, availability, lack of complications and exclusion of differential diagnoses. The most important criteria of chronic pancreatitis for ultrasonography, computed tomography and endoscopic retrograde pancreatography are listed in the *Cambridge classification system* (Table 7.4-1). The only drawback of ultrasonography is its limited sensitivity for the diagnosis of an uncomplicated early stage of chronic pancreatitis. The diagnostic criteria are the same for *computed tomography* (CT), the method being more expensive but less dependent on the investigator's skill and experience. CT scanning has probably the best diagnostic accuracy for pancreatic calcifications, a rather specific sign of advanced chronic pancreatitis [8]. In our hands, the major use of CT is for complicated chronic pancreatitis with specific questions concerning the presence of inflammatory masses, pseudocysts or calculi in the main pancreatic duct.

Endoscopic retrograde pancreatography (ERP) is the gold standard for the diagnosis and staging of chronic pancreatitis in the absence of histology. If the pancreatic duct and its side branches are displayed in high detail, certain abnormalities of pancreatograms can be considered highly specific findings for chronic pancreatitis. The current international definitions and criteria of pancreatographic diagnosis of chronic pancreatitis are the "heart" of the *Cambridge classification system* (Table 7.4-1). The accuracy of ERP is superior to that of transabdominal ultrasound and CT, but the technique is invasive and needs more and specialized training. Acute pancreatitis following ERP is reported in up to several percent of cases investigated [9]. Interpretation of pancreatograms may be difficult in the early follow-up period after acute pancreatitis (reversible or persistent or progressive damage?) and in the elderly (chronic pancreatitis or presbypancreas?) [10]. It seems still unlikely that *magnetic resonance pancreatography* (MRP) will be able to substitute for ERP in the diagnosis of mild chronic pancreatitis, since a sufficient visualization of the side branches will probably not be achieved [11, 12]. In complicated chronic pancreatitis, pancreatographic findings are often fundamental for therapeutic decision-making; and in selected cases, ERP and MRP findings may be complementary.

Table 7.4-1. Cambridge classification of chronic pancreatitis for endoscopic retrograde pancreatography, transabdominal ultrasonography and computed tomography. For endoscopic ultrasound, the same criteria may be applied (compare Table 7.4-2).

	ERCP	**Ultrasound or Computed Tomography (CT)**
Normal	Good quality study visualizing the whole gland without abnormal signs	
Equivocal	< 3 abnormal side branches	One abnormal sign from the following list: • main pancreatic duct 2–4 mm • gland enlarged 1- to 2-fold of normal • cavities < 10 mm • main pancreatic duct irregularity • focal acute pancreatitis • parenchymal heterogeneity • increased echogeneity of duct wall • contour irregularity of head/body
Mild	< 3 abnormal side branches	Two or more abnormal signs
Moderate	As "mild" plus abnormal main pancreatic duct	As "mild" (not differentiated)
Marked	As "moderate", plus one or more from the following list: • cavities > 10 mm • gland enlarged > 2-fold of normal • intraductal filling defects • calculi/pancreatic calcifications • duct obstruction (stricture) • severe main pancreatic duct dilatation or irregularity • contiguous organ invasion visible on ultrasound or CT	

An interesting but not yet sufficiently investigated and standardized diagnostic approach to chronic pancreatitis is the combination of imaging and stimulation of secretion. Sonographic or endosonographic measurement of main pancreatic duct caliber before and after *secretin stimulation* ("secretin test") has been promoted as a diagnostic tool in chronic pancreatitis, but its accuracy in early chronic pancreatitis is far from clear [13–15]. One important indication for the secretin test might be decision-making on sphincterotomy of the minor papilla in pancreas divisum, but this aspect must also be further investigated. Secretin stimulation is also increasingly being used in combination with MRP, either for better visualization of the pancreatic duct system or for noninvasive monitoring of stimulated secretion into the duodenum [16, 17]. The achievable pictures are fascinating, but results as to accuracy from different centers must be awaited.

Endoscopic ultrasound (EUS) is a promising tool for the diagnosis of chronic pancreatitis [15, 18–20]. The principal advantage of the method is that both parenchymal and ductal changes are visualized with a high frequency transducer that is placed in close proximity to the pancreas. Wiersema et al. have described and investigated positive predictive values of parenchymal and ductal signs of chronic pancreatitis detectable by EUS (Table 7.4-2) [18, 19]. Based on the necrosis-fibrosis sequence as crucial pathogenetic event in the development of chronic pancreatitis [3, 21], one might speculate that the detection of parenchymal necrosis or fibrotic septae by EUS might be achieved earlier in the course of the disease than detection of dilated side branches or irregularities of the main

Parenchymal features	PPV
• focal areas of reduced echogenicity	76%
• hyperechogenic foci (> 3 mm)	80%
• cysts	79%
• accentuation of lobular pattern	66%
Ductal features	
• irregular contour of MPD	90%
• dilatation of MPD	78%
• dilatation of side branches	80%
• increased echogenicity/thickness of MPD wall	80%
• calculi	100%
• narrowing	67%

MPD = Main Pancreatic Duct, PPV = Positive Predictive Value

Table 7.4-2. Criteria for the diagnosis of chronic pancreatitis by endoscopic ultrasound according to [20, 21]. At present, it may be assumed that these criteria have a high sensitivity for diagnosing an early stage of chronic pancreatitis, but their specificity can only be concluded from follow-up investigations in the future.

pancreatic duct by ERP. Our own experience supports this hypothesis. In Magdeburg we performed both ERCP and EUS in a large group of 130 patients with either pre-existing CP or a clinical history and symptoms suggestive of CP. There were 2 major findings:

1. EUS identified all cases of ERP stage 1, 2 and 3 according to the Cambridge classification system; and
2. there was a considerable subgroup of 32 patients with normal ERP but EUS signs of CP [22]. These patients are still under follow-up, and 53% of them have developed either ERP signs of CP or an abnormal secretin-ceruletide test during a median time of 18 months.

On the other hand, there are data on ERP and EUS in patients with alcoholic liver cirrhosis and no clinical history of CP, identifying a subgroup of alcoholics with normal ERP but parenchymal signs of CP on EUS [23]. These 18 subjects underwent a median follow-up of 22 months, and they developed no changes of EUS appearance and no abnormalities on ERP. So the open question that remains is how specific for CP or for progressive damage are parenchymal lesions on EUS in patients with alcohol abuse with or without a clinical history suggestive of CP. In the absence of histopathology, the specificity of EUS can only be concluded from follow-up investigations.

Exocrine pancreatic function tests

If exocrine pancreatic function tests are considered for the primary diagnosis of chronic pancreatitis, only the invasive duodenal intubation test following hormonal (secretin-ceruletide test) or test meal (Lundh test) stimulation might potentially diagnose the disease at an early stage. There are some data indicating that the combined use of ERP and a duodenal intubation test increases diagnostic accuracy, because abnormal findings may occur first in one or the other modality and because of unspecific ERP findings following severe acute pancreatitis and in the elderly [12, 24, 25]. There is evidence that age per se does not affect pancreatic function but pancreatic duct morphology [12, 24–26]. The use of pancreatic function tests should furthermore be advocated to complete the assessment of patients with chronic pancreatitis for grading the stage of disease and influence the decision on clinical managament, such as the need for pancreatic enzyme replacement. Knowledge of the degree of functional impairment may also contribute to the decision for either surgery or conservative management.

The *duodenal intubation test* with different modifications relating to the stimulation of secretion (secretin-ceruletide, secretin-CCK, Lundh test meal) is the gold standard for the detection of pancreatic insufficiency. Interlaboratory standardization of these tests has never been achieved, although the exogenous administration of the hormone secretin with either ceruletide or cholecystokinin (CCK 8) is favored by most clinical investigators. There is agreement that the doses of secretagogues to be used should provide maximal stimulation and be applied for a sufficiently long time (at least 60 up to 90 min) to uncover the pancreatic secretory reserve and thus allow better discrimination between normal and abnormal pancreatic function, especially in early stages of chronic pancreatitis. Following pancreatic stimulation, the output of pancreatic secretory products such as bicarbonate, proteases (chymotrypsin, trypsin), amylase and lipase is measured in duodenal juice aspirates. Which of these parameters might be most appropriate in detecting early pancreatic pathology has not been determined as yet [27–29].

Non-invasive (tubeless) pancreatic function tests available in clinical routine yield sufficient diagnostic accuracy in advanced chronic pancreatitis but their sensitivity in detection of the disease at an early stage is low. The principle of the *pancreolauryl test* (PLT) is based on the administration of a complex substrate which is hydrolized by the effect of a specific pancreatic enzyme with the release of a marker substance. This marker is then absorbed from the gut and detected and quantitated either in urine or serum [30]. In recent years the diagnostic accuracy of the PLT has been further increased in the serum test version [31, 32]. A continuing limitation of the PLT is that its results are influenced by a variety of abnormalities of the anatomical and functional integrity of the upper gastrointestinal tract. The *PABA test* is no longer available for clinical routine.

The low diagnostic value of fecal fat analysis [33] has prompted a search for individual enzymes in stool specimen with the aim of increasing diagnostic sensitivity. *Fecal chymotrypsin* measurements are easy to perform and still popular, but their diagnostic accuracy is unsatisfactory. Progress in diagnostic accuracy of fecal pancreatic enzyme analysis has been achieved through the development of an ELISA that detects human pancreatic elastase 1. In addition to elastase's high stability during intestinal transit, the commercially available assay detects exclusively human elastase and therefore does not interfere with simultaneous therapeutic pancreatic enzyme supplementation from porcine preparations. Although the *fecal elastase* test is superior to the fecal chymotrypsin test in the majority of investigations, its diagnostic value for the detection of chronic pancreatitis should not be overestimated [34–40]. In a prospective series of outpatients with abdominal pain of unknown etiology or due to CP, fecal elastase was not very accurate for the diagnosis of CP

1. because the number of abnormal test results in patients with early stages of the disease was too low (low sensitivity), and
2. because the number of abnormal test results in patients with various other gastrointestinal diseases, especially of the bowel, was too high (low specificity) [37].

The most recent data from Magdeburg based on the secretin-cerulein test confirm the low sensitivity (35%) of fecal elastase in mild to moderate exocrine insufficiency [41]. The major role of fecal elastase should be to monitor exocrine function in patients were CP was diagnosed by other means.

New noninvasive *breath tests* have been developed based on the administration of a radioactive ^{14}C- or more recently of a non-radioactive ^{13}C-labeled substrate. The substrate is administered orally and digested by a specific pancreatic enzyme, and the resulting $^{13}CO_2$ exhalation serves as a parameter of exocrine pancreatic function. The ^{13}C-mixed triglyceride [42, 43], triolein [44, 45] and hiolein [46] breath tests are based on the administration of lipids similar to the triglycerides found in the normal diet. The cholesteryl octanoate breath test utilizes a substrate which is metabolized by pancreatic cholesterol esterase [47, 48]. In summary, all these tests reveal reduced $^{13}CO_2$ exhalation and sometimes even a flat recovery curve in patients with steatorrhea. In patients with normal fat excretion or with mild exocrine insufficiency, the pattern of expired $^{13}CO_2$ is generally normal. Since these tests have a relatively high specificity in detecting deficient lipolytic activity, they may be used in the diagnostic work-up of patients with chronic diarrhea in order to rule out the presence of fat malabsorption. A further application is to monitor the efficiency of pancreatic enzyme supplementation if clinically indicated or for scientific purposes [49, 50]. These tests do not play a role in the diagnosis of early and moderate chronic pancreatitis. The same holds true for amylase as the specific enzyme tested in the ^{13}C-starch breath test [51, 52]. The future potential of these tests might be based on the development of ^{13}C labeled substrates split by specific pancreatic enzymes that are produced in much smaller amounts than amylase and lipase, thus probably allowing pancreatic damage to be detected at an earlier stage. The costs must also be further reduced before ^{13}C-breath tests can be considered for widespread use in clinical practice.

Endocrine pancreatic function tests

B-cell function tests have repeatedly been shown to be inappropriate for the diagnosis of chronic pancreatitis (poor sensitivity and poor specificity) [53]. The investigation of glucagon release following arginine infusion may help to distinguish different types of diabetes if necessary [53, 54]. Alterations of interdigestive and stimulated pancreatic polypeptide release in chronic pancreatitis have been described, but their clinical use for the diagnosis of chronic pancreatitis has not been pursued, and their diagnostic accuracy is probably unsatisfactory [55–57]. With regard to the clinical management of the patients, it seems appropriate to distinguish between normal and abnormal glucose tolerance and overt diabetes. At present, the role of endocrine pancreatic function tests is restricted to fasting blood sugar and (if normal) oral glucose tolerance tests as complementary tools for the staging of chronic pancreatitis.

Summary and clinical application

The current diagnostic approach to chronic pancreatitis is summarized in Figure 7.4-2 and sensitivities and specificities of the individual diagnostic procedures are given in Table 7.4-3. In a patient with chronic or recurrent abdominal pain, transabdominal ultrasonography remains the first choice to begin with. The further assessment of chronic pancreatitis should be based on the combination of imaging procedures and exocrine pancreatic function tests. If either the clinical case or the ultrasonographic finding is suggestive of chronic pancreatitis, we prefer to diagnose or exclude the disease by an invasive

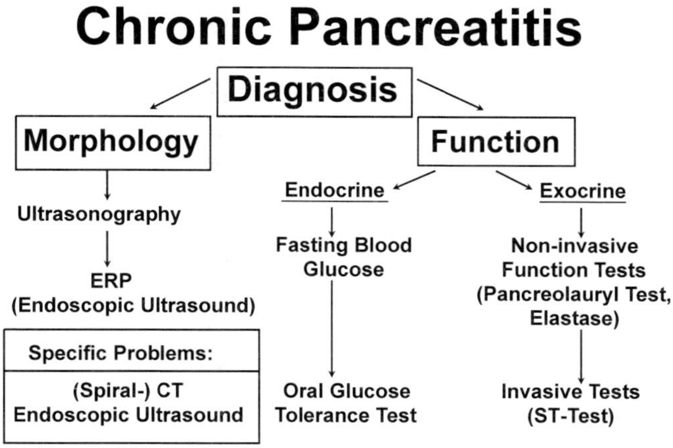

Figure 7.4-2. Flowchart for the diagnosis of chronic pancreatitis in a patient with a suggestive clinical history and abdominal pain of unknown etiology. Of course the procedure has to be adapted to specific problems and to the local availability of methods.

Diagnostic Procedure	Sensitivity	Specificity
Transabdominal ultrasound	48–90%	75–90%
Computed tomography	56–95%	85–90%
Endoscopic retrograde pancreatography	68–93%	89–97%
Endoscopic ultrasound	88–100% (?)	90–100% (?)
Fecal elastase	50–93%	62–93%
Pancreolauryl test	70–82%	70–87%
Secretin-ceruletide test	80–90%	90–95%

Table 7.4-3. Sensitivity and specificity ranges of the most important diagnostic procedures for the diagnosis of chronic pancreatitis in various investigations. The shortcomings of such data are the lack of a histologic gold standard and the highly variable inclusion of early and advanced stages of the disease.

imaging procedure (ERP and/or endoscopic ultrasound) together with a noninvasive and practicable exocrine pancreatic function test (pancreolauryl test or fecal elastase). In the case of alcoholic pancreatitis, a subcategory of subjects with probable chronic pancreatitis needs follow-up with the application of the same modalities in yearly intervals or depending on the clinical course. Other imaging procedures (for example computed tomography) or invasive exocrine pancreatic function tests (secretin-ceruletide test) are reserved for cases with specific problems. Endocrine pancreatic function is assessed by regular controls of fasting blood glucose levels and, if normal, by an oral glucose load (for example at primary diagnosis and following major events like severe acute attacks or operations).

References

1. Sarner M. Pancreatitis: definitions and classification. In: Go VLW, DiMagno EP, Gardner JD, Lebenthal E, Reber HA, Scheele GA, eds. The Pancreas. New York: Raven Press, 1993: 575–80.
2. Ammann RW. A clinically based classification system for alcoholic chronic pancreatitis: summary of an international workshop on chronic pancreatitis. Pancreas 1997; 14: 215–21.
3. Ammann RW, Heitz PU, Klöppel G. Course of alcoholic chronic pancreatitis: a prospective clinicomorphological long-term study. Gastroenterology 1996; 111: 224–31.
4. Sarner M, Cotten PB. Classification of pancreatitis. Gut 1984; 25: 756–9.

5. Singer MV, Gyr KE, Sarles H. Revised classification of pancreatitis. Gastroenterology 1985; 89: 683–90.
6. Adler G, Kropf J, Grobe E, Gressner AM. Follow-up of the serum levels of extracellular matrix components in acute and chronic pancreatitis. Eur J Clin Invest 1990; 20: 494–501.
7. Rau B, Steinbach G, Gansauge F, Mayer J, Gruenert A, Beger HG. The potential role of procalcitonin and interleukin 8 in the prediction of infected necrosis in acute pancreatitis. Gut 1997; 41: 832–40.
8. Malfertheiner P, Büchler MW, Stanescu A, Ditschuneit H. Pancreatic morphology and function in relationship to pain in chronic pancreatitis. Int J Pancreatol 1987; 2(1): 59–66.
9. Gottlieb K, Sherman S. ERCP and biliary endoscopic sphincterotomy-induced pancreatitis. Gastrointest Endosc Clin North Am 1998; 8: 87–114.
10. Forsmark CE, Toskes PP. What does an abnormal pancreatogram mean? Gastrointest Endosc Clin North Am 1995; 5: 105–23.
11. Merkle EM, Nüssle K, Glasbrenner B, Tomczak R, Preclik G, Rieber A, Adler G, Brambs HJ. MRCP – current status. Z Gastroenterol 1998; 36: 215–24.
12. Soto JA, Yucel EK, Barish MA, Chuttani R, Ferrucci JT. MR cholangio-pancreatography after unsuccessful or incomplete ERCP. Radiology 1996; 199: 91–8.
13. Bolondi L, Li Bassi S, Gaiani S, Santi V, Gullo L, Barbara L. Impaired response of main pancreatic duct to secretin stimulation in early chronic pancreatitis. Dig Dis Sci 1989; 34: 834–40.
14. Glaser J, Mann O, Pausch J. Diagnosis of chronic pancreatitis by means of a sonographic secretin test. Int J Pancreatol 1994; 15: 195–200.
15. Catalano MF, Lahoti S, Geenen JE, Hogan WJ. Prospective evaluation of endoscopic ultrasonography, endoscopic retrograde pancreatography, and secretin test in the diagnosis of chronic pancreatitis. Gastrointest Endosc 1998; 48: 11–7.
16. Manfredi R, Costamagna G, Veccioli A, Colagrande C, Spina S, Marano P. Dynamic pancreatography with magnetic resonance after functional stimulus with secretin in chronic pancreatitis. Radiol Med (Torino) 1998; 96: 226–31.
17. Matos C, Deviere J, Nicaise N, Braude P, Van Gansbeke D, Metens T, Struyven J, Cremer M. Magnetic resonance cholangiopancreatography (MRCP): a perspective on potential clinical applications. Acta Gastro-enterol Belg 1997; 60: 268–73.
18. Wiersema MJ, Hawes RH, Lehman GA, Kochman ML, Sherman S, Kopecky KK. Prospective evaluation of endoscopic ultrasonography and endoscopic retrograde cholangiopancreatography in patients with chronic abdominal pain of suspected pancreatic origin. Endoscopy 1993; 25: 555–64.
19. Wiersema MJ, Wiersema LM. Endosonography of the pancreas: normal variation versus changes of early chronic pancreatitis. Gastrointest Endosc Clin North Am 1995; 5: 487–96.
20. Buscail L, Escourrou J, Moreau J, Delvaux M, Louvel D, Lapeyre F, Tregant P, Frexinos J. Endoscopic ultrasonography in chronic pancreatitis: a comparative prospective study with conventional ultra-sonography, computed tomography, and ERCP. Pancreas 1995; 10: 251–7.
21. Klöppel G, Maillet B. Pathology of acute and chronic pancreatitis. Pancreas 1993; 8: 659–70.
22. Kahl S, Glasbrenner B, Leodolter A, Domínguez-Muñoz E, Malfertheiner P. Endoscopic ultrasound (EUS) or endoscopic retro-grade pancreatography (ERP) in the diagnosis of chronic pancreatitis (CP)? Endoscopy 1999; 31(Suppl 1): 31.
23. Hastier P, Buckley M, Francois E, Peten E, Dumas R, Caroli-Bosc FX, Delmont JP. A prospective study of pancreatic disease in patients with alcoholic cirrhosis: comparative diagnostic value of ERCP and EUS and long-term significance of isolated parenchymal abnormalities. Gastrointest Endosc 1999; 49: 705–9.
24. Gullo L. Direct panceatic function test (duodenal intubation) in the diagnosis of chronic pancreatitis. Gastroenterology 1986; 90: 799–800.
25. Lankisch PG, Seidensticker F, Otto J, Lubbers H, Mahlke R, Stockmann F, Fölsch UR, Creutzfeldt W. Secretin-pancreozymin test (SPT) and endoscopic retrograde cholangiopancreatography (ERCP): both are necessary for diagnosing or excluding chronic pancreatitis. Pancreas 1996; 12: 149–52.

26. Gullo L, Priori P, Daniele C, Ventrucci M, Gasbarrini G, Labo G. Exocrine pancreatic function in the elderly. Gerontology 1983; 29: 407–11.
27. Dürr GHK. The secretin-pancreozymin (caerulein)-test. Methodological problems. In: Gyr KE, Singer MV, Sarles H, eds. Pancreatitis. Amsterdam–New York–Oxford: Excerpta Medica, 1984: 261–6.
28. Lankisch PG. Function tests in the diagnosis of chronic pancreatitis. Critical evaluation. Int J Pancreatol 1993; 14: 9–20.
29. Gullo L. Direct pancreatic function tests in the diagnosis and staging of chronic pancreatitis. In: Malfertheiner P, Domínguez-Muñoz JE, Schulz HU, Lippert H, eds. Diagnostic Procedures in Pancreatic Disease. Berlin–Heidelberg: Springer-Verlag, 1997: 249–52.
30. Rünzi M, Layer P. Oral pancreatic function tests in the diagnosis and staging of chronic pancreatitis. In: Malfertheiner P, Domínguez-Muñoz JE, Schulz HU, Lippert H, eds. Diagnostic Procedures in Pancreatic Disease. Berlin–Heidelberg: Springer-Verlag, 1997: 253–60.
31. Malfertheiner P, Büchler MW, Müller A, Ditschuneit H. Fluorescein dilaurate (FDL) serum test – a rapid tubeless pancreatic function test. Pancreas 1987; 2: 53–60.
32. Domínguez-Muñoz JE, Malfertheiner P. Optimized serum pancreolauryl test for differentiating patients with and without chronic pancreatitis. Clin Chem 1998; 44: 869–75.
33. DiMagno EP, Go VL, Summerskill WH. Relations between pancreatic enzyme outputs and malabsorption in severe pancreatic insufficiency. N Engl J Med 1973; 288: 813–5.
34. Domínguez-Muñoz JE, Hieronymus C, Sauerbruch T, Malfertheiner P. Fecal elastase test: evaluation of a new noninvasive pancreatic function test. Am J Gastroenterol 1995; 90: 1834–7.
35. Stein J, Jung M, Sziegoleit A, Zeuzem S, Caspary WF, Lembcke B. Immunoreactive elastase I: clinical evaluation of a new noninvasive test of pancreatic function. Clin Chem 1996; 42: 222–6.
36. Löser C, Möllgaard A, Fölsch UR. Faecal elastase 1: a novel, highly sensitive, and specific tubeless pancreatic function test. Gut 1996; 39: 580–6.
37. Glasbrenner B, Schön A, Klatt S, Beckh K, Adler G. Clinical evaluation of the faecal elastase test in the diagnosis and staging of chronic pancreatitis. Eur J Gastroenterol Hepatol 1996; 8: 1117–20.
38. Amann ST, Bishop M, Curington C, Toskes PP. Fecal pancreatic elastase 1 is inaccurate in the diagnosis of chronic pancreatitis. Pancreas 1996; 13: 226–30.
39. Lankisch PG, Schmidt I, König H, Lehnick D, Knollmann R, Loehr M, Liebe S. Faecal elastase 1: not helpful in diagnosing chronic pancreatitis associated with mild to moderate exocrine pancreatic insufficiency. Gut 1998; 42: 551–4.
40. Gullo L, Ventrucci M, Tomassetti P, Migliori M, Pezzilli R. Fecal elastase 1 determination in chronic pancreatitis. Dig Dis Sci 1999; 44: 210–3.
41. Leodolter A, Kahl S, Domínguez-Muñoz JE, Gerards C, Glasbrenner B, Malfertheiner P. Comparison of two tubeless function tests in the Assessment of mild-to-moderate exocrine pancreatic insufficiency. Eur J Gastroenterol Hepatol 2000; 12: 1–4.
42. Ghoos YF, Vantrappen GR, Rutgeerts PJ, Schurmans PC. A mixed triglyceride breath test for intraluminal fat digestive capacity. Digestion 1981; 22: 239–47.
43. Vantrappen GR, Rutgeerts PJ, Ghoos YF, Hiele ML. Mixed triglyceride breath test: a noninvasive test of pancreatic lipase activity in the duodenum. Gastroenterology 1989; 96: 1126–34.
44. Newcomer AD, Hofmann AF, DiMagno EP, Thomas PJ, Carlson GL. Triolein breath test: a sensitive and specific test for fat malabsorption. Gastroenterology 1979; 76: 6–13.
45. Mylvaganam K, Hudson PR, Ross A, Williams CP. ^{14}C triolein breath test: a routine test in the gastroenterology clinic? Gut 1986; 27: 1347–9.
46. Lembcke B, Braden B, Caspary WF. Exocrine pancreatic insufficiency: accuracy and clinical value of the uniformly labeled ^{13}C-Hiolein breath test. Gut 1996; 39: 668–74.
47. Cole SG, Rossi S, Stern A, Hofmann AF. Cholesteryl octanoate breath test. Preliminary studies on a new noninvasive test of human pancreatic exocrine function. Gastroenterology 1987; 93: 1372–80.
48. Ventrucci M, Cipolla A, Ubalducci GM, Roda A, Roda E. ^{13}C labelled cholesteryl octanoate breath test for assessing pancreatic exocrine insufficiency. Gut 1998; 42: 81–7.

49. Mundlos S, Kuhnelt P, Adler G. Monitoring enzyme replacement treatment in exocrine pancreatic insufficiency using the cholesteryl octanoate breath test. Gut 1990; 31: 1324–8.
50. Adler G, Mundlos S, Kuhnelt P, Dreyer E. New methods for assessment of enzyme activity: do they help to optimize enzyme treatment? Digestion 1993; 54: 3–9.
51. Patel VP, Jain NK, Agarwal N, Gee Varghese PJ, Pitchumoni CS. Comparison of bentiromide test and rice flour breath hydrogen test in the detection of exocrine pancreatic insufficiency. Pancreas 1986; 1: 172–5.
52. Loser C, Mollgaard A, Aygen S, Hennemann O, Fölsch UR. ^{13}C-starch breath test – comparative clinical evaluation of an indirect pancreatic function test. Z Gastroenterol 1997; 35: 187–94.
53. Glasbrenner B, Von Tirpitz C, Malfertheiner P, Adler G. Endocrine pancreatic function in the diagnosis and staging of chronic pancreatitis. In: Malfertheiner P, Domínguez-Muñoz JE, Schulz HU, Lippert H, eds. Diagnostic procedures in pancreatic disease. Berlin–Heidelberg: Springer-Verlag, 1997: 303–9.
54. von Tirpitz C, Glasbrenner B, Mayer D, Malfertheiner P, Adler G. Comparison of different endocrine stimulation tests in nondiabetic patients with chronic pancreatitis. Hepato-Gastroenterol 1998; 45: 1111–6.
55. Owyang C, Scarpello JH, Vinik AI. Correlation between pancreatic enzyme secretion and plasma concentration of human pancreatic polypeptide in health and in chronic pancreatitis. Gastroenterology 1982; 83: 55–62.
56. Pieramico O, Nelson DK, Glasbrenner B, Malfertheiner P. Impaired interdigestive pancreatic polypeptide release: early hormonal disorder in chronic pancreatitis? Dig Dis Sci 1994; 39: 69–74.
57. Glasbrenner B, Domínguez-Muñoz JE, Nelson DK, Riepl RL, Büchler MW, Malfertheiner P. Relationship between postprandial release of CCK and PP in health and in chronic pancreatitis. Regul Pept 1994; 50: 45–52.

7.5 Complications of chronic pancreatitis and implications for classification

R. A. Prinz, H. Shedd Keith

Chronic pancreatitis results from progressive fibro-inflammatory changes in the gland that cause permanent morphologic and functional damage. Although this process can remain clinically silent most patients with chronic pancreatitis come to medical attention because of complications that stem from their disease. The complications of chronic pancreatitis can be classified in a number of ways. For example, complications may be due to functional alterations or morphologic abnormalities; they may be secondary to the effects of the disease on the gland itself or on the surrounding structures; and they may be divided into those that are treated medically and those that require surgical correction. As with any attempt to classify a disease or its complications, there will always be overlap or gray areas. Nevertheless these efforts can be worthwhile in that they increase our understanding of these complications and their overall relationship to the disease. By focusing on the complications of chronic pancreatitis, we are not minimizing other factors such as etiology, extent of disease, duct size and so forth that can be used to classify the disease itself but rather are emphasizing the clinical and therapeutic aspects with which physicians must deal.

The fibrosis and inflammation of chronic pancreatitis leads to various degrees of endocrine and exocrine dysfunction. These problems of pancreatic function are due to progressive morphologic changes within the gland. They are treated medically, since no operation can restore functioning endocrine and exocrine tissue that has already been destroyed by chronic pancreatitis.

The incidence of overt diabetes in chronic pancreatitis can range as high as 40–70%. The treatment of diabetes secondary to chronic pancreatitis differs little from the standard management of diabetes. Blood glucose levels should be monitored and controlled by regulating dietary intake and using oral hypoglycemic agents and insulin as needed. Chronic pancreatitis patients with diabetes may be particularly sensitive to insulin and prone to hypoglycemia. Continued alcohol ingestion, exocrine insufficiency, erratic oral intake because of postprandial pain and abnormal release of counter-regulatory hormones such as glucagon make these patients prone to hypoglycemia. Thus, it is prudent not to control blood glucose as tightly in chronic pancreatitis as in primary diabetes. Continuous online monitoring of glucose may play a role in improving diabetic management in these patients.

Pancreatic enzymes are needed for normal digestion. When their secretion is insufficient, steatorrhea, diarrhea and azotorrhea result. These problems typically occur late in the course of chronic pancreatitis because malabsorption does not occur until the pancreatic damage has reduced enzyme secretion to less than 10% of normal. The treatment of pancreatic exocrine insufficiency is medical. A sufficient amount of pancreatic enzymes must be given with oral replacement therapy to approximate 5% of normal maximal pancreatic lipase output. Pancreatic enzymes are highly sensitive to acid and pepsin inactivation. Efforts to prevent acid pepsin inactivation of orally administered pancreatic enzyme supplements may improve therapeutic efficacy. These include raising gastric and duodenal pH with antacids or H2-receptor antagonists or using pancreatic enzymes in enteric-pH-coated forms.

Abdominal pain is the most frequent complication of chronic pancreatitis that brings patients to clinical attention. It is the most difficult complication of this disease to classify since its presence may indirectly affect pancreatic function; its etiology may be due to morphologic changes both within the gland and in peripancreatic tissue; and its treatment may be both medical and surgical. Postprandial pain may influence or even exacerbate pancreatic endocrine and exocrine insufficiency by altering the amount and type of oral intake. The indirect effects or pain must be kept in mind when managing diabetes and exocrine malabsorption in chronic pancreatitis.

Although the exact etiology of pain in chronic pancreatitis remains unclear most would agree that morphologic changes within the gland or in peripancreatic tissue are responsible. Pain can be caused by fibrosis and stricture formation in the pancreatic duct which results in increased ductal and glandular pressure or by inflammatory cell infiltrates around pancreatic and peripancreatic nerves and ganglia. Since chronic pancreatitis consists of a wide spectrum of clinical, anatomic and functional findings, it is possible for both of these mechanisms to be active alone or in combination in different patients. Although pain is the common end result in chronic pancreatitis, these differences in its etiology may influence some choices in its management.

Pain control in chronic pancreatitis is initially managed medically. The first step is to eliminate any precipitating cause of the disease, the most common of which is alcohol. Although patient acceptance of abstinence is often limited, it should be strongly emphasized as a critical component of management. Non-specific pain control with analgesics is the most common method of pain management. Therapy should begin with salicylates, acetaminophen, or non-steroidal anti-inflammatory agents. Narcotics are often required for effective relief. Although there is a reluctance to administer these potentially addicting agents, they are often necessary to break a vicious cycle of incapacitating pain. Judicious use of narcotics requires careful monitoring so that the lowest effective dose is administered and the risk of abuse is minimized.

Medical treatment of pain in chronic pancreatitis includes oral administration of pancreatic enzymes. Normal pancreatic enzyme secretion is subject to feedback regulation. Cholecystykinin [CCK] stimulates pancreatic enzyme secretion. When pancreatic juice rich in proteases such as trypsin and chymotrypsin reaches the duodenal lumen, it inhibits CCK secretion, which then shuts off further pancreatic enzyme secretion. Exogenous administration of pancreatic enzymes has also been shown to decrease pancreatic enzyme secretion by this feedback inhibition. In patients with chronic pancreatitis, oral pancreatic enzyme therapy should decrease CCK levels, reduce pancreatic hyperstimulation and intraductal and intraparenchymal pressures and hopefully relieve pain.

Octreotide, a synthetic analog of the hormone somatostatin, can inhibit pancreatic secretion and has anti-nociceptive activity. These properties have suggested that it may be beneficial for pain control in chronic pancreatitis. Unfortunately, the limited studies with octreotide have yet to prove its benefit in chronic pancreatitis. Percutaneous celiac plexus nerve blocks can provide pain relief for patients with pancreatic disease. The benefit in chronic pancreatitis is limited in terms of achieving lasting pain relief.

The goal of surgery in chronic pancreatitis is to relieve pain while preserving as much endocrine and exocrine function as possible. Although a wide variety of operative procedures have been tried to achieve this goal, only pancreatic duct drainage and pancreatic resection have proven benefit in terms of pain relief. I have favored pancreatic duct drainage because it sacrifices the least amount of pancreatic endocrine and exocrine tissue. Side to side pancreaticojejunostomy is a safe procedure with an operative mortality ranging from 0–4% [1, 2]. Its associated complication rate ranges from 10–25%. Long-term studies have shown that 65–85% of patients will have substantial or complete relief of their pain. It is unusual for diabetes or steatorrhea to be worsened by this procedure although there is attrition in pancreatic function due to the natural course of this disease. Side to side pancreaticojejunostomy may sometimes require resection of tissue in the head of the gland to achieve adequate drainage [3]. Even with this modification it is a safe and effective way to treat patients with disabling pain from chronic pancreatitis who have a dilated pancreatic duct.

In theory, removal of the diseased portion of the gland should be the most certain way to relieve pain in chronic pancreatitis. The major drawback of resection is the greater chance for insulin-dependent diabetes and pancreatic exocrine insufficiency when enough tissue is removed to insure pain relief. Although the reported mortality of pancreatic resection is comparable to that of pancreatic duct drainage, the risk of morbidity including the development of diabetes and steatorrhea is higher. The choice of proximal or distal pancreatectomy and the magnitude of the resection are determined primarily by the location and extent of the disease. Distal pancreatectomy is appropriate for focal disease in the body and tail of the gland. This anatomic confinement of chronic pancreatitis is typical of a traumatic origin but almost never occurs in alcoholic or idiopathic disease.

Most often the morphologic changes of chronic pancreatitis are concentrated in the head of the gland and surgeons who favor resection have focused their attention on this area. In the United States, pylorus-preserving pancreaticoduodenectomy is the favored procedure. The operative mortality rate is similar to that of pancreatic duct drainage [0–4%] as is the likelihood of pain relief [65–85%] [4. 5]. However, the majority of patients will require subsequent insulin and pancreatic enzyme replacement. We use pylorus-preserving pancreaticoduodenectomy for chronic pancreatitis but usually limit it to those patients with smaller caliber ducts or in whom a pancreatic cancer cannot be ruled out.

Beger and co-workers have championed duodenal preserving resection of the pancreatic head as a resective procedure that conserves intestinal and pancreatic function [6]. Pain relief with this procedure is as good as other direct operations on the pancreas. There are still metabolic consequences since at least 25–50% of patients will become insulin-dependent diabetics and 50–75% will require pancreatic enzyme replacement after this operation. One randomized study comparing pylorus-preserving pancreaticoduodenectomy with duodenal preserving pancreatic head resection showed a trend toward better pain relief and lesser metabolic consequences with the latter procedure [7]. However, the small number of patients and limited follow-up in this study makes it uncertain whether this procedure has any real advantage over pylorus-preserving pancreaticoduodenectomy.

Total pancreatectomy should not be considered a primary operation for chronic pancreatitis. Removal of the entire gland has major metabolic consequences. It often leads to brittle diabetes in patients who are frequently noncompliant, addicted to alcohol and/or narcotics and have unreliable oral intake. It should only be considered after all medical and surgical options have been exhausted in patients who have the intelligence and dependability needed to manage brittle insulin-dependent diabetes mellitus.

Complications of chronic pancreatitis may affect the pancreas or surrounding structures. Pancreatic complications of this disease include the development of a pseudocyst, abscess, pancreatic fistula, ascites or an inflammatory mass which may be impossible to differentiate from a pancreatic carcinoma. These problems are usually secondary to an anatomic abnormality that is highly likely to require surgical correction. Pancreatic pseudocysts are quite common in chronic pancreatitis, with an incidence ranging from 30 to almost 50% [8]. Pseudocysts occurring in chronic pancreatitis are unlikely to resolve spontaneously. Likewise, percutaneous drainage is much less successful since an underlying pancreatic duct stricture is often present proximal to the cyst. We believe that both the pseudocyst and the underlying chronic pancreatitis should be treated whenever possible. Combined pancreatic duct and pseudocyst drainage does not increase the morbidity and mortality of surgical intervention and decreases the likelihood of persistent or recurrent pain or pseudocyst formation.

Pancreatic abscess is relatively unusual in chronic pancreatitis. When it occurs, it is often a complication of interventions such as surgery or percutaneous drainage. Open surgical drainage should be considered the standard therapy but percutaneous drainage can play a role in some patients.

Pancreatic fistula and ascites are uncommon problems in chronic pancreatitis. They usually stem from a stricture in the pancreatic duct associated with distal rupture of the duct or a concomitant pseudocyst. Both problems can follow interventions such as percutaneous drainage or can occur spontaneously. Pancreatic ascites is more likely to occur spontaneously while pancreatic fistula are more likely to follow interventions. These problems are unlikely to resolve until the underlying anatomic abnormalities are corrected by surgical drainage or resection.

An inflammatory mass larger than 4 cm may occur in the head of the gland in as many as 75% of patients requiring surgery for chronic pancreatitis [6]. The presence of a mass can raise the specter of a possible pancreatic carcinoma. It can be extremely difficult to differentiate pancreatic cancer and chronic pancreatitis. There is a great deal of overlap in the signs and symptoms of each disease. Abdominal pain, weight loss, associated diabetes and obstructive jaundice are commonly present in both of them. Even with a high index of clinical suspicion, pancreatic cancer is missed in 2–4% of patients undergoing pancreatic duct drainage for presumed chronic pancreatitis [1]. Whenever there is a possibility of an underlying pancreatic cancer, pancreatic resection should be performed since it is both diagnostic and therapeutic.

Chronic pancreatitis can cause complications in structures that are in direct continuity with the gland. These complications can affect the common bile duct, duodenum, spleen and adjacent vasculature. The most common complication of chronic pancreatitis affecting surrounding structures is obstruction in the intrapancreatic portion of the common bile duct. The anatomic basis for this complication is readily apparent since the common bile duct is completely ensheathed by the pancreas as it makes its way to the duodenum in over 85% of people. The fibrosis and inflammation of chronic pancreatitis produces a long smooth tapering obstruction of the entire intrapancreatic portion of the common bile duct. There is no evidence of "shouldering" and the proximal dilated duct takes on a bent knee appearance as it enters the pancreas. This type of stricture occurs in 3–45% of patients with chronic pancreatitis but causes obstructive jaundice in a smaller percentage. Jaundice from chronic pancreatitis typically waxes and wanes while that of pancreatic cancer is progressive. Operative intervention is usually recommended for these strictures because they can cause pain, cholestasis, cholangitis, liver abscess, or biliary cirrhosis. We believe it is prudent to treat both the common bile duct obstruction and pancreatic duct obstruction in these patients and favor internal drainage of both [9]. Other surgeons prefer pancreatic resection as the most appropriate means of dealing with this problem. Endoscopic stent placement has a limited role because of the prevalence of stent blockage and frequent need for stent replacement in this benign condition.

Duodenal obstruction from chronic pancreatitis can be functional or anatomic. Functional obstruction is secondary to inflammatory changes that cause edema and dismotility of the stomach and duodenum. These abnormalities resolve with conservative management of pancreatitis in 1–2 weeks. Fixed anatomic obstruction occurs when the fibrosis and adhesions cause a long stricture by impinging on the lumen, usually in the second and third portion of the duodenum. The diagnosis can be confirmed by upper GI radiography or endoscopy. The complication occurs in up to 15% of patients requiring operation for chronic pancreatitis. Again the underlying chronic pancreatitis should be treated when intervening for this complication. Combined drainage and resection are both acceptable approaches. Common bile duct and duodenal obstruction can occur concomitantly in these patients. We have utilized combined biliary, gastric and pancreatic duct drainage to treat this complex while others have favored resection [9].

Despite its proximity to the pancreas, the spleen is rarely involved in complications of chronic pancreatitis. Less than 2% of patients requiring surgery for chronic pancreatitis will have a splenic complication [10]. These include intrasplenic pseudocyst, abscess, infarction, subcapsulary hematoma and splenic rupture. Intrasplenic pseudocysts most often develop by direct expansion from pseudocysts in the tail of the gland. Treatment is usually surgical as has already been discussed for pseudocysts in general.

Splenic infarction is presumably rare in chronic pancreatitis although its exact prevalence is unknown. It usually comes to clinical attention as a cause of pain or as a site of secondary infection. Perisplenic adhesions secondary to repeated attacks of pancreatitis are thought to favor the develop of splenic rupture in chronic pancreatitis. This can occur spontaneously or with minimal abdominal trauma. Many of the splenic complications including hematoma and rupture are associated with splenic vein thrombosis. The resulting venous hypertension certainly plays a role in the pathogenesis of these complications. Rupture can present with circulatory collapse that requires urgent surgical intervention.

The vascular complications of chronic pancreatitis can be divided into venous and arterial. Although they are usually thought to occur infrequently, when patients with chronic pancreatitis are screened by modern imaging modalities such as duplex sonography or vascular CT as many as 20–45% will have a vascular complication [11]. Venous problems occur more commonly than arterial with splenic vein compression/thrombosis being the most frequent. Superior mesenteric and portal vein obstruction can also occur. The mechanism is secondary involvement of the veins by the surrounding fibro-inflammatory process of chronic pancreatitis as they pass through or in continuity with the pancreatic parenchyma. When these veins become occluded or obstructed venous blood is forced to return to lower pressure symptoms through collaterals. This results in the development of gastric and esophageal varices. The presence of varices does not necessarily require treatment unless the patients develop bleeding or require surgery in the area.

Splenectomy is curative for left-sided portal hypertension resulting from splenic vein thrombosis but it is less effective when the central portal venous system is involved [12]. A proximal or distal splenorenal shunt may not be possible because of concomitant splenic vein thrombosis, so a mesocaval shunt may be the best alternative. In good risk patients with splenic vein thrombosis, the long-term risk of variceal bleeding may exceed that of splenectomy and post splenectomy sepsis making elective surgery the preferred option.

The arterial complications of chronic pancreatitis include erosion or pseudo-aneurysm of the major vessels adjacent to the gland, including the splenic, gastroduodenal and hepatic arteries. Erosion and pseudo-aneurysm formation often occur in proximity with a pseudocyst. Bleeding can occur freely into the peritoneal cavity or into the stomach, duodenum, pancreatic duct or colon. Whenever a pseudo-aneurysm is detected it should be treated electively by either embolization or surgical excision. This is indicated because a ruptured pancreatic pseudo-aneurysm can carry a mortality of up to 50% [11].

This review of the complications of chronic pancreatitis serves to heighten our awareness of them. It is the complications of chronic pancreatitis and not the disease itself that require clinical attention. Attempts to classify them are worthwhile since they help us understand the pathogenesis, diagnosis and treatment of these problems. Proper management of these complications will enhance the quality of life of the patients and allow them to be productive members of society.

References

1. Prinz RA. Surgical options in chronic pancreatitis. Int J Panc 1993; 14(2): 97–105.
2. Prinz RA. Technique of lateral pancreaticojejunostomy. Dig Surg 1997; 14: 495–9.
3. Frey CF, Ho HS. Local resection of the head of the pancreas combined with longitudinal pancreaticojejunostomy. Dig Surg 1997;14: 148–53.
4. Sakorafas GH, Farnett MG, Nagorney DM et al. Pancreatoduodenectomy for chronic pancreatitis. Arch Surg 2000; 135: 517–24.
5. Traverso LW, Kozarek RA. Pancreatoduodenectomy for chronic pancreatitis. Ann Surg 1997; 226(4): 429–38.
6. Beger HG, Schlosser W, Friess HM, Büchler MW. Duodenum-preserving head resection in chronic pancreatitis changes the natural course of the disease. Ann Surg 1999; 230(4): 512–23.
7. Büchler MW, Friess H, Muller MW, Wheatley AM. Randomized trial of duodenum-preserving pancreatic head resection versus pylorus-preserving Whipple in chronic pancreatitis. Am J Surg 1995; 169: 65–70.
8. Munn JD, Aranha GV, Greenlee HB, Prinz RA. Simultaneous treatment of chronic pancreatitis and pancreative pseudocyst. Arch Surg 1987; 122: 662–7.
9. Prinz RA, Aranha GV, Greenlee HB. Combined pancreatic duct and upper gastrointestinal and biliary tract drainage in chronic pancreatitis. Arch Surg 1985; 120: 361–86.
10. Malka D, Hammel P, Levy P et al. Splenic complications in chronic pancreatitis: prevalence and risk factors in a medical-surgical series of 500 patients. Br J Surg 1998; 85(12): 1645–9.
11. Seiler CA, Boss MA, Czerniak A et al. Vascular complications in chronic pancreatitis. Dig Surg 1997; 14: 107–12.
12. Sakorafas GH, Sarr MG, Farles DR, Farnett MB. The significance of sinistral portal hypertension complicating chronic pancreatitis. Am J Surg 2000; 179: 129–33.

8 Difficult decision-making in chronic pancreatitis: An interactive workshop

8.1 Discussion

J. Mössner

First case: a 75-year-old female patient
Presented by P. Layer, M.D., Hamburg, Germany

History

A 75-year-old lady was admitted to our hospital due to slight abdominal pain. Since her later youth she had consumed moderate "social" amounts of alcohol, amounting to up to two glasses of wine per day, but she did not impress as an alcoholic. She lived under socially very stable conditions and she had been a moderate smoker for many years. Some 20 years ago, she suffered an episode of slight abdominal pain which persisted for about two to three weeks. At that time, the "early times" of ultrasound, we were able to detect a cystic mass in the transition zone between the pancreatic body and tail. The diagnosis was a suspected pseudocyst on the basis of beginning chronic pancreatitis. However, we were not quite sure, and we added the differential diagnosis of a congenital cyst which might be unrelated to the pain episode. As an alternative, the cyst could be causative for the pain, but there is no pancreatitis. No further workup was done. The further clinical course was uneventful. She had some ultrasound follow-ups every two to four years and essentially the cyst remained unchanged in its size. Ten years ago, the size of the cyst was documented with 4 cm in diameter and this size remained stable throughout the years. She had no bout or any manifestation of pancreatitis.

In the beginning of April 2000, however, she had to go to her primary care physician since she felt weak, easily tired, and a little bit depressed, but she had no pain. She had no leading symptom, her appetite was still preserved, and she had observed no weight loss and no changes in bowel habits.

Objective findings

A slight normocytic anemia was found. She had no other symptoms. The cystic mass was unchanged by ultrasound, again 4 cm in diameter. A CT scan verified a pancreatic pseudocyst, 4.5 cm in diameter. This was the first CT ever performed. In the liver, in segment 4, a small hemangioma was seen, but otherwise normal findings. However, it was noted that tumor markers were slightly elevated. The slight elevation of CEA was attributed to her smoking. However, CA 19-9 was 112 U/μl, which is threefold above the upper limit of normal. Because of these findings she was sent to a gastroenterologist who performed an esophagogastroduodenoscopy and a colonoscopy. Both procedures revealed normal findings. A repeat of the spiral CT scan using angiocontrast confirmed the pancreatic cyst with no further signs of a tumor or chronic pancreatitis. The contrast enhancement of the liver tumor was considered typical for a hemangioma.

The lady was sent to our hospital with the specific question of endoscopic retrograde cholangiopancreaticography (ERCP) and endosonography. The ERCP showed a normal main pancreatic duct and small duct. However, in the body/tail transition zone, an abrupt termination of contrast filling was seen at the location of the cyst. The pancreatic duct had no communication with the cyst. In the endosonography we confirmed the expected cystic mass 5 cm in diameter. No sonographic signs of a solid tumor or chronic pancreatitis were seen.

Dr. DiMagno, what diagnosis do you think the lady has? Which further diagnostic workup would you perform?

Commentary by the gastroenterologist E. P. DiMagno, M.D., Rochester, USA

First of all, this is a 4 cm cystic lesion between body and tail of the pancreas in a 75-year-old lady. She had no history of a pancreatic disease, no events of pancreatitis. I did look as close as I could at the CT scan and the ERCP and I did not see any evidence of pancreatitis. Thus, I am just going to discuss quickly the differential diagnosis of pancreatic cysts. And I think we should keep in mind that the differential diagnosis depends heavily upon what the cyst looks like on the images. I will make comments as I go along in that regard and the treatment really depends, particularly in this lady who has elevated tumor markers even though she smokes, on a malignant potential of the suspected lesions. I will present a rather simple classification of cystic neoplasms of the pancreas:

Serous cystadenomas are benign tumors. Mucinous cystic neoplasms belong to the class of cystadenomas which may develop into cystadenocarcinomas. There are ductal papillary mucinous tumors, also premalignant lesions, and there are other cystic lesions such as cystic endocrine tumors.

Andy Warshaw from Boston reported a series with cystic pancreatic lesions in 1995. About half of them were mucinous cystic neoplasms, about a third were serous, intraductal papillary mucinous tumors (IPMT) about 12, and others about 8. Now, let me just quickly run through the cystic neoplasms. First of all, serous or microcystic cystadenomas are glycogen-rich and frequently incidental findings, as in this patient. However, microcystic cystadenomas are multilocular and none of the lesions are greater than 2 cm. They have sort of a honey-comb appearance. They may have a central calcified scar and there is essentially no malignant potential. They may cause pressure effects. In endosonography you see these multiple, interloculated cysts. In the magnetic resonance imaging you can see the cyst and small lobules within the cystic lesion.

Next to mucinous cystic cystadenomas, which are a precursor of cystadenocarcinomas, you have to consider papillary mucinous tumors. Both need to be differentiated from pancreatic pseudocysts. Up to about 25% of lesions in some series thought to be mucinous cystadenomas turned out to be pancreatic pseudocysts and that is part of our differential diagnosis in this particular patient, a typical middle-age woman.

Now, what about the current assumptions with the mucinous cystic neoplasms? It is assumed that all mucinous cystic pancreatic neoplasms are overtly or potentially malignant and that mucinous cystadenocarcinomas are less aggressive and have a five-year survival of about 60–70%. Recently Michael Sarr in our institution looked at this particular issue again with the following questions: Are mucinous cystic neoplasms premalignant and does complete resection imply cure? He demonstrated a five-year survival after curative resection of the cystadenocarcinoma of 60% indeed. When we looked at these 84 cystic lesions, mucinous cystadenomas comprised 54 of the 84 and non-invasive proliferative lesions 23 out of 84. Mucinous cystadenocarcinomas are represented only in

6 of these patients, a fairly small number. Of this group of patients, all of them underwent resection. Five of 6 had a recurrence of the adenocarcinoma, mean follow-up about 10 years. A complete resection of non-invasive lesions implies cure. In these particular patients detailed follow-up surveillance is not necessary. However, the survival after curative resection of cystadenocarcinoma is really dismal. It matches that of an ordinary pancreatic ductal adenocarcinoma.

Now to our patient: We have a differential diagnosis between a mucinous cystic pancreatic neoplasm and a pseudocyst. Again I would like to mention that these neoplasms are primarily in women with no history of pancreatic pathology. Her lesion is not multicystic and has no internal septae and no surrounding reactions. Thus, I think this patient really fits into the group of mucinous cystadenoma/cystadenocarcinoma. There have been some attempts to try to differentiate between inflammatory serous cysts and mucinous cystadenoma, primarily by fine needle aspirating the tumor and measuring amylase, which is elevated in pseudocysts, and mucin stains, which are prominent in the mucinous cystadenocarcinomas. Furthermore, CEA levels are supposed to be elevated in the mucinous tumors.

In a small series of 39 patients who underwent endosonography and fine needle aspiration, the negative predictive value for malignancy, taking into consideration the image of the endosonography plus the aspiration and analysis of the contents, was only about 66% and the positive predictive value for malignancy was about 75%.

A few more points and I will be finished. What about IPMT? The hallmarks of the lesion are mucin being extruded from the dilated papilla and a widely dilated pancreatic duct throughout the pancreas. Our experience to date with 64 patients with IPMT: about half of them had malignancy and resection. Of the 34 patients who had no malignancy at resection, 15 had a Kausch-Whipple resection, 12 a distal pancreatectomy. So, there were 4 recurrences in these patients with initially benign lesions, and one had an invasive malignancy. There were 7 total pancreatectomies. Thus, all of them have been alive after surgery.

Finally, there are a sort of odd-ball types of cysts, mixed solid and cystic papillary neoplasms, usually in young women. These tumors are slow growing. They have an intermediate malignant potential and are usually very large bulky masses. This does not fit with the patient in our discussion. A neuroendocrine tumor is also unlikely in our patient. 80% of them are solid but some of them may have cysts.

I think, taking all together with the appearance of the lesion on the CT that we were shown and some of the points that I made, it is likely that our patient has a mucinous cystadenoma. I would be worried about a cystadenocarcinoma, primarily because of the elevated tumor markers, but there are other explanations for the elevation of the tumor markers, particularly CEA, because the patient is a smoker as was mentioned. What about the anemia? Mucinous cystadenomas rarely can actually fistulize and have a potential communication with the gastrointestinal tract and I wonder if that might not be what is going on in this particular patient.

Commentary by the surgeon J. R. Izbicki, M.D, Hamburg, Germany

I have a somewhat more simplistic approach to this patient as compared to Dr. DiMagno. I think we have to take into account two points: First the patient had no history of pancreatitis besides the known cystic lesion. Second, I am concerned about the morphological appearance of this tumor. It is a little dense in the CT scan. So, our approach would be to perform, just as was done in Dr. Layer's institution, an endosonography. I believe that endosonography has the highest sensitivity and specificity especially if you combine it with fine needle aspiration.

Our experience with fine needle aspiration is a little bit better than the Mayo experience. Our 78 patients had a positive predictive value of 100% and a negative predictive value of 86%. And, of course, this is mostly due to the quality of your cytologist. If the cytology has a poor quality then of course endosonography-guided fine needle aspiration will not give you these good results. I think especially for decision-making this is of utmost importance, because nowadays you have the possibility of submitting this patient to so-called limited resection, a middle pancreatic segmentectomy and reconstruction with a T-shape anastomosis. Thus, in case the lesion is benign, you can avoid subjecting the patient to a major surgical procedure such as pylorus-preserving duodenopancreatectomy or a classical Kausch-Whipple resection.

Questions to the audience and answers by the gastroenterologist Dr. DiMagno

Question 1: What is your opinion about diagnostic procedures to exclude or diagnose pancreatic carcinoma?

A) ERCP is a must and still has the highest sensitivity and specificity.
B) Endosonography has the highest sensitivity and is a must to be performed before surgery.
C) CT is the most reliable method of choice to differentiate between pancreatitis and resectability.
D) PET is the method of choice to differentiate between pancreatitis and carcinoma.
E) "All in one" MRT + MR-angiography + MR-cholangiopancreaticography is the method of choice.

DiMagno: I frankly did not like any of these answers. I actually answered C. I did not like B, because it says "it is a must to be performed before surgery". I do not think so. The role of the endosonography, at least as I see it, is if you cannot make a decision on other imaging tests, particularly the CT, and you continue to suspect that this is a carcinoma. In these circumstances the endosonography is really quite a good test. You can detect lesions less than 2 cm fairly easily. Positron emission tomography (PET) I do not think is in wide use. Magnetic resonance tomography (MRT), MR angiography etc. is, in my view, not as accurate at this point and ERCP we actually use very little. So I checked off C, but I did not particularly like any of these answers.

Question 2: What kind of further diagnostic procedures would you recommend in this patient?

A) The patient is already 75 years old and does not seem to be severely ill. I would wait and watch. In a patient with this age all methods are a waste of money since in case of carcinoma she cannot be cured.
B) I am convinced that the patient has pancreatic cancer, maybe a cystadenocarcinoma. She should be operated on without further diagnostic workup.
C) I would perform a drainage of the cyst and analyze the content of the cystic fluid (CA 19-9, malignant cells?).
D) I would perform a mini-laparoscopy to exclude peritoneal metastasis.
E) I would vote for other diagnostic options.

DiMagno: I selected B. I am not too convinced that this is absolutely certain. But I think the patient likely has a cystadenoma/cystadenocarcinoma, probably the latter. The reason I did not do the drainage of the cyst, I think I would still be rather convinced of that opinion regardless of what the cyst analysis would have shown. It is not that the analysis of the cyst material is not 100% correct, at least in our hands all the time you can see exceptions, for example increase of the amylase in mucinous cystadenomas. So, I would not be totally confident, so I selected B.

Question 3: What kind of other diagnostic options should be performed before considering surgery?
A) CT of chest and abdomen is a must.
B) The patient has anemia. I would perform a bone marrow examination.
C) The patient is a smoker. I would perform bronchoscopy.
D) The patient has slight anemia and an elevation of CA 19-9. She might have breast cancer. I would perform mammography.
E) Anemia in a 75-year-old patient without GI bleeding is a tumor sign. I would perform a PET scan.

DiMagno: Well, I did just ask Dr. Layer if she had a chest x-ray, and she had a chest x-ray done actually. So I don't think I would have done a CT of the chest. And I would have assumed for general medical reasons, she would have had a mammogram. So, I would have done none of these.

Commentary by Dr. Layer

We performed endosonography together with fine needle aspiration of the cyst. Cytology was negative. This was a surprise. However, we got tremendous tumor marker levels within the cystic fluid, more than 50 million CA 19-9 and 250 000 CEA. So, we strongly recommended the patient have an operation. She wanted to think about it. Three days later she gave confirmed consent. The surgeon wanted an actual reevaluation, especially of the CT, which was already four months old. The new CT scan showed multiple lesions in the liver. The former single liver lesion was obviously misinterpreted as hemangioma. A sonography-guided puncture of one of the liver lesions revealed an adenocarcinoma. Thus, one has to assume that a cystic adenoma that was benign for more than 20 years finally progressed rather rapidly to an adenocarcinoma. The patient received a palliative treatment with gemcitabine.

Discussion with the audience

Mössner: Most of us would have performed the surgery immediately.

DiMagno: I would have done the surgery immediately without knowing what the actual CT showed at the time of admission to hospital. My colleague, Michael Sarr is shaking his head.

Sarr: That CT was 4 months old!

DiMagno: Yes, I know, but I was acting on that CT as if that was a current CT.

Layer: That was the information we had, a real "life case".

DiMagno: At least, I thought in an older patient with a possible pseudocyst, it should be considered as we say "unexplained pancreatitis in an older patient". However, this may represent already primary carcinoma of the pancreas. I have seen several, where my only suspicion in an otherwise normal-appearing cyst was the fact that this was an older patient without a good explanation for an episode of pancreatitis. And these haven't necessarily been admitted with acute pancreatitis, but with the cyst. And, at least, with the aggressive nature of this lesion, I wonder if this might have been primary pancreatic carcinoma with a pseudocyst that then evolved into a metastatic process.

Layer: However, the pseudocyst was documented for about 20 years!

DiMagno: But I don't think it was a pseudocyst. I think it was a cystic adenoma.

Layer: However, there was no progression. Apparently this 4 cm "cyst" went on for at least 15 years.

DiMagno: It doesn't have to get larger, it can stay relatively stable. I think, if I am quoting Sarr correctly and he can correct me if I am wrong, I have heard him state that he has never seen a cyst adenoma become a cystadenocarcinoma.

Sarr: We haven't followed patients long enough to know that!

DiMagno: Well, we take them all out!

Sarr: We take them out! So, do you think this was a cyst? I mean, what is the lesson of this case? Is this a cystadenoma which became a cystadenocarcinoma or is this an incidental cyst of the pancreas that happened to develop a pancreatic lesion next to it? Are we any wiser?

DiMagno: The point I would make is: In a 55-year-old lady, at the time of the onset of the cyst with no previous history of pancreatitis and the appearance of the cyst, I think the number one diagnosis in your mind must be a cystadenoma/cystadenocarcinoma, and resection should have been done 20 years ago, instead of waiting! We don't know what the rate of progression is from cystadenoma to cystadenocarcinoma.

Mössner: I would like to ask our experts if there is any information that Doppler vascular studies are helpful in distinguishing a pseudocyst from a cystadenoma.

DiMagno: No, I haven't seen anything with a Doppler in a cyst. I would have done only a transabdominal ultrasonography and then surgical resection and avoided the puncture for the risk of seeding pancreatic cancer.

Layer: I agree. The problem with our patient is that she was very hesitant about having surgery unless we demonstrated to her the urgency, just by the findings. She had her ultrasound examinations long ago and she was used to it. Except for her sort of slight, very unspecific complaints, we would not have been able to convince her. I think the lesson from this case is: do not trust a lesion in the liver without further biopsy.

Second case: a 44-year-old female patient
Presented by P. Dîté, M.D., Brno, Czech Republic

History

10 years ago, 1990, an at that time 33-year-old female patient presented with the following symptoms: flatulence, indeterminate epigastric pain and fullness. During the next three years the severity of the symptoms increased. Different analgesics and prokinetics were prescribed by her doctor. In June 1993, an esophagogastroduodenoscopy was performed and histologically bulbitis and helicobacter pylori negative antral gastritis described. In the same year, the patient developed typically biliary colics. Stones in the gallbladder were detected by sonography. A laparoscopic cholecystectomy was performed. In December 1993, severe epigastric pain, nausea and hyperamylasemia developed twice,

lasting for some days. She was admitted to the local hospital and discharged after some days with the diagnosis "acute relapse of chronic pancreatitis".

One year later, 1994, the patient again developed severe abdominal pain and was admitted to our hospital. She was slightly underweight, body mass index 20. She reported that there was no history of pancreatitis in her family. She has two healthy children. She has smoked at least 10 cigarettes per day for the last 20 years. She does not consume alcohol daily, but confessed to alcoholic excesses on occasions. She was living in the area of Moravia, where many families prepare their own home plum brandy.

She complained about epigastric pain regularly after each meal combined with the need to vomit.

Objective findings

Progressive body weight loss, jaundice and enlargement of the liver developed. Serum bilirubin, gamma-Glutamyltransferase, and alcalic phosphatase were markedly elevated. Serum-glucose was normal. Serum amylase was only slightly elevated. Transabdominal sonography revealed an enlargement of the pancreatic head with a cyst. The CT scan confirmed typical signs of chronic pancreatitis with enlargement of the pancreatic head and a pseudocyst, 4 cm in diameter. In contrast, the CT scan performed one year earlier at the local district hospital was almost normal. The ERCP showed dilatation of the common bile duct with marked but regular narrowing proximal to the papilla of Vater. The main pancreatic duct was irregular and slightly dilated and had a connection to the pseudocyst. We recommended resection of the pancreatic head. However, the patient refused surgery. Both a biliary and a pancreatic drainage were performed using plastic stents. After the endoscopic procedure all symptoms were relieved.

However, some months later, the patient again experienced severe abdominal pain. Sonography demonstrated a pseudocyst in the pancreatic head which compressed the distal part of the common bile duct. During the following years we exchanged the biliary and pancreatic stents almost regularly. The patient still refused surgery. Symptom relief lasted for about two to three months after each stent renewal. Without endoscopic drainages the patient suffered pain relapses rather rapidly. In January 1995, she finally agreed to surgical therapy. A duodenum-preserving pancreatic head resection with pancreatico-gastroanastomosis was performed.

However, only 3 months later, the patient was again admitted to our institution due to epigastric pain, vomitus, fever, pruritus, and jaundice.

On ERCP, the papilla of Vater looked like a pseudotumor, enlarged and very fragile. A canulation of the bile and pancreatic duct was not feasible. A transhepatic biliary drainage into the duodenum was performed using the "rendez-vous" technique. After this procedure the patient felt quite well without any further symptoms.

In January 1997, about half a year later, we removed the stent from the biliary duct. ERCPs in yearly intervals showed no relapse of the bile duct stenosis. In 1998, the patient was still without pain, but reported some abdominal discomfort intermittently. Her appetite was good. The body weight increased by 11 kg. All routine laboratory values were normal. In 2000, the patient visited us again, because she thought that it was a good interval and a good time to visit her doctor. She had no symptoms, constant body weight, almost normal laboratory values. However, the oral glucose tolerance test revealed beginning diabetes.

A repeated CT scan displays a dilatation of the pancreatic duct in the remaining body and tail. On ERCP a slight stenosis of the common bile duct was still seen although there were no laboratory signs of cholestasis.

Questions to the audience and answers by the gastroenterologist A. Nowak, M.D., Katowice, Poland

Question 1: The patient had a stenosis of both the pancreatic and the bile duct. How would you have treated the patient initially?
A) Endoscopic drainage of both ducts.
B) Endoscopic drainage of biliary duct only.
C) Endoscopic drainage of the pancreatic duct only.
D) Surgery.
E) Medical treatment; wait and see.

Nowak: This patient presented with severe pain and typical complications of chronic pancreatitis. I voted for D. Only 3% of the audience voted for medical treatment only. Of course we have obstructive jaundice and we have severe pain. However, we must remember that in not severe cases medical therapy might also work. Surgery should be the method of choice in this special case. There is bile duct obstruction with jaundice and we can expect initial pain relief after surgery in about 80% of patients together with good long-term results. However, we have to accept the patient's refusal of surgery at this stage of her disease. For endoscopic drainage of the pancreatic duct only, there is one pro: pancreatic pain relief. However, in this patient we still have to consider the biliary duct obstruction which will not be resolved by pancreatic drainage. Furthermore, we have to consider the risk of complications after pancreatic stenting. According to Michele Cremer, Brussels, pancreatic stenting results in longstanding pain relief in more than 50% of patients with prepapillary stenosis of the main pancreatic duct. Only about 15% of patients need surgery. The complication rate of pancreatic duct stenting is about 10%. However, these positive results of Cremer are not reported by all. We have to consider perforations by the stent and stent migrations. Furthermore, we must consider secondary inflammations which might resolve after stent removal. Endoscopic drainage of the biliary duct only is another option. Pro: only relief of biliary obstruction, but several contras: pancreatic pain will not resolve by the drainage of the biliary duct only. Biliary complications in chronic pancreatitis such as cholangitis and cholestasis are seen in 10 to 45% of patients. Endoscopic biliary drainage is a very good option for short-term solutions. However, long-term results are rather disappointing. Complete resolution of bile duct obstruction is achieved only in 10%, partial improvement in 55%. Thirty per cent do not show any improvement during 10 months of follow-up. A further drawback is the need to exchange plastic stents every 8 to 12 weeks. Endoscopic drainage of both ducts showed especially good results in this particular case. Pro: both biliary obstruction and pancreatic pain will be relieved. However, long-term results are as bad as with biliary stenting alone. Thus, there is only one good option, i.e. surgery.

Commentary on Question 1 by the surgeon M. Schilling, M.D., Homburg/Saar, Germany

I will elaborate on this case later after we have discussed the next questions. This case is, as opposed to the last case, not so much a challenge in diagnostic terms, but rather in therapeutic terms. We would agree with Dr. Dîté and with most of the audience that this patient should have been operated on already initially. However, she refused surgery. Thus, you have to offer the patient different treatment modalities. My second point: if you do surgery you have to choose the right procedure. And if you choose the right procedure you have to do that right. That is a problem we have seen in this case and we probably should discuss this matter later.

A member of the audience: I suggest putting in a stent first. If you see pain relief, you go on with surgery. However, first you have to proof that the pain is really coming from the pancreatic duct stenosis.

A member of the audience: One comment from the point of view of an endoscopist: I believe this patient is very special. She not only had a pancreatic head tumor, but she had a pseudocyst. Therefore, it makes sense first to try to decompress the cyst and see whether this also leads to a decompression of the bile duct and pain relief. One may proceed to surgery later.

A member of the audience: I would like to raise another important point: This patient has a long history of chronic alcoholic pancreatitis. She had biliary duct stenosis, pancreatic duct stenosis and a pseudocyst. You always have to keep in mind that this is a patient who potentially has developed a malignant tumor. This patient should be seen by a surgeon first!

Question 2 to the audience: After initial failure of endoscopic treatment and the patient's agreement to surgery a pylorus-preserving resection of the pancreatic head was performed. However, pain did not disappear and stenosis of the bile duct relapsed. What kind of operation would you have recommended?

A) Biliodigestive anastomosis leaving the pancreas unattended.
B) Kausch-Whipple resection.
C) Duodenum-preserving pancreatic head resection.
D) Resection according to Frey.
E) Biliodigestive anastomosis and Roux-en-Y pancreaticojejunostomy.

Commentary on Question 2 by the surgeon Dr. Schilling

Let me first take you back to common bile duct stenosis in chronic pancreatitis. We know that common bile duct stenosis is prevalent in about 30%–45% of all patients who are presented to us with chronic pancreatitis. However, not all of the patients that have bile duct stenosis on ERCP have obstructive jaundice. And only one third of those patients who have bile duct stenosis on imaging have obstructive jaundice. Thus not all of these patients require decompression. Only 10% of all patients with common bile duct stenosis require permanent decompression of the common bile duct. In the majority of patients, due to acute inflammation of the pancreas, the stenosis may subside all by itself.

The patient in this case presented to us with bile duct stenosis and with pancreatic duct stenosis. In those cases we always teach our residents to consider pancreatic cancer. We all know that the incidence of pancreatic cancer in chronic pancreatitis increases over time, even more so in hereditary pancreatitis which was not the case in this patient.

The patient was treated by pancreatic head resection and, it was said, with pylorus-preserving pancreatic head resection. Let's go back to the original paper by Traverso and Longmeyer who described that procedure. You clearly see that they recommended bile duct drainage by performing hepaticojejunostomy. If the surgeon had done that in our case, the biliary obstruction in the further follow-up of the patient would not have occurred. However, the patient had two stenoses, a bile duct stenosis and a pancreatic duct stenosis. You can treat both of those problems with either the Kausch-Whipple resection, either pylorus-preserving or the classical procedure, which in that case would have probably been too much. You can treat this patient with a Kausch-Whipple resection or with the Beger procedure, the duodenum-preserving pancreatic head resection. The problem with that procedure, however, is that you really have to make sure that you drain the bile duct correctly. If you recall the ERCP, you have seen there was at least a 1-cm stenosis of the distal bile duct. In addition, there were a couple of stents put in that bile duct already. All the surgeons who have operated on such patients know that repeated stents cause severe strictures, they can cause inflammation around the bile duct, and it's rather difficult to perform pancreatic resections in these patients. If you decided for a Beger's procedure, which is perfectly fine in that case, you certainly have to take care of the cyst and of the pancreatic duct stenosis. You have to make sure that the biliary tract is open. In that case you certainly have to open the bile duct and you probably have to perform an internal biliary anastomosis. You can avoid all of that by going primarily to the Kausch-Whipple resection.

Question 3 to the audience: After surgery jaundice recurred and the patient was again treated by biliary duct stenting. The patient became pain-free and the stent was removed after several months. What is your strongest opinion in this situation?
A) I would rather have performed a second surgical procedure.
B) Leaving a biliary stent unattended is too dangerous and may cause biliary sepsis.
C) I would have done nothing. The patient would have become pain-free anyway.
D) There are no standard recommendations for treating chronic pancreatitis according to evidence-based medicine. Each case has to be treated individually.
E) A combination of endoscopic and surgical treatment according to the individual case should be stressed more in chronic pancreatitis.

Commentary on Question 3 by Dr. Nowak

I have voted, like most of our audience, for E. I think more endoscopic treatment should be tried. However, we know that there are no randomized studies comparing surgical with endoscopic treatments. The endoscopic treatment in this patient was, however, very successful. She became pain-free and free of jaundice. I would like to stress again that we still need good randomized trials for any type of therapy before we will be able to give treatment recommendations based on evidence.

Discussion on Question 3 with the Audience

A member of the audience: I would like to make two comments: First, if we look to the D and E answers, they are both underlined by the same philosophy. So, I conclude that more than 60% of the audience is very open-minded about the treatment of these patients. Second, regarding our particular patient, I think the clinical history shows very clearly that if the patient had not refused surgery at the beginning, a lot of money, time and stress could have been avoided!

Chairman: I would like to thank our experts and the audience for the interesting case presentations and for the lively and competent discussions. I would especially like to thank the representatives of the Knoll Company, Germany, who supported our interactive workshop and who made the electronic question and answer voting system possible.

9 Chronic pancreatitis, diabetes mellitus and nutrition

9.1 Pathogenesis and treatment of diabetes secondary to chronic pancreatitis

P. Diem

Introduction

Due to the close anatomical and functional links between exocrine and endocrine pancreas in the majority of patients suffering from chronic pancreatitis the exocrine tissue damage is associated with some form of endocrine dysfunction. Diabetes mellitus caused by pancreatic exocrine disease is a distinct metabolic and clinical form of diabetes which typically develops within the first 10 years after the initial diagnosis of chronic pancreatitis. In the United States and other Western countries [1, 2] diabetes secondary to chronic pancreatitis accounts for < 1% of all diabetes. The exact mechanisms whereby chronic pancreatitis leads to glucose intolerance and diabetes are not fully elucidated, but reduction of β-cell mass with blunted insulin responses to glucose plays a major role. Diagnosis, pathogenesis and clinical implications of diabetes secondary to chronic pancreatitis are discussed in this short review.

Prevalence and diagnosis

Depending on the population studied and on the diagnostic criteria used, the prevalence of impaired glucose tolerance and diabetes following pancreatitis varies considerably. Transient hyperglycemia is seen in up to 50% of patients with acute pancreatitis [2], but persistent diabetes develops in less than 5% unless further attacks occur [2]. On the other hand in patients with chronic pancreatitis the incidence of glucose intolerance and diabetes increases over time. The incidence of disturbances of glucose metabolism is also influenced by the underlying disease leading to the inflammatory process. Alcohol, for example, may lead to more severe pancreatic tissue damage, and thus is associated with a higher incidence of glucose intolerance [3]. Impaired glucose tolerance or diabetes has been found in 30–70% of patients with chronic pancreatitis and in up to 90% of patients with chronic calcifying pancreatitis [4–6]. Risk factors for the development of diabetes secondary to pancreatitis are:

- alcoholic pancreatitis [2],
- continuing alcohol abuse [7],
- severe exocrine insufficiency [7],
- family history of type 2 diabetes mellitus [8] and
- pancreatic surgery [8].

Actuarial analyses have shown that within 10 years [7] to 15 years [8] around 80% of patients with known chronic pancreatitis develop diabetes mellitus.

The suspicion that impaired glucose tolerance or diabetes is secondary to chronic pancreatitis is often based on a history of chronic pancreatitis (with a known cause). Pancreatic calcifications on plain radiography or steatorrhea corroborate the diagnosis. However, in some patients diabetes precedes first clinical symptoms of pancreatitis, often leading to initial misclassification. To confirm the diagnosis of diabetes fasting plasma glucose levels or 2h-glucose values during an oral glucose tolerance test may be used. Due to the specific pathogenesis of endocrine disease secondary to pancreatitis in these patients 2h-glucose values during an oral glucose tolerance test are more sensitive for detecting early metabolic disturbances or for diagnosing diabetes.

Pathogenesis of endocrine insufficiency

Any disease affecting the exocrine pancreas may also lead to diabetes. In chronic pancreatitis the inflammatory disease leads to progressive tissue damage with fibrosis and sclerosis. This process also affects the islets of Langerhans and the progression of fibrosis leads to reduction of β-cell mass. In addition fibrosis and sclerosis may impair pancreatic capillary circulation and diminish islet perfusion. This may lead to impaired delivery of secretagogues and blunted hormonal responses of the islets. The loss of β-cell mass associated with chronic pancreatitis accounts for reduced insulin secretion. The greater the reduction of endocrine tissue, the more insulin secretion is impaired and the more glucose tolerance is reduced [9–11]. This association between exocrine and endocrine dysfunction may suggest a causal relationship between inflammatory tissue damage and the development of diabetes mellitus. As long as 20–40% of β-cell mass is retained, fasting plasma glucose and insulin levels are often normal (or near-normal) and overt diabetes is rare. Nonetheless, at this stage of endocrine insufficiency insulin responses following ingestion of an oral glucose load are delayed and blunted. Only when around 80% of β-cells are destroyed does fasting hyperglycemia develop [9]. Abnormal glucose sensing does not seem to be present in patients with impaired glucose tolerance or diabetes. In contrast, chronic hyperglycemia, through its negative effects on β-cell function [12], may induce a vicious cycle and further aggravate the metabolic imbalance.

Chronic pancreatitis is frequently associated with reduced secretion of incretins (GIP, GLIP-1) affecting the entero-pancreatic axis and postmeal insulin secretion [13, 14]. However, normal incretin effects have been seen by others, despite exocrine disease [5]. Thus it remains unclear to what extent abnormal incretin secretion contributes to the development of hyperglycemia.

Obviously, in some patients, besides the inflammatory process, pancreatic surgery (pancreatoduodenectomy, distal pancreatectomy, total pancreatectomy) is an important pathogenetical element leading to additional β-cell loss.

Clinical characteristics and therapeutic considerations

The symptoms of diabetes caused by chronic pancreatitis are the same as in any other form of diabetes. However, this form of diabetes has a number of distinct clinical characteristics. Most typical are the wide fluctuations in plasma glucose levels. Coexistent exocrine deficiency, a history of antral resection, non-compliance (with diet and medical therapy), and a disposition to hypoglycemic reactions all contribute to labile metabolic control. Importantly, patients with diabetes caused by chronic pancreatitis are especially prone to frequent, severe and unpredictable hypoglycemic episodes. A number of factors contribute to this tendency (summarized in Table 9.1-1). In contrast to these problems of metabolic control the development of diabetic ketoacidosis and diabetic coma is relatively

Table 9.1-1. Factors contributing to the increased risk of hypoglycemia and metabolic instability in patients with diabetes caused by chronic pancreatitis.

- Glucagon deficiency and blunted glucagon responses to hypoglycemia (reduced number of α-cells)
- Malabsorption/maldigestion (steatorrhea)
- Accelerated intestinal transit, dumping syndrome
- Low carbohydrate intake
- Alcohol
- Non-compliance with diet and medical therapy

uncommon and mainly seen in situations of marked stress (infection, surgery). The risk of early microvascular diabetic complications seems comparable to other forms of diabetes (reviewed by Del Prato and Tiengo [8]). Less is known about the more advanced stages of diabetic complications (blindness, end-stage kidney disease) due to the high mortality – not associated with diabetes – of patients with chronic pancreatitis.

Appropriate therapy of patients with diabetes caused by chronic pancreatitis has to be individually tailored in order to address inherent instability of metabolic control. Initial and important steps are adequate nutrition and dietary recommendations. In some patients sulfonylureas may be used successfully and short acting agents have to be preferred in order to reduce the risk of hypoglycemia. However, sulfonylureas are often contraindicated due to coexistent liver disease. In these situations biguanides should also be avoided and are generally less useful since the major pathogenetic defect is lack of insulin. Following total pancreatectomy and in cases with more severe β-cell destruction insulin therapy is mandatory. Insulin therapy, however, is associated with a number of specific problems and often extreme lability of metabolic control (see Table 9.1-1). In patients with diabetes secondary to chronic pancreatitis or following partial pancreatectomy insulin requirements are not different from those in matched type 1 diabetics, whereas in totally pancreatectomized patients daily insulin requirements are clearly lower [8]. This seems to be particularly true during nighttime [15]. Rigorous self-monitoring of blood glucose (SMBG) [16], intensified insulin treatment with multiple injections of small amounts of insulin [17] and total pancreatectomy performed with preservation of duodenum and pylorus [18] all are likely to reduce the risk of hypoglycemia.

When defining individual treatment goals comorbidity, overall prognosis, age and metabolic instability have to be considered. Often an HbA_{1c} value of 7–8% will be acceptable. In order to achieve good metabolic control the patient's nutritional status has to be adequate (and if necessary improved). Alcohol abstinence and sufficient enzyme substitution are essential. These measures will reduce metabolic instability and together with optimal patient education, SMBG and an intensified insulin regimen will allow HbA_{1c} values < 8% in many patients [17, 18].

Summary

Endocrine insufficiency leading to impaired glucose tolerance or diabetes is a significant complication of chronic pancreatitis. Reduction of β-cell mass with blunted insulin responses to glucose plays a major role in the pathogenesis of endocrine insufficiency. In a considerable number of patients dietary measures are sufficient; in most other patients insulin is advocated. However, due to extreme metabolic lability treatment is often difficult. Optimal patient education, good nutritional status, alcohol abstinence, adequate enzyme substitution, self-monitoring of blood glucose and intensified insulin treatment are the cornerstones of successful metabolic control of diabetes secondary to chronic pancreatitis.

References

1. Vinik AI, Jackson WPU. Endocrine secretions in chronic pancreatitis. In: Podolsky S, Viswanathran M, eds. Secondary Diabetes: The Spectrum of the Diabetic Syndromes. New York: Raven Press, 1981: 165–89.
2. Banks S. Chronic pancreatitis: Clinical features and medical management. Am J Gastroenterol 1986; 81: 153–67.
3. Sarles H, Cros RC, Bidart JM, International Group for the Study of Pancreatic Diseases. A multicenter inquiry on the etiology of pancreatic diseases. Digestion 1979; 19: 110–25.
4. Larsen S. Diabetes mellitus secondary to chronic pancreatitis. Den Med Bull 1993; 40: 153–62.
5. Owyang C. Endocrine changes in pancreatic insufficiency. In: Vay Liang W Go et al., eds. The pancreas. Biology, Pathology and Disease. New York: Raven Press, 1993: 803–10.
6. Amman RW, Akovbiantz A, Largiader F, Schneller G. Course and outcome of chronic pancreatitis. Gastroenterology 1984; 86: 820–8.
7. Lankisch PG, Löhr-Hoppe A, Otto J, Creutzfeldt W. Natural course in chronic pancreatitis. Digestion 1993; 54: 148–55.
8. Del Prato S, Tiengo A. Pancreatic diabetes. Diab Rev 1993; 1: 260–85.
9. Vinik AI. Insulin secretion in chronic pancreatitis. In: Tiengo A, Alberti KGMM, Del Prato S, Vranic M, eds. Diabetes secondary to pancreopathy. Amsterdam: Excerpta Medica, 1988: 35–50.
10. Kalk WJ, Vinik AI, Jackson WPU, Bank S. Insulin secretion and pancreatic exocrine function in patients with chronic pancreatitis. Diabetologia 1979; 16: 355–8.
11. Moran A, Diem P, Klein DJ, Levitt MD, Robertson RP. Pancreatic endocrine function in cystic fibrosis. J Pediatr 1991; 118: 715–23.
12. Rossetti L, Giaccari A, De Fronzo RA. Glucose toxicity. Diabetes Care; 13: 610–30.
13. Ebert R, Creutzfeldt W. Reversal of impaired GIP and insulin secretion in patients with pancreatogenic steatorrhea following enzyme substitution. Diabetologia 1980; 19: 198–204.
14. Gomez-Cerezo J, Gorces MC, Codoceo R et al. Postprandial glucose-dependent insulinotropic polypeptide and insulin responses in patients with chronic pancreatitis with and without secondary diabetes. Regul Pept 1996; 67: 201–5.
15. Beyer J, Schulz G, Cordes U. A glucose-controlled insulin infusion system (Biostator) in pancreatectomized patients. In: Brunetti P, Alberti KGMM, Albisser M, Hepp KD, Massi Benedetti M, eds. Artificial Systems for Insulin Delivery. New York: Raven Press, 1983: 535–42.
16. Dresler CM, Fortner JG, McDermott K, Bajorunas DR. Metabolic consequences of (regional) total pancreatectomy. Ann Surg 1991; 214: 131–40.
17. Starke AAR, Cuppers HJ, Berger M. Therapeutic problems in diabetes secondary to pancreatopathy. In: Tiengo A, Alberti KGMM, Del Prato S, Vranic M, eds. Diabetes secondary to pancreopathy. Amsterdam: Excerpta Medica, 1988: 227–33.
18. Easter DW, Cuschieri A. Total pancreatectomy with preservation of the duodenum and pylorus for chronic pancreatitis. Ann Surg 1990; 214: 575–80.

9.2 New classes of antidiabetic drugs: New perspectives for diabetes mellitus treatment

B. Göke, R. Göke

Introduction

Diabetes mellitus (DM) is a group of metabolic diseases arising from defects in insulin secretion or action, and is characterized by hyperglycemia. One of the primary defects of type 2 diabetes is insulin resistance, which comprises hyperinsulinemia, hypertension, dyslipidemia (particularly increased triglycerides and reduced high-density lipoprotein [HDL] cholesterol), and impaired glucose tolerance [23, 59].

Prolonged hyperglycemia puts patients with type 2 DM at an increased risk of microvascular and macrovascular complications. The UK Prospective Diabetes Study (UKPDS) followed 3867 such patients for 10 years. This study confirmed that lowering blood glucose is beneficial in type 2 DM patients, leading to a reduction in the risk of development of retinopathy and nephropathy, and possibly of neuropathy. The overall rate of microvascular complications was reduced by 25% in patients receiving intensive compared with conventional therapy [74, 75]. Recommendations by the authors included intensive blood glucose lowering, and the use of combination therapies including the newer agents.

New treatment guidelines and criteria for diagnosis of type 2 DM, recently developed by the American Diabetes Association (ADA), aim for a fasting plasma glucose (FPG) range of 80–120 mg/dL and an HbA_{1C} of less than 7%. Although specific treatment goals acknowledge the importance of addressing multiple risk factors including hypertension, cardiovascular disease, dyslipidemia, and lifestyle factors [34], the main target of therapy remains correction of hyperglycemia using appropriate monotherapy or combination therapy with insulin or oral glucose-lowering agents.

Current therapy options include glucosidase inhibitors (e.g. acarbose, miglitol, voglibose), glinides (repaglinide, nateglinide), sulfonylureas, metformin, and the recently available thiazolidinediones, which are likely to have a major impact on future therapy.

Sulfonylureas

Sulfonylureas (SU) stimulate insulin release more or less independently from the prevailing glucose plasma levels and may also enhance the sensitivity of pancreatic β-cells to glucose, but rely on a degree of endogenous insulin secretion [2, 46, 56]. Despite clear differences in the potency of the various sulfonylureas, it has not been possible to demonstrate differences in clinical efficacy between them in lowering blood glucose during long-term therapy [24]. Sulfonylurea therapy is limited by hypoglycemic effects (which are potentially fatal), weight gain, and putative negative effects on cardiac and vascular smooth muscle.

Hypoglycemia is considered the most serious adverse effect of sulfonylurea therapy in type 2 DM [25, 46]. It can occur with any member of the sulfonylurea class, but the risk is higher with long-acting agents (e.g., glibenclamide, chlorpropamide), and newer agents cannot be assumed to be safer than older agents. The risk of hypoglycemia increases with age, other predisposing factors, and specific drug interactions.

Because of their action on ATP-sensitive K^+ channels, sulfonylureas may have deleterious effects on cardiac and vascular function [69]. During normal physiological conditions, sulfonylureas could block ATP-sensitive K^+ channels in both coronary and peripheral vascular smooth muscle cells, leading to increases in vasoconstriction, blood pressure, and coronary vascular resistance. During pathophysiological conditions (e.g. hypoxia, ischemia), sulfonylureas could block ATP-sensitive K^+ channels in myocardial cells, increasing contractility and oxygen uptake [69, 77]. This effect, combined with the vasoconstriction caused by the action of sulfonylureas on vascular ATP-sensitive K^+ channels, could result in further degeneration of myocardial function.

Glinides (meglitinides and D-phenylalanine derivatives)

Meglitinides are new short-acting insulin secretagogues. They are used in patients with overt type 2 diabetes as well as impaired glucose tolerance. Repaglinide (Prandin®), the first non-sulfonylurea insulin secretagogue and a benzoic acid derivative, regulates prandial and postprandial glucose levels by rapidly inducing insulin secretion after ingestion of a meal [22, 53]. It should be given three to four times a day before each meal; however, it offers a flexible regimen when a meal is missed; the corresponding dose has to be skipped [16]. Nateglinide (Starlix®), a D-phenylalanine derivative, was recently approved in Japan, Switzerland, the EU and Brazil. It particularly restores early-phase insulin secretion and controls prandial glucose spikes. The adverse effects of meglitinides and D-phenylalanine derivatives are hypoglycemia during the night, although much less than with SU, and weight gain.

α-Glucosidase inhibitors

Alpha-glucosidase inhibitors block the metabolism of digested polysaccharides and lower the amount of carbohydrates absorbed in a meal [9]. They inhibit enzymes involved in the conversion of disaccharides, polysaccharides, or complex sugars into monosaccharides in the brush border of the small intestine [29]. Acarbose, miglitol or voglibose tablets must be administered with the first bite of food to be effective, and demonstrate the greatest benefits when taken together with a high-carbohydrate meal. They do not cause weight gain and may even induce small weight losses in some patients [29]. These compounds may be especially considered as attractive for combination therapies with other drugs employing alternative means of action.

Metformin

Metformin, a biguanide, is an antihyperglycemic agent rather than a hypoglycemic agent. It lowers blood glucose concentration during hyperglycemia without causing hypoglycemia. Metformin improves the type 2 DM disease profile without affecting plasma insulin levels [52, 57]; it has no effect on pancreatic insulin secretion, but requires the presence of some insulin for therapeutic effect.

A number of mechanisms of action have been proposed for metformin, although none is completely understood. Metformin accumulates in the wall of the intestine and reduces glucose absorption, although this action does not account for most of its effect in patients with type 2 DM [42]. Other proposed actions include reduced glucose production by the liver, increased glucose uptake by tissues, and reduced insulin requirements for glucose disposal (increased insulin sensitivity) [20, 41, 42]. Studies in both lean and obese type 2 DM patients found that basal hepatic glucose output was significantly lower after metformin therapy [17, 55]. At the cellular level, metformin appears to act at the post-receptor level by increasing glucose transport across the cell membrane, similar to the effect generated by acute insulin administration. More specifically, metformin increases the amount of GLUT-4 glucose transporters in the plasma membrane [35, 39, 43].

Effects independent of the antiglycemic action of metformin include weight loss, decreased platelet aggregation, and a beneficial effect on plasma lipid profile [42]. Metformin can result in a 1% to 3% reduction in body weight, usually in the first 6 months of therapy. The mechanism for this weight loss is unclear, although increased thermogenesis, an anorectic effect, and increased energy expenditure have been suggested as possible mechanisms. A decrease in platelet aggregation without hypocoagulation can occur with metformin, with beneficial effects in peripheral vascular disease. The beneficial effects of metformin on plasma lipid profile include a reduction in plasma triglycerides, an increase in HDL-cholesterol, and a reduction in LDL-cholesterol [17, 37, 58, 79]. The clinical benefit of metformin on macrovascular outcomes was demonstrated by the results of the UKPDS, which showed a 36% reduction in all-cause mortality in diet-treated obese type 2 DM patients receiving metformin ($P = 0.011$) [74, 75].

Drug intolerance, gastrointestinal adverse events, and lactic acidosis are tolerability issues that limit the use of metformin. Less than 5% of patients are estimated to stop metformin therapy because of drug intolerance, and between 5% and 20% of metformin-treated patients experience adverse events [7, 46]. These adverse events include diarrhea (in up to 20% of patients), anorexia, abdominal discomfort, and a metallic taste. They are often transient and can be minimized by administration with food and by slowly increasing the dose. There have been individual reports of anemia attributable to impaired vitamin B_{12} and folate absorption, and vasculitis with pneumonitis.

Lactic acidosis is the most notorious and serious adverse effect of biguanide therapy, mainly phenformin, but it can also occur with metformin. Metformin causes a small increase in blood lactate concentrations after meals (possibly arising from the intestine), and a small but significant increase in other gluconeogenic precursors (pyruvate and alanine). Metformin may accumulate in patients with renal impairment, leading to pathological hyperlactatemia with acidosis. Metformin-associated lactic acidosis is much less common than that associated with phenformin, but is still sporadically reported, and the mortality rate is as high as 50% [10, 46]. The incidence of fatal metformin-associated lactic acidosis is approximately the same as that of fatal sulfonylurea-induced hypoglycemia [10, 38]. Metformin should also be used with caution in the elderly and advanced cardiovascular complications [38]; metformin is contraindicated in patients with impaired renal function.

Thiazolidinediones

The thiazolidinediones are a new class of oral agents for the treatment of type 2 DM, and constitute the only antidiabetic agents that directly affect insulin sensitivity. These compounds are likely to significantly improve current therapy strategies. These agents do not stimulate insulin secretion; instead, they enhance or partially mimic some insulin actions on glucose and lipid metabolism, resulting in a glucose-lowering effect caused by increased peripheral glucose disposal and reduced hepatic glucose output. The presence of sufficient insulin is necessary for thiazolidinedione activity.

The thiazolidinedione pioglitazone has been shown to improve insulin resistance and preserve pancreatic β-cell function in monotherapy and in combination with sulfonylureas and metformin [61]. Based on Homeostasis Model Assessment (HOMA) analysis, insulin resistance was significantly reduced from baseline during pioglitazone monotherapy, sulfonylurea combination, and metformin combination studies and compared to placebo ($p \leq 0.05$). Similarly, β-cell function also improved significantly compared to baseline in all studies.

Large-scale placebo-controlled clinical trials conducted in the United States and Europe indicate a dose-dependent reduction in HbA_{1c}, fasting blood glucose, hyperinsulinemia, and hypertriglyceridemia with these agents [26, 31, 33, 47, 54, 60, 68, 76].

At a molecular level, thiazolidinediones activate a specific nuclear hormone receptor, the peroxisome proliferator-activated receptor-γ (PPAR-γ), which is found primarily in adipose tissue, but also in smaller amounts in skeletal muscle, heart, liver, kidney, gut, macrophages, and vascular smooth muscle cells. When activated, the PPAR-γ complex changes the conformation in the promoter region of specific genes regulating lipid and glucose metabolism [73, 78]. Therefore, thiazolidinediones mimic specific effects of insulin on adipocytes, enhancing expression of genes encoding lipoprotein lipase, fatty acid transporter protein, and glucokinase.

Increased expression of insulin-sensitive genes is thought to be the primary mechanism for reduction of insulin resistance by thiazolidinediones. Additional mechanisms include lipid-lowering effects (e.g., lowering triglyceride and nonesterified fatty acid concentrations), increasing GLUT-4 production, increasing hepatic glucose disposal, decreasing hepatic glucose production, correcting TNF-α overproduction, and possibly altering leptin gene expression [6, 12, 70]. Thiazolidinediones can cause weight gain over time, which is associated with improved glycemic control. This weight increase can be at least partly ascribed to their insulinergic effects, and appears in its magnitude over time similar to SU therapy.

Thiazolidinediones may improve macrovascular (cardiovascular) risk factors; this, however, needs to be proven. The enhanced insulin sensitivity leads to improved glucose tolerance [11, 28, 40], reduced hyperinsulinemia [28, 63], significant reductions in both systolic and diastolic blood pressure [45, 72], and improvements in lipid profile [13, 14, 40].

Concern over the safety of the thiazolidinedione class was generated by liver toxicity caused by troglitazone. Newer thiazolidinediones (rosiglitazone, pioglitazone), however, do not appear to be associated with liver-related adverse events. The incidence in clinical trials was comparable to that with placebo; ≤ 3 X Upper Limit of Normal (ULN) liver enzyme elevations were reported by 0.50% rosiglitazone-treated patients versus 0.20% in placebo-treated patients and by 0.25% placebo-treated patients versus 0.26% in pioglitazone-treated patients [1, 5]. Because abnormal liver function is common in type 2 DM patients, frequent precautionary testing of liver function is recommended during thiazolidinedione therapy for the time being.

Safety issues associated with hemodilution, fluid retention, cardiac hypertrophy, and thrombocytopenia raised during preclinical studies with thiazolidinediones have proven to have little clinical significance [1, 5]. Dose-related reductions in hemoglobin and hematocrit, remaining within normal limits, have been observed with thiazolidinediones. These changes tended to stabilize within 10–14 weeks and did not lead to any discontinuations from the treatment. Dose-related edema has been reported and no patients withdrew from therapy due to this adverse effect. Respective incidences were similar with both thiazolidinediones: 3.1 % with pioglitazone [8] and 4.8% with rosiglitazone [5]. Importantly, edema appears not to be associated in clinical trials with increased cardiovascular events over time [8, 31, 33, 51, 54, 60, 68]. Although the complete mechanism of edema effects remains still unclear, edema may rather be a result of precapillary vasodilation, which also occurs with treatment with insulin or calcium channel blockers [19].

Other aspects of thiazolidinediones

Recently, ligands for the peroxisome proliferator-activated receptor-γ have been shown to inhibit the expression of various cytokines in monocytes, macrophages and colon cells, thereby attenuating inflammation in a mouse model of inflammatory bowel disease [71]. These ligands can increase or decrease colonocyte proliferation depending on the model system studied [49, 62, 66, 67]. Furthermore, very recent data suggests that ligands of the peroxisome proliferator-activated receptor-γ are potent enhancers of the tumor necrosis factor (TNF)-related apoptosis inducing ligand (TRAIL) induced apoptosis, at least in certain tumor cell lines [30]. Such findings make thiazolidinediones exiting new compounds for research and for the development of new treatments for metabolic and neoplastic diseases.

Conclusions

Thiazolidinediones represent a new therapeutic approach to directly targeting a major underlying cause of type 2 DM: insulin resistance. They exploit the normal homeostatic mechanisms that regulate glucose and lipid metabolism and therefore may have a beneficial effect on cardiovascular disease progression. First evidence shows that these agents possibly preserve pancreatic β-cell function. They may also, in theory, prevent the development of type 2 DM in prediabetic individuals, since insulin resistance occurs well before the disease manifests. In elderly patients, safety and compliance are major issues.

Thiazolidinediones may also prove useful as anti-inflammatory and/or anti-neoplastic agents.

References

1. Actos [package insert]. Lincolnshire, IL: Takeda Pharmaceuticals America, 2000.
2. Aguilar-Bryan L, Nichols CG, Wechsler SW, Clement JP 4th, Boyd AE 3rd, Gonzalez G, Herrera-Sosa H, Nguy K, Bryan J, Nelson DA. Cloning of the beta cell high-affinity sulfonylurea receptor: a regulator of insulin secretion. Science 1995; 268: 423–6.
3. Al-Salman J, Arjomand H, Kemp DG, Mittal M. Hepatocellular injury in a patient receiving rosiglitazone. A case report. Ann Intern Med 2000; 132: 121–4.
4. American Diabetes Association. Standards of medical care for patients with diabetes mellitus. Diabetes Care 1999; 22(Suppl 1): 32–41.
5. Avandia [package insert]. Philadelphia, PA: SmithKline Beecham Pharmaceuticals, 2000.
6. Bahr M, Spelleken M, Bock M, von Holtey M, Kiehn R, Eckel J. Acute and chronic effects of troglitazone (CS-045) on isolated rat ventricular cardiomyocytes. Diabetologia 1996; 39: 766–74.
7. Bailey CJ. Biguanides and NIDDM. Diabetes Care 1992; 15: 755–72.

8. Belcher G, Mathews D. Safety and tolerability of Pioglitazone. Exp Clin Endocrinol and Diabetes 2000. (In Process Citation.)
9. Brown DL, Britton D. New directions in type 2 diabetes mellitus: an update of current oral antidiabetic therapy. J Natl Med Assoc 1999; 91(7): 389–95.
10. Chan NN, Brain HP, Feher MD. Metformin-associated lactic acidosis: a rare or very rare clinical entity? Diabet Med 1999; 16: 273–81.
11. Chapman H, Clapham JC, Holder JC, Moore GBT, Piercy V, Smith SA et al. Rosiglitazone plus (3-adrenoceptor agonist treatment normalises glycaemia in C57B1/KsJ db/db mice. Diabetologia 1999; 42(Suppl 1): A181.
12. Ciaraldi TP, Huber-Knudsen K, Hickman M, Olefsky JM. Regulation of glucose transport in cultured muscle cells by novel hypoglycaemic agents. Metabolism 1995; 44: 976–81.
13. Colca JR, Dailey CF, Palazuk BJ, Hillman RM, Dinh DM, Melchior GW, Spilman CH. Pioglitazone hydrochloride inhibits cholesterol absorption and lowers plasma cholesterol concentrations in cholesterol-fed rats. Diabetes 1991; 40: 1169–674.
14. Cominacini L, Garbin U, Pastorino AM, Campagnola M, Fratta Pasini A, Davoli A, Rigoni A, Lo Cascio V. Effects of troglitazone on in vitro oxidation of LDL and HDL induced by copper ions and endothelial cells. Diabetologia 1997; 40: 165–72.
15. Cranmer H, Jones NP, Patwardhan R. Rosiglitazone is effective in both obese and non-obese patients with type 2 diabetes. Diabetologia 1999; 42(Suppl 1): A228.
16. Damsbo P, Marbury TC, Hatorp V, Clauson P, Muller PG. Flexible prandial glucose regulation with repaglinide in patients with type 2 diabetes. Diabetes Res Clin Pract 1999; 45(1): 31–9.
17. DeFronzo RA, Barzilai N, Simonson DC. Mechanism of metformin action in obese and lean noninsulin-dependent diabetic subjects. J Clin Endocrinol Metab 1991; 73: 1294–1301.
18. Diabetes Control and Complications Trial Research Group (DCCT). The effect of intensive treatment of diabetes on the development and progression of long-term complications in insulin-dependent diabetes mellitus. N Engl J Med 1993; 329: 977–86.
19. Dougall HT, McLay J. A comparative review of the adverse effects of calcium antagonists. Drug Saf 1996; 15: 91–106.
20. Dunn CJ, Peters DH. Metformin. A review of its pharmacological properties and therapeutic use in non-insulin-dependent diabetes mellitus. Drugs 1995; 49: 721–49.
21. European Diabetes Policy Group. A desktop to type 2 diabetes mellitus. Exp Clin Endocrinol and Diabetes 1999; 107: 390–420.
22. Evans AJ, Krentz AJ. Recent developments and emerging therapies for type 2 diabetes mellitus. Drugs R D 1999; 2(2): 75–94.
23. Expert Committee on the Diagnosis and Classification of Diabetes Mellitus. Report of the expert committee on the diagnosis and classification of diabetes mellitus. Diabetes Care 1999; 22(Suppl 1): 5–19.
24. Ferner RE, Chaplin S. The relationship between the pharmacokinetic and pharmacodynamic effects of oral hypoglycaemic drugs. Clin Pharmacokinet 1987; 12: 397–401.
25. Ferner RE, Neil HA. Sulphonylureas and hypoglycaemia. Br Med J (Clin Res Ed) 1988; 296: 949–50.
26. Fonseca VA, Valiquett TR, Huang SM, Ghazzi MN, Whitcomb RW. Troglitazone monotherapy improves glycemic control in patients with type 2 diabetes mellitus: a randomized, controlled study. The Troglitazone Study Group. J Clin Endocrinol Metab 1998; 83: 3169–76.
27. Forman LM, Simmons DA, Diamond RH. Hepatic failure in a patient taking rosiglitazone. Ann Intern Med 2000; 132: 118–21.
28. Fujiwara T, Okuno A, Yoshioka S, Horikoshi H. Suppression of hepatic gluconeogenesis in long-term troglitazone treated diabetic KK and C57BL/KsJ-db/db mice. Metabolism 1995; 44: 486–90.
29. Garvey WT. Diabetes mellitus in adults. In: Rakel RA, ed. Conn's Current Therapy 2000. Philadelphia, Pa: WB Saunders Company, 2000: 549–66.
30. Göke R, Göke A, Göke B, Chen Y. Regulation of TRAIL-induced apoptosis by transcription factors. Cellular Immunology 2000; 201: 77–82.

31. Göke B, Kleist P, Scherbaum W, und die Pioglitazon-Studiengruppe. Pioglitazon, die deutsche klinische Phase-II-Studie. Diab Stoffw 1999; 8(Suppl 1): 27–8.
32. Gomis R, Jones NP, Vallance SE, Patwardhan R. Low-dose rosiglitazone enhances glycemic control when combined with sulphonylureas in type 2 diabetes. Diabetologia 1999; 42(Suppl 1): A227.
33. Grunberger G, Weston WM, Patwardhan R, Rappaport EB. Rosiglitazone once or twice daily improves glycemic control in patients with type 2 diabetes. Diabetologia 1999; 42(Suppl 1): A4.
34. Haffner SM, Miettinen H. Insulin resistance implications for type II diabetes mellitus and coronary heart disease. Am J Med 1997; 103: 152–62.
35. Hamann A, Benecke H, Greten H, Matthaei S. Metformin increases glucose transporter protein and gene expression in human fibroblasts. Biochem Biophys Res Commun 1993; 196: 382–7.
36. Hirshberg B, Muszkat M, Marom T, Shalit M. Natural course of insulin edema. J Endocrinol Invest 2000; 23: 187–8.
37. Hollenbeck CB, Johnston P, Varasteh BB, Chen YD, Reaven GM. Effects of metformin on glucose, insulin and lipid metabolism in patients with mild hypertriglyceridaemia and non-insulin dependent diabetes by glucose tolerance test criteria. Diabetes Metab 1991; 17: 483–9.
38. Howlett HC, Bailey CJ. A risk-benefit assessment of metformin in type 2 diabetes mellitus. Drug Saf 1999; 20: 489–503.
39. Hundal HS, Ramlal T, Reyes R, Leiter LA, Klip A. Cellular mechanism of metformin action involves glucose transporter translocation from an intracellular pool to the plasma membrane in L6 muscle cells. Endocrinology 1992; 131: 1165–73.
40. Ikeda H, Taketomi S, Sugiyama Y, Shimura Y, Sohda T, Meguro K, Fujita T. Effects of pioglitazone on glucose and lipid metabolism in normal and insulin resistant animals. Arzneimittelforschung 1990; 40: 156–62.
41. Jackson RA, Hawa MI, Jaspan JB, Sim BM, Disilvio L, Featherbe D, Kurtz AB. Mechanism of metformin action in non-insulin-dependent diabetes. Diabetes 1987; 36: 632–40.
42. Klepser TB, Kelly MW. Metformin hydrochloride: an antihyperglycemic agent. Am J Health Syst Pharm 1997; 54: 893–903.
43. Klip A, Leiter LA. Cellular mechanism of action of metformin. Diabetes Care 1990; 13: 696–704.
44. Kinoshita J, Tanaka Y, Niwa M, Yoshii H, Takagi M, Kawamori R. Impairment of insulin-induced vasodilation is associated with muscle insulin resistance in type 2 diabetes. Diabetes Res Clin Pract 2000; 47: 185–90.
45. Kotchen TA, Reddy S, Zhang HY. Increasing insulin sensitivity lowers blood pressure in the fructose-fed rat. Am J Hypertens 1997; 10: 1020–6.
46. Krentz AJ, Ferner RE, Bailey CJ. Comparative tolerability profiles of oral antidiabetic agents. Drug Saf 1994; 11: 223–41.
47. Kumar S, Boulton AJ, Beck-Nielsen H, Berthezene F, Muggeo M, Persson B, Spinas GA, Donoghue S, Lettis S, Stewart-Long P. Troglitazone, an insulin action enhancer, improves metabolic control in NIDDM patients. Troglitazone Study Group. Diabetologia 1996; 39: 701–9.
48. Lebovitz HE. Insulin Secretagogues: Old and New. Diabetes Reviews 1999; 7(3): 139.
49. Lefebvre AM, Chen I, Desreumaux P, Najib J, Fruchart JC, Geboes K, Briggs M, Heyman R, Auwerx J. Activation of the peroxisome proliferator-activated receptor-γ promotes the development of colon tumors in C57 BL/6J-APC min/+ mice. Nature Medicine 1998; 4: 1053–7.
50. Lefebvre AM, Peinado-Onsurbe J, Leitersdorf I, Briggs MR, Paterniti JR, Fruchart JC, Fievet C, Auwerx J, Staels B. Regulation of lipoprotein metabolism by thiazolidinediones occurs through a distinct but complementary mechanism relative to fibrates. Arterioscler Thromb Vasc Biol 1997; 17: 1756–64.
51. Mathisen AL, Schneider R, Rubin C, Houser V. The effect of pioglitazone on glucose control and lipid profile in patients with type 2 diabetes. Diabetologia 1999; 42(Suppl 1): A227.
52. Nagi DK, Yudkin JS. Effects of metformin on insulin resistance, risk factors for cardiovascular disease, and plasminogen activator inhibitor in NIDDM subjects. A study of two ethnic groups. Diabetes Care 1993; 16: 621–9.

53. Nattrass M, Bailey CJ. New agents for type 2 diabetes. Baillieres Clin Endocrinol Metab. 1999; 13(2): 309–29.
54. Patel J, Miller E, Patwardhan R. Rosiglitazone improves glycaemic control when used as a monotherapy in type 2 diabetic patients. Diabet Med 1998; 15(Suppl 2): 37–8.
55. Perriello G, Misericordia P, Volpi E, Santucci A, Santucci C, Ferrannini E, Ventura MM, Santeusanio F, Brunetti P, Bolli GB. Acute antihyperglycemic mechanisms of metformin in NIDDM. Evidence for suppression of lipid oxidation and hepatic glucose production. Diabetes 1994; 43: 920–8.
56. Philipson LH, Steiner DF. Pas de deux or more: the sulfonylurea receptor and K^+ channels. Science 1995; 268: 372–3.
57. Prager R, Schernthaner G. Insulin receptor binding to monocytes, insulin secretion, and glucose tolerance following metformin treatment. Results of a double-blind cross-over study in type II diabetics. Diabetes 1983; 32: 1083–6.
58. Rains SG, Wilson GA, Richmond W, Elkeles RS. The effect of glibenclamide and metformin on serum lipoproteins in type 2 diabetes. Diabet Med 1988; 5: 653–8.
59. Reaven GM. Banting lecture 1988. Role of insulin resistance in human disease. Diabetes 1988; 37: 1595–1607.
60. Rebuck AS, Weill S, Patwardhan R: Rosiglitazone given once or twice daily is effective first-line treatment for type 2 diabetes mellitus. Diabetologia 1999; 42(Suppl 1): A231.
61. Rosenstock J. Improved insulin sensitivity and beta cell responsivity suggested by HOMA analysis of pioglitazone therapy. Diabetologia 2000; 43(EASD Suppl.). (in press.)
62. Saez E, Tontonoz P, Nelson MC, Alvarez GA, Ming UT, Baird SM, Thomazy V, Evans R. Activators of the nuclear receptor γ enhance colon polyp formation. Nature Medicine 1998; 4: 1058–61.
63. Saha AK, Kurowski TG, Colca JR, Ruderman NB. Lipid abnormalities in tissues of the KKA^y mouse: effects of pioglitazone on malonyl-CoA and diacylglycerol. Am J Physiol 1994; 267: E95–101.
64. Saltiel AR, Olefsky JM. Thiazolidinediones in the treatment of insulin resistance and type II diabetes. Diabetes 1996; 45: 1661–9.
65. Salzman A. Rosiglitazone is not associated with hepatotoxicity. Diabetologia 1999; 42(Suppl 1): A3.
66. Sarraf P, Mueller E, Jones D, King FJ, DeAngelo DJ, Partridge JB, Holden SA, Chen LB, Singer S, Fletcher C, Spiegelman BM. Differentiation and reversal of malignant changes in colon cancer through PPAR-γ. Nature Medicine 1998; 4: 1046–52.
67. Seed B. PPAR-γ and colorectal carcinoma: conflicts in a nuclear family. Nature Medicine 1998; 4: 1004–5.
68. Schneider R, Lessem J, Lekich H. Pioglitazone is effective in the treatment of patients with type 2 diabetes. Pioglitazone 001 Study Group. Diabetes 1999; 48(Suppl 1): A109.
69. Smits P, Bijlstra PJ, Russel FG, Lutterman JA, Thien T. Cardiovascular effects of sulphonylurea derivatives. Diabetes Res Clin Pract 1996; 31(Suppl): S55–9.
70. Spiegelman BM. PPAR-γ: adipogenic regulator and thiazolidinedione receptor. Diabetes 1998; 47: 507–14.
71. Su CG, Wen X, Bailey ST, Jiang W, Rangwala SM, Keilbaugh SA, Flanigan A, Murthy S, Lazar MA, Wu GD. A novel therapy for colitis utilizing PPARγ-ligands to inhibit the epithelial inflammatory response. J Clin Invest 1999; 104: 383–9
72. Suzuki M, Nomura C, Odaka H, Ikeda H. Effect of an insulin sensitizer, pioglitazone, on hypertension in fructose-drinking rats. Jpn J Pharmacol 1997; 74: 297–302.
73. Tontonoz P, Hu E, Graves RA, Budavari AI, Spiegelman BM. mPPAR-γ2: tissue-specific regulator of an adipocyte enhancer. Genes Dev 1994; 8: 1224–34.
74. UK Prospective Diabetes Study (UKPDS) Group. Intensive blood-glucose control with sulphonylureas or insulin compared with conventional treatment and risk of complications in patients with type 2 diabetes (UKPDS 33). Lancet 1998a; 352: 837–53.

75. UK Prospective Diabetes Study (UKPDS) Group. Effect of intensive blood-glucose control with metformin on complications in overweight patients with type 2 diabetes (UKPDS 34). Lancet 1998b; 352: 854–65.
76. Valiquett T, Balagtas C, Whitcomb R. Troglitazone dose-response study in patients with NIDDM. Diabetes 1996; 44(Suppl 1): 109.
77. Végh Á, Papp JG. Haemodynamic and other effects of sulphonylurea drugs on the heart. Diabetes Res Clin Pract 1996; 31(Suppl): 43–53.
78. Vidal-Puig AJ, Considine RV, Jimenez-Linan M, Werman A, Pories WJ, Caro JF, Flier JS. Peroxisome proliferator-activated receptor gene expression in human tissues. Effects of obesity, weight loss, and regulation by insulin and glucocorticoids. J Clin Invest 1997; 99: 2416–22.
79. Wu MS, Johnston P, Sheu WH, Hollenbeck CB, Jeng CY, Goldfine ID, Chen YD, Reaven GM. Effect of metformin on carbohydrate and lipoprotein metabolism in NIDDM patients. Diabetes Care 1990; 13: 1–8.

9.3 Clinical relevance of enteral nutrition: Better postoperative outcome?

U. Giger, M. Schäfer, L. Krähenbühl

Introduction

Due to its high mortality and morbidity rates, pancreatoduodenectomy (PD) was not considered an appropriate treatment modality for chronic pancreatitis and other benign pancreatic diseases in the 1950–80s. Even for pancreatic and periampullary cancer, medical and interventional therapies were developed to avoid PD [1]. However, over the last two decades, the mortality rate has rapidly decreased to < 5% in high volume centers focused on pancreatic surgery [2–9]. Therefore, PD and its main modifications (e.g. pylorus-preserving PD, duodenum-preserving pancreatic head resection) have gained new acceptance as treatment options for pancreatic cancer and chronic pancreatitis. In addition, the relief of symptoms related to chronic pancreatitis has proven to be excellent [10, 11].

Although the mortality rate after PD has dramatically decreased, the overall morbidity remains at a high level, ranging from 20–55% [11]. The most frequent surgical complication, which accounts for approximately 30–50%, is delayed gastric emptying. The incidence of other complications, such as pancreatic and biliary leakage, hemorrhage, and intra-abdominal abscess formation is reported to be < 5% [10,12, 13]. These complications generally provoke delayed intake of oral food, prolonged hospital stay, and thus increased health-care costs. Preoperatively, patients with chronic pancreatitis or pancreatic cancer often have malnutrition (> 50%) due to impaired food intake and endocrine and exocrine pancreas insufficiency as well as intractable abdominal pain. If malnutrition with depletion of body cell mass and impaired organ function remains undetected, then infectious complications, impaired wound healing, and prolonged rehabilitation are more likely to occur during the postoperative course.

The aim of the current review was to assess the clinical relevance of enteral nutrition on the patient's outcome after PD for chronic pancreatitis and pancreatic cancer.

Assessment of nutritional status

Nutritional status can be assessed using clinical, laboratory or nutritional index parameters. Thus, overall malnourished patients can be easily detected and categorized as "at risk" patients qualifying for possible preoperative treatment [14, 15]. Although the possibility of predicting the overall risk in severely malnourished patients is well established, accurately predicting the individual risk remains difficult. Evaluation of total body potassium, total body nitrogen or creatinine-height index is predominantly reserved for research settings. A detailed personal history with the assessment of weight loss and a thorough physical examination by an experienced physician represent a simple and reliable method. Epidemiological studies suggest that body weight loss and the clinical signs of negative energy and protein balance are associated with impaired outcome in hospitalized patients. Weight loss exceeding 10% of pre-illness weight within three months is usually related to a poor clinical outcome and indicates severe malnutrition [16–18].

Current research has not yet clearly identified biochemical parameters reflecting nutrition-specific pathways in different patient populations. The degree of visceral protein depletion can be estimated by determining the serum levels of albumin. Most investigators agree that low serum albumin levels (< 30 g/l) indicate an increased patient risk of morbidity and mortality. Serum albumin levels may therefore be used to identify patients needing nutritional support [19–21]. However, patients with concomitant liver or pancreatic disease may have disturbed albumin synthesis. Thus, for patients with chronic pancreatitis, decreased serum albumin levels may not sufficiently reflect a true malnourished status. Assessment of the nutritional status can also be performed by using the Nutritional Risk Index according to Buzby (1.519 × serum albumin) + 0.417 × (present weight/usual weight) × 100. A score of 97.5–100 indicates borderline malnourishment; 83.5–97.5 and < 83.5 indicate mild and severe malnutrition respectively [22]. The Nutritional Risk Index may be used to predict the risk of suffering from postoperative complications. Combining the Nutritional Risk Index with different clinical assessment indices [e.g. Subjective Global Assessment (SGA)], increases the sensitivity to identify patients who may develop postoperative complications [23, 24].

Preoperative nutritional deficiency

The reported prevalence of malnutrition ranges from 23–63% for surgical patients. Protein-energy malnutrition is the most common nutritional deficiency in hospitalized patients. As many as 5–10% of patients are classified as severely malnourished [16–18]. Brennan reported on 259 patients undergoing pancreatic resection for malignancy, the majority showed preoperative nutritional impairment with a significant weight loss (–6%) and a decreased serum albumin level. Jaundice was present in two thirds of the patients at the time of surgery [25]. Therefore the preoperative nutritional status should carefully be assessed to select "at risk" patients who may benefit from perioperative nutritional support. Identifying "at risk" patients remains difficult, because malnutrition itself is a continuum that starts with inadequate nutrient intake, followed by a progressive series of metabolic, functional and body compositional changes. At this point the presence of protein-energy malnutrition or specific nutrient deficiencies become deleterious and the increased mortality and morbidity continues to be a subject of research.

Enteral versus parenteral nutrition

Despite the large number of studies and widespread use of nutritional therapy, many topics of nutritional support remain controversial [26]. Artificial nutrition is based on two closely related concepts. First, nutrient depletion is associated with increased morbidity and mortality, particularly in surgical patients [14]. Second, the prevention and correction of nutrient depletion may minimize the morbidity- and mortality-related malnutrition [26].

The impact of preoperative artificial nutrition has been investigated in 395 malnourished patients who required either laparotomy or noncardiac thoracotomy. Patients were randomized to receive either pre- and postoperative parenteral nutrition or postoperative parenteral nutrition alone. The rates of major complications during the first 30 postoperative days were similar, as were the overall mortality rates. Severely malnourished patients who received pre- and postoperative parenteral nutrition had fewer noninfectious complications than controls with no concomitant increase in infectious complications. Patients with borderline or mild malnourishment who received parenteral nutrition had a significantly increased rate of infections. Preoperative parenteral nutrition should therefore be limited to severely malnourished patients and used for at least 7–10 days preoperatively [22, 27].

The enteral route is preferable to parenteral nutrition due to decreased costs and incidence of metabolic side effects [28]. Artificial nutrition in the postoperative period is used to reduce nutritional deficits that ordinarily develop in untreated patients during the period of starvation after surgery or for already severe preoperative malnourishment. The duration of postoperative starvation that can be tolerated without increasing morbidity and mortality is unknown but this period is influenced by the patient's preoperative nutritional status, the severity of operative stress, and the nature and severity of underlying disease. Total starvation for less than three days in normal-weight, healthy adults results in mainly glycogen and water losses (~ 2 kg; 2–3% of body weight) and only minor functional consequences. Functional deficits may become evident in healthy normal-weight adults who restrict their food intake for more than 15 days [19, 29, 30]. Due to severe illness, many hospitalized patients are hypermetabolic, and depletion of nutrient stores will proceed more rapidly during starvation. The functional consequences of total or partial starvation thus evolve more rapidly in stressed and catabolic patients compared to healthy individuals [19]. A maximum period of 5–7 days for a severely limited nutrient intake is the empirical absolute limit most investigators set for hospitalized and surgical patients. Those patients requiring preoperative nutritional support related to severe malnutrition, and those undergoing major surgery with a postoperative period of starvation exceeding 5–7 days, benefit from early postoperative nutritional support. First oral food intake after PD is reported to be expected after the 7–10th postoperative day. This delay in oral food intake is mainly related to delayed gastric emptying, characterized by persistent elevated gastric output. This complication is reported to occur in between 30% and 50% of patients following PD [10, 12]. Therefore patients undergoing PD fit well with the above quoted guidelines and may benefit from early postoperative nutritional support.

Clinical experience of the way of administering and formulating artificial nutrition after PD is still limited [28]. The value of routine postoperative total parenteral nutrition (TPN) following PD has been investigated in 259 patients undergoing major pancreatic resection, where 117 were randomized postoperatively either to receive or not to receive adjuvant TPN. TPN was started on the first postoperative day and continued until the oral food intake exceeded 1000 kcal/day. In the control group a standard dextrose-containing salt solution was administered until the postoperative intake exceeded 1000 kcal/day. The two groups were similar in baseline nutritional and biochemical parameters. The results of postoperative outcome are summarized in Table 9.3-1.

Significant differences in major complications in the group receiving TPN were observed. These included an increase in intra-abdominal abscess formation, increased incidence of peritonitis, and intestinal obstruction. The increase in infectious complications was not caused by catheter-related sepsis, but by an increase in intra-abdominal abscess formation. In addition, significant differences regarding minor complications and reoperation rates became evident. Further, the group receiving TPN showed an elevated risk for biliary and pancreatic fistulas, anastomotic breakdown and a prolonged hospital stay

Table 9.3-1. Postoperative total parenteral nutrition (TPN) after pancreas resection (from [19]).

	TPN (60)	Control (57)
Major complications (%)	45*	22
Minor complications (%)	38*	22
Reoperation (%)	10*	5
Mortality (%)	6	2
Mean hospital stay (days)	16	14

* $p < 0.05$

compared to the control group. In fact, morbidity was increased in patients receiving routine application of postoperative adjuvant parenteral nutrition. Therefore postoperative TPN for patients undergoing major pancreatic resection is not justified for routine use as long as there are no other indications for TPN such as severe malnutrition [25].

A major recent change in nutritional support is the realization that enteral feeding is more efficacious than TPN in certain conditions and that the enteral route is more physiological. The liver is not bypassed and hepatic ability to take up, process, and store the various nutrients for later release on nervous or hormonal command is maintained, as is gut mucosal integrity. When mucosal integrity is not protected, increased translocation of bacteria or their products may occur, or at least decreased bacterial clearance [31]. The initial study done by Alexander and coworkers documented improved survival and a lower rate of sepsis in burned pediatric patients who received most of their protein through the gastrointestinal tract [32]. Two further prospective randomized studies showed that in posttraumatic situations early gut feeding results in lower mortality and septic complication rates compared to TPN [33, 34]. Enteral nutrition seems to be superior to parenteral nutrition with respect to outcome, but the exact mechanism is still not clear. More recent experimental and clinical findings on intestinal motility and absorption [35, 36], the development of needle-catheter jejunostomy [37, 38], and the appearance of new diets have given impetus to the use of enteral feeding for early postoperative feeding, also for patients undergoing PD.

The exocrine pancreas is stimulated by the vagus nerve and the release of gastrointestinal hormones in response to food application [39]. The influence on pancreatic enzyme stimulation during enteral feeding with a needle-catheter jejunostomy has been studied in patients with chronic pancreatitis who underwent pylorus-preserving PD (PPPD). Patients were randomly assigned to either receive enteral feeding or TPN. Neither the amount of bicarbonate, amylase, chymotrypsin, and protein nor the secretion pattern showed any difference, independent of the method of nutritional support. Therefore the secretion of the exocrine pancreas is not stimulated by jejunal feeding [40], indicating that pancreatic fistula or anastomotic breakdown do not occur more frequently in patients fed enterally. No randomized data comparing enteral or parenteral feeding in patients who have had surgery for chronic pancreatitis exists. However, one randomized trial on patients who had had surgery for malignant pancreatic disease comparing the route of feeding has been published (Table 9.3-2). 100 patients were randomized into three different groups either receiving a standard enteral formula (SEN; n = 35), immunonutrition with an enteral formula enriched with arginine, omega-3 fatty acids, and RNA (IEN group; n = 33) or TPN (n = 32). All patients received perioperative octreotide 0.1 mg s.c., one dose one hour before surgery and three doses/day until first oral food diet consump-

	TPN (32)	SEN (35)	IEN (33)
Morbidity (%)	59*	40	34
Infection (sepsis score) (%)	25*	17	9
Delayed gastric emptying	10	5	6
Pancreas fistula (%)	10	10	6
Mortality (%)	6.2	0	3.3
Mean hospital stay (days)	19.3*	17.8	16.3

* $p < 0.05$

Table 9.3-2. Enteral vs. parenteral nutrition after pancreatic surgery (from [27]).

tion. Enteral feeding was delivered by a catheter-feeding jejunostomy, started 12 hours after surgery and steadily increased to full nutritional goal of 25 kcal/day on postoperative day 3. Comparing the three groups, morbidity was significantly lower in the IEN group versus patients receiving TPN. The incidence and severity of infectious complications (sepsis score) was significantly lower in IEN than SEN and TPN. Thus, overall hospital stay was significantly shorter in EIN. The most frequent noninfectious complications were pancreatic fistulas and delayed gastric emptying, which showed no significant difference among the three groups. Forty-two patients (61.8%) did not experience any side effects of enteral feeding and the full nutritional goal was achieved. Twenty-six (38.2%) had some complications related to enteral feeding, of which abdominal cramps and diarrhea were the most frequent. In these patients the nutritional regimen was reached between days 5 and 10 postoperatively. Overall, 84% reached the nutritional goal versus 96% in the TPN group, indicating that jejunostomy is feasible and represents a safe and effective access for patients who have undergone PD [28].

Postoperative enteral feeding in patients undergoing major gastrointestinal surgery is widely documented as beneficial [41–43]. Many effects on gastrointestinal secretion and motility induced by jejunal feeding are still unclear. Extensive studies in animals and healthy volunteers receiving jejunal feeding showed a delay of gastric emptying through the activation of gastroduodenal feedback mechanisms. This effect is partly mediated by cholecystokinin (CCK) [44–48]. On the basis of gastroduodenal inhibition mediated through CCK, the existence of an additional jejunogastric feedback that promotes gastroparesis and delayed gastric emptying through continuous negative feedback on gastric emptying by jejunal feeding has been hypothesized. Continuous enteral feeding is supposed to activate this jejunogastric feedback, and therefore this mechanism could be suppressed by a cyclic enteral nutrition pattern. The effect of cyclic enteral nutrition using SEN after PPPD on the incidence of delayed gastric emptying, the number of days until normal oral diet was tolerated, and length of hospital stay (LOS) was investigated by Van Berge Henegouwen and coworkers. Fifty-seven patients undergoing PPPD were prospectively randomized to either receive continuous enteral feeding (CON) or cyclic feeding (CYC) in which enteral nutrition was stopped for six hours during night. Enteral feeding was performed using a needle catheter jejunostomy. Nutrition was started on the first postoperative day with a gradual increase over the first four days to a maximum of 1500 kcal/day in the CON group and 1125 kcal/day in the CYC group. All patients received perioperative octreotide 100 μg, two times daily from one hour before surgery until six days after surgery. Analyzing the three different regimens, the number of days of nasogastric intubation and days of enteral feeding did not significantly differ in the two groups (CON 9.1 days; CYC 6.7; $p = 0.82$. CON 10.3; CYC 9.3; $p = 0.60$). But first day of normal diet was significantly earlier for the CYC group (15.7 vs. 21.2 days; $p < 0.05$). LOS was also reduced in the CYC group (21.4 vs. 17.5 days; $p < 0.05$). Neither the overall incidence of delayed gastric emptying (25%) nor the postoperative morbidity (35%) showed a difference between the two groups. According to these results, cyclic enteral nutrition is therefore the postoperative regimen of choice in patients undergoing major gastrointestinal surgery, especially pancreatic surgery [49]. However, further studies on the effect of enteral feeding and delayed gastric emptying are needed.

Discussion

The reduced mortality rate after pancreatic resections has been a major achievement in surgery over recent decades [2–8]. Mortality rates below 5% are a prerequisite for the performance of pancreatic resection today [10]. Low mortality rates have also been demonstrated in elderly patients, if preoperative risks are assessed carefully [9, 28, 50]. Preoperative risk assessment includes evaluation of the nutritional status. To identify these "at risk" patients, different concepts of assessment of nutritional status are used. The Nutritional Risk Index is a biochemical-anthropometric index using weight loss and serum albumin levels. Applied to a healthy population by Naber et al., the Nutrition Risk Index indicated malnutrition in only 1.9% of those < 70 years of age and 5.9% in those over 70 years. Those classified as malnourished were only grouped as mildly malnourished [15]. Therefore, the risk of well nourished patients being misclassified as severely malnourished, especially those below 70 years of age, is low. Based on the Veterans Study Group, perioperative parenteral nutrition only shows a significant reduction of non-infectious complications (5% vs. 43%; $p = 0.3$) in severely malnourished patients. Those categorized as either borderline or mildly malnourished suffered from increased infectious complications (14% vs. 6.4%; $p = 0.01$) [26]. Therefore, preoperative TPN should be limited to severely malnourished patients, whereas the two other groups are probably best treated by prompt surgery. In spite of this benefit for nutritional high-risk patients undergoing preoperative artificial feeding, the enteral route should be preferable whenever feasible due to lower costs and fewer metabolic side effects [27]. In fact, enteral feeding prevents alterations related to the unused GI tract during parenteral nutrition, such as villous atrophy with subsequent loss of the gut barrier and development of bacterial translocation. Especially in critically ill patients, the septic complications are lower in enterally fed patients [33–35]. Furthermore, enteral feeding enhances immunological competence [51]. In contrast, TPN is known to induce cholestasis, which can impair Kupffer cell clearance of bacteria, leading to increased systemic septic complications [25]. Unrelated to the route of preoperative nutritional support, enteral or parenteral, feeding for less than 7–10 days before surgery is useless and may be harmful.

The calorific requirement should be individually adapted to the patient's need, but approximately 30 kcal/kg/day should be provided and this has to be continued postoperatively until oral food intake reaches an adequate calorific load [28]. In patients who have had PD, delayed gastric emptying, fistulas and abscesses result in delayed oral food intake and increased metabolic demand, which ends in an elevated risk of undernutrition, prolonged hospital stay and high health costs. First oral food intake after PD is reported to be expected to occur after the 10th postoperative day [10, 12]. Therefore, these patients fit well for early postoperative nutritional support to avert the negative effects of starvation

[19, 28]. As outlined above, current data indicate that routine TPN after major gastrointestinal surgery is not recommended as a standard feeding regimen, because there is a significantly higher risk of major complications like intra-abdominal abscess formation, peritonitis and intestinal obstruction compared to single glucose administration. In addition, significantly increased reoperation rates, biliary and pancreatic fistulas and anastomotic breakdown with a prolonged hospital stay are more likely to occur [25]. Comparing patients who have undergone PPPD receiving TPN, SEN or IEN, those that received enteral nutrition showed superiority of early postoperative enteral feeding compared to TPN. Additionally, those patients receiving IEN showed a significantly lower morbidity rate than those receiving SEN and TPN [28]. However, whether immunonutritional diets should be routinely used in patients who have had pancreatic surgery needs further investigation. The mechanisms induced by enteral feeding on gastro-intestinal motility are not fully understood, but jejunal feeding is known to promote delayed gastric emptying by activating a partly CCK mediated negative gastro-duodenal feedback mechanism [44–48]. Following PD, an additional CCK regulated jejuno-gastric inhibition of gastric motility seems to support the development of delayed gastric emptying. Indeed, inhibition of this negative feedback mechanism by cyclic enteral feeding (CYC) seems to be superior to continuous enteral feeding (CON), allowing earlier normal oral food intake. Whether this effect is mainly related to reduced levels of serum CCK remains unclear [49]. However, CYC feeding seems to be superior to CON in patients undergoing major gastrointestinal surgery and should be performed whenever possible, but its use may be limited, when full energy and nitrogen requirements need to be achieved (malnourishment and catabolic patients).

Conclusion

The following recommendations can be given from the above outlined data. Evaluation of the preoperative nutritional status and "at risk" patients who may benefit from perioperative artificial nutrition is essential before performing major gastrointestinal surgery. Nutritional status assessment can be easily achieved with the Nutritional Risk Index and clinical parameters. Those patients classified as severely malnourished benefit from preoperative artificial support. Patients borderline or mildly malnourished are probably best treated by prompt surgery. Preoperative nutritional support should be done whenever possible by using the enteral route. TPN should only be used if not all or none of the nutritional support can be administered by the gut. Preoperative feeding has to be performed for at least 7–10 days. Caloric requirements should be approximately 30 kcal/kg/day. Jaundice (due to biliary obstruction) markedly impairs liver metabolism, digestion and absorption of nutrients and thus these patients require effective bile drainage before establishing a nutritional strategy. Early postoperative enteral feeding is beneficial and can be safely performed via a needle-catheter jejunostomy. Enteral feeding can be started within 12 hours postoperatively with increasing amounts delivered until the caloric goal is reached. If only some of the nutritional requirements can be given enterally, additional supply is provided parenterally. TPN should only be performed if enteral nutrition is technically not feasible, due to abdominal cramps and/or diarrhea. Immunonutrition seems to be superior to standard formulas. In well-nourished patients, or patients suffering from side effects of enteral feeding, CYC may be performed. Hypermetabolic and severely malnourished patients need continuous enteral feeding. Further studies and research are needed to evaluate new formulas and routes of administration to optimize artificial nutritional support to reduce complications, patient discomfort and health-care cost in patients undergoing pancreatic surgery.

References

1. Cameron L. Whipple or Pylorus Preservation? Ann Surg 2000; 231: 301–2.
2. Van Berge Henegouwen MI, Moojen TM, van Gulik TM, Rauwes EAJ, Obertop H, Gouma DJ. Postoperative weight gain after standard Whipple's procedure versus pylorus-preserving pancreatoduodenectomy: the influence of tumor status. Br J Surg 1998; 85: 922–6.
3. Neoptolemos JP, Russell RC, Bramhall S, Theis B. Low mortality following resection for pancreatic and periampullary tumors in 1026 patients: UK survey of specialist pancreatic units. UK Pancreatic Cancer Group. Br J Surg 1997; 84: 1370–6.
4. Watanapa P, Williamson RC. Surgical palliation for pancreatic cancer: developments during the past two decades. Br J Surg 1992; 79: 8–20.
5. Trede M, Saeger HD, Schwall G, Rumstadt B. Resection of pancreatic cancer-surgical achievments. Langenbecks Arch Surg 1998; 383: 121–8.
6. Cameron JL, Pitt HA, Yeo CJ, Lillemoe KD, Kaufmann HS, Coleman J. One hundred and forty-five consecutive pancreaticoduodenectomies without mortality. Ann Surg 1993; 217: 430–5.
7. Trede M, Schwall G, Saeger HD. Survival after pancreatoduodenectomy. 118 consecutive resections without an operative mortality. Ann Surg 1990; 211: 447–58.
8. Yeo CJ, Cameron JL, Sohn TA, Lillemoe KD, Pitt HA, Talamini MA. Six hundred and fifty consecutive pancreaticoduodenectomies in the 1990s: pathology, complications, and outcomes. Ann Surg 1997; 226: 248–57.
9. Fernandez-del Castillo C, Rattner DW, Warshaw AL. Standards for pancreatic resection in the 1990s. Arch Surg 1995; 130: 295–9.
10. Buchler MW, Friess H, Wagner M, Kulli C, Wagener V, Zgraggen K. Pancreatic fistula after pancreatic head resection. Br J Surg 2000; 87: 883–9.
11. Trede M, Carter DC. The complications of pancreatoduodenectomy and their management. In: Trede M, Carter DC, eds. Surgery of the Pancreas. Edinburgh: Churchill Livingstone, 1993: 629–44.
12. Jimenez RE, Fernandez-del Castillo C, Rattner DW, Chang YC, Warshaw AL. Outcome of pancreaticoduodenectomy with pylorus preservation or with antrectomy in the treatment of chronic pancreatitis. Ann Surg 2000; 231: 293–300.
13. DiCarlo V, Balzano G, Zerbi A, Villa E. Pancreatic cancer resection in elderly patients. Br J Surg 1998; 85: 607–10.
14. Dempsey DT, Mullen JL, Buzby GP. The link between nutritional status and clinical outcome: can nutritional intervention modify it? Am J Clin Nutr 1988; 47(Suppl 2): 352–6.
15. Naber TH, de Bree A, Schermer TRJ, Bakkeren J, Bär B, de Wild G, Katan MB. Specificity of indexes of malnutrition when applied to apparently healthy people: the effect of age. Am J Clin Nutr 1997; 65: 1721–5.
16. Bristian BR, Blackburn GL, Halowell E. Protein status of general surgical patients. JAMA 1974; 230: 858–60.
17. Bristian BR, Blackburn GL, Vitale J. Prevalence of malnutrition in general medical patients. JAMA 1976; 235: 1567–70.
18. Coats KG, Morgan SL, Bartolucci AA. Hospital-associated malnutrition: A reevolution years later. J Am Diet Assoc 1998; 93: 27–33.
19. Allison SP. The uses and limitations of nutritional support. Clin Nutr 1992; 11: 319–30.
20. Windsor JA, Hill G: Weight loss with physiologic impairment: A basic indicator of surgical risk. Ann Surg 1988; 201: 290–6.
21. Seltzer MH, Slocum BA, Catald-Betcher ML. Instant nutritional assessment: Absolute loss and surgical mortality. JPEN 1982; 6: 218–21.

22. The Veterans Affairs Total Parenteral Nutrition Cooperative Study Group. Perioperative total parenteral nutrition in surgical patients. N Engl J Med 1991; 325: 525–32.
23. Baker JP, Detsky AS, Wesson DE. Nutritional assessment: a comparison of clinical judgement and objective measurements. N Engl J Med 1982; 306: 969–72.
24. Detsky AS, Mc Laughlin JR, Baker JP. What is subjective global assessment of nutritional status? JPEN 1987; 11: 8.
25. Brennan MF, Pisters PWT, Posner M, Quesada O, Shike M. A prospective randomized trial of total parenteral nutrition after major pancreatic resection for malignancy. Ann Surg 1994; 220: 436–44.
26. Klein S, Kinney J, Jeejeebhoy KJ, Alpers D, Hellerstein M, Murray M, Twomey P. Nutrition support in clinical practice: review of published data and recommendations for future research directions. National Institute of Health, American Society for Parenteral and Enteral Nutrition, and American Society for Clinical Nutrition. JPEN 1997; 21: 133.
27. Di Carlo V, Gianotti L, Balzano G, Zebri A. Complications of pancreatic surgery and the role of perioperative nutrition. Dig Surg 1999; 16: 320–6.
28. Salis C, Paccagnella A, Vannucci A. Italian multicenter study for the evaluation of resources employed in artificial nutrition in hospitalised patients. Riv Ital Nutr Parenter Enter 1998; 16: 14–24.
29. Leiter LA, Marliss EB. Survival during fasting may depend on fat as well as protein stores. JAMA 1982; 248: 2306–7.
30. Keys A, Broezk J, Henschel A. The Biology of Human Starvation, vol 1, 2. Minneapolis: University Minnesota Press, 1950 (IV).
31. Gennari R, Alexander JW, Gianotti L, Eaves-Pyles T, Hartmann S. Granulocyte macro-phage colony-stimulating factor improves survival in two models of gut-derived sepsis by improving gut barrier function and modulating bacterial clearance. Ann Surg 1994; 56: 530.
32. Alexander JW, Mac Millan BG, Stinett JD, Ogle CK, Bozian RC, Fischer JE, Oakes JB Morris, Krummel R. Beneficial effects of aggressive protein feeding in severely burned children. Ann Surg 1980; 192: 505.
33. Moore FA, Moore EE, Jones TN. Benefits of immediate jejunostomy feeding after major abdominal trauma: A prospective randomized study. J Trauma 1986; 26: 874–81.
34. Moore FA, Moore EE, Jones TN. TEN vs. TPN following major abdominal trauma: reduction of septic morbidity. J Trauma 1989; 29: 916–23.
35. Glucksman DI, Kalser MH, Warren WD. Small intestinal absorption in the immediate postoperative period. Surgery 1966; 60: 1020–5.
36. Wells C, Rawlinson K, Tinckler L, Jones H, Saunders J. Postoperative gastrointestinal motility. Lancet 1964; 1: 4–14.
37. Delany HM, Garvey JW. Jejunostomy by a needle catheter technique. Surgery 1973; 73: 786–90.
38. De Gottardi A, Krähenbühl L, Farhadi J, Gernhardt S, Schäfer M, Büchler MW. Clinical experience of feeding through a needle catheter jejunostomy after major abdominal operation. Eur J Surg 1999; 165: 1055–60.
39. Singer MV. Neurohumoral control of pancreatic enzyme secretion in animals. In: GO VLW, Gardner JD, Brooks FP, Lebenthal E, DiMango EP, Scheele GA, eds. The exocrine pancreas: biology, pathology and disease. New York: Raven Press 1986: 315–31.
40. Bodoky Harsanyi GL, Pap AMD, Tihany TM, Flautner T. Effect of enteral nutrition on exocrine pancreatic function. Am J Surg 1991; 161: 44–148.
41. Hoover HC Jr, Ryan JA, Anderson EJ, Fischer JE. Nutritional benefit of immediate postoperative jejunal feeding of an elemental diet. Am J Surg 1980; 139: 153–9.
42. Moore FA, Feliciano DV, Andrassy RJL. Early enteral feeding, compared with parenteral, reduces postoperative septic complications: the results of a meta-analysis. Ann Surg 1992; 216: 172–83.
43. Beier-Holgersen R, Boesby S. Influence of postoperative enteral nutrition on postsurgical infections. Gut 1997; 39: 833–5.
44. Raybould HE, Tache Y. Cholecystokinin inhibits gastric motility and emptying via a capsaicin-sensitive vagal pathway in rats. Am J Physiol 1988, 255: 242–6.

45. Lin HC, Doty JE, Reedy TJ, Meyer JH. Inhibition of gastric emptying glucose depends on length of intestine exposed to nutrient. Am J Physiol 1989; 256: 404–11.
46. Debas HT, Farooq O, Grossman MI. Inhibition of gastric emptying is a physiological action of cholecystokinin. Gastroenterology 1975; 68: 1211–7.
47. Fraser R, Fone D, Horowitz M, Dent J. Choelcystokinin octapeptide stimulates phasic and tonic pyloric motility in healthy humans. Gut 1993; 68: 33–7.
48. Kleibeuker JH, Beekhuis H, Jansen JB. Cholecystokinin is a physiological hormonal mediator of fat-induced inhibition of gastric emptying in man. Eur J Clin Invest 1988; 18: 173–7.
49. Van Berge Henegouwen MI, Akkermans LMA, van Gulik TM, Masclee AAM, Moojen TM, Obertop H, Gouma D. Prospective randomized trial on the effect of cyclic versus continuous enteral nutrition on postoperative gastric function after pylorus-preserving pancreatoduodenectomy. Ann Surg 1997; 226: 677–87.
50. Sohn SF, Yeo CJ, Cameron JL, Lillemore KD, Talamini MA, Hruban RH. Should pancreaticoduodenectomy be performed in octogenarians? J Gastrointest Surg 1998; 2: 207–16.
51. Wilmore DW, Smith RJ, O'Dwyer ST. The gut: a central organ after surgical stress. Surgery 1988; 104: 917–23.

9.4 Antibiotic treatment in pancreatic disease

Ch. A. Seiler, B. M. Schmied, W. Uhl and M. W. Büchler

Introduction

Antibiotics play a crucial role in the non-surgical management of pancreatic diseases and its complications. Due to improvements in the staging of pancreatic disease, treatment has become easier and antibiotics can be administered more selectively with a better therapeutic effect and an improved outcome in morbidity and mortality [1–5]. Prophylactic administration of antibiotics without staging of the pancreatic disease has proven to be without effect, since the pathogenesis of chronic pancreatitis and the mild edematous form of acute pancreatitis is primarily based on inflammation of the tissue without primary bacterial contamination. Therefore, there is no need for prophylactic antibiotic treatment [6]. Antibiotic administration in pancreatic disease becomes important when secondary infection of the inflamed tissue occurs. In these cases selection of the drug should be adapted to the bacterial spectrum. The same regimen should be performed in patients with chronic pancreatitis with complications, such as cholangitis, infected pseudocyst, pancreatic abscess and intestinal bacterial overgrowth in pancreatic insufficiency [7, 8]. The treatment plan of chronic pancreatitis should therefore primarily focus on source control, punction and drainage of the infected areas and adequate antibacterial treatment.

The most challenging form of pancreatic disease with regard to diagnosis and treatment, including indication and timing of antibiotic (prophylactic) treatment, is acute pancreatitis. About 80% of patients with acute pancreatitis suffer from mild edematous acute inflammation of the pancreatic tissue, which is a self-limiting disease with a mortality of less than 1% when treated conservatively and symptomatically [9, 10]. About 20% of the patients with acute pancreatitis, however, suffer from a necrotizing form which is a life-threatening disease and when not adequately treated cumulates in sepsis and sepsis-related multiple organ systemic failure (MOF). This form of necrotizing pancreatitis has a significantly higher mortality rate of up to 50% [9, 11–15] compared to mild edematous pancreatitis. Multiorgan failure and sepsis are today the leading causes of death (> 80%) in severe acute pancreatitis. Therefore reduction or prevention of sepsis or septic complications in acute necrotizing pancreatitis is still the most promising option in order to reduce morbidity and mortality of acute necrotizing pancreatitis.

Once showing bacterial infection, chronic pancreatitis, pancreatic abscess or acute pancreatitis require an antibiotic regimen, which will be explained in detail using the example of acute necrotizing pancreatitis.

Incidence of pancreatic necrosis in acute pancreatitis

The presence of pancreatic and peripancreatic necrosis in severe acute pancreatitis is of clinical importance since the presence of significant necrotic areas (> 30% of the volume of the pancreas detected by CT-scan) is predictive for the severity of the disease and patients are prone to develop (septic) complications [14, 16, 17]. High blood levels of C-reactive protein (CRP) may predict the incidence of the development of pancreatic necrosis. Indeed, in about 46% (22 of 46 patients) pancreatic necrosis occurs within the first 24 hours after the onset of symptoms (Fig. 9.4-1) [14, 16, 17]. Forty-eight, 72 and 96 hours after the onset of the disease the incidence of pancreatic or peripancreatic necrosis increases to 70%, 97% and 100%, respectively. These data indicate that pancreatic and peripancreatic necrosis occur very early after the first clinical symptoms and that necrosis is fully established within the first four days of the disease. The necrotic tissue serves as an excellent medium for infectious colonization. Therefore this early development of pancreatic and peripancreatic necrosis represents a significant risk factor for a negative outcome of the disease and in addition harbors an increased risk of fatal infection.

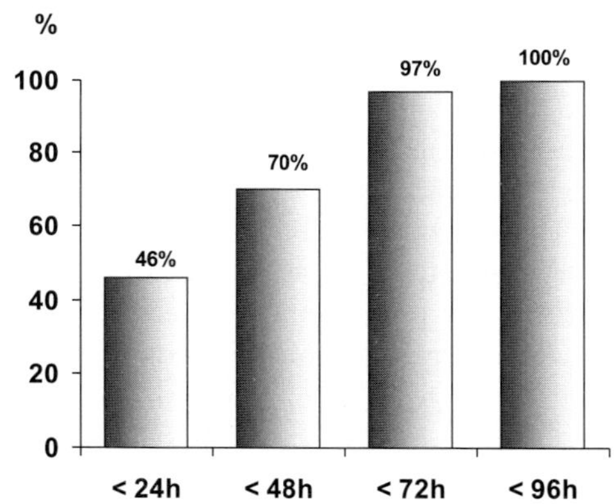

Figure 9.4-1. Incidence of pancreatic necrosis in acute pancreatitis over time.

Incidence of pancreatic infection

Pancreatic bacterial infection occurs in patients with pancreatic or peripancreatic necrosis. Several authors have examined its frequency in acute pancreatitis either by performing CT-guided fine needle aspiration of necrotic material or by analyzing smears taken during surgery [15, 18, 19]. Beger et al. [15] published data showing a correlation between acute pancreatitis and the infection rate in the natural course with the duration of the disease. In 24% of patients who were treated surgically because of pancreatic or peripancreatic necrosis, infected pancreatic necrosis (IPN) was found within the first week, increasing to 36% and 71% in the second and third week after the onset of the abdominal symptoms respectively (Fig. 9.4-2). Therefore, patients with acute necrotizing pancreatitis seem to have the highest risk for bacterial colonization of the necrotic areas during the third week after the onset of the disease. Interestingly, during the fourth week the role of infection declined to 32%. Overall, the time-independent infection rate was 39.4%. Other studies such as those of Bassi et al. [18] and Gerzof et al. [19] presented similar results, but showing in addition an incidence of retroperitoneal infection of 60% and 63% respectively.

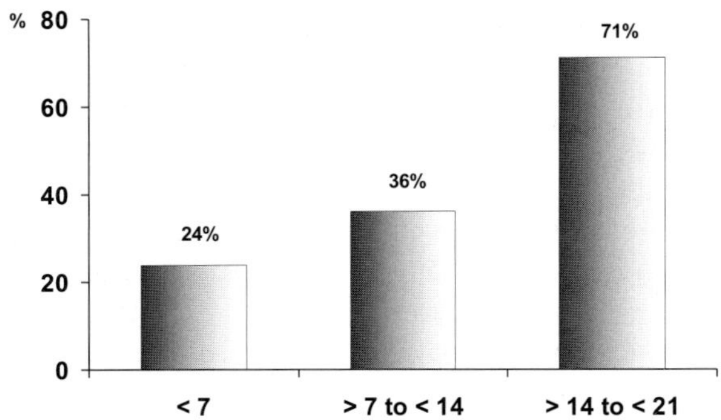

Figure 9.4-2. Incidence of infectious contamination of necrotic areas in acute pancreatitis over time.

Pathways of bacteria into pancreatic necrosis and spectrum of bacteria in infected pancreatic necrosis

The origin and transmission of bacteria through the body into the pancreas is of considerable clinical relevance. Though various animal studies have been performed in order to find a more conclusive answer, the source and pathway of pancreatic infection still remain uncertain [16, 20–24]. The following routes of infection through which bacteria can reach the pancreas are of importance:

1. Hematogenous (blood circulation).
2. Ascending infection (from the duodenum through the main pancreatic duct).
3. From the portal vein and liver (via the biliary tract).
4. Translocation (colonic migration of bacteria via the lymphatics).

Although there is evidence that the pancreatic juice shows protective intrinsic anti-bacterial activity [25, 26], this natural barrier seems to fail in the diseased pancreas and allows bacterial colonization of the gland. The bacterial spectrum in infected pancreatic or peripancreatic necrosis (IPN) has been analyzed by several authors [15, 18, 19]. Due to the natural course of the disease the spectrum of bacteria colonizing the necrotic areas mainly reflects the intestinal flora comprising primarily gram-negative (about two thirds of the cases) but also gram-positive germs, as well as anaerobes (Table 9.4-1). Most frequently it is Escherichia coli (26%) followed by Pseudomonas (16%) Staphylococcus aureus (15%), and others. Fungi may be responsible in about 5–7% of IPN, increasing with the length of the disease and especially after long-lasting antibiotic treatment [15, 18]. In 60–87% of IPN it is a monoinfection, whereas in 13–40% the necrotic areas are colonized by multiple germs.

Escherichia coli	26%
Pseudomonas aeroginosa	16%
Staphylococcus aureus	15%
Klebsiella	10%
Proteus	10%
Streptococcus faecalis	4%
Enterobacter	2–3%
Various anaerobes	16%

60–87% are monoinfections

Table 9.4-1. Spectrum of bacteria in infected pancreatic necrosis (IPN).

Influence of pancreatic infection on morbidity and mortality

Some 20% of the patients suffering from acute pancreatitis develop severe disease with a reported mortality rate of up to 50% even in specialized centers [11–13]. With a mortality rate of 40–80%, infection of necrotic areas of the pancreas is the leading cause of death in severe acute pancreatitis [15, 27]. The influence of bacterial infection on morbidity and mortality in necrotizing pancreatitis has been examined in 204 patients with severe pancreatitis in our institution [28] and has been compared with the results of a similar study performed a couple of years earlier [29] in Ulm, Germany. Details are shown in Table 9.4-2. There is a significant increase in morbidity, hospital stay, and morbidity in patients with infected (severe) pancreatic necrosis compared to patients with sterile pancreatic necrosis. These results indicate that infection of the pancreatic necrosis is indeed the most important prognostic factor in severe acute pancreatitis, with a mortality rate of up to 80% [15, 27]. Infection of pancreatic or peripancreatic necrosis can be detected by a single fine needle aspiration successfully, which represents a rapid, safe and highly sensitive technique performed with computer tomography (CT) or ultrasound (US) assistance. The immediate analysis of the gram stain is completed by *in vitro* culture [19].

In conclusion, bacterial infection of necrotic areas in acute necrotizing pancreatitis is a life-threatening situation. Therefore, in order to reduce morbidity or mortality effectively, the therapy of choice is to prevent bacterial contamination of pancreatic necrosis in acute pancreatitis.

Table 9.4-2. Influence of pancreatic necrosis on hospital stay, morbidity, and mortality.

	Sterile necrosis 58% / 66%	Infected necrosis 42% / 34%
Hospital stay (mean) days	45 / 24	64 / 85
Mortality	11% / 3.5%	20% / 24%
Morbidity (preoperative)		
• **pulmonary**	56% / 47%	72% / 93%
• **renal**	28% / 5%	45% / 28%
• **shock**	13% / 9%	30% / 5%

n = 170, Uhl et al. [29]
n = 204, Büchler et al. [28]

Pancreatic penetration of antibiotics

Due to some type of "pancreas-blood barrier" as described by Burns and co-workers [30], intravenously applied antibiotics are taken up into the pancreas selectively. Based on this knowledge and following the evaluation standards of antibiotic treatment protocols, a number of broad spectrum antibiotics were investigated for their pharmacokinetics and the ability to penetrate healthy and diseased human pancreatic tissue [31–33]. Based on the evidence that antibiotics first have to penetrate the pancreas, second in a high concentration, and third have to cover a broad spectrum of bacteria found in IPN (Table 9.4-1), an efficacy factor was defined. The efficacy factor includes 1) the type and frequency of bacteria found in infected pancreatic necrosis, 2) the tissue concentration of the antibiotics and c) the percentage of inhibited bacterial strains according to the mini-

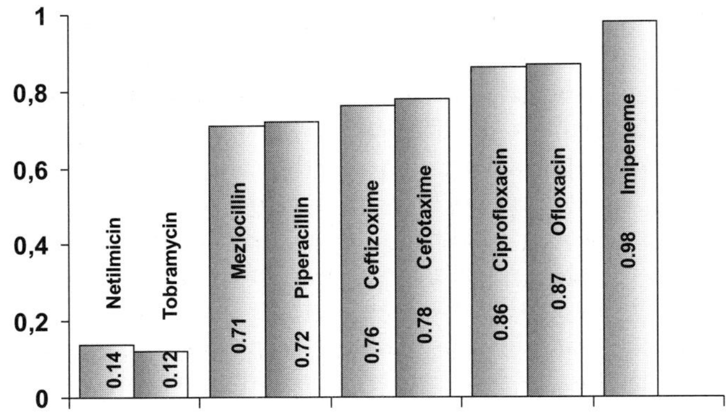

Figure 9.4-3. Efficacy factor of antibiotics used for treatment of infected pancreatic necrosis.

mal antibiotic inhibitory concentration. An efficacy factor of 1 equals a complete inhibition of all bacteria relevant for infected pancreatic necrosis. Figure 9.4-3 summarizes the efficacy factor of a selection of antibiotic classes: The efficacy factor of aminoglycosides is very low, about 0.12; it is higher in chinolons and cephalosporines (0.71–0.87) but highest and close to 1 (0.98) for Imipeneme. Metronidazole was not included in this analysis because of its limited activity on anaerobic germs only. However, these anti-anaerobic drugs showed good penetration capacity. Therefore, Metronidazole should be used only in combination with antibiotics covering the aerobic spectrum.

Prevention of infected pancreatic necrosis

Prevention of infection of pancreatic necrosis in acute pancreatitis was already the subject of research more than 20 years ago, when there were three randomized studies including some 350 patients focusing on prophylactic antibiotic treatment in acute pancreatitis [34–36]. Surprisingly none of the studies could show a beneficial effect of prophylactic antibiotic therapy on the clinical course in acute pancreatitis. However, the antibiotic regimen used at that time was Ampicillin, which has a low pancreatic tissue concentration and in addition only partly covers the spectrum of bacteria found in pancreatic necrosis. Most of the patients included in this study suffered only from mild edematous pancreatitis, which is reflected by the fact that the mortality rate was less than 1%. Pederzoli et al. [37] demonstrated for the first time in 1993, in an Italian multicenter randomized trial including 74 patients with acute necrotizing pancreatitis, a significant reduction of pancreatic sepsis after prophylactic treatment with Imipeneme/Cilastatin. The antibiotics were given three times a day (1.5 g/die) for a period of 14 days and were started within the first 72 hours after the onset of the disease. In the antibiotic treatment group the incidence of pancreatic sepsis decreased from 30% (untreated control group) to about 12% (Imipeneme treated subset; $p < 0.01$). However, no significant reduction in the incidence of need for surgery, multi-organ failure and mortality was achieved. Because this study was performed with a low number of patients (33 vs. 41) and insufficient randomization of the two groups, further studies are required to clarify this issue. According to the findings of Isenmann et al. [14, 38] better results probably could have been achieved by an adequate antibiotic treatment immediately after the onset of the disease. Similar findings have been described in an animal model of acute pancreatitis [39]. In a Scandinavian non-blinded randomized prospective study depicting a total of 30 patients with mostly alcohol-induced necrotizing pancreatitis the antibiotic therapy with Cefuroxime (4.5 gr/die) showed a significant reduction of infectious complications of 24% (54% in the control group vs 30% in the treated group; $p < 0.01$) and significant reduction of mortality (23% in the control vs. 3% in the Cefuroxime group; $p < 0.05$) [38, 40]. However, the low number of patients included in the study and change of the treatment protocol during the study ask for careful interpretation of the results.

Similar results were presented by Frey et al. [41]. In a retrospective review of 180 patients divided into three chronological patient cohorts (1982–1989 no antibiotic treatment, 1990–1992 non-protocol antibiotics and 1993–1996 Imipeneme 1.5 g/die) they demonstrated significant reduction of pancreatic infection from 96% (no antibiotic treatment) to 45% (non-protocol antibiotic treatment) and 27% (Imipeneme treatment). In this publication the antibiotic treatment did not significantly affect the mortality. At present, however, according to yet unpublished results of a follow-up study performed by the same group, the reduction of the mortality in the Imipeneme group became significant.

The Dutch researchers Luiten et al. published an interesting trial on topical antibiotic prophylaxis with selective decontamination of the digestive tract (SDD) in a multicenter randomized controlled trial including 102 patients with severe acute pancreatitis [42]. Fifty of a total of 102 patients were treated with oral and rectal application of SDD consisting of Colistin sulfate, Norfloxacin, and Amphothericin B combined with short term iv. substitution of Cefotaxime 1.5g/die until the bacterial cultures from oral and rectal smears became sterile. The SDD treatment resulted in a statistically significant reduction in mortality (35% in the untreated control group vs. 22% in the SDD treated group; $p < 0.05$) and in a significant reduction of bacterial contamination of the necrotic pancreas (38% vs. 18%; $p < 0.05$). Furthermore, the incidence of surgical intervention decreased from 3.1 (0–29) in the control group to 0.9 (0–17) in the SDD treated group ($p < 0.05$). However, no effect was achieved on early mortality (< 2 weeks). Although the follow-up in this study was longer than in the other trials (40 days) and the surgical concept differed from those in the other publications the most important question still remains whether the significant differences are due to the topical application of SDD or to the short duration of the iv. antibiotics. Infection rates and mortalities of all six studies are summarized in Table 9.4-3.

Table 9.4-3. Prevention of infected pancreatic necrosis.

	Infection %	Mortality %
Pederzoli et al. 1993 [37]		
Imipeneme vs Placebo	30 vs 12*	7 vs 12
Sainio et al. 1995 [40]		
Cefuroxin vs Placebo	40 vs 30	3 vs 23*
Luiten et al. 1995[42]		
SDD vs Placebo	38 vs 18*	22 vs 35
Delcenserie et al. 1996 [44]		
Ceftazidim/Amikacin Metronidazole vs Placebo	58 vs 0*	9 vs 29
Schwarz et al. 1997 [45]		
Offaxacin/Metronidazole vs Placebo	53 vs 61	0 vs 15
Bassi et al. 1999 [46]		
Imipeneme vs Pefloxacin	44 vs 20*	10 vs 24

* $p < 0.05$

In summary, an antibiotic regimen in acute necrotizing pancreatitis seems to reduce septic complications and mortality. However, information for the prevention of bacterial infection of the necrotic pancreas is still scarce and not uniform. To establish a treatment concept further data based on adequate clinical trials are required.

Strategies for antibiotic usage

Based on the presented data there is evidence that antibiotic treatment significantly decreases complications in acute necrotizing pancreatitis. To summarize the actual knowledge and to attempt to promote a possible treatment plan for acute necrotizing pancreatitis, the treatment strategies should be based on the following seven thoughts:

1. Prophylactic antibiotic treatment is indicated in patients with a necrotic area of at least 30% diagnosed with CT scan or with an increase of the CRP serum level to 150 mg/l or more (no necessity of antibiotic treatment in about 80% of all patients with mild acute pancreatitis) [15, 18, 19, 29].
2. The drug has to be administered as early as possible in severe disease [14, 16, 34].
3. The antibiotic regimen has to cover all possible pathways of infection [16, 20–24].
4. The administered antibiotics have to cover the entire bacterial spectrum including Escherichia coli, Pseudomonas, Staphylococcus aureus, Klebsiella, Proteus, Streptococcus faecalis, Enterobacter etc. (Table 9.4-1) [15, 18, 19].
5. In order to achieve an optimal antibiotic tissue concentration and a maximal inhibition of bacterial growth in the pancreas [31–33, 43], the efficacy factor of the antibiotic regimen should be as close as possible to 1.0.
6. The antibiotic treatment should be administered for at least 14 days, preferably even longer since infection of the pancreas often occurs after day 14 (Fig. 9.4-2) [15, 18, 19].
7. Application of topical antibiotic regimens (small bowel decontamination = SDD) is effective and in combination with iv. antibiotics may even enhance the overall protective effect. With inclusion of SDD, fungal infection as one of the major Achilles heels of longtime antibiotic treatment is already treated prophylactically [42].

Final conclusion

Based on our own data [28] showing that the incidence of bacterial infection in acute necrotizing pancreatitis is significantly greater than in the mild edematous form and therefore negatively affects morbidity and mortality, we recommend prophylactic antibiotic treatment of these patients according to the seven points summarized above. The selected drugs have to cover a broad spectrum of bacteria due to the heterogeneity of the bacterial contamination in this disease. It should be administered during a relatively long period of time due to the fact that even after 14 days of antibiotic treatment the risk of infection of the necrotic areas is still significantly increased. The effectiveness of prophylactic administration of antimycotic drugs still remains to be proven with further studies. There is still an evident and crucial need for more sufficient data based on prospective controlled trials of adequate statistical power. Consequently maximal effort has to be focused on this issue, since mortality and morbidity from untreated acute necrotizing pancreatitis is still significant all over the world and even today still presents a tremendous socio-economic problem in Western countries.

References

1. Dervenis C, Johnson CD, Bassi C, Bradley E, Imrie CW, McMahon MJ, Modlin I. Diagnosis, objective assessment of severity, and management of acute pancreatitis. Santorini consensus conference. Int J Pancreatol 1999; 25: 195–210.
2. Schoenberg MH, Rau B, Beger HG. New approaches in surgical management of severe acute pancreatitis. Digestion 1999; 60: 22–6.
3. Uhl W, Isenmann R, Büchler MW. Infections complicating pancreatitis: diagnosing, treating, preventing. New Horiz 1998; 6: 72–9.
4. Wyncoll DL. The management of severe acute necrotising pancreatitis: an evidence-based review of the literature. Intensive Care Med 1999; 25: 146–56.
5. Baudin F, Ozier Y. Early antibiotic treatment in acute necrotising pancreatitis [letter; comment] [see comments]. Lancet 1995; 346: 1374–5.
6. Uhl W, Vogel R, Büchler MW. [Surgical therapy of severe acute pancreatitis]. Schweiz Med Wochenschr 1997; 127: 805–11.
7. Trespi E, Ferrieri A. Intestinal bacterial overgrowth during chronic pancreatitis. Curr Med Res Opin 1999; 15: 47–52.
8. Baril NB, Ralls PW, Wren SM, Selby RR, Radin R, Parekh D, Jabbour N, Stain SC. Does an infected peripancreatic fluid collection or abscess mandate operation? Ann Surg 2000; 231: 361–7.
9. Büchler MW, Binder M, Friess H. Role of somatostatin and its analogues in the treatment of acute and chronic pancreatitis. Gut 1994; 35: 15–9.
10. Banks PA. Acute pancreatitis: medical and surgical management. Am J Gastroenterol 1994; 89: 78–85.
11. Karimgani I, Porter KA, Langevin RE, Banks PA. Prognostic factors in sterile pancreatic necrosis [see comments]. Gastroenterology 1992; 103: 1636–40.
12. Bradley EL, Allen K. A prospective longitudinal study of observation versus surgical intervention in the management of necrotizing pancreatitis. Am J Surg 1991; 161: 19–24; discussion 24–5.
13. Beger H, Büchler MW, Malfertheiner P. Standards in pancreatic surgery. Berlin, Heidelberg: Springer Verlag 1993.
14. Isenmann R, Büchler MW, Uhl W, Malfertheiner P, Martini M, Beger HG. Pancreatic necrosis: an early finding in severe acute pancreatitis. Pancreas 1993; 8: 358–61.
15. Beger HG, Bittner R, Block S, Büchler MW. Bacterial contamination of pancreatic necrosis. A prospective clinical study. Gastroenterology 1986; 91: 433–8.
16. Schwarz M, Büchler M, Thomsen J, Friess H, Isenmann R, Beger H. Pancreatic infection in experimental acute pancreatitis. Digestion 1993; 54: A119.
17. Friess H, Silva J, Isenmann R, Büchler M. Acute pancreatitis: The role of infection. Dig Surg 1996; 151: 357–61.
18. Bassi C, Falconi M, Girelli R, Nifosi F, Elio A, Martini N, Pederzoli P. Microbiological findings in severe pancreatitis. Surg Res Commun 1989; 5: 1–4.
19. Gerzof SG, Banks PA, Robbins AH, Johnson WC, Spechler SJ, Wetzner SM, Snider JM, Langevin RE, Jay ME. Early diagnosis of pancreatic infection by computed tomography-guided aspiration. Gastroenterology 1987; 93: 1315–20.
20. Widdison A, Karanjia N, Reber H. Routes of spread of bacteria to the pancreas in acute necrotizing pancreatitis. Pancreas 1990; 5: A736.
21. Widdison A, Karanjia N, Alvarez C, Reber H. The association between pancreatic infection and the severity of acute pancreatitis. Gastroenterology 1991; 100: A304.
22. Medich DS, Lee TK, Melhem MF, Rowe MI, Schraut WH, Lee KK. Pathogenesis of pancreatic sepsis. Am J Surg 1993; 165: 46–50; discussion 51–2.
23. Lange JF, van Gool J, Tytgat GN. The protective effect of a reduction in intestinal flora on mortality of acute haemorrhagic pancreatitis in the rat. Hepatogastroenterology 1987; 34: 28–30.
24. Wells CL, Rotstein OD, Pruett TL, Simmons RL. Intestinal bacteria translocate into experimental intra-abdominal abscesses. Arch Surg 1986; 121: 102–7.

25. Mett H, Gyr K, Zak O, Vosbeck K. Duodeno-pancreatic secretions enhance bactericidal activity of antimicrobial drugs. Antimicrob Agents Chemother 1984; 26: 35–8.
26. Rubinstein E, Mark Z, Haspel J, Ben-Ari G, Dreznik Z, Mirelman D, Tadmor A. Antibacterial activity of the pancreatic fluid. Gastroenterology 1985; 88: 927–32.
27. Bradley ELD. Antibiotics in acute pancreatitis. Current status and future directions. Am J Surg 1989; 158: 472–7; discussion 477–8.
28. Büchler M, Gloor B, Müller CA, Friess H, Seiler CA, Uhl W. Acute necrotizing Pancreatitis: Treatment strategies according to the status of infection. Ann Surg 2000 (accepted for publication).
29. Uhl W, Schrag H, Wheatley A, Büchler M. The role of infection in acute pancreatitis. Dig Surg 1994; 11: 214–9.
30. Burns GP, Stein TA, Kabnick LS. Blood-pancreatic juice barrier to antibiotic excretion. Am J Surg 1986; 151: 205–8.
31. Bergan T. Kinetics of tissue penetration. Scand J Infect 1978; Dis. 14(Suppl 14): 36–46.
32. Schentag JJ, Gengo FM. Principles of antibiotic tissue penetration and guidelines for pharmacokinetic analysis. Med Clin North Am 1982; 66: 39–49.
33. Büchler MW, Malfertheiner P, Friess H, Bittner R, Vanek E, Schlegel P, Beger HG. The penetration of antibiotics into human pancreas. Infection 1989; 17: 20–5.
34. Finch WT, Sawyers JL, Schenker S. A prospective study to determine the efficacy of antibiotics in acute pancreatitis. Ann Surg 1976; 183: 667–71.
35. Craig RM, Dordal E, Myles L. Letter: The use of ampicillin in acute pancreatitis. Ann Intern Med 1975; 83: 831–2.
36. Howes R, Zuidema GD, Cameron JL. Evaluation of prophylactic antibiotics in acute pancreatitis. J Surg Res 1975; 18: 197–200.
37. Pederzoli P, Bassi C, Vesentini S, Campedelli A. A randomized multicenter clinical trial of antibiotic prophylaxis of septic complications in acute necrotizing pancreatitis with Imipeneme. Surg Gynecol Obstet 1993; 176: 480–3.
38. Barie PS. A critical review of antibiotic prophylaxis in severe acute pancreatitis. Am J Surg 1996; 172: 38–43.
39. Foitzik T, Fernandez-del Castillo C, Rattner O, Ferraro M, Warshaw A. Prevention of pancreatic infection in experimental acute necrotizing pancreatitis. Int J Pancreatol 1994; 16: A317.
40. Sainio V, Kemppainen E, Puolakkainen P, Taavitsainen M, Kivisaari L, Valtonen V, Haapiainen R, Schroder T, Kivilaakso E. Early antibiotic treatment in acute necrotising pancreatitis [see comments]. Lancet 1995; 346: 663–7.
41. Ho HS, Frey CF. The role of antibiotic prophylaxis in severe acute pancreatitis. Arch Surg 1997; 132: 487–92; discussion 492–3.
42. Luiten EJ, Hop WC, Lange JF, Bruining HA. Controlled clinical trial of selective decontamination for the treatment of severe acute pancreatitis. Ann Surg 1995; 222: 57–65.
43. Büchler M, Malfertheiner P, Friess H, Isenmann R, Vanek E, Grimm H, Schlegel P, Friess T, Beger HG. Human pancreatic tissue concentration of bactericidal antibiotics. Gastroenterology 1992; 103: 1902–8.
44. Delcenserie R, Yzet T, Ducroix JP. Prophylactic antibiotics in treatment of severe acute alcoholic pancreatitis. Pancreas 1996; 13: 198–201.
45. Schwarz M, Isenmann R, Meyer H, Beger HG. [Antibiotic use in necrotizing pancreatitis. Results of a controlled study]. Dtsch Med Wochenschr 1997; 122: 356–61.
46. Bassi C, Falconi M, Caldiron E, Salvia R, Sartori N, Butturini G, Contro C, Marcucci S, Casetti L, Pederzoli P. Assessment and treatment of severe pancreatitis. Protease inhibitor. Digestion 1999; 60: 5–8.

10 Conservative treatment of chronic pancreatitis

10.1 Treatment of pain in chronic pancreatitis: Inhibition of enzyme secretion

Ph. P. Toskes

Abdominal pain is a predominant symptom in patients with chronic pancreatitis, yet the management of this abdominal pain is frustrating for both patients and physicians. The multiple potential etiologies of the pain in patients with chronic pancreatitis contributes to the management problems. The pathogenesis of the pain is quite ill understood. Table 10.1-1 lists some of the more important causes of the abdominal pain in patients with chronic pancreatitis. In all likelihood, chronic pancreatitis is not one disease but has many forms, and yet clinicians have often tried to approach all patients with chronic pancreatitis in the same manner. It has not been generally appreciated by non-experts in the management of chronic pancreatitis that the approach to the patient with large duct alcohol-induced chronic pancreatitis is vastly different from that to the patient with small duct idiopathic chronic pancreatitis. The approach to diagnosing these patients, the clinical course of these patients, and the prognosis of these patients differ greatly [12]. The discussion will focus on those patients who make up a subset of patients with chronic pancreatitis and abdominal pain, that being those patients with small duct chronic pancreatitis not related to alcohol-induced disease.

Table 10.1-1. Causes of abdominal pain in chronic pancreatitis.

- Pseudocyst
- Hypertension of main pancreatic duct
- Hypertension of small ducts
- Inflamed foci
- Neutral inflammation
- Stenosis of common bile duct
- Stenosis of duodenum

It seems reasonable to approach the patient with abdominal pain and suspected chronic pancreatitis in the following manner. After other causes of abdominal pain have been appropriately excluded, particularly dysmotility syndromes, a CT scan of the pancreas should be performed. If no abnormalities are found, a hormone stimulation test (secretin, cholecystokinin) should be done. Invariably, if the pain is related to chronic pancreatitis, the hormone stimulation test will be abnormal. If the hormone stimulation test confirms the clinical impression of chronic pancreatitis, a trial of non-enteric coated pancreatic enzymes is indicated for four to six weeks. If relief in pain is achieved, no further steps need to be taken. The clinical course of patients receiving pancreatic enzymes for pain has not yet been fully defined. It is our habit to stop the enzymes if a patient has been pain-free for six months while on enzymes. When that is done, about 50% of the patients stay pain-free and no further therapy has to be given. The other 50% of patients seem to relapse quickly and they must be put on pancreatic enzymes indefinitely. It is as if putting the patients' pancreas to rest, if you will, by the administration of exogenous enzymes allows the altered feedback mechanism to someway be corrected. Many patients do not want to go off enzymes even though they are pain-free because their previous experience with pancreatitis has been so detrimental to them and their well-being.

Fortunately, this therapy is virtually without side effects and well tolerated by patients. The only drawback has been the need for patients to take large numbers of pancreatic enzymes, but that inconvenience has been somewhat diminished by the recent approval by the FDA of an enhanced conventional enzyme preparation which now requires that the patient take half the number of tablets needed before. Table 10.1-2 details the currently available pancreatic enzyme preparations that have been utilized in clinical practice with some frequency in the United States. The enzymes fall into two categories, conventional non-enteric coated enzymes and enteric-coated enzymes. The enteric-coated enzymes allow the physicians to give the patient much fewer capsules and are ideal for the treatment of steatorrhea but not satisfactory for the treatment of abdominal pain.

Table 10.1-2. Frequently utilized pancreatic enzyme preparations.

	Protease* (X 1000)	Lipase* (X 1000)
Non-enteric-coated		
Viokase 8 (Axcan Scandipharm, Birmingham, Alabama)	30	8
Viokase 16 (Axcan Scandipharm, Birmingham, Alabama)	60	16
Kuzyme HP (Schwartz, Milwaukee, WI)	30	8
Cotazym (Organon, East Orange, NJ)	30	8
Enteric-Coated		
Creon 5 (Solvay, Marietta, GA)	18.75	5
Creon 10 (Solvay)	37.5	10
Creon 20 (Solvay)	75	20
Pancrease MT4 (McNeil Pharmaceuticals, Ft. Washington, PA)	12	4
Pancrease MT10 (McNeil Pharmaceuticals)	30	10
Pancrease MT16 (McNeil Pharmaceuticals)	48	16
Ultrase 12 (Scandipharm, Birmingham, AL)	39	12
Ultrase 18 (Scandipharm)	58.5	18
Ultrase 20 (Scandipharm)	65	20
Cotazym-S (Organon)	20	5

* United States Pharmacopea units per tablet or capsule.
Manufacturers and their locations follow names of drugs.

Conventional enzymes are preferred for the treatment of pain since the feedback inhibition principle by which these enzymes relieve pain is operative only in the proximal small intestine, most predominantly in the duodenum. Experimental studies in rats using selective extirpation of various segments of the small intestine have supported this concept. Likewise, in patients who have had a gastrojejunostomy we have been unable to demonstrate suppression of pancreatic secretion by perfusing the jejunum with pancreatic proteases, in contrast to the suppression that is seen of both secretion and elevated CCK levels in the blood when serine proteases are perfused into the duodenum [2, 3].

The enteric-coated enzymes appear to open their enteric coat and release their enzymes often when they go beyond the duodenum and do not effect feedback inhibition appropriately. The conventional or non-enteric coated enzymes that escape destruction by acid in the stomach always deliver their proteases into the duodenum and in a positive way effect feedback control of pancreatic secretion, decrease CCK levels and reduce abdominal pain. Since it is imperative that as much proteases as possible be delivered into the duodenum, a proton-pump inhibitor should be given with the conventional enzyme preparation. If the results of pancreatic enzyme therapy are unsatisfactory an endoscopic retrograde cholangiopancreatography (ERCP) should be performed looking for inflammatory strictures or other lesions that might be corrected with surgery. Endoscopic ultrasonography could be substituted for ERCP, but the reliability of EUS in detecting early changes of chronic pancreatitis is yet to be defined [4]. Certainly EUS can detect abnormalities associated with big duct chronic pancreatitis.

Drainage of a pseudocyst, if found, often brings dramatic relief of pain. If no pseudocyst exists, two patterns of abnormality are usually present: 1) some patients have minimal or no abnormalities on ERCP and an abnormal hormone stimulation test and 2) others have dilated ducts or strictures or both detected by ERCP. Traditionally the abnormalities in the latter group have been thought to be amenable to surgery. The findings of the ERCP have largely dictated the surgical approach and the surgical procedure of choice has been drainage of the main pancreatic duct.

Treatment of the former group, i.e. those with normal ducts on ERCP, has been completely unsatisfactory but the appropriate enzyme preparation in such a patient may relieve pain. It appears that pharmacological doses of proteases may inhibit pancreatic exocrine secretion by putting the pancreas at rest while affording pain relief. These clinical observations fit with a large amount of experimental data in animals which indicate that the amount of serine proteases (trypsin, chymotrypsin, elastase) within the lumen of the proximal duodenum exerts a controlling influence on pancreatic exocrine secretion – a feedback control mechanism. This feedback mechanism appears to be mediated through inhibition of cholecystokinin (CCK) by serine proteases [5].

After the ingestion of a meal, CCK-releasing factor (CCK-RF) is released in cells within the proximal small intestine; CCK-RF (1–5 K molecular weight) is stimulated by fat and protein and is catabolized by serine proteases [6]. CCK-RF then stimulates the release of CCK from the duodenum into the circulation. This results in pancreatic acinar cell stimulation and pancreatic enzyme production. Also, gastric acid produced in response to a meal induces secretin release from the duodenum into the circulation. This results in stimulation of pancreatic ductal cells to produce an increased volume of bicarbonate; this together with enzymes promotes digestion. The presence of serine proteases in the proximal duodenum increases the amount of CCK-RF available and this lowers CCK levels, placing the pancreas at rest.

In the normal physiologic state, ingested proteins are broken down by serine proteases. CCK-RF is also broken down by these proteases. It stimulates the release of only normal amounts of CCK into the circulation. In the patient with chronic pancreatitis with either relative or absolute deficiency in pancreatic proteases, there is an excessive amount of CCK-RF in the duodenum. This promotes the release into the blood of elevated levels of CCK which continually stimulates the pancreas, perhaps leading to inflammatory changes in the small ducts and abdominal pain. The administration of exogenous pancreatic enzymes to patients with chronic pancreatitis may restore the catabolism of CCK-RF in the duodenum, thus lowering blood CCK levels. Lowering blood CCK levels may lessen pancreatic stimulation and decrease abdominal pain.

As shown in Table 10.1-3, there have been five placebo-controlled double-blind studies evaluating the effect of pancreatic enzymes on the abdominal pain associated with chronic pancreatitis [2, 3, 7, 8, 9]. The two that have been positive utilized conventional, i.e. non-enteric-coated pancreatic enzymes and the three that have been negative utilized enteric-coated pancreatic enzymes. Our ongoing extensive clinical experience supports these studies. The patients whose pain responds best to pancreatic enzymes are those with mild-to-moderate exocrine insufficiency (abnormal secretin stimulation test results, no steatorrhea) and minimal to no change on ERCP.

Author	Enzyme Used	Response
Ihse [2]	Conventional	Yes
Toskes [3]	Conventional	Yes
Worning [7]	Enteric-coated	No
Mossner [8]	Enteric-coated	No
Malesci [9]	Enteric-coated	No

Table 10.1-3. Pancreatic enzymes and pain relief placebo-controlled trials.

Thus, the type of pancreatic enzyme utilized is an important influence on the effectiveness of therapy. Recent studies from our laboratory have demonstrated that non-enteric coated enzymes regularly deliver more proteases into the proximal duodenum than do enteric-coated enzymes. Enteric-coated enzymes also fail to lower blood CCK levels or provide pain relief in patients with painful chronic pancreatitis [10]. Table 10.1-4 compares these two types of enzyme preparation. Thus, in attempting to decide how to use pancreatic enzymes for the treatment of pain via feedback inhibition of pancreatic exocrine secretion it is important to select an appropriate patient and to use the appropriate enzyme formulation. Patients with severe pancreatic insufficiency (those with steatorrhea) failed to respond to enzyme therapy, for feedback suppression cannot be restored. Those with mild-to-moderate impairment of the exocrine function of the pancreas will demonstrate a remarkable decrease in abdominal pain if they are treated with conventional or non-enteric coated pancreatic enzymes.

Criteria	Conventional	Enteric-coated
Release of proteases in duodenum	Yes	No
Lower CCK level	Yes	No
Decrease exocrine secretion	Yes	No
Reduce pain	Yes	No

Table 10.1-4. Conventional versus enteric-coated enzymes.

In those patients with severe pancreatic insufficiency who have failed to respond to pancreatic enzymes, surgery, particularly ductal compression, has been the accepted medical therapy, but this surgery is far from perfect. The ductal decompression may provide short-term pain relief in up to 80% of patients, although long-term results are closer to 50% [11]. Employing this feedback inhibition principle, the somatostatin analog octreotide has been demonstrated, in a multi-center randomized placebo-controlled pilot study involving 91 patients, to decrease abdominal pain in 65% of those patients with severe chronic pancreatitis, especially if the pain was constant [12]. In the open-labeled phase of the study, 31% of the patients became totally pain-free. Octreotide was utilized because it lowered blood CCK levels and decreased pancreatic secretion. Whether these salutary effects on pain with octreotide are due to its effect on exocrine secretion and lowering of blood CCK or to the antinociceptive activity of octreotide remains to be fully clarified.

It is incumbent upon the clinician to be familiar with this principle of feedback inhibition of pancreatic exocrine secretion so the principle may be applied to the management of appropriate patients with chronic pancreatitis who have severe abdominal pain. Again, it should be stressed that the use of pancreatic enzymes to relieve abdominal pain in patients with severe pancreatic exocrine insufficiency already manifesting steatorrhea is apt to be met with failure. It is in the patients who have small duct disease who have not yet developed steatorrhea that this enzyme therapy will be most beneficial.

What potential therapies are under consideration that may give even more effective pain control in these patients with chronic pancreatitis? Enhanced enzyme formulations are under consideration with a combination of free proteases for pain relief and enteric-coated lipase for improving fat absorption. Such a preparation would be an ideal single agent to treat the two main problems that patients with chronic pancreatitis manifest, that is, abdominal pain and maldigestion. A long-acting form of octreotide is now available but has not yet been evaluated in the treatment of the pain of chronic pancreatitis. Studies are planned utilizing this form of long-acting octreotide. All of these studies have suggested that a 20 mg dose of this depot form of octreotide would be effective for approximately 28 days. Finally, new CCK antagonists are available which can be taken by mouth and are selective CCK receptor antagonists. Information existing in our laboratory suggests that such CCK antagonists are effective in blunting pancreatic secretion and effecting CCK homeostasis. Such CCK antagonists have not been taken into the clinical area for placebo-controlled trials as yet.

References

1. Toskes PP. Update on diagnosis and management of chronic pancreatitis. Curr Gastroenterol Rep 1999: 145–53.
2. Isaksson G, Ihse I. Pain reduction by an oral pancreatic enzyme preparation in chronic pancreatitis. Dig Dis Sci 1983; 28(2): 97–102.
3. Slaff J, Jacobson D, Tillman CR, Curington C, Toskes P. Protease-specific suppression of pancreatic exocrine secretion. Gastroenterology 1984; 87(1): 44–52.
4. Chowdhury RS, Bhutani MS, Mishra G, Forsmark CE, Toskes PP: Comparative analysis of pancreatic function testing versus morphological assessment (by EUS) for the evaluation of chronic unexplained abdominal pain (UAP). Gastro 2001; 120: A647.
5. Owyang C, Louie DS, Tatum D. Feedback regulation of pancreatic enzyme secretion: suppression of cholecystokinin release by trypsin. J Clin Invest 1986; 77: 2042–7.

6. Shetzline MA, Liddle RA. Neurohormonal control of the exocrine pancreas. Curr Opin Gastroenterol 1999; 15: 380–4.
7. Halgreen H, Pedersen NT, Worning H. Symptomatic effect of pancreatic enzyme therapy in patients with chronic pancreatitis. Scand J Gastroenterol 1986; 21: 104–8.
8. Mössner J, Seckmus R, Meyer J et al.: Treatment of pain with pancreatic extracts in chronic pancreatitis: Results of a prospective placebo-controlled multi-center trial. Digestion 1992; 53: 54–66.
9. Malesci A, Gaia E, Fioretta A et al.: No effect of long-term treatment with pancreatic extract on recurrent abdominal pain in patients with chronic pancreatitis. Scand J Gastroenterol 1995; 30: 392–8.
10. Campbell D, Jadunandan I, Curington C et al.: Alcoholic and idiopathic patients with painful chronic pancreatitis do not experience suppression of CCK levels or pain relief following treatment with enteric-coated pancreatin (abstract). Gastroenterology 1992; 102: A259.
11. Moosa AR. Surgical treatment of chronic pancreatitis: An overview. Br J Surg 1987; 74(8): 661–7.
12. Toskes PP, Forsmark CE, DeMeo MT et al.: A multicenter controlled trial of octreotide for the pain of chronic pancreatitis. Pancreas (in press).

10.2 Treatment of pancreatic exocrine dysfunction

Th. Arendt, U. R. Fölsch

Introduction

Pancreatic enzyme extracts have been used for exactly 100 years now to improve maldigestion of nutrients due to pancreatic insufficiency [1]. The number of patients suffering from pancreatic exocrine insufficiency has risen in western countries [2]. Important reasons are i) an increase in alcohol consumption and thereby in the incidence of chronic pancreatitis [2] and ii) the increase in mean life expectancy to 35–40 years in patients with cystic fibrosis [3].

Background physiology

The pancreas releases more than two liters of secretion rich in enzymes and bicarbonate daily. The quantity of enzymes secreted by acinar cells is approximately ten times the amount of enzymes or proenzymes needed to ensure normal digestion of ingested food [4]. Protein secretion per gram of tissue exceeds that of any other organ [5], more than 85% of this protein content being made up of enzymes [6]. In contrast to the proteolytic enzymes, the non-proteolytic enzymes such as lipase are secreted in active form. Physiological loss of pancreatic exocrine enzyme activity during aboral transit along the intestinal lumen is due to degradation by proteases such as chymotrypsinogen [7, 8]. Whereas pancreatic acinar cells are responsible for protein synthesis and secretion, duct cells secrete bicarbonate and water, which have a profound influence on duodenal luminal pH.

Background pathophysiology

In patients with exocrine pancreatic insufficiency, digestion of fat is more impaired than carbohydrate and protein digestion. This is due to a number of reasons (Table 10.2-1):

Table 10.2-1. Reasons for earlier and more severe impairment of fat digestion in patients with pancreatic insufficiency compared to protein and carbohydrate digestion.

- Earlier impairment of pancreatic lipase synthesis and secretion
- More rapid and complete inactivation of lipase in the acidic duodenum due to impaired bicarbonate output
- Proteolytic degradation of lipase occurs earlier during aboral transit than that of amylase and proteases
- Impairment of pancreatic bicarbonate secretion decreases duodenal pH, thereby resulting in precipitation of glycine conjugated bile acids and further deterioration of fat digestion
- Extrapancreatic sources of lipase (such as lingual and gastric lipase) are not able to compensate for loss of pancreatic lipase activity

a) as pancreatic insufficiency progresses, lipase activity in pancreatic secretions diminishes at a faster rate than that of other enzymes [9] and cystic fibrosis [10]; b) proteolytic degradation of lipase occurs earlier during aboral transit than that of amylase and proteases [11]; c) lipase is more easily destroyed than the other pancreatic exocrine enzymes at acidic pH [12]. This is crucial because the course of pancreatic exocrine insufficiency is characterized by a substantial reduction in bicarbonate secretion, a decrease in duodenal pH [13] and thereby an increase in inactivation of lipase by gastric acid; d) moreover, decrease of duodenal pH due to impairment of pancreatic bicarbonate secretion results in the precipitation of glycin-conjugated bile acids and thereby in a further deterioration of fat digestion; e) extrapancreatic sources of lipase (such as lingual and gastric lipase) are not able to compensate for the loss in pancreatic lipase activity in pancreatic exocrine insufficiency [14], whereas loss of both pancreatic protease and amylase activity is more easily compensated for by enteral peptidases, proteases, and salivary amylase.

For all these reasons, steatorrhea is the leading symptom in patients with pancreatic exocrine insufficiency and frequently persists even despite supplementation of large doses of pancreatic enzymes (up to 2,500 units lipase/kg/meal) [15], whereas azotorrhea (protein malabsorption) can usually be corrected with this therapy. It has even been suggested that azotorrhea in patients with exocrine pancreatic insufficiency on adequate enzyme supplementation requires exclusion of a protein-losing enteropathy or concomitant liver disease [16].

Pharmacology

In order to correct fat maldigestion in pancreatic exocrine insufficiency, the goal of the therapy is to ensure that optimal amounts of lipase reach the duodenum together with the delivered food. With the currently available pancreatic enzyme supplement preparations this goal is frequently not achieved [17, 18].

There are two major problems associated with the delivery of an optimal amount of lipase into the duodenum (Table 10.2-2):

Table 10.2-2. Problems associated with delivery of an optimal amount of lipase into the duodenum.

• Inactivation of porcine or bovine pancreatic enzymes by gastric acid
• Asynchronous gastroduodenal passage of pancreatic enzymes and food

1. *Gastric acid.* Lipase used in pork or bovine pancreatic enzyme supplement preparations is inactivated by gastric acid comparable to the human enzyme. Due to acid degradation of lipase, only 8% of the enzyme activity supplemented is recovered at the ligament of Treitz [18]. Therefore, enteric coating of enzyme supplements was developed, which prevents the destruction of lipase in the acidic environment of the stomach. Coated enzyme supplements are released from the preparations when pH rises above pH = 5. However, duodenal pH depends among other factors (such as the bicarbonate secretion of the intestine, gastric and bile acid delivery into the duodenum) upon the bicarbonate secretion of the pancreas. A reduced pancreatic secretion of bicarbonate leads to a slower increase in duodenal pH and may thus result in an enzyme supplement release from coated preparations too far distally in the intestine for optimal digestion.

2. Asynchronous gastroduodenal passage of enzyme preparations and food is another major problem associated with pancreatic enzyme supplementation. Numerous studies have shown that the size of particles of stomach content determines the speed of gastroduodenal transit [19, 20]. Available enteric coated microspheres are less than 2 mm in diameter because particles with a diameter > 2 mm have been shown to enter the duodenum more slowly than smaller particles [19, 20]. The microsphere formulation has been further improved by the development of so-called mini-microspheres (0.7–1.6 mm) which have a still smaller diameter than conventional microspheres (1–2 mm), but contain identical amounts of lipase. However, in a currently published double-blind, crossover study it was demonstrated that the two formulations (0.7–1.6 mm and 1–2 mm) were equivalent with regard to the improvement of fat malabsorption [21].

Indications for pancreatic exocrine enzyme supplementation

Supplementation of pancreatic enzymes is indicated in patients with pancreatic exocrine insufficiency (irrespective of the cause of pancreatic dysfunction) (Table 10.2-3) when weight loss and steatorrhea develop. Enzymes are also supplemented when steatorrhea occurs without weight loss. Though there are no studies to demonstrate when to begin enzyme supplementation in patients without weight loss, stool fat excretion > 15 g/d has generally been accepted as an indication for therapy. Hyperoxaluria, another complication of steatorrhea, only rarely results in the development of nephrolithiasis [22]. Therefore, though not formally studied, exocrine enzyme supplementation may also be used in patients who present with pancreatic exocrine insufficiency, hyperoxaluria, and nephrolithiasis. Complaints such as diarrhea and severe meteorism, which may be associated with exocrine pancreatic insufficiency, have also been taken as an indication for pancreatic enzyme supplementation. Treatment of pain associated with chronic pancreatitis and meteorism is another interesting indication which could be tried in individual cases without having convincing evidence to strongly support this [23, 24].

Table 10.2-3. Indications for pancreatic exocrine enzyme supplementation.

- Steatorrhea > 15 g/d
- Continuous weight loss
- Malabsorption of proteins and carbohydrates (rare)
- Dyspepsia, meteorism, diarrhea
- Pain (?)

Preparations of pancreatic exocrine enzymes

Four types of pancreatic exocrine enzyme preparations are currently available (Table 10.2-4): i) Rapid release enzyme preparations from porcine or bovine pancreas in unprotected powder, tablet, capsule or granule form; ii) enzyme preparations used in combination with acid reducing compounds; iii) enteric-coated enzyme tablets; iv) enteric-coated enzyme microspheres, v) stable lipases of microbial origin.

Table 10.2-4. Pancreatic enzyme preparations.

I.	**Uncoated preparations**
	• Powder
	• Film-coated tablets
	• Granules
II.	**Enteric-coated preparations**
	• Granules
	• Tablets
	• Microspheres
	• Minimicrospheres
III.	**Fats**
	• Acid-resistant enzymes of microbial origin

Rapid release unprotected preparations

Conventional pancreatin preparations without any acid protection were used for the first time one hundred years ago [1]. Due to their inactivation by gastric acid, enormous dosages of enzymes are required in order to achieve a diminution in nutrient loss, whereas other patients respond only poorly to this therapy. Therefore, these preparations should only be used in patients with pancreatic exocrine insufficiency who present with hypo- or achlorhydria. In this subgroup of patients, comparatively low costs and the optimal mixing and simultaneous passage into duodenum of enzymes together with food are advantageous [25].

Enzyme preparations in combination with acid reducing compounds

Antacids capable of protecting enzyme supplements from inactivation by acid must maintain the gastric pH above 4.0 for at least 90 min [26]. In general, most acid-reducing or neutralizing agents decrease fat malabsorption to a varying degree when administered together with enzymes. Furthermore, it has been shown that the sole administration of omeprazole for 14 days in Japanese patients reduced the daily fat excretion to some extent by improving upper small intestine pH levels following the elevation of gastric pH levels [27]. Sodium bicarbonate has only a marginal effect in decreasing nutrient loss in CF, but leads to heavy meteorism due to carbon dioxide production [28]. In children, antacids are generally unacceptable because of their unpalatability and bulk [17]. Studies on the effect of H_2-receptor antagonists showed contradictory results. Cimetidine supplementation has been shown to eliminate steatorrhea [29], to decrease it [30], or to have no effect [31]. The proton pump inhibitor omeprazole reduced fecal fat excretion in patients with CF when given with enzymes in the form of enteric-coated microspheres [32]. However, though additional administration of H_2-receptor antagonists or proton pump inhibitors decreases fecal nutrient loss, their routine use is not justified for a number of reasons: i) the need for additional medications is likely to increase noncompliance; ii) there is a substantial increase in costs; iii) the effects of acid-reducing therapy are too variable. Finally, the safety of long-term administration of these drugs, especially in children, has not been firmly established [17].

Enteric-coated tablets

These preparations are ineffective for decreasing fat excretion due to erratic enzyme release. Due to their large size, tablets do not synchronously leave the stomach with the food ingested, or they dissolve too late during passage along the intestine or may even pass intact through the gut [26, 33]. Their use is strongly discouraged.

Enteric-coated microspheres

A special polymer coating protects the pancreatic enzymes in these preparations at low pH. A significant release of enzymes occurs only at a pH at least as high as 4.5. Thus, less inactivation of the preparation by acid and pepsin occurs in the stomach. There is no need for simultaneous administration of antacids, H_2-receptor antagonists or proton pump inhibitors. Due to their small size, there is synchronous passage of microspheres with the meal into the duodenum and a more even distribution of the enzymes in chyme compared to enteric coated tablets. It is likely that this results in better patient compliance because fewer tablets are needed [17]. However, microencapsulation results in a considerable increase in costs. Moreover, there are considerable differences in the diameter of the microspheres and in their physical nature due to differences in the manufacturing process [17]. This results in considerable differences in the dissolution characteristics of the various preparations dependent both on pH and bile salt concentrations [34, 35]. However, it has not been shown that differences in the dissolution characteristics of the various enteric-coated microsphere preparations result in detectable clinical differences [36, 37], though it might be possible that stool fat determinations are too inaccurate to detect potential differences. Overall, the superiority of enteric-coated microsphere preparations over conventional enzyme preparations with regard to decrease in stool fat excretion is firmly established [38].

Stable lipase of microbial origin

In contrast to human, porcine and bovine pancreatic lipase, certain bacterial and fungal lipases (e.g., prepared from *Rhizopus arrhizus*) are resistant against acid denaturation and (in part) proteolytic digestion. Acid- and protease-stable lipase preparations of fungal origin are in clinical use in some countries. Controlled clinical trials have shown that these preparations improve steatorrhea, but no superiority over enteric-coated microsphere preparations has been demonstrated to date [39, 40]. Decreased lipolytic activity of fungal lipase in the presence of bile acids has been put forward as a possible explanation [18].

Effects of pancreatic exocrine enzyme supplementation

Pancreatic exocrine enzyme supplements improve steatorrhea and consecutively prevent weight loss in patients with pancreatic exocrine insufficiency due to chronic pancreatitis [9, 18], pancreatic cancer [41], pancreatic resection [42], and cystic fibrosis [15, 27, 32, 36–40]. Improvement of nutrition has also been shown in some studies in patients with pancreatic exocrine dysfunction associated with gastric surgery [43, 44]. In patients with cystic fibrosis, pancreatic exocrine insufficiency has been shown to be associated with a faster decline in pulmonary function [45] and it is likely that pancreatic exocrine enzyme supplementation increases survival in these patients [17].

Side effects of pancreatic exocrine enzyme supplementation

Pancreatic exocrine enzyme supplements have very few side effects. The superb tolerance of these preparations has been shown in studies of more than 28,000 patients [46, 47]. Side effects include sourness of mouth, perianal irritation, abdominal pain, diarrhea/abdominal distension, constipation in infants, hyperuricemia, allergic reactions to pork protein, hypersensitivity reactions following inhalation and fibrosing colonopathy in cystic fibrosis patients [17, 25].

Hyperuricemia and uricosuria associated with pancreatic exocrine enzyme supplementation are generally believed to result from the high purine content of the enzyme preparations which are metabolized to uric acid and excreted by the kidneys [48]. However, in cystic fibrosis patients, there was no relationship between the amount of pancreatic enzymes ingested and hyperuricemia, but a direct relationship between the severity of disease and hyperuricemia suggesting that the increased metabolism and inflammatory cell turnover in these patients was causative in producing hyperuricemia.

Pancreatic exocrine enzyme preparations may cause allergic responses. Porcine extracts are known to contain more than 25 potentially antigenic proteins and 96% of cystic fibrosis patients have been shown to develop serum IgG directed against porcine trypsin within 4.2 years of therapy [49]. Allergic responses such as bronchospasm, nasal irritation and coughing may also be induced in nurses who prepare the preparations, particularly when powdered pancreatic extracts are used which may be inadvertently inhaled [50].

In patients with cystic fibrosis, a strong relationship has been described between high daily doses of enzyme supplements and the development of fibrosing colonopathy [51]. Therefore, it has been recommended that the maximum dose of lipase should not exceed 10,000 units lipase/kg per day, or 2,500 units of lipase/kg per meal [52].

References

1. Gockel M. Über Erfolge mit "Pankreon", einem neuen, gegen Magensaft widerstandsfähigen Pankreaspräparat. Centralblatt für Stoffwechsel und Verdauungskrankheiten 1900; 11.
2. Worning H. Incidence and prevalence of chronic pancreatitis. In: Beger HG, Büchler MW, Ditschuneit H, eds. Chronic pancreatitis. Berlin: Springer-Verlag, 1990.
3. FitzSimmons SC. The changing epidemiology of cystic fibrosis. J Pediatrics 1993; 122: 1–9.
4. DiMagno EP, Go VLW, Summerskill WHJ. Relations between pancreatic enzyme output and malabsorption in severe pancreatic insufficiency. N Engl J Med 1973; 288: 813–5.
5. Rinderknecht H. Pancreatic secretory enzymes in the exocrine pancreas. In: Go VL, et al., eds. The exocrine pancreas: biology, pathobiology, and diseases. New York: Raven Press, 1986: 163–83.
6. Desnuelle P, Figarella C. Biochemistry. In: Howat HAT, Sarles H, eds. The exocrine pancreas. Philadelphia: WB Saunders, 1978: 86–112.
7. Layer P, Go VLW, DiMagno EP. Fate of pancreatic enzymes during small intestinal aboral transit in humans. Am J Physiol 1986; 251: G475–80.
8. Thiruvengadam R, DiMagno EP. Inactivation of human lipase by proteases. Am J Physiol 1988; 255: G476–81.
9. DiMagno EP, Clain JE, Layer P. Chronic pancreatitis. In: Go VLW et al., eds. The pancreas: biology, pathobiology, and diseases. 2nd ed. New York: Raven Press, 1993: 665–706.
10. DiMagno EP, Malagelada JR, Go VLW, Moertel CG. Fate of orally ingested enzymes in pancreatic insufficiency: comparison of two dosage schedules. N Engl J Med 1977; 296: 1318–22.
11. Doty JE, Fin AS, Meyer JH. Alteration in digestive function caused by pancreatic disease. Surg Clin North Am 1989; 69: 447–65.
12. Roy CC, Weber AM, Lepage G, Smith L, Leby E. Digestive and absorptive phase anomalies associated with the exocrine pancreatic insufficiency of cystic fibrosis. J Pediatr Gastrenterol Nutr 1988; 7(Suppl 1): S1–7.
13. Youngberg CA, Berardi RR, Howatt WF, Hyneck ML, Amidon GL, Meyer JH, Dressman JB. Comparison of gastrointestinal pH in cystic fibrosis and healthy subjects. Dig Dis Sci 1987; 32: 472–80.

14. Abrams CK, Hamosh M, Hubbard VS, Dulta SK, Hamosh P. Lingual lipase in cystic fibrosis: Quantitation of enzyme activity in the upper small intestine of patients with exocrine pancreatic insufficiency. J Clin Invest 1986; 73: 374–82.
15. Brady MS, Rickard K, Yu P, Eigen H. Effectiveness and safety of small versus large doses of enteric-coated pancreatic enzymes in reducing steatorrhea in children with cystic fibrosis: a prospective randomized study. Pediatr Pulm 1991; 10: 79–85.
16. Regan PT, Phillips SF, DiMagno EP. Pancreatic insufficiency and Menetriers disease: report of a case with clinical response to pancreatic enzyme replacement. Am J Dig Dis 1978; 23: 759–62.
17. Lebenthal E, Rolston DK, Holsclaw DS Jr. Enzyme therapy for pancreatic insufficiency: Present status and future needs. Pancreas 1994; 9: 1–12.
18. Layer P, Holtmann G. Pancreatic enzymes in chronic pancreatitis. Int J Pancreatol 1994; 15: 1–11.
19. Meyer JH, Elashoff J, Porter-Fink V, Dressmann J, Amidon GL. Human postprandial gastric emptying of 1–3 millimeter spheres. Gastroenterology 1988; 94: 115–1325.
20. Kühnelt P, Mundlos S, Adler G. Einfluß der Pelletgröße eines Pankreasenzympräparates auf die duodenale lipolytische Aktivität. Z Gastroenterol 1991; 29: 417–21.
21. Haln U, Löser Ch, Löhr M, Katschinski M, Mössner J. A double-blind, randomized, multicentre, crossover study to prove equivalence of pancreatic minimicrospheres versus microspheres in exocrine pancreatic insufficiency. Aliment Pharmacol Ther 1999; 13: 951–7.
22. Grendell JH, Cello J. Chronic pancreatitis. In: Sleisinger MH, Fordtran JS, eds. Gastrointestinal disease. Pathophysiology, diagnosis, management. Philadelphia: WB Saunders, 1993: 1654–81.
23. Adler G. Enzymsubstitution zur Behandlung der Schmerzen bei chronischer Pankreatitis. Dtsch med Wschr 1988; 113: 1075–9.
24. Fölsch UR. Pankreasenzym-Präparate zur Schmerztherapie bei chronischer Pankreatitis. Dt Ärztebl 1989; 86: 604–5.
25. Löser C, Fölsch UR. Differentialtherapie der exokrinen Pankreasinsuffizienz – Aktuelle Aspekte und zukünftige Perspektiven der Substitutionstherapie mit Pankreasenzymen. Z Gastroenterol 1995; 33: 715–22.
26. Graham DY. Enzyme replacement therapy of exocrine pancreatic insufficiency in man. Relation between in vitro enzyme activities and in vivo potency in commercial pancreatic extracts. N Engl J Med 1977; 296: 1314–7.
27. Nakamura T, Arai Y, Tando Y, Terada A, Yamada N, Tsujino M, Imamura K, Machida K, Kikuchi H, Takebe K. Effect of omeprazole on changes in gastric and upper small intestine pH levels in patients with chronic pancreatitis. Clin Ther 1995; 17: 448–59.
28. Durie PA, Bell L, Linton W, Corey ML, Forstner GG. Effect of cimetidine and sodium bicarbonate on pancreatic replacement therapy in cystic fibrosis. Gut 1980; 21: 778–86.
29. Regan PT, Malagelada JR, DiMagno EP, Glanzman SL, Go VLW. Comparative effects of antacids, cimetidine and enteric coating on the therapeutic response to oral enzymes in severe pancreatic insufficiency. N Engl J Med 1977; 297: 854–8.
30. Lankisch PG, Lembcke B, Göke B, Creutzfeldt W. Therapy of pancreatogenic steatorrhea: Does acid protection of pancreatic enzymes offer any advantage? Z Gastroenterol 1986; 24: 753–7.
31. Staub JL, Sarles H, Soule JC, Galmiche HP, Capron JP. No effect of cimetidine on the therapeutic response to oral enzymes in severe pancreatic insufficiency. N Engl J Med 1981; 304: 1364–5.
32. Heijerman HG. Lamers CB, Bakker W. Omeprazole enhances the efficacy of pancreatin (pancrease) in cystic fibrosis. Ann Intern Med 1991; 114: 200–1.
33. Meyer J. The ins and outs of oral pancreatic enzymes. Editorial. N Engl J Med 1977; 296: 1347–8.
34. Littlewood JM, Kelleher J, Walters MP, Johnson AW. In vivo and in vitro studies of microsphere pancreatic supplements. J Pediatr Gastroenterol Nutr 1988; 7(Suppl 1): S18–S21.
35. Whitehead AM. Study to compare the enzyme activity, acid resistance and dissolution characteristics of currently available pancreatic enzyme preparations. Pharm Weekbl (Sci) 1988; 10: 12–6.

36. Williams J, MacDonald A, Littlewood JM, Robinson T, Walter MP. Two enteric-coated microspheres in cystic fibrosis. Arch Dis Child 1990; 65: 594–7.
37. Beverly DW, Kelleher J, MacDonald A, Littlewood JM, Robinson T. Walter MP. Comparison of four pancreatic extracts in cystic fibrosis. Arch Dis Child 1987; 62: 564–568.
38. Mischler EH, Parrell S, Farrell PM, Odell GB. Comparison of effectiveness of pancreatic enzyme preparations in cystic fibrosis. Am J Dis Child 1982; 136: 1060–3.
39. Griffin SM, Alderson D, Farndon JR. Acid resistant lipase as replacement therapy in chronic pancreatic exocrine insufficiency: A study in dogs. Gut 1989; 30: 1012–5.
40. Zentler Munro PL, Assoufi BA, Balasubramanian K, Cornell C, Benoliel D, Northfiled TC, Hodson ME: Therapeutic potential and clinical efficacy of acid-resistant fungal lipase in the treatment of pancreatic steatorrhea due to cystic fibrosis. Pancreas 1992; 7: 311–9.
41. Bruno MJ, Haverkort EB, Tijssen GP, Tytgat GNJ, van Leeuwen DJ. Placebo-controlled trial of enteric coated pancreatin microsphere treatment in patients with unresectable cancer of the pancreatic head region. Gut 1998; 42: 92–6.
42. Neoptolemos JP, Ghaneh P, Andren-Sandberg A, Bramhall S, Patankar R, Leibeukter JH, Johnson CD. Treatment of pancreatic exocrine insufficiency after pancreatic resection. Results of a randomized, double-blind, placebo-controlled, crossover study of high vs. standard dose pancreatin. Int J Pancreatol 1999; 25: 171–80.
43. Bruno MJ, Borm JJ, Hoek FJ, Delzenne B, Hofmann AF, de Goreij JJ, van Royen EA, van Gulik TM, de Wit LT, Gouma DJ, van Leeuwen DJ, Tytgat GN. Comparative effects of enteric-coated pancreatin microsphere therapy after conventional and pylorus-preserving pancreatoduodenectomy. Br J Surg 1997; 84: 953–6.
44. Friess H, Bohm J, Muller MW, Glasbrenner B, Riepl RL, Malfertheiner P, Büchler MW. Maldigestion after total gastrectomy is associated with pancreatic insufficiency. Am J Gastroenterol 1996; 91: 341–7.
45. Gaskin K, Gurwitz D, Durie P, Corey M, Levinson H, Forstner G. Improved respiratory prognosis in cystic fibrosis patients with normal fat absorption. J Pediatr 1982; 100: 857–62.
46. Gretzmacher I, Rüther HG. Maldigestion. A clinical picture observed in daily practice. Therapiewoche 1983; 33: 676–82.
47. Zorn J. Erfahrungen bei der Substitutionstherapie mit einem neuen Pankreasferment-Präparat pflanzlicher Herkunft. Fortschr Med 1978; 96: 1941–3.
48. Stapleton FB, Kennedy J, Nousia-Arvanitakis S, Linshw MA. Hyperuricemia due to high-dose pancreatic extract therapy in cystic fibrosis. N Engl J Med 1976; 29: 246–8.
49. Couper R, Lichman S, Cleghorn G, del Castillo V, Durie P. Serum immunoglobulin G directed against porcine trypsin in pancreatic insufficient cystic fibrosis patients receiving pancreatic enzyme supplements. Pancreas 1991; 6: 558–63.
50. Lipkin GW, Vidkers DW. Allergy in cystic fibrosis nurses to pancreatic extract. Lancet 1987; 1: 392.
51. Lebenthal E. High strength pancreatic exocrine enzyme capsules associated with colonic strictures in patients with cystic fibrosis: "more is not necessarily better". Pediatr Gastroenterol Nutr 1994; 18: 423–5.
52. Borowitz DS, Grand RJ, Durie P, and the Consensus Committee. Use of pancreatic enzyme supplements for patients with cystic fibrosis in the context of fibrosing colonopathy. J Pediatrics 1995; 127: 681–4.

10.3 Exocrine pancreatic insufficiency: Current and future treatment

E. P. DiMagno

Natural history of malabsorption

Malabsorption is the clinical hallmark of severe exocrine pancreatic insufficiency. It occurs when exocrine pancreatic secretion is less than 10% of normal [1]. Common causes of exocrine pancreas-associated malabsorption are chronic pancreatitis, pancreatic cancer and cystic fibrosis. The etiology of chronic pancreatitis predicates the rate of developing exocrine insufficiency [2]. In chronic pancreatitis due to alcohol, exocrine insufficiency develops a median of 13 years after onset of disease [3]. On the other hand, some patients with idiopathic chronic pancreatitis develop exocrine insufficiency much more slowly. We have found that idiopathic chronic pancreatitis comprises of two groups: early onset (onset of disease < 36 yr old) and late onset. The phenotype of the groups differs. For example, exocrine insufficiency develops very slowly in the early-onset group (28 yr after onset of disease compared to 17 yr in the late-onset group). Similarly, calcification and endocrine insufficiency develop at different rates among the 3 groups of chronic pancreatitis. Calcification and endocrine insufficiency develop a median of 9 and 20 yr in alcoholic chronic pancreatitis, 25 and 28 yr in early-onset idiopathic chronic pancreatitis and 19 and 12 yr in late-onset idiopathic chronic pancreatitis. Seventy-five to 80% of patients with pancreatic cancer [3] and cystic fibrosis have exocrine insufficiency.

Treatment of exocrine pancreatic insufficiency

Nutritional

Resting energy expenditure is high in chronic pancreatitis. It is 33% above the value predicted by the Harris and Benedict formula [4]. Hypermetabolism occurs in 49% of stable outpatients with alcoholic chronic pancreatitis and 65% of undernourished patients [5]. However, most patients with pancreatic insufficiency maintain weight and strength due to a good appetite, high caloric intake and ingesting pancreatic enzymes. Rarely are other measures needed to achieve or maintain an acceptable nutritional state. Severely malnourished patients usually have a complication such as exacerbation of chronic pancreatitis, pancreatic ascites, or symptomatic pseudocysts. In these situations, enteral feedings or total parenteral nutrition may be needed for extended periods of time to prepare a patient for surgery and in the postoperative period.

Treatment with enzymes

Standard pancreatin treatment consisting of doses of eight tablets with each of 4 meals a day, each meal consisting of 25 g of fat, will abolish azotorrhea and reduce but not totally correct steatorrhea [6]. Most patients on this regimen achieve satisfactory nutritional status and become relatively asymptomatic. In symptomatic patients, occasionally reduction in fat intake effectively alleviates symptoms. However, reducing fat intake may paradoxically reduce the efficiency of fat absorption and decrease the coefficient of fat absorption, at least in dogs with exocrine pancreatic insufficiency (see below).

Porcine lipase, the lipase in commercial preparations, rarely abolishes pancreatic steatorrhea due to chronic pancreatitis or cystic fibrosis because lipase is inactivated within the gastrointestinal tract by acid [6, 7] and proteases [8, 9]. Therapies that have been used to reduce pancreatic steatorrhea in addition to porcine lipase include increasing survival of lipolytic activity by neutralizing acid with antacids [10], reducing acid secretion with H_2 blockers [7, 11] or with omeprazole [12], using enteric-coated microsphere formulations [13, 14] to protect enzymes from denaturation, or using lipases that are resistant to acid denaturation. Some antacid-antisecretory strategies correct steatorrhea in a minority of patients, but they are not popular because they require taking multiple medications and are expensive.

Enteric coated microsphere formulations do not abolish steatorrhea in most patients because there is not appropriate mixing of lipolytic activity within the preparation with food. Adequate mixing does not occur because the large pellet size in some preparations (> 1 mm) interferes with gastric emptying and the optimum pH for dissolution of the coatings, which is necessary to release enzymes, is not present in the upper small intestine. The overall effect of these problems causes the food to empty from the stomach without enzymes and the enzymes are liberated very distally in the small intestine after the major portion of the meal has traversed the small intestine [15]. Although microencapsulated preparations containing high doses of lipase may correct steatorrhea in some patients [16], these preparations have been withdrawn from the US market because they are associated with colonic strictures in children with cystic fibrosis who ingest large numbers of capsules [17, 18].

Thus, in patients with persistent symptoms, adding an H_2 blocker [7,11] or omeprazole [12] to standard pancreatin treatment will abolish steatorrhea in 40–50% of patients (Fig. 10.3-1) and alleviate troublesome diarrhea. Similar results have also been achieved with bicarbonate [10]. If symptoms and steatorrhea continue, special intraluminal studies may be necessary to determine if intraluminal conditions are present for certain dose

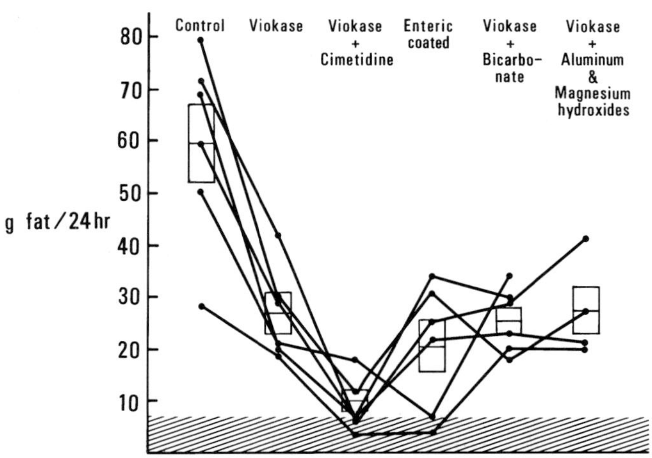

Figure 10.3-1. Effects of various treatments on fecal fat excretions (g/24 hr) in patients with chronic pancreatitis. The pancreatin used in these studies was Viokase. Modified from Regan PT, Malagelada J-R, DiMagno EP, Glanzman SL, Go VLW. Comparative effects of antacids, cimetidine, and enteric coating on the therapeutic response to oral enzymes in severe pancreatic insufficiency. N Engl J Med 1977; 297: 854–858.

schedules to be effective or that intraluminal conditions have been altered by adjunctive therapy. For example, when gastric pH is greater than 4 for approximately 2 hr postprandially, altering the dose schedule from 8 tablets with meals to 2 tablets hourly may alleviate steatorrhea. Alternatively, if administration of a standard dose of an H_2 blocker or proton pump inhibitor does not keep the gastric pH greater than 4, either more should be given or, if intraluminal conditions are relatively acidic (<4) for a long time postprandially, microencapsulated preparations may be effective [19].

Assessment of treatment of exocrine insufficiency

Occasionally persistent symptomatic steatorrhea is a problem despite optimum treatment with pancreatic enzymes. In this instance, a simple diagnostic maneuver is to test various adjuvant regimens (addition of cimetidine, ranitidine or omeprazole, antacids or using microencapsulated enteric coated preparations) with two stage fecal fat or triolein breath tests. If symptoms of steatorrhea persist, intragastric and intraduodenal pH measurements during adjuvant treatments may be necessary so that dose adjustments can be made to alkalize the upper gastrointestinal tract.

Novel lipases and other potential measures to improve treatment

Novel lipases

The characteristics of an ideal lipase for treatment of exocrine pancreatic insufficiency includes resistance to denaturation by acid and proteolytic digestion and maintenance of lipolytic activity within the lumen of the upper small intestinal tract. Acid resistant lipases that might be useful to treat pancreatic insufficiency are fungal and gastric lipase but they are inactivated by physiologic bile acid concentrations existing in the lumen of the small intestine [20] and fungal lipase was found to be ineffective in alleviating steatorrhea. In addition to resisting acid denaturation and proteolytic digestion, the formulation should promote appropriate mixing of lipolytic activity with the fat content of the meal during aboral transit.

A novel bacterial lipase isolated from *Burkholderia plantarii*, previously called *Pseudomonas glumae* [21] may improve treatment of steatorrhea. We showed that in vitro the lipolytic activity of bacterial lipase survives better than porcine lipase in human gastric juice at conditions most likely present postprandially (pH approximately 3–4 and nutrients present) [22]. We also showed that in human duodenal juice survival of the lipolytic activity of bacterial lipase was much greater than the lipolytic activity of porcine lipase under the conditions to simulate those found postprandially in patients with exocrine pancreatic insufficiency [22]. Importantly we also demonstrated that bacterial lipase was active in the presence of physiologic concentrations of bile acids. These findings prompted the hypothesis that bacterial lipase may be an ideal lipase for treatment of exocrine pancreatic insufficiency and superior to porcine lipase in alleviating pancreatic steatorrhea.

Experimental treatments

Diet. The nutrient composition of the diet may be important in the treatment of pancreatic steatorrhea. This hypothesis arises because nutrients increase the survival of pancreatic enzymes during storage [23], during incubation in human duodenal juice [24] and during intestinal transit in normal humans [25]. For example, incubating lipase in duodenal juice containing a normal postprandial concentration of lipolytic activity (250 IU/mL) or at concentrations found in pancreatic insufficiency (25 IU/mL) with protein and fat prevents loss of lipolytic activity but carbohydrate does not and nutrients increase survival of pancreatic lipolytic activity during duodenal-ileal transit in normal humans. These studies suggest that diets with high fat content might increase survival of lipolytic activity and increase fat absorption in pancreatic insufficiency.

Diet and enzymes. In canine exocrine insufficiency, we showed that 300,000–600,000 IU of lipolytic activity as powdered bacterial lipase (120 mg), the total normal amount of lipolytic activity secreted for 6 hr postprandially, corrects steatorrhea, particularly when given with meals containing a high proportion of fat as calories [26] (Fig. 10.3-2). Pancreatin also corrects steatorrhea at these doses of lipolytic activity, but giving 300,000 IU of lipolytic activity requires administering 18 g of pancreatin, a highly impractical dose, compared to only 120 mg of bacterial lipase. Therefore, human pancreatic steatorrhea might be abolished by giving large amounts of lipolytic activity as bacterial lipase with high fat content meals. These data may lead to revision of treatment of human pancreatic insufficiency; these studies in dogs show that administration of mg amounts of bacterial lipase may abolish steatorrhea without use of any adjuvant therapy. Therefore, the regimen of high fat diets with porcine lipase should be evaluated in humans with pancreatic steatorrhea.

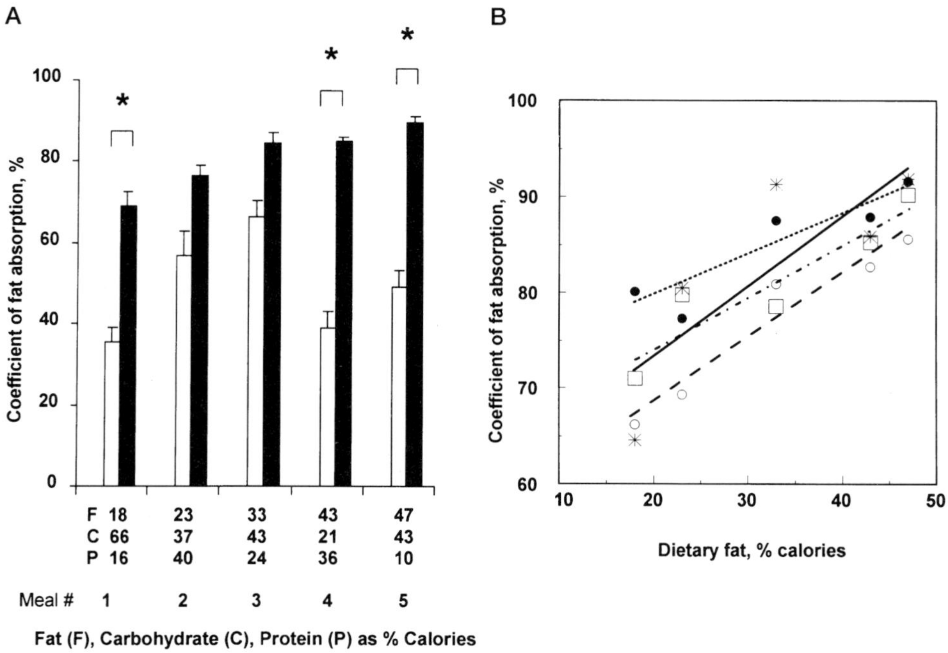

Figure 10.3-2A, B. Effects of bacterial lipase on coefficient of fat absorption with different diets in each of four dogs. **A:** Response to no treatment (□) or 300,000 IU powder bacterial lipase (■) with different diets (horizontal axis, ascending order of percentage of fat calories in meals). Values are mean ± SE. *$p < 0.01$. **B:** Each combination of symbol and line is one of four dogs. r = 0.835-0.977 for the four dogs ($p = 0.002$ for slopes vs. 0). With permission from [26].

Formulation of enzymes. In dogs we have tested different formulations of bacterial lipase and found that encapsulation of any formulation (powder, microtablets enteric coated microtablets) reduces fat absorption [27]. Of the formulations, powder reduces steatorrhea greater than all other formulations. Also in dogs we found that powder pancrealipase improves fat absorption better than tablets. These findings should be investigated in persons with pancreatic steatorrhea. In the meantime, powder porcine pancrealipase might be effective in patients who are symptomatic and cannot be controlled with usual formulations. The increased fat absorption with a high fat diet and powder is due to improved mixing of the lipids in the diet with the lipase in the powder formulation [28].

We believe it is important to abolish steatorrhea. For example, in cystic fibrosis correction of malabsorption may decrease morbidity, induce more normal growth and increase survival since children with cystic fibrosis who do not have exocrine pancreatic insufficiency have a slower decline of pulmonary function [29]. Our canine studies provide data to potentially support the ingestion of high caloric, high fat meals in exocrine pancreatic insufficiency, especially for the children with cystic fibrosis who need better nutritional management to enhance growth and development and perhaps reduce morbidity and mortality.

References

1. DiMagno EP, Go VLW, Summerskill WHJ. Relations between pancreatic enzyme outputs and malabsorption in severe pancreatic insufficiency. N Engl J Med 1973; 288: 813–5.
2. Layer P, Yamamoto H, Kalthoff L, Clain JE, Bakken LJ, DiMagno EP. The different courses of early and late onset idiopathic and alcoholic chronic pancreatitis. Gastroenterology 1994; 107: 1481–7.
3. Perez MM, Newcomer AD, Moertel CG, Go VLW, DiMagno EP. Assessment of weight loss, food intake, fat metabolism, malabsorption, and treatment of pancreatic insufficiency in pancreatic cancer. Cancer 1983; 52: 346–52.
4. Dickerson RN, Vehe KL, Mullen JL, Feurer ID. Resting energy expenditure in patients with pancreatitis. Crit Care Med 1991; 19: 484–90.
5. Hebuterne X, Hastier P, Peroux JL, Zeboudj N, Delmont JP, Rampal P. Resting energy expenditure in patients with alcoholic chronic pancreatitis. Dig Dis Sci 1996; 41: 533–9.
6. DiMagno EP, Malagelada JR, Go VLW, Moertel CG. Fate of orally ingested enzymes in pancreatic insufficiency: comparison of two dosage schedules. N Engl J Med 1977; 296: 1318–22.
7. Regan PT, Malagelada JR, DiMagno EP, Glanzman SL, Go VLW. Comparative effects of antacids, cimetidine, and enteric coating on the therapeutic response to oral enzymes in severe pancreatic insufficiency. N Engl J Med 1977; 297: 854–8.
8. Thiruvengadam R, DiMagno EP: Inactivation of human lipase by proteases. Am J Physiol 1988; 255: G476–81.
9. Thiruvengadam R, Zinsmeister AR, DiMagno EP. Is human lipase survival during aboral intestinal transit dependent upon intraluminal chymotrypsin (CT) activity and bile acid concentrations (BAC)? Dig Dis Sci 1987; 32: 1189.
10. Graham DY. Pancreatic enzyme replacement: the effect of antacids or cimetidine. Dig Dis Sci 1982; 27: 485–90.
11. Saunders JH, Drummond S, Wormsley KG. Inhibition of gastric secretion in treatment of pancreatic insufficiency. Br Med J 1977; 1: 418–9.
12. Heijerman HG, Lamers CB, Bakker W. Omeprazole enhances the efficacy of pancreatin (pancrease) in cystic fibrosis. Ann Intern Med 1991; 114: 200–1.
13. Dutta SK, Rubin J, Harvey J. Comparative evaluation of the therapeutic efficacy of a pH sensitive enteric coated pancreatic enzyme preparation with conventional pancreatic enzyme therapy in the treatment of exocrine pancreatic insufficiency. Gastroenterology 1983; 84: 476–82.

14. Layer P et al. Enzyme pellet size and luminal nutrients digestion in pancreatic insufficiency. Digestion 1992; 52: 100.
15. Guarner L, Rodriguez R, Guarner F, Malagelada JR. Fate of oral enzymes in pancreatic insufficiency. Gut 1993; 34: 708–12.
16. Malesci A, Mariani A, Mezzi G. Bocchia P, Basilisco M. New enteric-coated high- lipase pancreatic extract in the treatment of pancreatic steatorrhea. J Clin Gastroenterol 1994; 18: 32–5.
17. Smyth RL, van Velzen D, Smyth AR, Lloyd DA, Heaf DP. Strictures of ascending colon in cystic fibrosis and high-strength pancreatic enzymes. Lancet 1994; 343: 85–6.
18. Taylor CJ. Colonic strictures in cystic fibrosis. Lancet 1994; 343: 615–6.
19. DiMagno EP. Medical treatment of pancreatic insufficiency. Mayo Clin Proc 1979; 54: 435–42.
20. Zentler-Munro PL, Assoufi BA, Balasubramanian K, Cornell S, Benoliel D, Northfield TC, Hodson ME. Therapeutic potential and clinical efficacy of acid-resistant fungal lipase in the treatment of pancreatic steatorrhoea due to cystic fibrosis. Pancreas 1992; 7: 311–9.
21. Cleasby A, Garman E, Egmond MR, Batenburg M. Crystallization and preliminary x-ray study of a lipase from Pseudomonas glumae. J Mol Biol 1992; 224: 281–2.
22. Raimondo M, DiMagno EP. Lipolytic activity of bacterial lipase survives better than that of porcine lipase in human gastric and duodenal content. Gastroenterology 1994; 107: 231–5.
23. Kelly DG, Sternby B, DiMagno EP. How to protect human pancreatic enzyme activities in frozen duodenal juice. Gastroenterology 1991; 100: 189–95.
24. Kelly DG, Bentley KJ, Sandberg RJ, Zinsmeister AR, DiMagno EP. Do nutrients and bile in human duodenal juice affect the survival of lipase activity? Gastroenterology 1988; 94: 222.
25. Holtmann G, Kelly DG, Sternby B, DiMagno EP: Survival of human pancreatic enzymes during small bowel transit: effect of nutrients, bile acids, and enzymes. Am J Physiol 1997; 273: G553–8.
26. Suzuki A, Mizumoto A, Sarr MG, DiMagno EP: Bacterial lipase and high fat diets in canine exocrine pancreatic insufficiency: a new therapy of steatorrhea? Gastroenterology 1997; 112: 2048–55.
27. Chung JP, Metzger A, Asakura N, Sarr MG, DiMagno EP. Effects of doses and formulations of bacterial lipase (BL) on gastric emptying, delivery of lipolytic activity (LA) and steatorrhea in canine exocrine insufficiency. Pancreas 1997; 15: 432.
28. Chung JP, Metzger A, Asakura N, Sarr MG, DiMagno EP. Different mixing of chyme and lipolytic activity (LA) in powder and microtablet formulations of bacterial lipase (BL) during GI transit explains variable correction of canine pancreatic steatorrhea. Gastroenterology 1998; 114: A448.
29. Gaskin K, Gurwitz D, Durie P, Covey M, Levison H, Forstner G. Improved respiratory prognosis in cystic fibrosis patients with normal fat absorption. J Pediatr 1982; 100: 857–62.

10.4 An integrated approach to the non-operative treatment of pain in chronic pancreatitis

St. Kahl, B. Glasbrenner, H.-U. Schulz, P. Malfertheiner

Introduction

Chronic pancreatitis is an evolutive disease with a progressive destruction of pancreatic parenchyma due to inflammation, necrosis, and consequent biosynthesis of fibrotic tissue. Regardless of its etiology, chronic pancreatitis is characterized by disabling pain, and progressive loss of exocrine and endocrine tissue and complications due to involvement of surrounding organs.

Most commonly pain brings the patients to the attention of either gastroenterologists or surgeons. Pain significantly reduces patients' quality of life.

While exocrine insufficiency and diabetes mellitus are the domain of nonsurgical treatment, pain and complications of chronic pancreatitis may also be treated surgically.

The specific cause of pain in an individual patient may be difficult to determine, and there are at least two major concepts for the pathogenesis of pain. Taking this into account no single therapy would be expected to work in all patients. Randomized, controlled trials comparing different treatment options and strategies are not available. Non-operative treatment (a combination of medical therapy and interventional endoscopy) is generally the first line therapy in patients with painful chronic pancreatitis. There is a wide spectrum of different therapeutic interventions which must be integrated into an individual treatment concept. In this chapter we focus on specific problems of nonoperative interventions against pancreatic pain.

Causes of pain

Pain is the leading symptom in chronic pancreatitis, and presents a heterogeneous pattern ranging from a few relapses per year to continuous pain.

Two mechanisms are commonly suggested for the generation of pain in the absence of local complications: 1) Ductal and intraparenchymal hypertension [1–4] and 2) inflammatory changes of pancreatic parenchyma with involvement of pancreatic nerves [5, 6].

Increased intrapancreatic pressure

In this model at least one stenosis of the main pancreatic duct leads to increased intrapancreatic pressure [4] which furthermore causes dilatation of main pancreatic duct and side branches upstream of the stenotic segment [1, 2]. The hypertension model was advanced by the theory that increased ductal and parenchymal pressure may lead to reduced capillary blood flow with accumulation of acidic metabolites and decrease of pancreatic interstitial pH [3].

Based on this theory those options which reduce the intrapancreatic pressure (inhibition/suppression of pancreatic secretion, interventional endoscopy) may lead to a significant reduction of pancreatic pain.

Inflammation

A significant invasion of inflammatory cells into pancreatic parenchyma and pancreatic nerves in chronic pancreatitis is well documented [5]. These cells discharge inflammatory mediators and therefore a significantly increased amount of inflammatory mediators in pancreatic parenchyma and pancreatic nerves is found in patients who have pain [6]. This is the rationale for medical, analgesic and anti-inflammatory, treatment.

Medical treatment options against pancreatic pain

There are three general medical treatment options which may be combined with or supported by interventional methods (therapeutic endoscopy and lithotripsy; see Table 10.4-1).

• Diet (stop alcohol intake)
• Analgesics
• Inhibition/suppression of pancreatic secretion

Table 10.4-1. Medical treatment options for painful chronic pancreatitis.

Diet and alcohol abstinence

The first step in pain management consists of the complete avoidance of alcohol. The benefit of alcohol abstinence in reducing pancreatic pain has not been firmly established. Total abstinence from alcohol as only measure achieves pain relief in up to 50% of patients, but this effect appears restricted to those with mild to moderate disease [7]. Other than this, there are no specific dietary measures that have been found to be effective in preventing pancreatic pain.

Analgesics

Prior to using analgesics, any complication which may be responsible for pain (e.g. pseudocysts, compression of adjacent visceral structures) needs to be excluded. There are no prospective, randomized, controlled studies which compare the efficacy of different drugs or different drug treatment regimens for treatment of pain in patients with chronic pancreatitis. The recommendations for analgesic treatment given here are based on the consensus report of the German society of gastroenterology [8] and on our own experience.

Analgesics should be administered by one physician who assumes full responsibility. Analgesic drug treatment should begin with non-narcotic agents (e.g. paracetamol, nonsteroidal anti-inflammatory drugs). In a further step opioids are often required. Type and doses of analgesic drugs required vary between patients. Treatment should be adapted to individual needs with the lowest drug doses necessary to control pain and should be increased stepwise, according to recommendations of WHO [9] (see Table 10.4-2). In this context it is indispensable to register the individual pain intensity by a visual analogue scale to find the required type and dosage of analgesics. Available analgesics and dosages are listed in Table 10.4-3.

Table 10.4- 2. WHO schema for analgesic treatment. Adapted from [9].

Step	Analgesics and additional drugs	Preparations
I Moderate pain	Peripheral analgesics	Paracetamol, Metamizol
II Strong pain *(step I ineffective)*	Peripheral analgesics + Central effective analgesic	Paracetamol, Metamizol + Pentacocine
IIIa Stronger pain *(step II ineffective)*	Mild opioids	Tramadol, Tilidin
IIIb*	Neuroleptica antidepressants	Levopromacin Clomipramin
IV Strongest pain *(step III ineffective)*	Opioids	Buprenorphine Morphium

* To add neuroleptica and/or antidepressants to any step in this scheme (not only step III) may be helpful, see text.

Table 10.4-3. Available analgesics for pain treatment in chronic pancreatitis. Adopted from [8].

Generic name	Daily dosage	Maximum dosage
Paracetamol	2–3 × 500–1,000 mg	4,000 (6,000) mg
Metamizol	1–4 × 500–1,000 mg	4,000 (6,000) mg
Tramadol	Up to 4 × 100 mg 2–3 × 200 mg (retard)	400 (600) mg
Buprenorphine	3–4 × 0.2–0.4 mg	Maximum single dose 6–9 µg/kg BW
Pentacocine	6–7 × 50 mg	360 mg
Tilidin	3 × 50–200 mg	600 mg
Morphine	Individual daily dosage	As required
Levopromacin	3–5 × 10 mg	300 mg
Clomipramin	1 × 50–100 mg	

Inflammatory cells within the pancreas play an important role in chronic pancreatitis, especially when they affect nerves [5]. We suspect in these patients with pain mainly caused by inflammation and by invasion of inflammatory cells, anti-inflammatory drugs (NSAIDs or selective COX_2-inhibitors) may be most useful. If NSAIDs are used regularly, proton pump inhibitors should to be added.

Often a coexisting depression lowers the visceral pain threshold in individual patients. In these cases an antidepressant can be useful (see Table 10.4-3). Additionally to the effect on the depression, antidepressants have an effect on pain and potentiate the effect of opiates.

Suppression/inhibition of pancreatic secretion

Enzymes. There are six studies available that have evaluated the effect of oral pancreatic enzymes in reducing pain in chronic pancreatitis [10–15].

The idea behind this approach is that pancreatic secretion is regulated by CCK and CCK-releasing peptide, which is destroyed by trypsin from basal pancreatic secretion. In exocrine pancreatic insufficiency with decreasing amounts of enzymes in pancreatic secretion there is less denaturation of CCK-releasing peptide with increasing amounts of CCK, which then stimulates pancreatic secretion. The precise mechanism of pancreatic pain induced by CCK stimulation is unclear. One possible mechanism may be an increasing pancreatic volume flow that leads to increased intrapancreatic pressure.

Only two of six randomized prospective trials showed that enzymes are effective in reducing pain in patients with chronic pancreatitis [10, 11] (see Table 10.4-4). These two studies used an enzyme preparation in tablets, the remaining four used microspheres which do not release pancreatic enzymes in the duodenum [12–15]. Therefore they could not interfere with the negative feedback mechanism. It is unclear if enzymes would still be helpful in patients with severe exocrine insufficiency, when the volume flow is decreased.

	No effect on pain	With effect on pain
Enzymes	Halgreen, 1986 [14] Larvin, 1991 [12] Mössner, 1992 [13] Malesci, 1995 [15]	Slaff, 1984 [11] Isaksson, 1983 [10]
Inhibition of pancreatic secretion	Malfertheiner, 1992 [19] Malfertheiner, 1995 [18]	Schmalz, 1992 [69] Toskes, 1993 [20] Toskes, 1994 [21]

Table 10.4-4. Effect of different medical treatment options on pain caused by chronic pancreatitis.

Although a meta-analysis [16] of the six published studies on enzymes for pain treatment concluded that there is no positive effect of pancreatic enzyme preparations on pain this is inconclusive because of heterogeneity of study populations and significant differences in drug preparations. Therefore the effect of pancreatic enzyme preparations on pain remains uncertain.

Suppression of enzyme production: Somatostatin. Somatostatin has a profound inhibitory effect on pancreatic secretion[17]. This has been used for treatment of pseudocysts. If somatostatin was used for pain treatment the small number of studies showed different effects on pain [18–21] (see Table 10.4-4).

Additional studies are necessary to evaluate the effects of somatostatin and its analogue octreotide on pain in patients with chronic pancreatitis and to clarify which patients may benefit.

Interventional procedures

From studies of the natural history we know that between 30% and 60% of patients will ultimately undergo surgery [22]. This suggests that medical treatment is effective in a substantial proportion of patients with painful chronic pancreatitis. The disease course of chronic pancreatitis may be improved by the combination of medical therapy and interventional procedures.

In patients with strictures of the common bile duct or of the main pancreatic duct with resulting significant outflow obstruction or with pseudocysts, interventional endoscopy is of potential benefit. In cases with calculi in the main pancreatic duct additional lithotripsy may be helpful.

Stenting of stenosis of the common bile duct

Stenosis of the common bile duct occurs in 10 to 40% of patients with chronic pancreatitis [27]. Indications for interventions at the common bile duct are listed in Table 10.4-5) [23]. In those cases with stenosis of the common bile duct and pain as leading symptom, pain may result from increased common bile duct pressure.

- Significant cholestasis
- Cholangitis
- Prevention of secondary biliary cirrhosis
- Differentiation of pain causes (stenosis of distal common bile duct vs. pancreatitis)

Table 10.4-5. Indications for interventional endoscopy at common bile duct [23].

There are several studies which reported on the efficacy of interventional endoscopy in common bile duct stenosis. There is conclusive evidence that a clinical benefit of nonoperative procedures occurs only in one third of the patients during a three-year follow-up period. In shorter follow-up the effect is less [24–29] (see Table 10.4-6). Our own experience shows that patients with inflammatory masses due to acute bouts of inflammation benefit from common bile duct stents whereas those with advanced fibrosis are not candidates for interventional endoscopy.

Author	Patients (n)	Follow-up period	Definite clinical benefit (%)
Deviere, 1990 [24]	25	12	14.4
Kohler, 1992 [28]	12	36	33
Huibregtse, 1994 [29]	52	33	32
Barthet, 1994 [25]	19	12	10.5
Smits, 1996 [26]	58	49	28
Riemann, 1996 [27]	17	36	33

Table 10.4-6. Common bile duct stenosis in chronic pancreatitis: Interventional endoscopy.

Stenting of stenosis of the main pancreatic duct

Endoscopic stent placement within the main pancreatic duct has been reported to be effective in improving pain associated with chronic pancreatitis. This may be the case if pain is mainly caused by significant outflow obstruction in the pancreatic duct. Indications for stent placement in the main pancreatic duct are listed in Table 10.4-7.

- Dominant strictures
- Occlusion due to calcifications
- Fistulae
- Drainage of pancreatic pseudocysts
- Symptomatic stenosis of papillae

Table 10.4-7. Indications for stent placement into main pancreatic duct in chronic pancreatitis.

Stents can be inserted safely and in a follow-up of approximately 2 to 3 years an improvement of pain has been reported [30–33] (see Table 10.4-8). It needs to be considered that stent placement can induce further alterations of main pancreatic duct [34–41] (see Table 10.4-9). In cases with normal pancreatic duct stent placement may induce ductal changes as in chronic pancreatitis [42]. But there are no controlled data suggesting that stent placement intensifies destruction of the main pancreatic duct more than the natural course of the disease.

The benefit of interventional endoscopy to drain the main pancreatic duct for pain management remains uncertain in the absence of prospective, randomized, controlled studies.

Author	Patients (n)	Follow-up (months)	Definite clinical benefit (%)
Cremer, 1991 [33]	76	37	94
Smits, 1995 [70]	51	34	82
Ponchon, 1995 [30]	23	12	91
Binmoeller, 1995 [32]	93	59	64

Table 10.4-8. Results of endoscopic stent placement for chronic pancreatitis.

Author	Patients (n)	Additional duct changes after stent placement (% of n)
Kozarek, 1990 [34]	38	36
Defus, 1990 [35]	36	83
Rossos, 1992 [36]	33	29
Burdick, 1992 [37]	26	61
Lehmann, 1993 [38]	34	50
Smith, 1996 [39]	61	82
Eisen, 1994 [40]	69	33
Sherman, 1996 [41]	16	56

Table 10.4-9. Influence of stent placement into main pancreatic duct on further duct alterations.

Lithotripsy and interventional endoscopy for pancreatic duct stones

In cases with main pancreatic duct stenosis and obstructing calculi within the duct a combination of interventional endoscopy and lithotripsy was reported to improve pancreatic pain. The reduction in pain correlated with the elimination of obstructing pancreatic stones and a decrease of the main pancreatic duct dilatation [31, 43–50] (see Table 10.4-10).

Adamek et al. reported that there is no significant difference in improvement of pain, need of analgesics or improvement of body weight between patients with successful or unsuccessful lithotripsy for pancreatic duct stones in a follow-up period of up to 92 months [50].

Further studies are required to establish the effect of these interventions on pancreatic pain.

Table 10.4-10. Clinical results of interventional endoscopy and lithotripsy.

Author	Patients (n)	Complete stone clearance (%)	Improvement of pain (%)
Delhaye, 1992 [43]	123	58	85
Sauerbruch, 1992 [44]	24	41	50
Schneider, 1994 [45]	50	60	62
Van der Hul, 1994 [46]	17	41	59
Johanns, 1996 [47]	35	46	85
Smits, 1996 [31]	53	79	74
Ohara, 1996 [48]	32	75	79
Costamagna, 1997 [49]	35	74	
Adamek, 1999 [50]	80	54	76

Interventional therapy for pancreatic pseudocysts

For the nonoperative treatment of symptomatic pseudocysts there are several different treatment procedures [51–68]. Selection of the procedure type depends on the anatomical situation (e.g. compression of stomach or duodenum), morphological findings (e.g. communication of the cyst with pancreatic duct) and the expertise and technical equipment of the gastroenterologist or endoscopist who is in attendance on the patient.

Evaluating the published papers dealing with nonoperative treatment of patients with symptomatic pseudocysts we have to recognize the lack of standardized methods for the evaluation of the results of these different interventions.

Taking this into account the success rates of different pseudocyst drainage procedures range from 26% to 100%. A higher success rate is more often seen with the more complex invasive procedures (see Table 10.4-11).

Summary, integration and conclusion

Medical therapy and interventional procedures are cornerstones of non-operative treatment strategies in patients with painful chronic pancreatitis. There are still no prospective, randomized controlled trials comparing the efficacy of different medical or inter-

Table 10.4-11. Pseudocysts: Results of interventional endoscopy.

Type of intervention	Requirements	References	Success rate
Transcutaneous puncture	No connection to pancreatic ductal system	Schwerk, 1989 [51] Grosso, 1989 [52]	29–58%
Transcutaneous drainage	No connection to pancreatic ductal system	Schwerk, 1989 [51] Grosso, 1989 [52] Barkin, 1991 [56] D'Agostino, 1993 [55] Pavlovsky, 1998 [54]	62–93%
Transcutaneous drainage + somatostatin		Barkin, 1991 [56] D'Agostino, 1993 [55]	87–100%
Cystogastric drainage (transcutaneous-transgastral puncture)	Direct contact of cyst to the dorsal gastric wall	Hancke, 1985 [53] Heyder, 1992 [57] Sever, 1998 [58]	Approx. 75%
Endoscopic pseudocystostomy	Impression of gastric or duodenal wall by pseudocysts	Cremer, 1989 [59] Sahel, 1991[60] Binmoeller, 1995 [61] Dohmoto, 1995 [52] Pfaffenbach, 1998 [64] Beckingham, 1999 [65]	62–88%
Endoscopic transpapillary drainage	Connection of pseudocyst to main pancreatic duct	Dohmoto, 1992 [63] Smits, 1995 [66] Barthet, 1995 [67] Catalano, 1995 [68] Binmoeller, 1995 [61]	69–77%

ventional methods or the combination of both for pain treatment. This is the crucial point which makes it impossible to recommend a specific procedure as gold standard or first line therapy. Based on our current knowledge the best way is to make a decision based on an individual patient's symptoms, on his pancreatic and biliary morphology (ERCP, EUS, CT), pancreatic function, and quality of life. The resulting therapeutic concept should take into consideration all medical and interventional methods.

Further extensive studies are necessary for the evaluation of treatment options in painful chronic pancreatitis.

References

1. Ebbehoj N, Borly L, Bulow J, Rasmussen SG, Madsen P. Evaluation of pancreatic tissue fluid pressure and pain in chronic pancreatitis. Scand J Gastroenterol 1990; 25: 462–6.
2. Ebbehoj N, Borly L, Bulow J et al. Pancreatic tissue fluid pressure in chronic pancreatitis. Scand J Gastroenterol 1990; 25: 1046–51.
3. Patel AG, Toyama MT, Alvarez C, Nguyen TN, Ashley SW, Reber HA. Pancreatic interstitial pH in human and feline chronic pancreatitis. Gastroenterology 1995; 109: 1639–45.
4. Manes G, Büchler MW, Pieramico O, Di Sebastiano P, Malfertheiner P. Is increased pancreatic pressure related to pain in chronic pancreatitis? Int J Pancreatol 1994; 15: 113–7.
5. Bockman DE, Büchler MW, Malfertheiner P, Beger HG. Analysis of nerves in chronic pancreatitis. Gastroenterology 1988; 94: 1459–69.
6. Büchler MW, Weihe E, Friess H et al. Changes in peptidergic innervation in chronic pancreatitis. Pancreas 1992; 7: 183–92.

7. Gullo L, Barbara L, Labo G. Effect of cessation of alcohol use on the course of pancreatic dysfunction in alcoholic pancreatitis. Gastroenterology 1988; 95: 1063–8.
8. Mössner J, Keim V, Niederau C et al. [Guidelines for therapy of chronic pancreatitis. Consensus Conference of the German Society of Digestive and Metabolic Diseases. Halle 21–23 November 1996]. Z Gastroenterol 1998; 36: 359–67.
9. World Health Organization. Cancer pain relief and palliative care: Report on a WHO expert committee. 1990. Geneva Switzerland, World Health Organization.
10. Isaksson G, Ihse I. Pain reduction by an oral pancreatic enzyme preparation in chronic pancreatitis. Dig Dis Sci 1983; 28: 97–102.
11. Slaff J, Jacobson D, Tillman CR, Curington C, Toskes PP. Protease-specific suppression of pancreatic exocrine secretion. Gastroenterology 1984; 87: 44–52.
12. Larvin M, McMahon MJ, Thomas WEG. Creon (enteric coated Pancreatic microspheres) for the treatment of pain in chronic pancreatitis: A double-blind, randomized, placebo-controlled, crossover study. Gastroenterology 1991; 100: A283.
13. Mössner J, Secknus R, Meyer J, Niederau C, Adler G. Treatment of pain with pancreatic extracts in chronic pancreatitis: results of a prospective placebo-controlled multicenter trial. Digestion 1992; 53: 54–66.
14. Halgreen H, Pedersen NT, Worning H. Symptomatic effect of pancreatic enzyme therapy in patients with chronic pancreatitis. Scand J Gastroenterol 1986; 21: 104–8.
15. Malesci A, Gaia E, Fioretta A et al. No effect of long-term treatment with pancreatic extract on recurrent abdominal pain in patients with chronic pancreatitis. Scand J Gastroenterol 1995; 30: 392–8.
16. Brown A, Hughes M, Tenner S, Banks PA. Does pancreatic enzyme supplementation reduce pain in patients with chronic pancreatitis: a meta-analysis. Am J Gastroenterol 1997; 92: 2032–5.
17. Lembke B, Creutzfeldt W, Schleser S, Ebert R, Shaw C, Koop I. Effect of somatostatin analogue sandostatin (SMS 201-995) on gastrointestinal, pancreatic, and biliary function and hormone release in normal men. Digestion 1987; 36: 108–24.
18. Malfertheiner P, Mayer D, Büchler MW, Domínguez-Muñoz JE, Schiefer B, Ditschuneit H. Treatment of pain in chronic pancreatitis by inhibition of pancreatic secretion with octreotide. Gut 1995; 36: 450–4.
19. Malfertheiner P, Mayer P, Schiefer B, Büchler MW, Ditschuneit H. Does inhibition of pancreatic secretion alleviate chronic pain in chronic pancreatitis? Gastroenterology 1992; 102: A277.
20. Toskes PP, Forsmark CE, DeMeo MT. A multicentre controlled trial of octreotide for the pain of chronic pancreatitis. Pancreas 1993; 8: 774.
21. Toskes PP, Forsmark CE, DeMeo MT. An open-label trial of octreotide for the pain of chronic pancreatitis. Gastroenterology 1994; 106: A326.
22. Ammann RW, Akovbiantz A, Largiader F, Schueler G. Course and outcome of chronic pancreatitis. Longitudinal study of a mixed medical-surgical series of 245 patients. Gastroenterology 1984; 86: 820–8.
23. Smith MT, Sherman S, Lehman GA. Endoscopic management of benign strictures of the biliary tree. Endoscopy 1995; 27: 253–66.
24. Deviere J, Devaere S, Baize M, Cremer M. Endoscopic biliary drainage in chronic pancreatitis. Gastrointest Endosc 1990; 36: 96–100.
25. Barthet M, Bernard JP, Duval JL, Affriat C, Sahel J. Biliary stenting in benign biliary stenosis complicating chronic calcifying pancreatitis. Endoscopy 1994; 26: 569–72.
26. Smits ME, Rauws EA, van Gulik TM, Gouma DJ, Tytgat GN, Huibregtse K. Long-term results of endoscopic stenting and surgical drainage for biliary stricture due to chronic pancreatitis. Br J Surg 1996; 83: 764–8.
27. Riemann JF, Maier M, Kohler B. Interventionelle endoskopische Therapie der chronischen Pankreatitis. In: Hahn EG, Riemann JF, eds. Klinische Gastroenterologie. Stuttgart, New York: Thieme Verlag, 1996: 1170–5.
28. Kohler B, Riemann JF. Therapie des Verschlußikterus bei chronischer Pankreatitis. Endoskopie heute 1992; 5: 15–8.

29. Huibregtse K, Smits ME. Endoscopic management of diseases of the pancreas. Am J Gastroenterol 1994; 89: S66–S77.
30. Ponchon T, Bory RM, Hedelius F et al. Endoscopic stenting for pain relief in chronic pancreatitis: results of a standardized protocol. Gastrointest Endosc 1995; 42: 452–6.
31. Smits ME, Rauws EA, Tytgat GN, Huibregtse K. Endoscopic treatment of pancreatic stones in patients with chronic pancreatitis. Gastrointest Endosc 1996; 43: 556–60.
32. Binmoeller KF, Jue P, Seifert H, Nam WC, Izbicki J, Soehendra N. Endoscopic pancreatic stent drainage in chronic pancreatitis and a dominant stricture: long-term results. Endoscopy 1995; 27: 638–44.
33. Cremer M, Deviere J, Delhaye M, Baize M, Vandermeeren A. Stenting in severe chronic pancreatitis: results of medium-term follow-up in seventy-six patients. Endoscopy 1991; 23: 171–6.
34. Kozarek RA. Pancreatic stents can induce ductal changes consistent with chronic pancreatitis. Gastrointest Endosc 1990; 36: 93–5.
35. Derfus GA, Geenen JE, Hogan WJ. Effect of endoscopic pancreatic duct stent placement on pancreatic ductal morphology. Gastrointest Endosc 1990; 36: A206.
36. Rossos PG, Kortan P, Haber GB. Complications associated with pancreatic duct stenting. Gastrointest Endosc 1992; 38: A252.
37. Burdick JS, Geenen JE, Venu RP. Ductal morphological changes due to pancreatic stent therapy – a randomized controlled study. Am J Gastroenterol 1992; 87: A155.
38. Lehman GA, Sherman S, Nisi R, Hawes RH. Pancreas divisum: results of minor papilla sphincterotomy. Gastrointest Endosc 1993; 39: 1–8.
39. Smith MT, Sherman S, Ikenberry SO, Hawes RH, Lehman GA. Alterations in pancreatic ductal morphology following polyethylene pancreatic stent therapy. Gastrointest Endosc 1996; 44: 268–75.
40. Eisen G, Coleman S, Troughton A, Cotton PB. Morphological changes in the pancreatic duct after stent placement for benign pancreatic disease. Gastrointest Endosc 1994; 40: A107.
41. Sherman S, Hawes RH, Savides TJ et al. Stent-induced pancreatic ductal and parenchymal changes: correlation of endoscopic ultrasound with ERCP. Gastrointest Endosc 1996; 44: 276–82.
42. Alvarez C, Robert M, Sherman S, Reber HA. Histologic changes after stenting of the pancreatic duct. Arch Surg 1994; 129: 765–8.
43. Delhaye M, Vandermeeren A, Baize M, Cremer M. Extracorporeal shock-wave lithotripsy of pancreatic calculi. Gastroenterology 1992; 102: 610–20.
44. Sauerbruch T, Holl J, Sackmann M, Paumgartner G. Extracorporeal lithotripsy of pancreatic stones in patients with chronic pancreatitis and pain: a prospective follow-up study. Gut 1992; 33: 969–72.
45. Schneider HT, May A, Benninger J et al. Piezoelectric shock wave lithotripsy of pancreatic duct stones. Am J Gastroenterol 1994; 89: 2042–8.
46. van der Hul R, Plaisier P, Jeekel J, Terpstra O, den Toom R, Bruining H. Extracorporeal shock-wave lithotripsy of pancreatic duct stones: immediate and long-term results. Endoscopy 1994; 26: 573–8.
47. Johanns W, Jakobeit C, Greiner L, Janssen J. Ultrasound-guided extracorporeal shock wave lithotripsy of pancreatic ductal stones: six years' experience. Can J Gastroenterol 1996; 10: 471–5.
48. Ohara H, Hoshino M, Hayakawa T et al. Single application extracorporeal shock wave lithotripsy is the first choice for patients with pancreatic duct stones. Am J Gastroenterol 1996; 91: 1388–94.
49. Costamagna G, Gabbrielli A, Mutignani M et al. Extracorporeal shock wave lithotripsy of pancreatic stones in chronic pancreatitis: immediate and medium-term results. Gastrointest Endosc 1997; 46: 231–6.
50. Adamek HE, Jakobs R, Buttmann A, Adamek MU, Schneider AR, Riemann JF. Long-term follow-up of patients with chronic pancreatitis and pancreatic stones treated with extracorporeal shock wave lithotripsy. Gut 1999; 45: 402–5.

51. Schwerk WB, Gorg K, Gorg CH, Richter G, Rothmund M. [Percutaneous puncture and drainage of pancreatic pseudocysts]. Z Gastroenterol 1989; 27: 432–7.
52. Grosso M, Gandini G, Cassinis MC, Regge D, Righi D, Rossi P. Percutaneous treatment (including pseudocystogastrostomy) of 74 pancreatic pseudocysts. Radiology 1989; 173: 493–7.
53. Hancke S, Henriksen FW. Percutaneous pancreatic cystogastrostomy guided by ultrasound scanning and gastroscopy. Br J Surg 1985; 72: 916–7.
54. Pavlovsky M, Perejaslov A, Chooklin S, Dovgan Y. Current management of pancreatic pseudocysts. Hepatogastroenterology 1998; 45: 846–8.
55. D'Agostino HB, van Sonnenberg E, Sanchez RB, Goodacre BW, Villaveiran RG, Lyche K. Treatment of pancreatic pseudocysts with percutaneous drainage and octreotide. Work in progress. Radiology 1993; 187: 685–8.
56. Barkin JS, Reiner DK, Deutch E. Sandostatin for control of catheter drainage of pancreatic pseudocyst. Pancreas 1991; 6: 245–8.
57. Heyder N, Gunter E, Hahn EG. [Endoscopic-sonographic control of cystogastric catheter drainage of pancreatogenic fluid collections]. Z Gastroenterol 1992; 30: 553–7.
58. Sever M, Vidmar D, Surlan M, Pleskovic A, Visnar-Perovic A. Percutaneous drainage of pancreatic pseudocyst into the stomach. Surg Endosc 1998; 12: 1249–53.
59. Cremer M, Deviere J, Engelholm L. Endoscopic management of cysts and pseudocysts in chronic pancreatitis: long-term follow-up after 7 years of experience. Gastrointest Endosc 1989; 35: 1–9.
60. Sahel J. Endoscopic drainage of pancreatic cysts. Endoscopy 1991; 23: 181–4.
61. Binmoeller KF, Seifert H, Walter A, Soehendra N. Transpapillary and transmural drainage of pancreatic pseudocysts. Gastrointest Endosc 1995; 42: 219–24.
62. Dohmoto M, Rupp KD, Hunerbein M, Schlag PM. [Endoscopic drainage of pancreatic pseudocysts]. Dtsch Med Wochenschr 1995; 120: 1647–51.
63. Dohmoto M, Rupp KD. Endoscopic drainage of pancreatic pseudocysts. Surg Endosc 1992; 6: 118–24.
64. Pfaffenbach B, Langer M, Stabenow-Lohbauer U, Lux G. [Endosonography-controlled transgastric drainage of pancreatic pseudocysts]. Dtsch Med Wochenschr 1998; 123: 1439–42.
65. Beckingham IJ, Krige JE, Bornman PC, Terblanche J. Long-term outcome of endoscopic drainage of pancreatic pseudocysts. Am J Gastroenterol 1999; 94: 71–4.
66. Smits ME, Rauws EA, Tytgat GN, Huibregtse K. The efficacy of endoscopic treatment of pancreatic pseudocysts. Gastrointest Endosc 1995; 42: 202–7.
67. Barthet M, Sahel J, Bodiou-Bertei C, Bernard JP. Endoscopic transpapillary drainage of pancreatic pseudocysts. Gastrointest Endosc 1995; 42: 208–13.
68. Catalano MF, Geenen JE, Schmalz MJ, Johnson GK, Dean RS, Hogan WJ. Treatment of pancreatic pseudocysts with ductal communication by transpapillary pancreatic duct endoprosthesis. Gastrointest Endosc 1995; 42: 214–8.
69. Schmalz MJ, Soergel KH, Johanson J. The effect of octreotide acetate (Sandostatin) on the pain of chronic pancreatitis. Gastroenterology 1992; 102: A290.
70. Smits ME, Badiga SM, Rauws EA, Tytgat GN, Huibregtse K. Long-term results of pancreatic stents in chronic pancreatitis. Gastrointest Endosc 1995; 42: 461–7.

10.5 Nutrition in chronic pancreatitis

R. Meier

Abstract

In the late course of chronic pancreatitis weight loss is often seen due to reduced calorie intake (pain, persistent alcohol intake) and a reduction of pancreatic enzyme secretion resulting in maldigestion with steatorrhea and azotorrhea.

Nutritional interventions depend on the degree of maldigestion and nutritional status.

Most of the patients can be managed by dietary recommendation and pancreatic enzyme supplements. Ten to 15% need additional polymeric or semielemental oral supplements. Enteral nutrition is necessary in less than 5% when severe maldigestion and malnutrition cannot be managed orally. It can also be of benefit before and after surgery. Parenteral nutrition is indicated on rare occasions in patients with small bowel obstruction or when a complicated fistula is present.

Introduction

Alcohol is the etiologic factor in 60–70% of patients with chronic pancreatitis. Other causes of chronic pancreatitis are much less common (pancreatic duct obstruction, pancreas divisum, hereditary or tropical pancreatitis). Between 15 and 35% of patients have no apparent underlying disease (idiopathic chronic pancreatitis) (Table 10.5-1) [1].

The morphologic changes include edema, acute inflammation and necrosis, superimposed on a background of chronic changes that include fibrosis, calcification, inflammation, and a loss of exocrine tissue. Ductal elements may be dilated, and intraductal protein plugs, which may be calcified, can be seen [2, 3]. During the course of chronic pancreatitis enzyme secretion is gradually decreased, resulting in maldigestion with steatorrhea and azotorrhea when more than 90% of pancreatic tissue is destroyed.

Table 10.5-1. Etiology of chronic pancreatitis.

Alcoholic	(60–70%)
Obstructive	
Hereditary	
Tropical	
Idiopathic	(15–35%)

Physiology and pathophysiology of pancreatic secretion

Digestion of nutrients and absorption of individual food components are complex and co-ordinated processes in humans which require multiple and interactive gastrointestinal functions including secretory, absorptive, motor and circulatory mechanisms. The normal human pancreas secretes, besides other non-enzyme proteins, more than 10 different enzymes together with water and bicarbonate. These enzymes are secreted in excess; they hydrolyze macronutrients (especially lipids, proteins and carbohydrates) within the intestinal lumen. Postprandially, regulation of human pancreatic secretion should be seen as a part of an overall integrated motor-secretory response [4]. Moreover, while a meal is the most important physiologic stimulus, pancreatic secretion also occurs in the fasting (interdigestive) state in a precisely regulated and coordinated fashion.

The pancreatic response is influenced by the physical properties and composition of the meal. A mixed solid-liquid meal induces a longer response than homogenized or liquid meals with a comparable energy content [5]. In both instances, the rate of gastric emptying and thus duodenal delivery of stimulatory nutrients are the key factors determining the duration of pancreatic secretion. The proportions of fat, carbohydrate and protein content within a meal also influence the duration and enzyme composition of the pancreatic response in humans [6]. The most important mechanism inducing postprandial human pancreatic secretion is the presence of nutrients within the duodenal lumen (intestinal phase of stimulation). Mediation of postprandial stimulation of human pancreatic secretion by duodenal nutrients involves the activation of neural pathways, in particular vagal-cholinergic reflexes, and the release of regulatory peptides, in particular cholecystokinin (CCK) with a tight interaction of the neural and humoral systems. Under normal conditions the site of maximal nutrient digestion and absorption is the proximal small intestine, but enzymatic degradation of chyme continues during small intestinal transit, a process, which is partly determined by the intraluminal presence of pancreatic enzymes. Not only lumenal pancreatic but also mucosal brush-border enzymes are involved in the postduodenal digestion of protein and carbohydrates. Moreover, human pancreatic lipase is less stable than other pancreatic enzymes against acid denaturation in the duodenum and during subsequent small intestinal transit, because it is rapidly destroyed by pancreatic proteases, in particular by the chymotrypsin present in chyme [7, 8]. The loss of the endocrine function of the pancreas, particularly insulin and glucagon secretion, has important implications for nutritional management as well.

Malnutrition and chronic pancreatitis

In the late course of chronic pancreatitis malnutrition is common. Malnutrition is one of the major predictors of outcome. The severity of malnutrition is directly correlated with complications. The two principle factors in malnutrition are depletion of nutrients and increased metabolic activity. Persistent alcohol intake, pain after a meal and maldigestion are the main contributors to malnutrition. Resting energy expenditure (REE) is increased in up to 65% in patients, especially when there are already signs of malnutrition [9]. Maldigestion is a late complication of chronic pancreatitis and depends on the underlying disease. The medium latency between onset of first symptoms and signs of maldigestion is about 8 to 9 years in alcoholic chronic pancreatitis and more than 15 years in idiopathic non-alcoholic chronic pancreatitis [10]. Weight loss is strongly associated with maldigestion of fat. Clinical steatorrhea resulting from exocrine insufficiency occurs only when over 90% of the pancreatic secretory function is lost [11]. Steatorrhea is more severe and develops earlier than overt maldigestion of protein and carbohydrates [4, 12]. Several mechanisms are involved. Lumenal lipid digestion within the small intestine depends on the combined action of pancreatic lipase and its cofactors, such as colipase and bile acids. There are no triglyceride-digesting enzyme systems within the intestinal brush-border. Furthermore, a low gastric lipase secretion has been found in patients with alcoholic chronic pancreatitis [13]. The loss of pancreatic lipase cannot be completely compensated by other mechanisms. This is in contrast to protein and carbohydrate digestion. Protein digestion is initiated by intragastric proteolytic activity, continued by intestinal brush-border peptidases, and is maintained even in the absence of lumenal pancreatic proteolytic activity [14]. Similarly, carbohydrate digestion is maintained by the salivary amylase and by brush-border oligosaccharidases [15]. Lipid digestion can be further decreased when bile acids are not secreted in a sufficient amount. Since the pancreatic bicarbonate secretion is also diminished in exocrine pancreatic insufficiency, postprandial intraduodenal pH may fall below 4. Lipase is more sensitive against acid destruction than other enzymes; as a consequence, the small residual quantities of lipase secreted to the duodenum may be further inactivated by low intralumenal pH [4]. Lumenal lipase degradation occurs more rapidly than that of other enzymes due to its greater instability against proteolysis. As a result, lipase is available for a shorter time period for digestive action during small intestinal transit, not only in healthy individuals but, more relevantly, in patients with exocrine pancreatic insufficiency [16].

Chronic maldigestion is therefore the major cause of progressive nutritional and metabolic impairment in patients with chronic pancreatitis, resulting in progressive weight loss. In addition, maldigestion may be associated with malabsorption of lipid-soluble vitamins A, D, E and K [17].

Nutritional assessment and nutritional intervention

Nutritional interventions depend on the degree of maldigestion (steatorrhea) and the nutritional status. It is therefore important to assess the nutritional status in these patients.

Nutritional assessment

Nutritional assessment is easy to perform. Weight loss over time, body mass index, anthropometry and laboratory values are useful parameters (Table 10.5-2) [18]. Furthermore, several nutritional screening scores [subjective global assessment (SGA), nutritional risk index (NRI), minimal nutritional assessment (MNA)] are available to select patients with nutritional deficiencies who are at increased risk of developing complications [19–23].

Table 10.5-2. Nutritional assessment.

• Weight loss > 10% in 6 months	
• Weight loss > 5% in 1 month	
• Body mass index < 20	
• Anthropometry	
• Biochemical parameters	
– Serum albumin	< 30 g/l
– Serum transferrin	< 1.5 g/l
– Serum praealbumin	< 10 mg/l
– Total lymphocyte count	< 1,500 cells/mm^3

General nutritional intervention

According to the literature about 80% of the patients can be managed by dietary recommendation and pancreatic enzyme supplements, 10–15% need oral supplements (polymeric or semielemental), 5% need enteral tube feeding and around 1% need total parenteral nutrition (TPN).

The main principles of nutritional therapy in chronic pancreatitis are to reduce steatorrhea and to supply adequate amounts of calories. Treatment of exocrine insufficiency starts with dietary recommendation and pancreatic enzyme supplementation [24].

Dietary recommendations begin with total abstinence from alcohol. Furthermore an adequate amount of calories should be given. Frequent meals are the cornerstone to increase the caloric need. Table 10.5-3 and Table 10.5-4 show the recommendation for patients without and with signs of malnutrition. The diet should be rich in carbohydrates and proteins. The intake of carbohydrates should be limited when an overt diabetes mellitus is present. A protein diet of 1.0–1.5g per kg body weight per day is mostly sufficient and well tolerated. To reach the necessary caloric goal, fat must also be given. In general, 30–40% of the calories given as fat are well tolerated, especially when they are rich in vegetable fats. When no weight gain can be achieved and steatorrhea persists, medium chain triglycerides (MCT) may be used to increase fat absorption because minimal digestion is required [25]. MCT are absorbed directly across the small bowel into the portal vein, even in the absence of lipase, colipase and bile salts. Unfortunately MCTs have a lower energy density than LCTs (8.3 kcl/g), they are unpalatable and cause adverse effects such as cramps, nausea and diarrhea. A slow increase in MCTs is recommended according to the tolerance of the patient. The diet should be low in fiber, because fiber may absorb enzymes and delay the absorption of nutrients. Fat soluble vitamins (A, D, E, K), vitamin B_{12} and other micronutrients should be supplemented if serum levels indicate a deficiency [26].

Table 10.5-3. Nutritional intervention in patients with chronic pancreatitis with steatorrhea and no malnutrition.

• Frequent meals (4–5 times a day) with adequate enzyme supplementation	
– 30–35 kcal/kg BW/day	
– proteins:	100–150 g/day
– fat:	50–80 g/day
– ch:	rest
– low fiber	

Table 10.5-4. Nutritional intervention in patients with chronic pancreatitis with steatorrhea and malnutrition.

• Frequent meals (6–7 times a day) with adequate enzyme supplementation	
– 40–45 kcal/kg BW/day	
– proteins	80–120 g/day
– fat:	50–60 g/day
– ch:	rest
– low fiber	
– fat soluble vitamins	
• When no weight gain and steatorrhea persist	
– MCT:	80–120 g/day
– essential fatty acids:	1–3% linol acid

It is well known that patients with chronic pancreatitis have an increased production of free radicals (oxidative stress); furthermore, antioxidants (vitamins D, C und E, selenium and methionine) have been prescribed to relieve pain in patients with chronic pancreatitis [25]. The prescription of antioxidants is safe and inexpensive, but the effects have to be confirmed in large, well-controlled studies.

An adequate quantity of exogenous pancreatic enzymes can correct protein maldigestion and improve steatorrhea [7]. Enzyme preparations vary in the amount of porcine lipase they contain. The specific dose for a particular patient is difficult to define and depends on the degree of exocrine insufficiency. Each patient needs to be supplemented in a individual way. Weight control, symptomatic relief of diarrhea, and a decrease in 72-hour fecal fat excretion are practical end points of the therapy. It is important to give enzymes together with the meal to ensure adequate mixing. If steatorrhea cannot be controlled the addition of H2-histamine receptor antagonists or proton-pump inhibitors can be tried. Blocking acid secretion reduces duodenal acid load, thus preventing inactivation of lipase by low gastric and duodenal pH [27]. If this regimen is not effective, enteric-coated preparations can be helpful. These preparations are only effective if pancreatic enzymes are delivered to the upper small intestine with ingested food. Enteric-coated preparations are not significantly better than non-enteric preparations for reducing steatorrhea. Microincapsulated preparations containing large amounts of lipase have been withdrawn from the market because of reports of colonic strictures in children with cystic fibrosis [28]. Patients with gastrectomy require a powdered form of enzyme supplementation to promote a rapid dissolution of the extract.

Indications for enteral nutrition

There are 4 main indications for enteral nutrition in chronic pancreatitis:

1. When a patient is not able to eat (pain or pyloro-duodenostenosis due to an enlarged pancreatic head or pseudocyst formation).
2. Progressive weight loss despite an adequate dietary regimen.
3. Acute complications (acute flare of chronic pancreatitis or fistulas).
4. Before and after surgery.

Enteral nutrition should be instituted with a tube introduced into the jejunum.

For progressive weight loss despite an adequate dietary regimen, a nasojejunal tube or a percutaneous endoscopic gastrostomy with a jejunal loop (PEG-J) is recommended. Semielemental diets are well tolerated, especially when they are continuously given overnight. Unfortunately there are no controlled data available and present outcome data are solely based on case reports.

The use of early enteral feeding in patients with a severe, acute flare of chronic pancreatitis can reduce the incidence of nosocomial infections, the duration of systemic inflammatory response and severity [29, 30]. A semielemental diet or an immuno-enhancing diet is safe. Little data are available documenting the benefit of nasojejunal tube feeding with a semielemental diet in patients with pancreatic fistulas [31].

Enteral nutrition can also be very important in patients before pancreatic surgery, especially when signs of malnutrition are present. The severity of malnutrition predicts the outcome in these patients. To support such a regimen, there are only data from patients with general abdominal surgery showing that preoperative enteral nutrition with a semielemental or an immuno-enhancing diet improves outcome by reducing postoperative, infectious complications, translating into a reduction in the length of hospital stay [32–35]. Furthermore, it is well established that patients benefit from early enteral nutrition by fine-needle catheter jejunostomy (FNJ) or nasojejunal (NJ) tube after major abdominal surgery. Several studies with semielemental diets or an immuno-enhancing diet have demonstrated that early postoperative enteral nutrition may improve outcome [36–39].

Indications for parenteral nutrition

Total parenteral nutrition is very seldom necessary in patients with chronic pancreatitis. TPN must be instituted when gastric emptying is blocked, when the patients need gastric decompression, when a tube cannot be introduced into the jejunum or when a complicated fistula is present. There are no reported series of patients with chronic pancreatic insufficiency who have been treated with intravenous nutrition.

In summary, dietary modification, pancreatic enzyme supplements and sometimes fat soluble vitamins are the cornerstones of nutritional management in patients with chronic pancreatitis. Enteral nutrition is not often necessary. Enteral nutrition can be useful in patients with severe maldigestion and malnutrition, when dietary regimens fail or before and after pancreatic surgery. Adequate tubes and diets are available. Jejunal application of semielemental diets or immuno-enhancing diets are well tolerated. These recommendations are still empirical, because prospective trials with patients with chronic pancreatitis using enteral feeding protocols are lacking.

References

1. Steer ML, Waxman I, Freedman S. Chronic pancreatitis. NEJM 1995; 332: 1482–90.
2. Singer MV, Gyr KE, Sarles H. Revised classification of pancreatitis: report of the Second International Symposium on the Classification of Pancreatitis in Marseille, France, March 28–30, 1984. Gastroenterology 1985; 89: 683–5.
3. Samer M, Cotton PB. Classification of pancreatitis. Gut 1984; 25: 756–9.
4. DiMagno EP, Layer P. Human exocrine pancreatic enzyme secretion. In: Go VLW et al., ed. The Pancreas. 2nd ed. Biology, Pathobiology, and Diseases. New York: Raven Press, 1993: 275–300.
5. Malagelada JR, Go VLW, Summerskill WHJ. Different gastric pancreatic and biliary responses to solid-liquid or homogenized meals. Dig Dis Sci 1979; 24: 101–10.
6. Boivin M, Lanspa SJ, Zinsmeister AR, Go VLW, DiMagno EP. Are diets associated with different rates of human interdigestive and postprandial pancreatic enzyme secretion. Gastroenterology 1990; 99: 1763–71.
7. DiMagno EP, Malagelada JR, Go VLW, Moertel CG. Fate of orally ingested enzymes in pancreatic insufficiency: comparison of two dosage schedules. NEJM 1977; 296: 1318–22.
8. Layer P, Go VLW, DiMagno EP. Fate of pancreatic enzymes during aboral small intestinal transit in humans. Am J Physiol 1986; 251: G475–80.
9. Hebuterne X, Hastier P, Peroux JL et al. Resting energy expenditure in patients with alcoholic chronic pancreatitis. Dig Dis Sci 1996; 41: 533–9.
10. Layer P, Yamamoto H, Kalthoff L, Clain JE, Bakken LJ, DiMagno EP. The different courses of early- and late-onset idiopathic and alcoholic chronic pancreatitis. Gastroenterology 1994; 107: 1481–7.
11. Latifi R, McIntosh JK, Dudrick SJ. Nutritional management of acute and chronic pancreatitis. Surg Clin North Am 1991; 71: 579–95.
12. Lanspa SJ, Chan ATH, Bell JS III, Go VLW, Dickson ER, DiMagno EP. Pathogenesis of steatorrhea in primary biliary cirrhosis. Hepatology 1985; 5: 837–42.
13. Wojdemann M, Sternby B, Larsen S, Olsen O. Cephalic phase of lipolysis is impaired in pancreatic insufficiency: role of gastric lipase. Scand J Gastroenterol 2000; 35: 204–11.

14. DiMagno EP, Malagelada JR, Go VLW. Relationship between alcoholism and pancreatic insufficiency. NY Acad Sci 1975; 252: 200–7.
15. Layer P, Zinsmeister AR, DiMagno EP. Effects of decreasing intraluminal amylase activity on starch digestion and postprandial gastrointestinal function in humans. Gastroenterology 1986; 91: 41–8.
16. Layer P, von der Ohe MR, Holst JJ, Jansen JBMJ, Grandt D, Holtmann G, Goebell H. Altered postprandial motility in chronic pancreatitis: role of malabsorption. Gastroenterology 1997; 112: 1624–34.
17. DiMagno EP, Clain JE, Layer P. Chronic pancreatitis. In: Go VLW et al., ed. The Pancreas. 2nd ed. Biology, Pathobiology, and Diseases. New York: Raven Press, 1993: 665–706.
18. Heymsfield SB. Nutritional assessment by anthropometric and biochemical methods. In: Shils ME, ed. Modern Nutrition in Health and Disease. Philadelphia: Lea & Febiger, 1994: 812–41.
19. Detsky AS, Smalley PS, Chang J. Is this patient malnourished? JAMA 1994; 271: 54–8.
20. Veterans Affairs Total Parenteral Nutrition Cooperative Study Group. Perioperative TPN in surgical patients. NEJM 1991; 325: 525–32.
21. Guigoz Y, Vellas BJ, Garry PJ. Assessing the nutritional status of the elderly: the Mini Nutritional Assessment as part of the geriatric evaluation. Nutr Rev 1996; 54: S59–65.
22. Vellas B, Guigoz Y. The Mini Nutritional Assessment. Facts, research and intervention in geriatrics. 4th ed. Paris: Springer & Serdi Publ Co., 1997.
23. Vellas B, Guigoz Y. Nutritional assessment as part of the geriatric evaluation. In: Rubenstein LZ, Bernabei R, Wieland D, eds. Geriatric assessment technology: state of the arts. Milan: Kutiz Publ Co., 1995: 179–86.
24. DiMagno EP. Medical treatment of pancreatic insufficiency. Mayo Clin Proc 1979; 54: 435–42.
25. Scolapio JS, Malhi-Chowla N, Ukleja A. Nutrition supplementation in patients with acute and chronic pancreatitis. Gastroenterol Clin North Am 1999; 28: 695–706.
26. Havala T, Shronts E, Cerra F. Nutritional support in acute pancreatitis. Gastroenterol Clin North Am 1989; 18: 525–42.
27. Heijerman HG, Lamers CB, Bakker W. Omeprazole enhances the efficacy of pancreatin (Pancrease) in cystic fibrosis. Ann Intern Med 1991; 114: 200–1.
28. Smyth RL, Van Velzen D, Smyth AR et al. Strictures of ascending colon in cystic fibrosis and high-strength pancreatic enzymes. Lancet 1994; 343: 85–6.
29. McClave SA, Greene LM, Snider HL, Makk LJK, Cheadle WG, Owens NA et al. Comparison of the safety of early enteral vs parenteral nutrition in mild acute pancreatitis. JPEN 1997; 21: 14–20.
30. Hamvas J, Pap A. The role of jejunal feeding in the treatment of acute necrotizing pancreatitis and in recurrence of chronic pancreatitis with severe necrosis. Orv Hetil 1998; 139: 945–9.
31. Botta D, Gauthier AP. Indications of enteral nutrition in pancreatic disorders. Ann Gastroenterol Hepatol 1988; 24: 335–8.
32. Wachtler P, Hilger RA, König W, Bauer KH, Kemen M, Köller M. Influence of a pre-operative enteral supplement on functional activities of peripheral leukocytes from patients with major surgery. Clin Nutr 1995; 14: 275–82.
33. Braga M, Gianotti L, Cestari A, Vignali A, Pellegatta F, Dolci A, Di Carlo V. Gut function and immune and inflammatory responses in patients perioperatively fed with supplemented enteral formulas. Arch Surg 1996; 131: 1257–65.
34. Gianotti L, Braga M, Fortis C, Soldini L, Viganali A, Colombo S, Radaelli G, Di Carlo V. A prospective, randomized clinical trial on perioperative feeding with arginine-, omega-3 fatty acid-, and RNA-enriched enteral diet: Effect on host response and nutritional status. JPEN 1999; 23: 314–20.
35. Braga M, Gianotti L, Radaelli G, Vignali A, Mari G, Gentilini O, Di Carlo V. Perioperative immunonutrition in patients undergoing cancer surgery: Results of a randomized double-blind phase 3 trial. Arch Surg 1999; 134: 428–33.
36. Braga M, Gianotti L, Vignali A, Cestari A, Bisagni P, Di Carlo V. Artificial nutrition after major abdominal surgery: Impact of route of administration and composition of the diet. Crit Care Med 1998; 26: 24–30.

37. Gianotti L, Braga M, Vignali A, Balzano G, Zerbi A, Bisagni P, Di Carlo V. Effect of route of delivery and formulation of postoperative nutritional support in patients undergoing major operations for malignant neoplasms. Arch Surg 1997; 132: 1222–30.
38. Bodoky G, Pap A, Harsanyi L, Flautner L, Tihanyi T. The effect of early postoperative jejunal feeding on the exocrine function of the pancreas. Orv Hetil 1990; 131: 1861–2, 1865–6.
39. Bodoky G, Harsanyi L, Pap A, Tihanyi T, Flautner L. Effect of enteral nutrition on exocrine pancreatic function. Am J Surg 1991; 161: 144–8.

11 100th anniversary of pancreatic enzyme treatment

11.1 100 years of pancreatic enzyme substitution

M. A. Rudmann

The Solvay group of pharmaceutical companies is proud to celebrate the unique event of "100 years of expertise in the manufacturing and development of *pancreatic enzymes*" with its brands Pankreon® and Creon®.

The year 2000 marks the beginning of a new century and of "real modernity", an exceptional year of celebration and a moment of reflection. Reflection about the achievements of the last century since 1900 and the challenges for the next hundred years.

This chapter contains a short summary of 2500 years of medical history and research into the exocrine pancreas with insights into first achievements and periods of scientific stagnation.

The history of pancreatin, with first therapeutic attempts more than one hundred years ago, until today and the history of Solvay's brands Pankreon® and Creon® are also covered, completed by a short outlook into future technologies and therapeutic options.

2500 years of medical history

One of the earliest recorded remarks about digestion was made by *Empedocles of Agrigent* in the 5th century BC. He thought that food was converted in the body by decay.

Hippocrates, born in 460 BC on the island of Cos, probably did not contribute much to knowledge about the pancreas. However, the name "*pan kreas*", meaning something like *all flesh,* results from the Hippocratic idea that all glands in the body are completely flesh.

Herophilos and *Erasistratos* (~300 BC), the first anatomists to systematically examine human corpses, described the pancreas and Herophilos even coined the term "duodenum". Another contemporary scientist, *Eudemus,* may have already made the assumption that *"a certain fluid flows from it [the pancreas] into the intestines that is similar to saliva and promotes digestion"*, an assumption that was lost and forgotten for the next 1800 years.

Galen, who lived from 129–199, was one of the most powerful "opinion leaders" of his time and the scientific founder of ancient medicine. His conclusion that the pancreas or the *"beautiful* flesh", as he called it, played a protective role for neighboring organs and vessels (this assumption was already promoted by Aristotle, 384–322 BC) "paralyzed" scientific progress in studying the function of this organ for several hundred years [1].

In addition, further progress was impossible due to the powerful position of the Middle Ages Church and Councils (Council of Tours in 1163: *the church spills no blood*) in the Middle Ages and therefore many scientific disciplines remained theoretical and speculative.

Theophrast von Hohenheim (1493/94–1541), better known as *Paracelsus,* was the first to turn away from Galen's teaching of the bodily humors as the cause of diseases and promote drugs, for example from medicinal herbs, and chemicals (iron, arsenic) with a specific effect for specific diseases. *Andreas Vesal* (1514–1564), the founder of scientific anatomy, discovered various errors made by Galen and published *"De humani corporis fabrica"* in 1543, one of the most significant contributions to medicine.

It took another one hundred years with descriptions of the pancreas as a kind of cushion (e.g. by Fallopia) or sponge before *Johann Georg Wirsüng* described the excretory duct of the pancreas *(ductus Wirsungianus)* in 1642. One year earlier in Padua, an outstanding center of education at that time, Moritz Hofmann had found a kind of duct in the middle of the pancreas in animals. However, an explanation for this discovery in animals and humans was not found.

Progress in physics and chemistry changed thinking and theories substantially in the 17th century. *François de le Boë Sylvius* came to the conclusion that the pancreas was a secretory gland, and he was the first to make a distinct connection between pancreatic juice and digestion.

With these achievements, the pancreas had to be regarded as an important organ and interest in it increased enormously. However, pancreas research faced another setback with Brunner's conclusion after complete removal of the organ: The pancreas is not essential because its removal had no substantial consequences. But his experiments were incomplete and like others after him he did not take into account the reserve capacity of the gland.

François Magendie (1783–1855), the founder of experimental pharmacology and one of the fathers of experimental physiology, clearly recognized that in the medicine of the time hardly anything was based on definite knowledge. He was the first to describe *pancreatic juice* as alkaline and with a high protein content.

Progress initiated by awards for the best scientific contribution, for example from the Académie française in 1823 concerning digestion, was again blocked by increasing national feeling in Europe, creating contradictory results and positions instead of cooperation.

A few isolated observations were made by scientists like Eberle, on artificial pancreatic juice, Berzelius, on catalysis, Mialhe, on ptyalin and Kuntzmann, who first described a connection between fatty stools and pancreatic disease in 1820.

Claude Bernard (1813–1878) deserves credit for having drawn the right conclusions from what had been demonstrated and from his own experiments and clearly rejected unproven theories and doctrines: the gland has universal function in digestion due to the fact that pancreatic juice acts on "all three categories of food".

Bernard and Corvisart succeeded in isolating a "protein-like body" from pancreatic juice by precipitation with alcohol and called it pancreatin. They were always convinced of the necessity to isolate the active agent from the pancreas in order to demonstrate its effect.

First therapeutic attempts with pancreatin Formation of the pharmaceutical industry

In 1859 the Dutch practitioner *Joseph Alexander Fles* had to treat a diabetic patient with steatorrhea. Fles was fully aware of Bernard's results and consequently organized glands from calves, minced them and pounded the pulp with water which had to be taken by the patient with every meal. The treatment had no impact on diabetes but steatorrhea was completely controlled and Fles published the first therapeutic use of *"pancreatin"* as a case report in 1864. In the Ukraine another practitioner, *Alexander Jakulovic Danilevsky* prepared an artificial pancreatic juice in 1861/62 and observed that free hydrochloric acid inhibited the effect of protein "digestion".

Meanwhile physiologists had identified and introduced into terminology *"zymogen"* (Heidenhain), *"enzymes"* and *"trypsin"* (Kühn).

Parallel to the various new findings of the basic disciplines and the first therapeutic attempts of a few practitioners, several apothecaries had started to produce medicines to serve the increasing demands. In consequence, apothecaries, who traditionally had prepared medicine, became manufacturers.

In 1843 *William Brockedon* in England received the first patent for a process to produce tablets, an important step towards more convenient presentation forms.

This dynamic process towards "professional" manufacturing of medicines and pancreatic extracts continued, although diagnostic procedures were still lacking or underdeveloped.

The formation of the *"pharmaceutical industry"* began around the middle of the 19th century with the aim and the need to offer medicines for a cheaper price and with consistent quality in reasonable quantity.

Langdon-Down reported the successful treatment of a patient with a commercially available pancreatin preparation for the first time in 1869. At that time Savory & Moore in London was one of the companies producing such products, but they were very expensive and unsuitable.

This unsatisfactory situation induced an engaged practitioner, *Hermann Engesser*, to develop a kind of "acid-stable" pancreatin preparation which could be produced "on a large scale, *stored easily … and could be offered in a more appetising form*". The result was a powder and later on tablets which were manufactured by Keller Bros until 1930.

In fact, all of the available pancreatin preparations were judged completely ineffective by relevant opinion leaders because the preparations contained only zymogen or were not acid protected, although practical experience showed the opposite, at least in isolated cases.

Meanwhile surgery had made substantial progress due to Lord Joseph Lister's antiseptic principle with carbolic acid and surgeons were becoming more and more interested in the pancreas.

In 1881 Bilroth carried out the first stomach resection, in 1883 *Carl Gussenbauer* performed the first surgical operation on the pancreas, and in 1889 *Joseph Freiherr von Mering and Oscar Minkovski* were the first to perform a complete removal of the pancreas in animals. The connection between pancreatic disease and diabetes already postulated earlier was now confirmed because all animals without exception developed the typical symptoms of diabetes mellitus.

With the refined surgical techniques at hand, Minkovski asked one of his students to investigate the influence of the removal on the utilization of food. *Abelmann* in 1890 clearly demonstrated that dogs without a pancreas could not absorb fat but fat absorption increased by feeding with pig pancreas or the administration of commercial pancreatin.

One problem remained: the problem of passing pancreatic enzymes through the stomach in such a way that they did not lose their effectiveness.

The history of Pankreon®

Two chemists, *Franz Thomas* and *Wilhelm Weber*, developed a process for the production of an acid-stable pancreatin and filed a patent which became effective on April 22, 1900. (Fig. 11.1-1: Rhenania patent specification) Both of them were working for the Chemi-

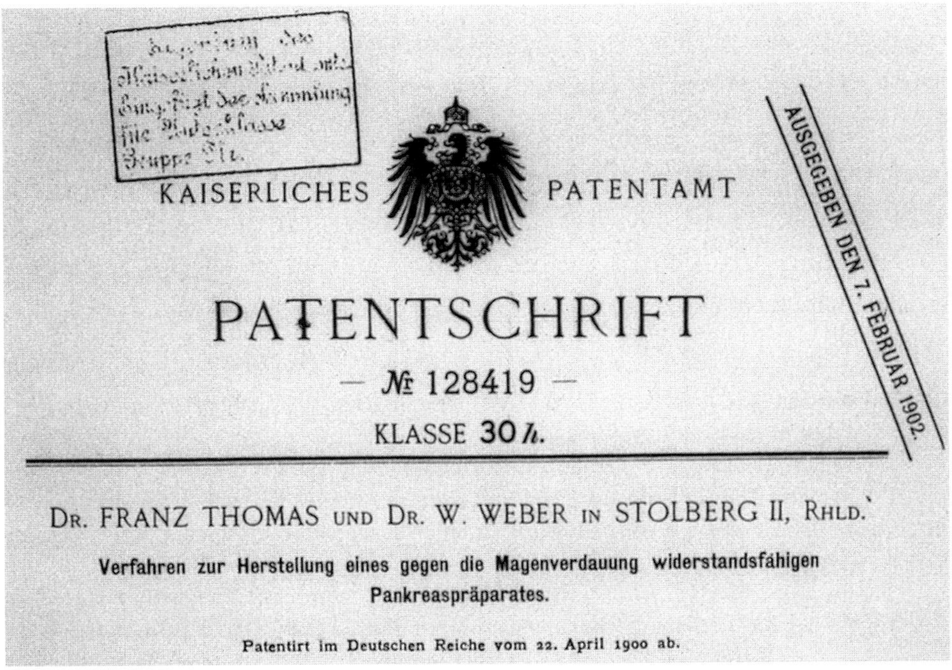

KAISERLICHES PATENTAMT

AUSGEGEBEN DEN 7. FEBRUAR 1902.

PATENTSCHRIFT

— № 128419 —

KLASSE 30 *h*.

DR. FRANZ THOMAS UND DR. W. WEBER IN STOLBERG II, RHLD.

Verfahren zur Herstellung eines gegen die Magenverdauung widerstandsfähigen Pankreaspräparates.

Patentirt im Deutschen Reiche vom 22. April 1900 ab.

Figure 11.1-1. Rhenania patent specification (April 1900).

sche Fabrik Rhenania AG in Aachen, a small company that had had some experience in the manufacture of pancreatin from pig pancreas since 1897. As described in Patent No. 128419, pancreatin was combined with tannin and due to the already existing know-how, the first acid-protected pancreatic enzyme preparation was obtained: "*Pankreon*".

The most important product of Rhenania, founded in 1855, in the early years was soda, manufactured by the Leblanc process. The company developed very successfully until 1861, when the Belgian *Ernest Solvay* [2] filed a patent for his process for the manufacture of ammonia soda, a process that proved to be considerably more economical. In the 1880s Solvay took over other factories in Germany, while many others were converted from Leblanc's method to the new Solvay process.

This development was certainly one of the reasons for the general manager of Rhenania, the pharmacist *Robert Hasenclever*, to build a more diversified company with engagement in the prosperous pharmaceutical business.

Mathias Gockel, a practicing gastroenterologist, presented his therapeutic results with Pankreon® at the 72nd assembly of the *Society of German Natural Science Researchers and Doctors* in September 1900. Fifty-nine per cent of his patients suffering predominantly from gastric disease (25 out of 34 cases) showed positive treatment results in terms of substantial weight gain, an objective parameter [3].

The publication of his results in the "*Centralblatt für Stoffwechsel & Verdauungskrankheiten*" (Central Journal of Metabolic & Digestive Diseases) in the 1st October issue in 1900 (Fig. 11.1-2: Gockel's article in the "Central Journal") created a lot of positive feedback from several colleagues, also in pancreatogenic steatorrhea. Rhenania had made Pankreon® available to physicians even before its market launch.

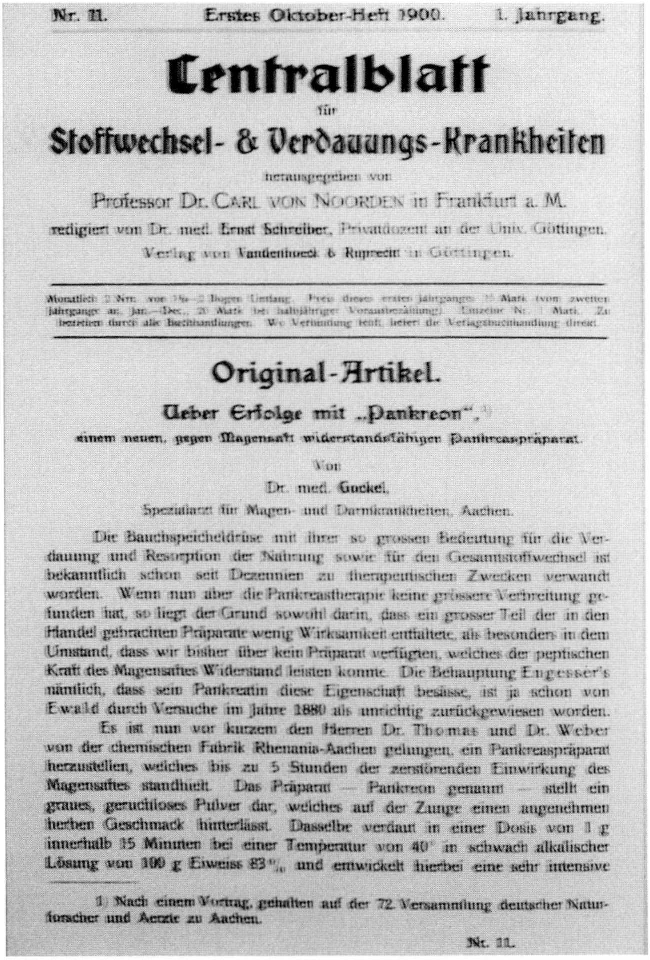

Nr. 11. Erstes Oktober-Heft 1900. 1. Jahrgang.

Centralblatt

für

Stoffwechsel- & Verdauungs-Krankheiten

herausgegeben von

Professor Dr. CARL VON NOORDEN in Frankfurt a. M.

redigiert von Dr. med. Ernst Schreiber, Privatdozent an der Univ. Göttingen.

Verlag von Vandenhoeck & Ruprecht in Göttingen.

Monatlich 2 Nrn. von 1½–2 Bogen Umfang. Preis dieses ersten Jahrganges 15 Mark (vom zweiten Jahrgange an, Jan.—Dec., 20 Mark bei halbjähriger Vorausbezahlung). Einzelne Nr. 1 Mark. Zu beziehen durch alle Buchhandlungen. Wo Verbindung fehlt, liefert die Verlagsbuchhandlung direkt.

Original-Artikel.

Ueber Erfolge mit „Pankreon", [1]

einem neuen, gegen Magensaft widerstandsfähigen Pankreaspräparat.

Von

Dr. med. Gockel,

Spezialarzt für Magen- und Darmkrankheiten, Aachen.

Die Bauchspeicheldrüse mit ihrer so grossen Bedeutung für die Verdauung und Resorption der Nahrung sowie für den Gesamtstoffwechsel ist bekanntlich schon seit Dezennien zu therapeutischen Zwecken verwandt worden. Wenn nun aber die Pankreastherapie keine grössere Verbreitung gefunden hat, so liegt der Grund sowohl darin, dass ein grosser Teil der in den Handel gebrachten Präparate wenig Wirksamkeit entfaltete, als besonders in dem Umstand, dass wir bisher über kein Präparat verfügten, welches der peptischen Kraft des Magensaftes Widerstand leisten konnte. Die Behauptung Engesser's nämlich, dass sein Pankreatin diese Eigenschaft besässe, ist ja schon von Ewald durch Versuche im Jahre 1880 als unrichtig zurückgewiesen worden.

Es ist nun vor kurzem den Herren Dr. Thomas und Dr. Weber von der chemischen Fabrik Rhenania-Aachen gelungen, ein Pankreaspräparat herzustellen, welches bis zu 5 Stunden der zerstörenden Einwirkung des Magensaftes standhielt. Das Präparat — Pankreon genannt — stellt ein graues, geruchloses Pulver dar, welches auf der Zunge einen angenehmen herben Geschmack hinterlässt. Dasselbe verdaut in einer Dosis von 1 g innerhalb 15 Minuten bei einer Temperatur von 40° in schwach alkalischer Lösung von 100 g Eiweiss 83%, und entwickelt hierbei eine sehr intensive

1) Nach einem Vortrag, gehalten auf der 72. Versammlung deutscher Naturforscher und Aerzte zu Aachen.

Nr. 11.

Figure 11.1-2. Gockel's article in the "Central Journal" (October 1900).

In 1907 *Julius Bence* reported on two severely underweight diabetes patients with very fatty stools whose symptoms were very well controlled with Pankreon®.

The editor of the Central Journal of Metabolic & Digestive Diseases, Carl von Noorden, who was very critical of new preparations, certified in 1908 that only Pankreon® could be considered an effective preparation. Moreover, he concluded that " … the probability of pancreatic disease becomes evident by the effect of the preparation" [4].

In 1909 Sorensen investigated the influence of hydrogen ions on the activity of enzymes and introduced the pH (Abbreviation for *potentia hydrogenii*) value to describe this effect. The pH scale (0–7 acid, 7–14 alkaline) has been in use since 1924.

Although various *pharmacopoeia* already existed (e.g. the German Pharmacopoeia since 1872), there were considerable differences in quality between the available pancreatic enzyme preparations because quality control did not exist.

This situation started to change in 1930 when Rojahn and Müller examined preparations for their enzyme content. They analyzed eleven preparations and found that some did not contain all three enzymes (lipase, amylase, protease) and some only small quantities. Pankreon® proved to be the best preparation with a sufficiently high concentration of enzymes even after acid treatment, although Pankreon® was at this time a so-called conventional preparation, i.e. tablets without enteric coating.

In 1941 Heinz Büter confirmed these findings summarizing that Pankreon® had the lowest tablet weight, but the highest enzyme levels of the eleven preparations tested.

With the success of Pankreon®, the decision-makers within Rhenania were encouraged to move the manufacture from Stolberg near Aachen to a new production plant in Altona in 1901. Several additional patents were filed and granted within the following years to improve the technology and the manufacturing process.

Rhenania expanded by taking over other companies (in 1920 the Verein Chemischer Fabriken in Mannheim, in 1925 Kunheim & Co in Berlin) and moved its administration to Berlin.

However, a further partnership was needed in preparation for future challenges and identified in the Kaliwerk Neustaßfurt-Friedrichshall. Agreements were signed and the new company, Kali-Chemie AG, was founded in 1928 with its office in the administration building of Rhenania-Kunheim in Berlin.

At the end of 1935 Krause-Medico GmbH in Munich, the manufacturer of Pankreas-Dispert, and the Chemische Fabrik Güstrow AG were taken over by Kali-Chemie, an important step in consolidating technology, know-how and the pharmaceutical sector.

In March 1945 the complete destruction of the administration office in Berlin forced Kali-Chemie AG to move to Sehnde near Hanover.

In 1951 Kali-Chemie AG obtained new administration buildings and laboratories directly in Hanover, supplemented by a production plant in Neustadt near Hanover in 1960 and research facilities in 1966.

The Solvay company also suffered from the consequences of the Second World War, and the plants and branches in East Germany were lost. In order to reinforce its presence in Germany and to diversify its business, the Solvay group acquired a majority share in Kali-Chemie AG in 1953.

In the same year (1953) Balzer and Werner confirmed the high quality of Pankreon® as one of the preparations, beside Combizym® and Festal®, that deliver large quantities of active pancreatic enzymes to the gastrointestinal tract.

The comparison of different products, at least in terms of enzyme content, became much more reliable with the introduction of the FIP (Fédération Internationale Pharmaceutique) units, a standardized method of measuring enzyme concentration and activity.

Kali-Chemie AG carefully observed the needs of its customers and introduced new galenic formulations to the market: Pankreon® for children, a pink powder with pancreatin and taste correctives in 1960; and Pankreon® granulate (non enteric-coated) to overcome the poor mixing of tablets with the chyme and the problem of delayed dissolution of some coated tablet preparations.

Traditionally, Pankreon® contained substantial excess of enzymes to guarantee that sufficient amounts could reach the small intestine despite destruction from acid with the disadvantage that high doses had to be taken.

Modern pancreatic enzyme substitution: Present and future

With the acquisition of companies like Duphar in The Netherlands, Reid-Rowell in the United States of America and Unione Chimica Medicamenti in Italy, Solvay strengthened its position and strategy to become a global pharmaceutical company in the 1980s [2]. In the 1990s all the subsidiary companies, including the Japanese one, changed their names to Solvay and the headquarters in Hanover became "Solvay Pharmaceuticals" in 1997.

This development enabled Solvay to improve the pancreatic enzyme preparations and the manufacturing process to meet international standards and needs.

The so-called "acetone process" (1900–1966), defattening and dehydration with acetone, had the major disadvantage of a high loss of enzyme activity. With the subsequent "freeze-drying" process (1967–1988) it was possible to reduce the loss of activity to < 5% but the problem of an unsatisfactory high germ count per gram of pancreatin remained.

Continuous efforts to improve the quality of the manufactured pancreatin and to meet the requirements of, for example, the American pharmacopoeia have resulted in a new technique, the "T-Process" (1977–1999). This process, based on counter-current extraction of enzymes with dichloromethane followed by spray-drying, made it possible not only to produce a high-quality, fiber-free pancreatin without pathogenic germs but to increase lipase activity to > 50,000 FIP-units per gram.

These achievements in terms of manufacturing capability combined with close cooperation with health professionals, patient associations and universities have resulted in a new generation of pancreatic enzyme preparations: *Creon*® (in some countries Kreon®), the successor to Pankreon®, made available in 1983.

Since 1995 an additional "fine tuning" of the high-quality pancreatin became reality with the "precipitation process", with the advantage of complete control of the enrichment and the degree of activation of enzymes and a lipase activity of > 90,000 FIP units per gram. This process does not contain a chemical transformation step but does contain a partial enzymatic digestion step *(hydrolysis)* [5].

Pancreas glands are removed from healthy pigs in certified slaughterhouses after veterinary inspection (Fig. 11.1-3), stored at –20°C and delivered to the manufacturing plant in an uninterrupted freezing chain. The enzyme content of the *pig pancreas* is similar to

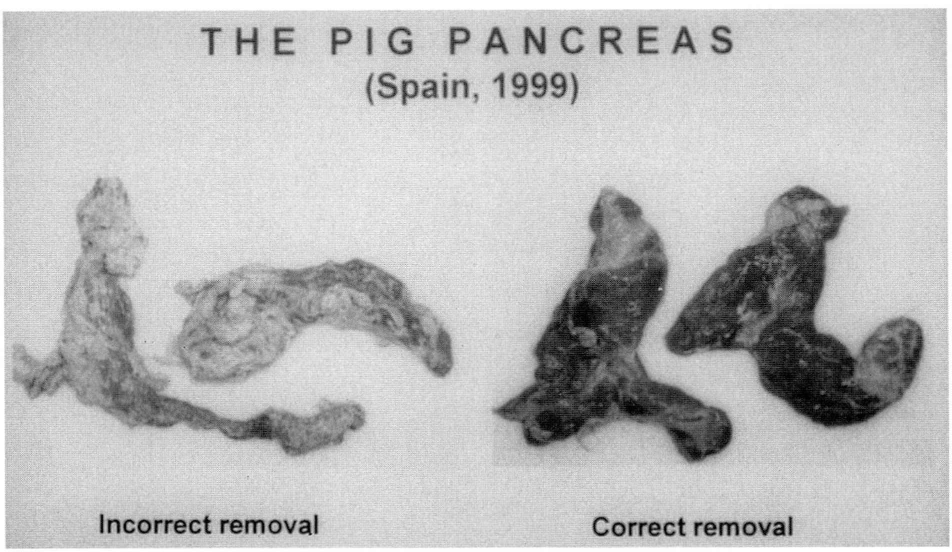

Figure 11.1-3. Removed pancreata of the pig.

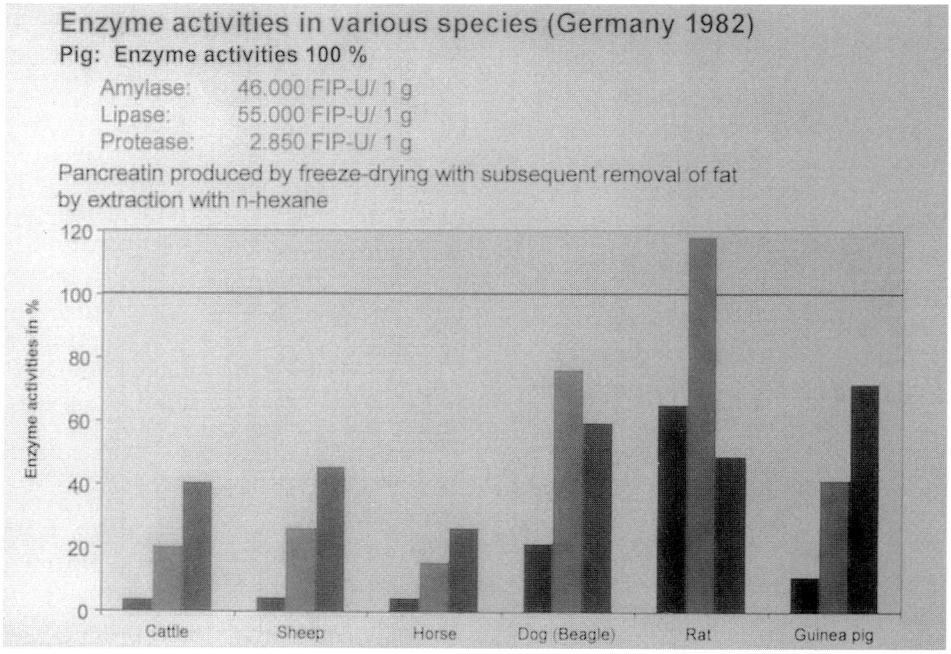

Figure 11.1-4. Enzyme activities (%) in different animal species.

that of humans and has a reasonable size compared to other species (Fig. 11.1-4), qualifying it as the preferred source for raw material currently.

The frozen pancreas glands are milled and suspended in a mixture of water, sodium bicarbonate and isopropyl alcohol. To initiate hydrolysis, a liquid starter (high trypsin content) is added; calcium hydroxide is used for enzyme stabilization. Hydrolysis is stopped by increasing the concentration of isopropyl alcohol and reducing the temperature to prevent prolonged hydrolysis.

Fibers are separated and the dissolved enzymes are precipitated out by a further increase in the isopropyl alcohol concentration, while the low-molecular weight proteins remain in solution.

Various separation and washing steps follow before the moist pancreatin is dried in a vacuum dryer until a residual moisture content of $< 3.5\%$ by weight is reached (Fig. 11.1-5).

Extrusion, rounding, spheronizing and coating of the spheres complete the process before the particles are filled into hard gelatin capsules of different size or sachets.

The plant of today produces for more than 70 countries worldwide and according to the rules of "Good Manufacturing Practice" (GMP) to the satisfaction of relevant authorities such as the Food and Drug Administration (FDA).

The general prerequisites for modern pancreatic enzyme preparation are quality, safety and (cost-)effectiveness.

Quality has to be guaranteed with regard to the absence of contamination, stability and enzyme content (according to a specific pharmacopoeia for the most relevant enzymes *lipase,* amylase and proteases). Enzymes are sensitive proteins and their activity dimin-

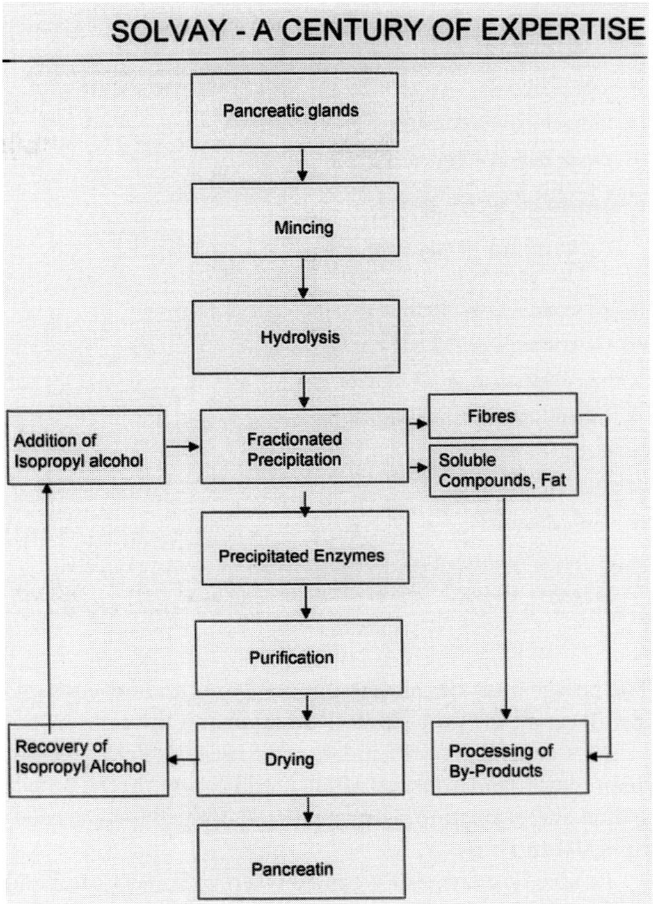

Figure 11.1-5. Block diagram of the manufacturing process.

ishes under biological conditions. To preserve the declared activity over a prolonged period or up to the end of shelf life, pancreatin and pancreatic enzyme products must be stored under cool and anhydrous conditions.

The safety aspect is particularly important in view of the patient population treated – newborns, children and the elderly. Pancreatic enzyme preparations are considered non-toxic and safe and are associated with only a few non-serious adverse events (incidence < 1 per cent). Unlike other preparations with a Eudragit coating, Creon® brands are not associated with the development of fibrosing colonopathy [6–8].

Pharmacoeconomic studies are currently underway while the effectiveness of Creon® brands has been demonstrated in numerous controlled clinical investigations.

Exogenous pancreatic enzymes are indicated to correct the symptoms of maldigestion and malabsorption due to *pancreatic exocrine insufficiency* (PEI) caused by various diseases and conditions (Table 11.1-1). It is a cornerstone of treatment in inherited diseases like cystic fibrosis [9], in different forms of pancreatitis [10, 11] and after surgical intervention [12–14]. Epidemiological and clinical data are or being generated to elucidate the clinical relevance of pancreatic enzyme substitution in other diseases associated with PEI such as diabetes mellitus [15, 16].

Diseases and conditions causing pancreatic exocrine insufficiency (PEI)
• Cystic fibrosis
• Shwachman syndrome
• Acute pancreatitis
• Chronic pancreatitis – Tropical calcifying pancreatitis – Hereditary pancreatitis – The aging pancreas ("senile pancreatitis")
• Pancreatic resection due to pancreatic cancer
• Gastric surgery
Other diseases associated with PEI
• Inflammatory bowel disease
• Celiac disease
• Diabetes mellitus
• Liver disease
• Acquired immune deficiency syndrome
• Sjögren's disease

Table 11.1-1. List of diseases and conditions associated with pancreatic exocrine insufficiency.

The dosage must be calculated individually and depends on the severity of the disease or insufficiency, the post-surgical situation and the composition of food.

As a general recommendation, at least 30,000 units of lipase need to be given with main meals. Underdosing, which is still common, can be avoided by regular stool fat collection and evaluation. The calculation of the dosage needed should not be based only on clinical symptoms.

Pancreatic enzymes have to be taken with every meal and snack. They have to be taken during the meal, either in one portion shortly after the beginning of food intake or divided into two or three portions over the food intake, and not before (except in small children) or after a meal or snack.

Creon® brands are available in a number of different presentation forms and strengths to meet the needs of all age groups (for example *Kreon® für Kinder* with 5,000 European Pharmacopoeia (Ph.Eur.) units lipase or the standard formulation with 10,000 Ph.Eur. units of lipase). High-strength preparations with a lipase content of 20,000, 25,000 or 40,000 international units have been made available since the early 1990s and have marked a substantial advance in the treatment of, for example, cystic fibrosis adults or pancreatectomized patients with improved treatment adherence due to a reduction in the daily number of capsules [17–19].

The ultimate aim of enzyme replacement therapy is to target a sufficient quantity of active pancreatic enzymes to the proximal duodenum. Modern preparations are therefore "designed" or formulated to meet this therapeutic need as follows:

Multi-unit dose aspect

The superiority of multiple-unit dose preparations over single-unit dose preparations such as tablets has been documented [20, 21]. Multiple-unit dose preparations contain hundreds of encapsulated enteric-coated microspheres or, more recently, *minimicros-*

pheres which are now considered the enzyme treatment of choice [22]. For Creon 10,000 Minimicrospheres®, available since 1996, a substantial reduction of 50% (in volume) of the original capsule size was made possible by the new manufacturing process (see above).

After release from the hard gelatin capsule (capsule dissolves within 1–2 minutes after contact with fluids under physiological conditions), the high number of particles achieves an even distribution within the stomach and allows thorough mixing with the chyme, the larger surface area increasing the digestion potency.

Sphere size

Several publications have demonstrated the importance of particle size for high enzymatic duodenal availability during the digestive phase. To leave the stomach and pass the pylorus together with food, particles must be 1.4 ± 0.3 mm in diameter [23].

Smaller spheres (1.0–1.2 mm) seem to be 25 per cent more effective than larger ones (1.8–2.0 mm) [24, 25]. These findings have been confirmed by additional investigations [26, 27] and have provided the basis for the development of minimicrospheres. The majority of the minimicrospheres have a diameter of around 1 mm with a range between 0.7 and 1.6 mm (Fig. 11.1-6), which is currently considered optimal [28].

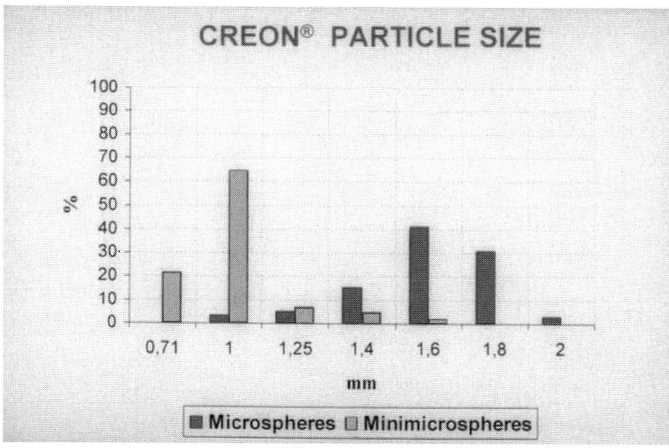

Figure 11.1-6. Distribution of the size of microspheres and minimicrospheres.

Acid protection

Pancreatic lipase is very acid-labile and irreversibly inactivated at a pH < 4.0. Enteric-coated preparations are therefore preferred to acid-sensitive (conventional) preparations for treating forms of pancreatic insufficiency [29, 30]. All Creon® brands are enteric-coated with hydroxymethylcellulose phthalate (HP55), ensuring a resistance to acid of 98 per cent [31, 32].

Dissolution characteristics

Effective enzyme preparations must demonstrate a very rapid release of enzymes (> 80 per cent) as soon as pH 5.5 has been reached. Creon® ensures a very steep release of more than 90 per cent at pH 5.5 or above after 45 minutes, and appears to be superior to competitors in this respect [33]. Similar results have also been demonstrated *in vitro* with Creon® 25,000 (Fig. 11.1-7: Release characteristics of lipase activity [33].

Creon® brands are today the most prescribed enzyme preparations worldwide and certainly among the most extensively documented.

Although 90–95% of patients with pancreatic exocrine insufficiency achieve adequate symptom control with the modern formulations, further improvements in terms of coating and particle size are under investigation, including a water-soluble pancreatin.

Alternatives to porcine pancreatin such as gastric lipase, fungal enzymes and microbial enzymes may be future options for the treatment of poor or non-responders or patients who have objections to medicine derived from pigs for religious or other reasons.

Solvay will develop and offer reliable and high-quality treatment options to satisfy the medical need of its customers for the next hundred years.

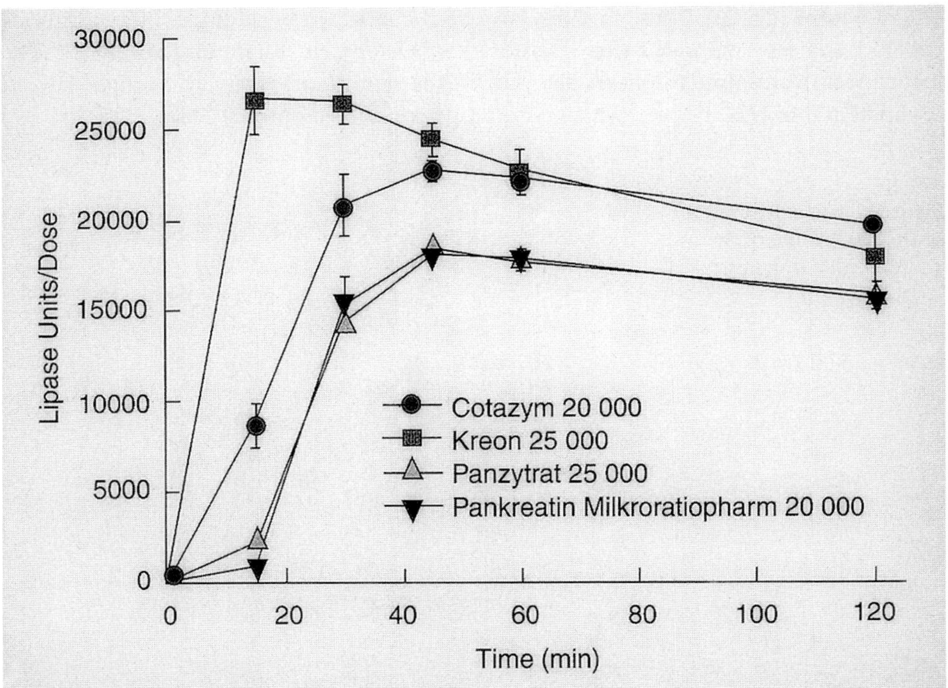

Figure 11.1-7. Release characteristics of lipase activity [33].

References

1. Rudmann MA, ed. The Magic Potions in the Belly Gland [Kuhlmann H. Die Zauberstoffe im Wampenbries]. Hanover: Solvay Pharmaceuticals GmbH, 2000.
2. Rapaille M. Solvay. Ein Mann und sein Werk [Solvay. A man and his work]. Brussels: Didier Hatier, 1991.
3. Gockel M. Über Erfolge mit "Pankreon", einem neuen, gegen Magensaft widerstandsfähigen Pankreaspräparat [On success with "Pankreon", a new pancreatic preparation resistant to gastric juice]. Centralblatt für Stoffwechsel- und Verdauungskrankheiten 1900; 11: 251–56.

4. Von Noorden C. Zur Diagnostik der Pankreaserkrankungen [On the diagnosis of pancreatic disease]. Klinisch-therapeutische Wochenschr 1908; 35: 929–34.
5. Peschke G. Solvay Pharmaceuticals GmbH (data on file), 2000.
6. Smyth RL et al. Fibrosing colonopathy in cystic fibrosis: results of a case-control study. The Lancet 1995; 346: 1247–51.
7. Prescott P, Bakowski MT. Pathogenesis of fibrosing colonopathy: the role of methacrylic acid copolymer. Pharmacoepidemiol Drug Saf 1999; 8: 377–84.
8. Bansi DS et al. Fibrosing colonopathy in an adult owing to overuse of pancreatic enzyme supplements. Gut 2000; 46: 283–85.
9. Littlewood JM, Wolfe SP. Control of malabsorption in cystic fibrosis. Paediatr Drugs 2000; 3: 205–22.
10. Apte MV et al. Chronic pancreatitis: complications and management. J Clin Gastroenterol 1999; 29: 225–40.
11. Mohan V et al. Oral pancreatic enzyme therapy in the control of diabetes mellitus in tropical calculous pancreatitis. Int J Pancreatol 1998; 24: 19–22.
12. Van Hoozen CM et al. Efficacy of enzyme supplementation after surgery for chronic pancreatitis. Pancreas 1997; 14: 174–80.
13. Neoptolemos JP et al. Treatment of pancreatic exocrine insufficiency after pancreatic resection. Int J Pancreatol 1999; 25: 171–80.
14. Brägelmann R et al. The effect of pancreatic enzyme supplementation in patients with steatorrhoea after gastrectomy. Eur J Gastroenterol Hepatol 1999; 11: 231–7.
15. Kitagawa M et al. Evaluating exocrine function tests for diagnosing chronic pancreatitis. Pancreas 1997; 15: 402–8.
16. Rathmann W et al. Pancreatic exocrine insufficiency and type 2 diabetes are strongly associated. Diabetol 42 (Suppl 1) A 1999; 82: 297.
17. George DE et al. Comparison of two pancreatic enzyme supplements in patients with cystic fibrosis. Adv Ther 1990; 7: 109–18.
18. Friesen C, Prestidge C. Comparison of a high-strength pancreatic enzyme preparation and a standard-strength preparation in cystic fibrosis. Adv Ther 1995; 12: 236–44.
19. Braden B et al. Monitoring pancreatin supplementation in cystic fibrosis patients with the ^{13}C-Hiolein® breath test: evidence of normalized fat assimilation with high-dose pancreatin therapy. Z Gastroenterol 1997; 35: 123–9.
20. Lankisch PG. Conservative treatment of chronic pancreatitis. Digestion 1987; 37(Suppl 1): 47–55.
21. Vyas H et al. A comparison of enteric coated microspheres with enteric coated tablet pancreatic enzyme preparations in cystic fibrosis: A controlled study. Eur J Pediatr 1990; 149: 241–3.
22. Layer P, Holtmann G. Pancreatic enzymes in chronic pancreatitis. Int J Pancreatol 1994; 15: 1–11.
23. Meyer JH et al. Human postprandial gastric emptying of 1–3 millimeter spheres. Gastroenterol 1988; 94: 1315–25.
24. Kühnelt P, Mundlos S, Adler G. Einfluß der Pelletgröße eines Pankreasenzympräparates auf die duodenale lipolytische Aktivität [The size of enteric-coated microspheres influences the intraduodenal lipolytic activity]. Z Gastroenterol 1991; 29: 417–21.
25. Mundlos S, Kühnelt P, Adler G. Monitoring enzyme replacement treatment in exocrine pancreatic insufficiency using the cholesteryl octanoate breath test. Gut 1991; 31: 1324–8.
26. Layer P et al. Enzyme pellet size and luminal nutrient digestion in pancreatic insufficiency. Digestion 1992; 52: 100.
27. Norregard P et al. Gastric emptying of pancreatin granules and dietary lipids in pancreatic insufficiency. Aliment Pharmacol Ther 1996; 10: 427–32.
28. Lippold BC. What is the ideal size for enteric-coated pancreatic preparations? Drugs made in Germany 1998; 41: 52–6.
29. Beverley DW et al. Comparison of four different pancreatic extracts in cystic fibrosis. Arch Dis Child 1987; 62: 564–8.

30. Stead RJ et al. Treatment of steatorrhoea in cystic fibrosis: A comparison of enteric coated microspheres of pancreatin versus non-enteric coated pancreatin and adjuvant cimetidine. Aliment Pharmacol Ther 1988; 2: 471–82.
31. Whitehead AM. Study to compare the enzyme activity, acid resistance and dissolution characteristics of currently available pancreatic enzyme preparations. Pharm Weekbl (Sci) 1988; 10: 12–6.
32. Atkinson SN. A comparative study of enzyme activity, acid resistance and dissolution characteristics of four enteric coated microsphere preparations of pancreatin. Eur J Clin Res 1991; 1: 37–45.
33. Hüwel S, Behrens R, Spener F. Pankreasenzyme: Präparate im Vergleich [Pancreatic enzymes: Comparison of preparations]. PZ 1996; 37: 33–42.

11.2 Therapy of pancreatic exocrine insufficiency: New experimental data

P. C. Gregory, R. Tabeling, C. Fassmann, J. Kamphues

Summary

Studies have been made of total and prececal digestion/absorption of nutrients in ileo-cecal re-entrant fistulated control minipigs fed a high-fat diet. The results were compared with those in similarly prepared, pancreatic exocrine insufficient (PEI; pancreatic duct ligated) minipigs with and without administration of enteric-coated pancreatin (Creon® 10,000 mms™) or an uncoated, highly stable, bacterial lipase. Complete PEI resulted in lowered intestinal pH, and a very severe and roughly equal malabsorption of fat and protein, and a more moderate (load-dependent) malabsorption of starch. Protein malabsorption was observed in fecal samples, but the real degree of malabsorption could only be measured at the ileum; starch malabsorption could only be determined at the level of the ileum – in both cases due to the extensive nature of hindgut fermentation, which partially compensates for poor prececal digestion. In contrast, fecal fat excretion tended to be greater than ileal fat excretion in PEI minipigs, presumably due to microbial fat synthesis. Administration of the bacterial lipase caused, at best, a similar improvement of fat absorption as pancreatin, even though the bacterial lipase could function throughout the GI tract while pancreatin had first to be released from its enteric-coating. It remains to be tested whether there is any added benefit if it is administered together with pancreatin. Bacterial lipase had no influence on the malabsorption of protein and starch. Administration of Creon (8–24 caps/meal) normalized the coefficient of starch absorption and caused a dose-dependent improvement of those of fat and protein. Creon supplementation also reversed the small intestinal bacterial overgrowth observed in untreated PEI minipigs. By extrapolation of the dose-response curves it was estimated that around 1 million FIP U/meal lipase would have had to be administered to normalize fat digestion following the 75 g fat meal in the PEI minipig. Since PEI results in malabsorption of protein, starch and fat, the optimum therapy must improve digestion/absorption of all these nutrients. Therefore, for the present, pancreatin remains the therapy of choice in PEI.

Introduction

Pancreatic exocrine insufficiency (PEI) is a common complication in patients with chronic pancreatitis. In the 1970s studies performed by DiMagno and co-workers [1] established that insufficiency occurs progressively in alcoholic, chronic pancreatitis (CP) patients and that symptoms of PEI such as steatorrhea and azotorrhea only appear after some 90% of the secretory capacity of the pancreas is lost (as judged by the response to a maximal stimulus of secretin plus cerulein/CCK). It has furthermore been claimed that lipase activity becomes insufficient before protease or amylase activity [2] in alcoholic chronic pancreatitis. Therapy with pancreatin has been successful in improving symptoms of PEI, but nevertheless complete normalization of fat digestion has proved difficult to achieve in many of these patients [3] whether by administration of large doses of enzymes or co-administration of acid secretion blockers, which may not only improve fat digestion but can also severely reduce protein digestibility [4]. This has raised interest in looking for other lipases, e.g. microbial lipases with wider stability and activity properties, as new therapeutic alternatives (or as add-on) to pancreatin.

It has therefore been necessary to develop an animal model of PEI to investigate the changes occurring due to PEI and the problems with therapy. The pancreatic duct ligated minipig was chosen as the model of induced PEI. The pigs were also fitted with an ileocecal re-entrant fistula to allow determination of prececal digestibility. Subsequently, studies have been made of the efficacy of a highly potent bacterial lipase to treat PEI-induced malabsorption.

Methods

Surgical preparation

Digestibility studies were performed in groups of 3–6 female Göttingen minipigs (Ellegaard, 20–30 kg at surgery). The pigs were sedated with Tilest® (Tiletamin/Zolazepam; i.m.) and intubated. Thereafter they were anaesthetized with a mixture of halothane, nitrous oxide and oxygen and following a mid-line laparotomy they were fitted with an ileocecal, re-entrant titanium fistula, which was exteriorized on the right flank. In addition, in one group of animals the pancreatic duct was carefully isolated and ligated (PEI; pancreatic exocrine insufficient); no ligation was performed in control animals. The pigs were prophylactically treated with antibiotics (Tardomyocel®, Benzylpenicillin, Dihydrostreptomycin) and with an analgesic (Tramal®, Tramadol). The pigs were given at least 4 weeks to recover from the surgery before studies began.

Preliminary studies of the influence of duct ligation on intestinal pH and enzyme activity were made in German Landrace (male & female) and female Göttingen minipigs prepared as above, but with simple T-fistulae implanted in the duodenum or jejunum and ileum respectively.

Experimental protocol

Pigs were fed two meals per day (250 g/meal in 500 ml H_2O, of a finely milled high-fat diet [30.1% fat, 24.9% starch, 14.9% protein], plus 0.625 g/meal Cr_2O_3 [Aldrich], as a marker), at 08.00 and 20.00 h. PEI pigs were additionally administered different doses of enzyme supplements (pancreatin [Creon® 10,000 MMS™, 0, 8, 16 or 24 capsules; i.e. PEI-0, PEI-8, PEI-16, PEI-24 respectively], or the equivalent FIP units of bacterial lipase with each meal). At least 7 days adaptation were allowed with each change of enzymes or of diet before any measurements were made. Then, all feces were collected for 5 days, after which ileal chyme was collected on ice for 12h on 3 successive days. Samples for enzyme activity analysis were stored at –80°C, all other samples were stored at –20°C until analysis.

The doses of bacterial lipase administered were selected according to the actual lipase activities measured in the Creon® capsules immediately before the study was performed.

Analytical procedure

The frozen samples as well as the original diet were freeze-dried and were analyzed for dry matter, crude fat, crude protein, starch and sugar [5] and Cr_2O_3 content [6]. In brief, dry matter was estimated by weight after 8 h at 103°C; crude protein was determined via Kjeldahl analysis of nitrogen content (crude protein = nitrogen × 6.25]; crude fat was determined gravimetrically after boiling for 30 min in concentrated HCl, followed by a 6-h extraction with petrol ether; starch was analyzed polarimetrically after acid hydolysis; sugar was estimated gravimetrically; and Cr_2O_3 was oxidized to chromate and chromium content estimated via extinction at 365 nm. Lipopolysaccharides (LPS), constituents of the cell wall of gram-negative bacteria (used as a marker for gram-negative bacteria), were measured in frozen fecal or ileal samples by the Limulus-Test®.

Pancreatic lipase, trypsin, chymotrypsin and α-amylase activity were determined in the ileal samples by a modification of the microtiter method of Lainé et al. [7], with a Biomek 1000.

Coefficient of absorption (apparent digestibility)

The coefficient of whole GIT absorption (CA) of each food component was estimated according to the formula:

$$\text{CA }(\%) = \frac{\text{g/day in feed} - \text{g/day in feces}}{\text{g/day in feed}} \times 100$$

Coefficient of prececal absorption (CPA) of each nutrient was estimated by marker method:

$$\text{CPA }(\%) = \frac{\%\ Cr_2O_3 \text{ in feed}}{\%\ Cr_2O_3 \text{ in chyme}} \times \frac{\% \text{ nutrient in chyme}}{\% \text{ nutrient in feed}} \times 100$$

Estimation of % maximal lipase efficacy

A rough approximation of the dose of lipase necessary for maximal fat digestion was estimated by extrapolation (to 100%) of the log dose-response curve, according to the observed coefficient of fat absorption (CFA), and using Excel 5.0:

$$\%\text{ effect at dose y} = \frac{\text{CFA (PEI-y)} - \text{CFA (PEI-0)}}{\text{CFA Control} - \text{CFA (PEI-0)}} \times 100$$

Statistics

Means and standard deviations were calculated using Excel 5.0. Statistical procedures were performed with the SAS® Software programme. Treatment effects were tested by analysis of variance. Independent samples were checked with the t-test for independent observations (control vs PEI-0), dependent samples with the t-test for dependent observations (PEI-0 vs PEI-8, PEI-16, PEI-24, etc.).

Results

The influences of pancreatic duct ligation and the effects of pancreatic enzyme supplementation with pancreatin in these animals have been described elsewhere in full [8, 9] and will only be briefly outlined here.

Influences of pancreatic duct ligation

General observations. Ligation of the pancreatic duct caused complete pancreatic exocrine insufficiency, with undetectable trypsin, chymotrypsin and amylase activities at the ileum. In contrast, low lipase activity, approx. 3% of control values, was regularly recorded at the ileum and low chymotrypsin activity (0.3 ± 0.7 U/g), about 2% of control values (12.8 ± 5.6 U/g), was recorded in the feces. Weight gain stopped abruptly, after pancreatic duct ligation, in German Landrace pigs and despite a normal feed intake the body weight remained relatively constant/fell slightly over a period of 10 weeks. They showed few outward signs of digestive disturbance. Even when fed the 30% fat diet neither PEI pigs nor minipigs developed more than transient diarrhea. In the first few days on this diet the pigs/minipigs produced foul-smelling, watery feces but within a few days the smell disappeared and the feces became more solid again, albeit still softer and more formless than in controls.

Quality of intestinal chyme. Duct ligation resulted in a lowering of duodenal pH, by approx. 2 units, in German Landrace pigs, in both the pre- and the postprandial period (7.0 ± 1.1, to 4.3 ± 0.9, and 6.8 ± 1.2 to 4.8 ± 0.9 for controls and PEI respectively). In the Göttingen minipigs, preprandial jejunal (6.0 ± 0.6) and 0–12 h postprandial ileal pH (7.3 ± 0.4) in PEI minipigs were almost 0.5 units lower than in control minipigs (6.4 ± 0.6, and 7.8 ± 0.4) respectively. Following pancreatic duct ligation, there was a dramatic > 20-fold increase in the LPS concentration (from 29 ± 12 to 634 ± 254 μg LPS/g ileal chyme, and from 85 ± 25 to 2700 ± 797 μg LPS/g DM of feces) and a 40 to 100-fold increase in the total daily amount of LPS entering the hindgut or excreted in the feces respectively.

Coefficient of absorption. There was an especially large fall in the coefficient of absorption of whole GIT absorption of fat and a smaller but nevertheless still considerable reduction in the coefficient of absorption of dry matter and protein in the PEI minipigs compared to the controls (Table 11.2-1). In contrast, the coefficient of starch digestion

Table 11.2-1. Coefficient of whole GIT absorption in control vs PEI minipigs ± pancreatin.

Pig group	Dry matter	Fat	Protein	Starch
Control	87.5 ± 3.3[a]	95.5 ± 0.9[a]	89.9 ± 3.3[a]	99.2 ± 0.3
PEI 0 caps	62.5 ± 3.4[b]	31.5 ± 8.1[b]	56.9 ± 2.6[b]	99.1 ± 0.2
PEI 8 caps	68.7 ± 3.6[c]	51.7 ± 12.5[c]	69.3 ± 2.5[c]	98.5 ± 0.3
PEI 16 caps	73.0 ± 3.5[c,d]	61.1 ± 7.2[c]	74.5 ± 4.1[c,d]	98.3 ± 0.1
PEI 24 caps	77.8 ± 4.0[d]	68.5 ± 6.8[c]	81.8 ± 3.3[d]	98.5 ± 0.2

Values are mean ± SD; significant differences ($P < 0.05$) are indicated by different superscripts (a,b,c,d).

Values were determined after a 5-day total feces collection from 3 PEI minipigs (given 0, 8, 16 or 24 capsules Creon® 10,000 MMS™/meal) and 3 control minipigs, fed twice daily (08.00 and 20.00 h) for 7–10 days prior and during collection 250 g/meal (30% fat, 25% starch, 15% protein, 0.625 g Cr_2O_3) in 500 ml water. Feces were stored at –20°C, freeze-dried and samples analyzed for dry matter, fat, protein and starch content. Coefficient of absorption of each nutrient was calculated according to the formula:

$$\text{Coefficient of absorption (\%)} = \frac{\text{g/day in feed} - \text{g/day in feces}}{\text{g/day in feed}} \times 100$$

was around 99% in both groups of minipigs. Pancreatic duct ligation had even more dramatic effects upon prececal digestion. The most severe effects were on the reduction of the coefficient of absorption of protein and fat. The absorption of dry matter was also strongly reduced, coincident with a rise in dry matter content of ileal chyme from 14.4 ± 0.8 to 21.3 ± 0.9%. On the other hand, starch digestion was only moderately reduced (Table 11.2-2).

Table 11.2-2. Coefficient of prececal absorption in controls vs PEI minipigs ± pancreatin.

Pig group	Dry matter	Fat	Protein	Starch
Controls	78.9 ± 1.5[a]	95.2 ± 0.4[a]	79.0 ± 3.2[a]	97.4 ± 0.2[a]
PEI 0 caps	42.7 ± 0.2[b]	43.0 ± 9.0[b]	27.4 ± 7.8[b]	87.7 ± 6.2[a.b]
PEI 8 caps	59.9 ± 0.1[c]	69.8 ± 3.7[b]	53.4 ± 4.2[c]	95.2 ± 1.3[b]
PEI 16 caps	66.1 ± 2.9[c.d]	78.2 ± 9.2[b.c]	63.5 ± 2.3[d]	95.8 ± 0.2[b]
PEI 24 caps	68.1 ± 2.7[d]	83.3 ± 5.7[c]	66.2 ± 6.6[c.d]	96.3 ± 0.6[b]

Values are mean ± SD; significant differences ($P < 0.05$) are indicated by different superscripts (a, b, c, d).
Ileal chyme was collected on ice for 12 h on 3 successive days, following the 5 day feces collection, in 3 PEI minipigs (given 0, 8, 16 or 24 capsules Creon® 10,000 MMS™/meal) and 3 control minipigs, fed twice daily (08.00 and 20.00 h) 250 g/meal (30% fat, 25% starch, 15% protein, 0.625 g Cr_2O_3) in 500 ml water. Ileal samples were frozen at –20°C and freeze-dried before analysis for dry matter, fat, protein, starch and chrome (see methods). Coefficient of prececal absorption (CPA) of each nutrient was estimated by marker method:

$$\text{CPA (\%)} = \frac{\%\ Cr_2O_3 \text{ in feed}}{\%\ Cr_2O_3 \text{ in chyme}} \times \frac{\% \text{ nutrient in chyme}}{\% \text{ nutrient in feed}} \times 100$$

Influence of pancreatin in PEI minipigs fed a 30% fat diet

Quality of intestinal chyme. Following pancreatin administration there appeared to be a reduction in gram-negative intestinal bacterial content. Thus, after 24 caps Creon®/meal, the ileal LPS values were completely normalized (30.5 ± 31.7 µg/g), while the fecal LPS content was more moderately reduced (1980 ± 1093 µg/g DM). Ileal pH was moderately increased after pancreatin therapy (e.g. mean 12h pH of 7.55 ± 0.23 with 16 capsules Creon®/meal), to reach mid-way between untreated PEI and control values.

Coefficient of absorption. Administration of pancreatin (8–24 caps/meal) caused a dose-related improvement in coefficient of whole GIT absorption of protein ≥ dry matter >> fat absorption, without achieving the same levels seen in control minipigs (Table 11.2-1). In contrast, pancreatin (8–24 caps/meal) produced a dose-related improvement in coefficient of prececal absorption of fat = dry matter = protein, without achieving control levels. Starch absorption was normalized already at the lowest dose of pancreatin (Table 11.2-2).

Influence of bacterial lipase on digestibility of a 30% fat diet in PEI minipigs

Administration of bacterial lipase (112,000 and 336,000 FIP units/meal) resulted in the formation of hard fecal pellets and caused a strong, dose-related increase in coefficient of whole GIT absorption of fat and thereby also of dry matter absorption (Fig. 11.2-1) and surprisingly, a small improvement in coefficient of protein absorption was also observed.

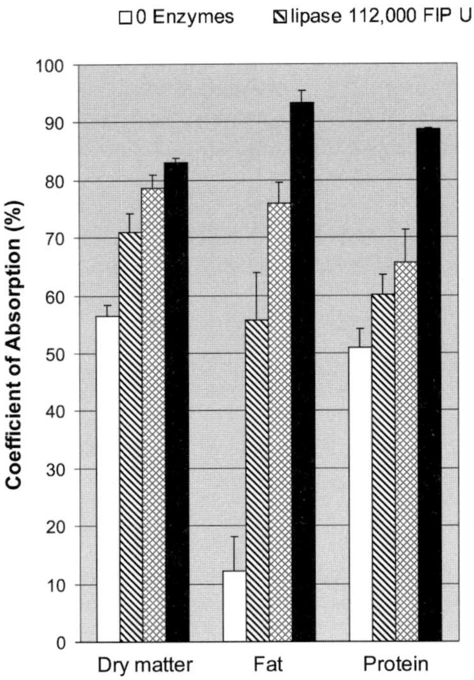

Figure 11.2-1. Coefficient of whole GIT absorption: Influence of bacterial lipase.
Values (mean ± SD) were determined after a 5-day total feces collection from 6 PEI minipigs (given 0; 112,000 or 336,000 FIP U bacterial lipase/meal) and 3 control minipigs, fed for 10 days prior to and during collection twice daily (08.00 and 20.00 h) 250 g/meal (30% fat, 25% starch, 15% protein) in 500 ml water. Sample preparation and calculations as in Table 11.2-1.

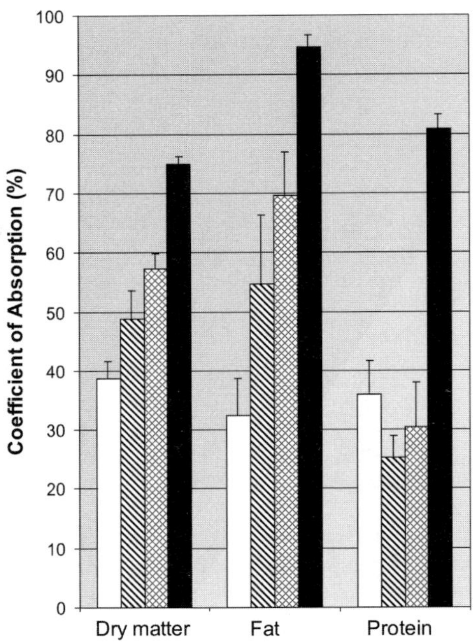

Figure 11.2-2. Coefficient of prececal absorption: Influence of bacterial lipase.
Ileal chyme was collected on ice for 12 h on 3 successive days, following the 5-day feces collection, in 6 PEI minipigs (given 0; 112,000 or 336,000 FIP U bacterial lipase/meal) and 3 control minipigs, fed twice daily (08.00 and 20.00 h) 250 g/meal (30% fat, 25% starch, 15% protein, 0.625 g Cr_2O_3) in 500 ml water. Sample preparation and calculations as described in Table 11.2-2.

The bacterial lipase caused similar improvement in the coefficient of prececal fat absorption, but did not affect the coefficient of prececal absorption of protein (Fig. 11.2-2). It had no effect on coefficient of starch absorption (86.7 ± 9.2; 79.5 ± 1.1; 81.4 ± 4.8% at 0; 112,000 & 336,000 FIP U/meal respectively).

Estimation of lipase dose for maximal fat digestion

The log dose-response for pancreatic lipase was linear over the doses tested (Fig. 11.2-3). By extrapolation it was calculated that a dose of between 890,545 FIP U/meal (prececal) and 1,100,394 FIP U/meal (fecal values) would bring the 100% effect (i.e. reach control CFA values). With bacterial lipase it was estimated that the 100% effect would be reached after administration of between 866,991 FIP U/meal (fecal values) and 2,107,625 FIP U/meal (ileal values).

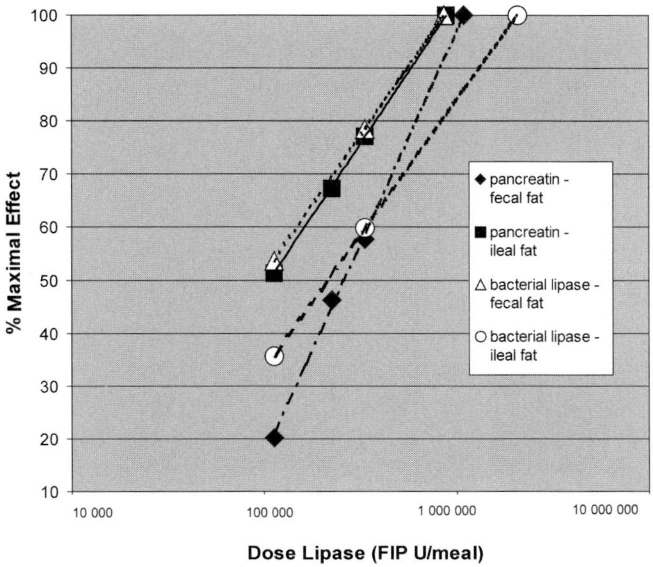

Figure 11.2-3. Log dose-response of lipase in PEI minipigs (extrapolation to 100% effect). The doses of pancreatic and bacterial lipase which would have been necessary for maximal fat digestion have been estimated by extrapolation (to 100%) of the log dose-response curve, according to the observed ileal and fecal coefficient of fat absorption (CFA), and using Excel 5.0:

$$\% \text{ effect at dose y} = \frac{\text{CFA (PEI-y)} - \text{CFA (PEI-0)}}{\text{CFA Control} - \text{CFA (PEI-0)}} \times 100$$

Thus, 100% maximal effect represents the CFA seen in control minipigs; 0% that in untreated PEI minipigs.

Discussion

Pancreatic duct ligation caused a complete pancreatic exocrine insufficiency in the minipig. This led to a severe fall in duodenal pH, similar to what has been observed in human PEI [10], but only a slight fall in jejunal and ileal pH as well as small intestinal bacterial overgrowth. Interestingly, pancreatin therapy reversed the bacterial overgrowth, perhaps by a direct antibiotic effect [11] or indirectly by removing bacterial substrate, and partly corrected the fall in ileal pH. The ileal pH may therefore be at least partly dependent upon the degree of bacterial fermentation and on the content of unabsorbed nutrients (e.g., fatty acids). Pancreatic secretions clearly play an important role in preventing small intestinal bacterial overgrowth.

Severe disturbances of fat and protein together with a more moderate disturbance of starch digestion were observed in the PEI minipig. Presumably as a result of the extensive hindgut fermentation of unabsorbed nutrients, malabsorption of starch could only be detected at the level of the ileum, while prececal malabsorption of protein was also considerably greater than malabsorption measured in the feces. Conversely, malabsorption of fat appeared to be slightly greater when measured in the feces than at the ileum, a finding which has been sporadically observed previously in control pigs (e.g. 12). This apparent hindgut fat synthesis in the PEI minipigs is still under investigation, but it has been reported that the hindgut microflora may cause such findings [13], i.e. the bacterial content of fat combined with the increase in the hindgut microflora population in the PEI minipigs could give rise to an apparent fat synthesis within the hindgut. In this context it should be noted that most fecal protein is of bacterial rather than dietary origin [14]. It is interesting to speculate as to whether microbial fat synthesis might contribute to the problem of normalizing fat excretion in some PEI patients.

The present study showed, similar to human PEI, that it is also difficult to normalize fat absorption with pancreatin therapy in PEI minipigs. By extrapolation of the dose-response curve it could be estimated that normalization of fat absorption with this meal might only be achieved after administration of some 1 million FIP lipase units/meal. This figure is only an approximation and certainly the dose of enzymes required for normalization depends upon the dietary fat load, which was very high in the present study (75 g fat/meal), but it does indicate that higher doses of lipase than hitherto expected may be needed in order to completely normalize fat absorption. No determination has been made of the pancreatic secretion rate in the minipig, but in 17–25 kg pigs a lipase secretion rate of about 650,000 lipase units/12 h was reported [15]. If similar rates of secretion occur in the minipig, it would appear that around 100% (of normal secretion rate) pancreatic lipase may have to be returned to the PEI minipig fed a high-fat diet if digestion/absorption of fat is to be completely normalized. Similar results have also been observed in dogs with induced PEI [16]. This does not easily reconcile with the human data that symptoms of PEI only occur after approx. 90% loss of pancreatic secretory capacity [1]. One factor which might play a role here is that lipase is rapidly inactivated during small intestinal transit [17]. Another potential problem, that of delayed release of lipase from the enteric-coated microspheres due to low intestinal pH, is unlikely to have been a major problem in these studies, since already in the jejunum (1 m from pylorus) the pH was sufficiently high to allow rapid enzyme release (release is rapid at pH > 5.5). Furthermore, the pancreatin used was administered in enteric-coated minimicrospheres of a size (sieve fraction 0.7–1.6 mm) which should be optimal for mixing and emptying with the meal [18], and so inappropriate emptying of the enzymes relative to the meal is also unlikely to have been a factor here. Moreover, studies in which uncoated pancreatin was infused direct into the duodenum showed that steatorrhea was far from abolished in CP patients with PEI even with infusion of up to 40% of the normal rate of pancreatic lipase secretion [19]. Finally, administration of the lipase inhibitor Orlistat (tetrahydrolipstatin; 120 mg tid) causes about 30% malabsorption of dietary fat [20] despite inhibiting postprandial duodenal lipolysis by only 70% at most, depending on the meal [21]. This leaves some uncertainty regarding the validity of the secretin/CCK-induced maximal pancreatic secretory capacity as a relevant marker for physiological postprandial pancreatic secretion, which appears to be largely under neural control [22], and/or regarding the accuracy of the fecal fat excretion test. In any event it seems clear that complete normalization of steatorrhea in PEI can require supplementation by far more than 10% and perhaps even 100% of the normal enzyme secretion in patients with a high fat intake.

The findings with bacterial lipase therapy can best be discussed in the light of the results with pancreatin therapy. The bacterial lipase was selected on the basis of *in vitro* studies which demonstrated a profile superior to that of pancreatic lipase: it is resistant to protease inactivation (to both gastric and pancreatic proteases), and moreover is stable and active over a wide pH range (pH 4–9) and is not markedly influenced by bile salts. It was therefore administered without any enteric coating, allowing activity already in the stomach and throughout the intestine. Disappointingly, it did not produce a markedly better efficacy than pancreatin, but rather the coefficient of fat absorption was similar to that observed with pancreatin. The studies with bacterial lipase were performed in different individuals and under slightly different conditions than those with pancreatin, which prevents a direct comparison of efficacy. However, extrapolation of the dose-response curves for bacterial lipase suggests that normalization of fat absorption might have been achieved with administration of between 890,000 and 2,100,000 lipase units/meal according to fecal or ileal curves respectively. Therefore the bacterial lipase at best shows similar efficacy to pancreatin. The reasons why it is not superior to pancreatin remain to be determined, but some gastric inactivation of the lipase may occur over time, since it is rapidly denatured at pH 3, a pH which has been observed at the pyloric antrum of pigs 6 h after feeding [23]. Unexpectedly, there were signs of a dose-dependent reduction in fecal nitrogen excretion with bacterial lipase. However, the prececal nitrogen values were completely unaffected by bacterial lipase administration, and therefore it is clear that the lipase had no real effect on protein absorption.

It has been suggested that lipase deficiency occurs before that of protease or amylase in CP [2], and by implication these patients only require lipase supplementation. However, earlier loss of lipase was clearly evident in only 2 of the 17 patients reported in that study [2], while a parallel, similar reduction of lipase and trypsin was seen in the other 15 patients. Furthermore, from other reports it can be seen that the level of fat excretion correlates in almost identical manner to maximal stimulated output of lipase or trypsin [1], and even of amylase [24]. Determination of pancreatic enzymes in pure pancreatic juice showed that output of all enzymes measured was lower in CP, and that in most (9/12) patients there was an approximate equal reduction in maximum stimulated output of amylase, chymotrypsin and lipase [25]. Similarly, duodenal incremental output of lipase, amylase, trypsin and chymotrypsin were all equally reduced in 11 CP pts following a duodenally perfused liquid meal [26], while interdigestive output of pancreatic enzymes also appear to be reduced in parallel in CP compared to controls [27]. It can therefore be concluded that deficiency of protease and amylase can be expected to usually accompany lipase deficiency in PEI, and require supplementation. Certainly, the present pig studies also indicate that protein digestibility may be more seriously affected in PEI than generally realized, and moreover that it may be just as difficult to normalize absorption of protein as that of fat, but that the true degree of protein malabsorption can only be seen if measured at the level of the ileum. This confirms recent studies using ^{13}C- ^{15}N- and ^{2}H-labeled proteins combined with urine and fecal collections and a breath test in man, in which it was observed that protein absorption may be far from complete even in healthy controls and that protein malabsorption is probably far more widespread and more severe than is generally recognized in PEI but that the fecal nitrogen test may be too insensitive to demonstrate this [28, 29]. Notwithstanding, in the few studies in which it was measured, even with this test it could be demonstrated that PEI also causes protein malabsorption in most untreated CP patients with steatorrhea [30–34]. Indeed from these studies plus patients cited in these studies in which both intake and excretion of fat and protein were reported (n = 32), the mean coefficient of fat absorption was 52% and of protein was 62%. The observation that mild steatorrhea (91–93% CFA) may precede azotorrhea in CP [29] is as likely to reflect the insensitivity of the fecal nitrogen test as any lack of protease insufficiency.

Lastly, the present study re-emphasizes that malabsorption of starch cannot be determined from fecal samples, due to the avid microbial fermentation of undigested carbohydrates. Indeed, in earlier pig studies it could be shown that there is a load-dependent malabsorption of starch in the ileum in PEI minipigs (i.e. coefficient of ileal starch absorption of 88%, 62% in PEI pigs fed 25%, 55% starch diets respectively, compared to > 97% in controls), despite fecal values of 99% starch absorption in all animals [9]. A similar situation can be expected in CP patients with PEI, and although difficult to quantify, by using the H_2 breath test [35–38] or measuring fecal excretion of short-chain fatty acids [39] it has been possible to indirectly demonstrate that most CP patients with PEI probably suffer from starch malabsorption. Since PEI results in malabsorption of protein, starch and fat, the optimum therapy must improve digestion/absorption of all these nutrients. Therefore, for the present, pancreatin remains the therapy of choice in PEI, although it remains to be tested whether addition of bacterial lipase to pancreatin might improve therapy still further.

References

1. DiMagno EP, Go VLW, Summerskill WHJ. Relations between pancreatic enzyme outputs and malabsorption in severe pancreatic insufficiency. N Engl J Med 1973; 288: 813–5.
2. DiMagno EP, Malagelada JR, Go VLW. Relationship between alcoholism and pancreatic insufficiency. Ann NY Acad Sci 1975; 252: 200–7.
3. Löser C, Fölsch UR. Differentialtherapie der exocrinen Pankreasinsuffizienz – Aktuelle Aspekte und zukünftige Perspektiven der Substitutionstherapie mit Pankreasenzymen. Z Gastroenterol 1995; 33: 715–22.
4. Evenepoel P, Claus D, Geypens B, Maes B, Hiele M, Rutgeerts P, Ghoos Y. Evidence for impaired assimilation and increased colonic fermentation of protein, related to gastric acid suppression therapy. Aliment Pharmacol Ther 1998; 12: 1011–9.
5. Naumann C, Bassler R. Die chemische Untersuchung von Futtermitteln. 3 Aufl. Darmstadt: VDLUFA-Verlag, 1993.
6. Petry H, Rapp W. Zur Problematik der Chromoxidbestimmung in Verdauungsversuchen. Z Tierphysiol 1970; 27: 181–189.
7. Lainé J, Beattie M, LeBel D. Simultaneous kinetic determinations of lipase, chymotrypsin, trypsin, elastase, and amylase on the same microtiter plate. Pancreas 1993; 8: 383–6.
8. Tabeling R, Gregory P, Meil J, Kamphues J. Studies on nutrient digestibilities (precaecal and total) in pancreatic duct ligated pigs and the effects of enzyme substitution. J Anim Physiol a Anim Nutr 1999; 82: 251–63.
9. Gregory PC, Tabeling R, Kamphues J. Growth and digestion in pancreatic duct ligated pigs. Effect of enzyme supplementation. In: Pierzynowski SG, Zabielski R, eds. Biology of the Pancreas in Growing Animals. Elsevier Science BV, 1999: 381–93.
10. Gregory PC. Gastrointestinal pH, motility/transit and permeability in cystic fibrosis. J Paediatr Gastroenterol & Nutr 1996; 23: 513–23.
11. Pierzynowski SG, Sharma P, Sobczyk J, Garwacki S, Barej W, Weström B. Comparative study of antibacterial activity of pancreatic juice in six mammalian species. Pancreas 1993; 8: 546–50.
12. Dierick NA, Vervaeke IJ, Decuypere JA, Henderickx HK. Bacterial protein synthesis in relation to organic matter digestion in the hindgut of growing pigs; contribution of hindgut fermentation to total energy supply and growth performances. J Anim Physiol Anim Nutr 1990; 63: 220–35.
13. Mason VC, Just A. Bacterial activity in the hind-gut of pigs. 1. Its influence on the apparent digestibility of dietary energy and fat. Z Tierphysiol 1976; 36: 301–10.
14. Stephens AM, Cummings JH. The microbial contribution to human faecal mass. J Med Microbiol 1980; 13: 45–56.

15. Botermans JAM, Hedemann MS, Sörhede-Winzill M, Erlanson-Albertsson C, Svendsen J, Evilevitch L, Pierzynowski SG. The effect of feeding time (day versus night) and feeding frequency on pancreatic exocrine secretion in pigs. J Anim Physiol a Anim Nutr 2000; 83: 24–35.
16. Suzuki A, Mizumoto A, Sarr MG, DiMagno EP. Bacterial lipase and high-fat diets in canine exocrine pancreatic insufficiency: a new therapy of steatorrhea? Gastroenterol 1997; 112: 2048–55.
17. Layer P, Go VLW, DiMagno EP. Fate of pancreatic enzymes during small intestinal aboral transit in humans. Am J Physiol 1986; 251: G475–80.
18. Meyer JH, Ohashi H, Jehn D, Thomson JB. Size of liver particles emptied from the human stomach. Gastroenterol 1981; 80: 1489–96.
19. Zerega J, Lerner S, Meyer JH. Duodenal instillation of pancreatin does not abolish steatorrhea in patients with pancreatic insufficiency. Dig Dis Sci 1988; 33: 1245–9.
20. Guercolini R. Mode of action of orlistat. Int J Obes Relat Metab Disord 1997; 21(Suppl 3): S12–23.
21. Carriere F, Renou C, Ransac S, Lopez V, De Caro J, Ferrato F, De Caro A, Lengsfeld H, Verger R, Laugier R. Effect of orlistat on lipolysis following standard test meals. (abstr). Gastroenterol 1999; 116: A543.
22. Adler G, Nelson DK, Katschinski M, Beglinger C. Neurohormonal control of human pancreatic exocrine secretion. Pancreas 1995; 10: 1–13.
23. Kamphues J. Untersuchungen zu Verdauungsvorgängen bei Absetzferkeln in Abhängigkeit von Futtermenge und -zubereitung sowie von Futterzusätzen. Habil.-Schr., Hannover, Tierärztl Hochsch, 1987.
24. Nakamura T, Takebe K, Kudoh K, Ishii M, Imamura K, Kikuchi H, Kasei F, Tandoh Y, Yamada N, Arai Y, Terada A, Machida K. Steatorrhea in Japanese patients with chronic pancreatitis. J Gastroenterol 1995; 30: 79–83.
25. Harada H, Hayashi T, Ono A, Yamamoto N, Ikubo I, Shundo T, Negron A, Mishima K, Kimura I. Analysis of human pure pancreatic juice in chronic pancreatitis and cancer of the pancreas. Gastroenterol Japonica 1978; 13: 461–7.
26. Katschinski M, Schirra J, Bross A, Göke B, Arnold R. Duodenal secretion and fecal excretion of pancreatic elastase-1 in healthy humans and patients with chronic pancreatitis. Pancreas 1997; 15: 191–200.
27. Pieramico O, Domínguez-Muñoz JE, Nelson DK, Böck W, Büchler MW, Malfertheiner P. Interdigestive cycling in chronic pancreatitis: altered coordination among pancreatic secretion, motility and hormones. Gastroenterol 1995; 109: 224–30.
28. Evenepoel P. Study of protein assimilation and fermentation using stable isotope techniques. Thesis for Doctor of Medical Sciences; Catholic University of Leuven, 1997.
29. Evenepoel P, Claus D, Geypens B, Hiele M, Geboes K, Rutgeerts R, Ghoos Y. Amount and fate of egg protein escaping assimilation in the small intestine of humans. Am J Physiol 1999; 277: G935–43.
30. Beazell JM, Schmidt CR, Ivy AC. The diagnosis and treatment of achylia pancreatica. JAMA 1941; 116: 2735–9.
31. Dornberger GR, Comfort MW, Wollaeger EE, Power MH. Total fecal solids, fat and nitrogen. IV. A study of patients with chronic relapsing pancreatitis. Gastroenterol 1948; 11: 691.
32. DiMagno EP, Malagelada JR, Go VLW, Moertel CG. Fate of orally ingested enzymes in pancreatic insufficiency. Comparison of two dosage schedules. N Engl J Med 1977; 296: 1318–22.
33. Van Hoozen CM, Peeke PG, Taubeneck M, Frey CF, Halsted CH. Efficacy of enzyme supplementation after surgery for chronic pancreatitis. Pancreas 1997; 14: 174–80.
34. Regan PT, Malagelada JR, DiMagno EP, Glanzmann SL, Go VLW. Comparative effects of antacids, cimetidine and enteric coating on the therapeutic response to oral enzymes in severe pancreatic insufficiency. N Engl J Med 1977; 297: 854–8.
35. Kerlin P, Wong L, Harris B, Capra S. Rice flour, breath hydrogen, and malabsorption. Gastroenterol 1984; 87: 578–85.
36. Nordgaard I, Rumessen JJ, Gudmand-Høyer E. Assimilation of wheat starch in patients with chronic pancreatitis. Scand J Gastroenterol 1992; 27: 412–6.

37. Keshavarzian AS, Dutta SK. Carbohydrate malabsorption in alcoholic pancreatic insufficiency. The effect of pancreatic enzyme therapy on intestinal transit time. J Clin Gastroenterol 1988; 10: 528–32.
38. Ladas SD, Giorgiotis K, Raptis SA. Complex carbohydrate malabsorption in exocrine pancreatic insufficiency. Gut 1993; 34: 984–7.
39. Nakamura T, Tabeke K, Terada A, Kudoh K, Yamada N, Arai Y, Kikuchi H. Short-chain carboxylic acid in the feces in patients with pancreatic insufficiency. Acta Gastro-Enterol Belg 1993; 56: 326–31.

11.3 Exocrine pancreatic insufficiency in diabetes mellitus

J.-M. Löhr

The endocrine pancreas, i.e. the islets of Langerhans and the exocrine pancreas, the acini, are closely linked to each other both anatomically and physiologically [27]. Derived from different parts of the embryonic mesoderm, the two compartments are intimately related in the mammal organism. The acknowledgement of a functional relationship between the endocrine and exocrine pancreas was long in coming, as was the unraveling of the function of the pancreas *per se*, including the detection of the endocrine cells and their correlation to disease. In recent decades, it has been well recognized that pathological conditions in the exocrine tissue can cause impairment of the endocrine function and vice versa. The pancreatic diseases that may cause diabetes mellitus of more than transient nature include all forms of chronic pancreatitis (alcohol-induced, hereditary, tropical, autoimmune), cystic fibrosis, hemochromatosis, surgical resections, and pancreatic cancer. Impairment of the exocrine function in diabetic patients is also well known.

Historical

The first description of the pancreatic gland was a milestone in medical history. However, we still do not know exactly who the author was. Most likely, it was one of the ancient Greeks, Hippocrates or Herophilus or Eudemus. We know when it might have happened: during the fourth century B.C. They called it παγ κρεας (body of flesh). The term Diabetes mellitus was also coined by the Greeks, presumably during the sixth century B.C. The link between the pancreas and diabetes was left to be found centuries later by Mering und Minkowski, during the 19th century.

At that time, knowledge about diseases connected to the pancreas was spreading. Pemberton (1810) described cachexia in patients having pain and an "altered" pancreas upon autopsy; Kuntzmann (1820) recognized the relation between fatty stools and pancreatic disease. Claessen (1842) in his monograph *"Die Krankheiten der Bauchspeicheldrüse"* suggested that the pancreas was an organ absolutely necessary for life [4].

In the middle of the 19th century, Claude Bernard in his seminal monograph *"Mémoires sur le pancréas"* figured out that pancreatic juice not only emulsified fats but could break them down into fatty acids. He emphasized the universal function of the pancreas for digestion and on the basis of his experiments he asserted that the pancreas had a threefold capacity for digesting sugar, protein, and fat. Together with Corvisart, Bernard (1859) achieved the ethanol extraction of pancreatic juice that could be restituted with water to an active digestive substance encompassing all the properties of natural pancreatic juice. This substance was called *pancreatin* [21].

At about the same time, another pioneer entered the stage. The Dutch physician Fles was called for consultation to a diabetic patient who suffered from severe diarrhea. He stated (1859): *"Ich glaubte aber nun hier einen Fall vor mir zu haben, in dem die Anwendung des Pancreasaftes versucht zu werden verdiente. Die Controversen, die Bernard's Ver-*

suche hervorgerufen, durften mich wenigstens nicht zurückhalten. Die günstige Wirkung des täglichen Gebrauchs von Kalbspancreas auf den Allgemeinzustand war wirklich merkwürdig. Die so schnell vorgeschrittene Abmagerung stand stille; die Extremitäten bekamen wieder eine mehr runde Form." And further on: "*Wir sahen beinahe ein ganzes Jahr lang, wie bei einem Manne, der so gut wie keine Fette und die Eiweisskörper nur theilweise verdaute, der tägliche Gebrauch von Kalbspancreas-Extract alle Fette aufgenommen und die Muskelbündel zum grössten Theile verdaut wurden. Wenn man bedenkt, dass der Kranke sehr grosse Mengen Fett einnahm, welche durch ein Pancreas täglich absorptionsfähig gemacht wurden, und weiter, dass jedesmal, wenn das Mittel ausgesetzt wurde, das Fett uncenweise in den Faeces zurückgefunden wurde, so geht daraus stringent hervor, dass Bernard Recht hatte, als er die hohe Bedeutung des Pancreassaftes für die Fettdigestion, nach Eberle, wiederum hervorhob.*" [6]. Thus the first reported patient ever treated with pancreatic enzymes also suffered from diabetes mellitus. This will be the topic of the following review.

Exocrine pancreatic insufficiency in diabetes mellitus

Insulin is a so-called trophic hormone [45], i.e. it stimulates the intermediate energy metabolism [31, 32]. A question that long puzzled scientists was the purpose of the islets of Langerhans in the pancreas in mammals. Fish and other lower vertebrates have a separate insulin-producing organ [43]. In other words, "why are the islets of Langerhans" [14]? The addition of insulin to isolated pancreatic acini in tissue culture upregulated amylase mRNA [20] (Fig. 11.3-1). Glucose-induced insulin secretion increases the content of amylase (+25%) and total protein (+40%) in rats; making the animals diabetic led to reverse results, i.e. a reduction by 30% [1]. Vascular shortcuts on the capillary level direct the blood from the islets of Langerhans to the surrounding acini [2], thus forming the anatomical basis for what is called the endo-exo axis [15]. Acini in the close vicinity of the islets profit from this intimate relationship and produce more amylase and lipase [1], a phenomenon called the "halo effect". While the vanishing of insulin-producing B-cells is an autoimmune process with insulitis as the morphological hallmark [9] and circulating antibodies against islets (ICA) [25], there is evidence that this autoimmune process may be directed directly against the exocrine pancreas, thus contributing to exocrine pancreatic impairment [19]. Further support for the supposition that the insulin-producing cells and the acini are the cause of exocrine pancreatic insufficiency is given by the fact

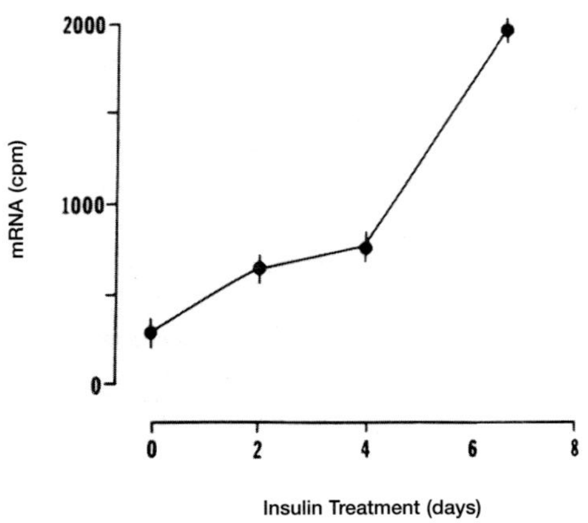

Fig. 11.3-1. Increase in amylase mRNA in isolated rat acini in response to insulin treatment. From [20] with permission of the author.

that bicarbonate secretion is the same in patients with insulin-dependent diabetes mellitus and controls [12]. However, this was recently challenged by a more accurate investigation cannulating the pancreatic duct rather than collecting duodenal juice [16]. It should be emphasized that secondary diabetes may also develop in long-standing chronic pancreatitis; the numbers are said to be as high as 90% in chronic calcifying pancreatitis after disease durations of more than a decade [38]. For that reason, minimal diagnostic tests are mandatory, as outlined below. This may be important since there are some hints that endoscopic therapy in chronic pancreatitis, e.g. stenting or lithotrypsy, may improve not only exocrine but also endocrine pancreatic function [29].

The growth of the pancreas is dependent on age, with increasing volumes during adolescence and reduction in the elderly [39]. In diabetics, the pancreatic gland appears to be smaller than in healthy individuals of the same age (Fig. 11.3-2) [10, 26]. This is the result of an exocrine atrophy [8] that seems to be accentuated around the islets, in particular those lacking insulin-producing B-cells [26] (Fig. 11.3-2). This exocrine atrophy can be quantified: parenchymal volume (both volume density and absolute mass), number of nuclei/0.5 mm^2 and the nucleus-to-cytoplasm ratio are reduced in diabetes by one third to half of the numbers in non-diabetic controls [26].

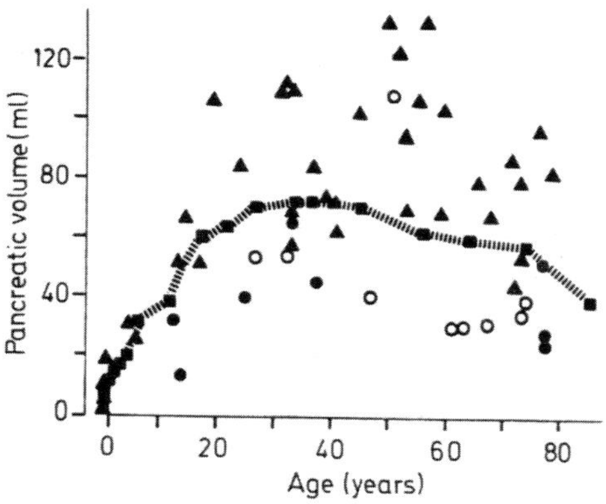

Fig. 11.3-2. Volume of the pancreas in 18 patients wih chronic type 1 diabetes (○ insulin negative; (●) insulin positive) compared with that of 45 control subjects (▲) and the means according to Rössle (■) [39]. Gland volumes are 89.9 ± 22.6 ml (controls) vs. 56.3 ± 16.7 ml (diabetes). From [26] with permission of the author.

Early reports in patients with diabetes mellitus already suggested exocrine pancreatic insufficiency both in type 1 and in type 2 diabetes mellitus [5, 7, 22] (Table 11.3-1). Employing a modified secretin-cholecystokinin test analyzing pure pancreatic juice, pancreatic juice flow, protein output and HCO_3 content were reduced in type 2 diabetics whereas responses to IV glucose for blood sugar levels, insulin and C-peptide were comparable with healthy controls [16].

The availability of an easily manageable pancreatic function test, the fecal elastase-1 test [40, 41], prompted investigations of exocrine pancreatic insufficiency on a broader scale, including patients with diabetes mellitus. These studies revealed that a considerable number of patients with both type 1 and type 2 diabetes mellitus have a reduced fecal elastase-1. The largest study in 526 patients and age- and sex-matched controls revealed that 11.8% of the type 2 diabetics had fecal elastase-1 levels below 100 μg/g stool versus 3.8% of the "healthy" controls [37]. Considering the relative insensitivity of this test for mild to moderate exocrine pancreatic insufficiency [24], about 10% of the patients still

Table 11.3-1. Impairment of exocrine pancreatic function in diabetes mellitus.

Author	Year	Number of patients	Percentage of patients with reduction of exocrine pancreatic function	Test
Type 1 diabetes mellitus (IDDM)				
Pollard [36] (cit. Hardt [13])	1943	13	61	n. a.
Chey [3] (cit. Hardt [13])	1963	47	55	n. a.
Vacca [42] (cit. Hardt [13])	1964	22	73	n. a.
Frier [7]	1976	20	80	SP
Lankisch [22]	1982	53	43	SP
Lorini [30]	1990	21	57	PABA
Hardt [13]	1999	39	74	FE, CT
Wagner (adapt. from Hardt [13])	1999	87	59	FE
Type 2 diabetes mellitus (NIDDM)				
Chey [3]	1963	13	15	n. a.
Vacca [42]	1964	33	73	n. a.
Hardt [13]	1999	77	36	FE, CT
Wagner (cit. Hardt [13])	1999	349	59	FE
Rathmann [37]	1999	526	12	FE
Diabetes mellitus unspecified				
Kitagawa [17]	1997	24	17	SP
Klör [18]	1998	436	42	FE

n. a. = not assessed by [13], SP = secretin-pancreozymin test, FE = fecal elastase-1 test, CT = chymotrypsin

remain with significantly reduced fecal elastase-1 (i.e. below 100 µg/g stool), suggestive of severe exocrine pancreatic insufficiency. This shows that type 2 diabetes mellitus increases the risk of exocrine pancreatic insufficiency (OR 3,8) [37]. However, it was not possible to predict a worse glycemic control of the parameters of exocrine pancreatic impairment from static measurement [30].

Based on these results it was suggested that enzyme substitution in diabetic patients with proven exocrine pancreatic insufficiency – particularly malnourished juvenile type 1 diabetes mellitus – would lead to an increase in body weight (BMI) and normalization of general development; however, large-scale prospective randomized clinical trials are lacking. In a small-scale study, there was only a tendency towards smaller oscillations of blood glucose after pancreatin treatment [11]. Therefore, it is reasonable to suggest that glycemic homeostasis is more easily achieved if resorption of nutrition's becomes more reliable and predictable during exogenous enzyme supplementation [35]. This is supported by a study in patients with diabetes mellitus due to tropical calculous pancreatitis where postprandial plasma glucose levels were reduced after induction of enzyme therapy, as was the glycosylated hemoglobin (HbA_{1c}) [33].

There are no data supporting enzyme supplementation in all diabetic patients regardless of their state of exocrine pancreatic function. It is strongly recommended that in

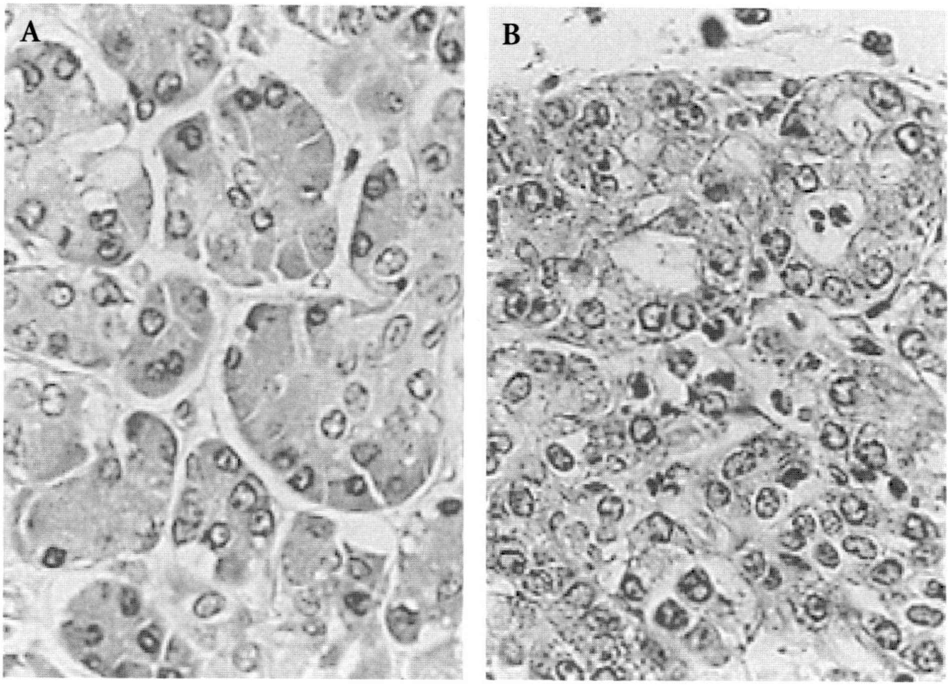

Fig. 11.3-3A, B. Histological appearance (H&E stain) of a normal exocrine pancreas (**A**) and the exocrine pancreas of a patient with long-standing type 1 diabetes (**B**).

all cases of diabetic patients suspected to suffer from exocrine pancreatic insufficiency a minimal diagnostic work-up should be employed after ruling out other more common causes of diarrhea in diabetes mellitus [44]. Isolated reduction of fecal elastase-1 or chymotrypsin for that matter cannot be taken as an imperative rationale for treating diabetic patients with enzyme supplements. Rather, clinical symptoms such as progressive weight loss and steatorrhea should be additionally present [23]. The treatment of exocrine pancreatic insufficiency is then not different from established algorithms [28, 34].

References

1. Adler G, Kern HF. Regulation of exocrine pancreatic secretory process by insulin. Horm Metab Res 1975; 7: 290–6.
2. Bonner-Weir S. The microvasculature of the pancreas, with emphasis on that of the islets of Langerhans. In: Go VLW, DiMagno EP, Gardner JD, Lebenthal E, Reber HA, Scheele GA, eds. The pancreas. Biology, pathobiology, and disease. New York, NY: Raven Press, 1993: 759–68.
3. Chey WY, Shay H, Shuman CR. External pancreatic secretion in diabetes mellitus. Ann Intern Med 1963; 59: 812–21.
4. Claessen H. Die Krankheiten der Bauchspeicheldrüse. Köln, 1842.
5. Domschke W, Tympner F, Domschke S, Demling L. Exocrine pancreatic function in juvenile diabetics. Am J Dig Dis 1975; 20: 309–12.
6. Fles JA. Ein Fall von Diabetes mellitus mit Atrophie der Leber und des Pancreas. Arch f Holländ Beitr Natur- und Heilkunde 1864; III: 187–205.

7. Frier BM, Saunders JH, Wormsley KG, Bouchier IA. Exocrine pancreatic function in juvenile-onset diabetes mellitus. Gut 1976; 17: 685–91.
8. Gepts W. Pathology of the pancreas in juvenile diabetes. Diabetes 1965; 14: 619–33.
9. Gepts W. Islet changes in human diabetes. In: Cooperstein SJ, Watkins D, eds. The islets of Langerhans. London: Academic Press, 1981: 321–56.
10. Gilbeau J, Poncelet V, Libon E, Deruc G, Heller FR. The density, contour and thickness of the pancreas in diabetics. Am J Radiol 1992; 159: 527–31.
11. Glasbrenner B, Malfertheiner P, Kerner W, Scherbaum WA, Ditschuneit H. Einfluß von Pankreatin auf den Diabetes mellitus bei chronischer Pankreatitis. Z Gastroenterol 1990; 28: 275–9.
12. Gröger G, Keller J, Kenter M, Schweflinghaus C, Cherian L, Goebell H, Layer P. Exocrine pancreatic secretion is altered in patients with insulin-dependent diabetes mellitus. Pancreas 19(4), 1999.
13. Hardt PD, Kloer HU. Diabetes mellitus and exocrine pancreatic disease. In: Johnson CD, Imrie CW, eds. Pancreatic disease: towards the year 2000. London: Springer Verlag, 1999: 235–41.
14. Henderson JR. Why are the islets of Langerhans? Lancet 1969; ii.
15. Henderson JR, Daniel PM, Fraser PA. The pancreas as a single organ: the influence of the endocrine upon the exocrine part of the gland. Gut 1981; 22: 158–67.
16. Kim KH, Lee HS, Kim CD, Chun HJ, Song CW, Um SH, Ryu HS, Hyun JH. Evaluation of pancreatic exocrine function using pure pancreatic juice in noninsulin-dependent diabetes mellitus. J Clin Gastroenterol 2000; 31(1): 51–4.
17. Kitagawa M, Naruse S, Ishiguro H, Nakae Y, Kondo T, Hayakawa T. Evaluating exocrine function tests for diagnosing chronic pancreatitis. Pancreas 1997; 15: 402–8.
18. Klör HU. Pankreasinsuffizienz bei Diabetes und Gallensteinleiden. Ärztliche Praxis 1998; 70: 1–4.
19. Kobayashi T, Nakanishi K, Kajio H, Morinaga S, Sugimoto T, Murase T et al. Pancreatic cytokeratin: an antigen of pancreatic exocrine cell autoantibodies in type 1 (insulin-dependent) diabetes mellitus. Diabetologia 1990; 33: 363–70.
20. Korc M, Owerbach D, Quinto C, Rutter WJ. Pancreatic islet-acinar cell interaction: amylase messenger RNA levels are determined by insulin. Science 1981; 213: 351–3.
21. Kuhlmann H. Die Zauberstoffe im Wampenbries. Hannover: Solvay, 1999.
22. Lankisch PG, Manthey G, Otto J, Koop H, Talaulicar M, Willms B et al. Exocrine pancreatic function in insulin-dependent diabetes mellitus. Digestion 1982; 25: 211–6.
23. Lankisch PG, Nauck M. Diabetes und chronische Pankreatitis. Dtsch Ärztebl 2000; 97: A-1894.
24. Lankisch PG, Schmidt I, König H, Knollmann R, Löhr M, Liebe S. Faecal elastase-1: not helpful in diagnosing chronic pancreatitis with mild to moderate exocrine pancreatic insufficiency. Gut 1998; 42: 551–4.
25. Lernmark A. Islet cell antibodies. Diabet Med 1987; 4: 285–92.
26. Löhr M, Klöppel G. Residual insulin positivity and pancreatic atrophy in relation to duration of chronic type 1 (insulin-dependent) diabetes mellitus and microangiopathy. Diabetologia 1987; 30: 757–62.
27. Löhr M, Klöppel G. Topographische Anatomie des Pankreas. In: Riemann JF, Hahn EG, eds. Klinische Gastroenterologie. Stuttgart: Thieme Verlag, 1995: 1090–6.
28. Löhr M, Schneider HT. Exokrine Pankreasinsuffizienz. Bremen: Unimed Verlag, 2000. (in press.)
29. Löhr M, Schneider HT, Farnbacher M, May A, Hahn EG, Fleig WE et al. Endoskopische Therapie von Komplikationen bei der chronischen Pankreatitis. Z Gastroenterol 1997; 35: 437–48.
30. Lorini R, Cortona L, Scotta MS, Melzi d'Eril GV, Severi F. Exocrine pancreatic function in children and adolescents with insulin-dependent diabetes mellitus. Diabetes Res Clin Pract 1990; 8: 263–7.
31. Malaisse WJ. Insulin release: the fuel concept. Diab Metab 1983; 9: 313–20.
32. Malaisse WJ. Regulation, pertubation, and correction of metabolic events in pancreatic islets. Acta Diabetol 1996; 33: 173–9.

33. Mohan V, Poongothai S, Pitchumoni CS. Oral pancreatic enzyme therapy in the control of diabetes mellitus in tropical calculous pancreatitis. Int J Pancreatol 1998; 24: 19–22.
34. Mössner J, Keim V, Niederau C, Buchler M, Singer MV, Lankisch PG et al. Leitlinien zur Therapie der chronischen Pankreatitis. Konsensuskonferenz der Deutschen Gesellschaft für Verdauungs- und Stoffwechselkrankheiten. Halle, 21.–23. November 1996. Z Gastroenterol 1998; 36: 359–67.
35. Ogbonnaya KI, Arem R. Diabetic diarrhea. Pathophysiology, diagnosis, and management. Arch Intern Med 1990; 150: 262–7.
36. Pollard H, Miller L, Brewer W. External secretion of the pancreas and diabetes. Am J Dig Sci 1943; 10: 20–1.
37. Rathmann W, Icks A, Haastert B, Giani G, Curran S, Mitchell J, Hennings S, Wareham NJ. Pancreatic exocrine insufficiency and type 2 diabetes are strongly associated. Diabetes 1999; 42(Suppl 1): A356–97.
38. Raue G, Keim V. Sekundärer Diabetes bei chronischer Pankreatitis. Z Gastroenterol 1999; 37(Suppl 1): 4–9.
39. Rössle R. Beiträge zur Kenntnis der gesunden und kranken Bauchspeicheldrüse. Beitr Pathol Anat Allg Pathol 1921; 69: 163–84.
40. Scheefers-Borchel U, Scheefers H, Arnold R, Fischer P, Sziegoleit A. Pankreatische Elastase-1: Parameter für die chronische und akute Pankreatitis. Lab Med 1992; 16: 427–32.
41. Stein J, Jung M, Bienek U, Scheefers H, Lembcke B, Caspary WF. Fäkale Pankreas-Elastase 1 (E1). Ein neuer zuverlässiger Parameter zur Diagnose der exokrinen Pankreasinsuffizienz. Z Gastroenterol 1993; 31: 543–50.
42. Vacca JB, Henke WJ, Knight WA. The exocrine pancreas in diabetes mellitus. Ann Intern Med 1964; 61: 242–7.
43. van Noorden S, Falkner S. Gut-islet endocrinology – some evolutionary aspects. Invest Cell Pathol 1980; 3: 21–35.
44. von der Ohe M. Diarrhea in patients with diabetes mellitus. Eur J Gastroenterol Hepatol 1995; 7: 730–6.
45. Williams JA, Goldfine ID. The insulin-pancreatic acinar axis. Diabetes 1985; 34: 980–6.

12 Endoscopic treatment of chronic pancreatitis: Impact on long-term outcome

12.1 Pancreatic cysts: Somatostatin and drainage

L. Gullo

Pancreatic pseudocysts are one of the most frequent complications of chronic pancreatitis [1–3]; they often cause persistent pain and require prompt treatment, in order to relieve pain as well as to prevent the development of additional complications [4, 5]. Until recently, the only treatment possible has been surgical drainage or resection of the cyst. In the last few years various alternative procedures have been developed, including echo- or CT-guided external percutaneous drainage and internal drainage by endoscopic techniques [6–9]. All of these procedures, however, can be performed only in specialized centers, are invasive and not without risk [7–9]. In this paper, I will report mainly on my personal experience with the medical treatment with octreotide of pancreatic pseudocysts complicating chronic pancreatitis.

Since pancreatic secretions are the primary constituent of pancreatic pseudocysts [10], recently we investigated the possibility of treating them medically with the somatostatin analog octreotide [11], a potent inhibitor of exocrine pancreatic secretion [12–15]. Seven consecutive patients with chronic pancreatitis who were admitted to our hospital because of persistent abdominal pain were studied. Four patients had an intrapancreatic pseudocyst, 2 a large extrapancreatic one, and the remaining patient had one intra- and one extrapancreatic pseudocyst. The maximal diameter of the pseudocysts ranged from 5 to 14 cm, with an average of 8 cm.

The treatment plan consisted of subcutaneous administration of octreotide (Sandostatin, Sandoz Spa, Milan, Italy) 0.1 mg 3 times daily (every 8 h) for 2 weeks. Since octreotide also suppresses the pancreatic secretion stimulated by a meal [12, 14, 15], patients were permitted a normal diet during treatment. No other drugs were administered concurrently except pancreatic extracts during meals, insulin (in 2 patients), and analgesics as needed.

In 3 patients, there were no significant changes in the size of the pseudocysts during treatment with octreotide. In the remaining 4, however, there was a decrease in size of the pseudocysts which was already evident in the sonogram done after 1 week of treatment. After 2 weeks, pseudocyst size was further decreased to dimensions ranging from 29 to 52%, average 42%, of the initial pretreatment values. In these 4 patients octreotide was then continued for an additional 45 days and the pseudocyst disappeared completely in all of them. In one of these 4 patients the pseudocyst regrew, reaching a new maximal diameter of 11 cm about 3 months later; a second course (50 days) of octreotide was then administered, at the end of which the cyst had completely disappeared.

Regarding pain, octreotide had no significant effect in the 3 patients in whom the size of the pseudocyst remained unchanged. In the 4 patients in whom there was a decrease in size of the pseudocysts during octreotide administration and then a disappearance at the end of treatment, pain disappeared completely within 3–5 days of the start of treatment.

Since this initial study, another one has been performed in which 14 patients with chronic pancreatitis and pancreatic pseudocyst were studied [16]. All had persistent ab-

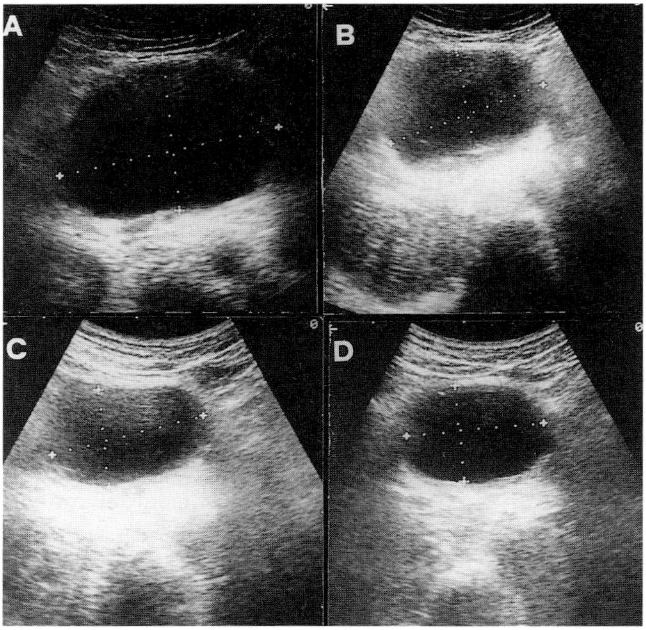

Figure 12.1-1A–D. Abdominal ultrasound of a patient with chronic pancreatitis and persistent pain. **A,** a pseudocyst of the head of the pancreas is seen (diameters, 12 × 8 cm). **B, C,** and **D**: after 1, 2, and 3 weeks, respectively, of octreotide treatment, the size of the pseudocyst progressively decreased (diameters, 7.6 × 5 cm, in D). After 2 months of treatment the pseudocyst disappeared completely.

dominal pain. The maximal diameter of the pseudocysts ranged from 5 to 14 cm, with an average of 7.5 cm. Octreotide was administered at the same dosage as in the previous study. After one week of treatment, octreotide had no significant effect on the size of the pseudocyst and on pain in 6 of the 14 patients and the drug was discontinued. In the remaining 8 patients, pain disappeared completely after 2–5 days of treatment with octreotide. In these 8 patients, repeat ultrasound showed a reduction in the size of the pseudocyst which reached an average of 25%, with respect to the initial size, after 1 week. In all cases, the disappearance of pain occurred concomitant with the reduction in the volume of the pseudocyst. Octreotide administration was then continued for 6–8 weeks, at home, leading to resolution of the pseudocyst in 6 and almost complete resolution in the remaining 2. Figure 12.1-1 shows one of these cases.

In 3 of the 6 patients with pancreatic pseudocyst which did not respond to octreotide treatment, perioperatory wirsungography showed that the pseudocyst communicated with a grossly abnormal Wirsung duct, which was irregularly dilated in the body and tail portion of the gland and markedly narrowed in its cephalic tract.

These results suggest that suppression of pancreatic secretion with octreotide can favorably influence the course of symptomatic pseudocysts complicating chronic pancreatitis. In assessment of these findings, however, the question arises whether the decrease in size of pseudocysts following octreotide administration happened spontaneously rather than as an effect of the peptide. We feel that this was not the case, for several reasons. First of all, spontaneous resolution of pseudocysts is a frequent occurrence in acute pancreatitis, whereas in chronic pancreatitis it is rare [4, 5, 10, 17, 18]. Moreover, it should be noted that spontaneous resolution has been observed mainly in pseudocysts which are asymptomatic, generally small in size (< 4–5 cm) and recently formed [4, 5, 19–21]; none of these traits characterized the pseudocysts treated by us. Second, in our patients the decrease in pseudocyst size occurred promptly following the initiation of treatment, reaching a percent decrease of about 30–40% within 1 week. To our knowledge, there are no data in the literature demonstrating that the size of the pseudocysts, especially if chronic, can decrease spontaneously to this degree in such a brief period of time. Finally, the fact that in 1 patient the pseudocyst reappeared after suspension of octreotide and again disappeared with renewed administration of the peptide is strongly suggestive of a causal effect of octreotide.

From a clinical point of view, it is worth stressing that the decrease in size of the pseudocysts was accompanied by a complete disappearance of pain, even when it had been severe. Similar pain relief is observed when cysts have been successfully drained by surgery or other invasive procedures [2, 4, 21].

The reason why octreotide had no effect on pain in 9 of the 21 patients with pseudocysts is not clear, but it seems related to the fact that there was no reduction in cyst size in these patients. Indeed, in 6 of these in whom a cysto-jejunostomy was performed soon after this study, surgical drainage of the cyst resulted in the immediate disappearance of pain. In 5 of these 6 patients, the pseudocyst communicated with the Wirsung duct which was narrowed in its cephalic tract, distal to the cyst. It is possible that octreotide was ineffective in reducing the size of the cyst in these patients because of this obstacle to the flow of pancreatic juice into the duodenum.

The external percutaneous drainage of pancreatic pseudocysts has been utilized mainly in the past [6, 22–25]. Several studies have been published on this therapeutic technique. However, the results varied considerably [6, 22–25]. Moreover, in most of these studies there is a clear preponderance of pseudocysts due to acute pancreatitis and it is difficult to draw conclusions concerning the pseudocysts due to chronic pancreatitis. Generally, only few patients with this last disease have been treated, the clinical characteristics of the pseudocysts and of the patients were usually not well defined, and there are no long-term controls of the results. The reported percentages of favorable results in patients with chronic pancreatitis vary greatly, with a mean of about 50% [22–25]. At present, this external percutaneous drainage is used mainly in pseudocysts due to acute pancreatitis while it has been almost abandoned in pseudocysts due to chronic pancreatitis.

In conclusion, my experience [11, 16] indicates that octreotide can be useful in the treatment of symptomatic pseudocysts complicating chronic pancreatitis, at least in a subgroup of patients in whom the pseudocyst does not communicate with the Wirsung duct. It should be underlined that this treatment is quite simple: the peptide is administered by subcutaneous injection and patients may eat normally, so treatment could even be carried out at home. The treatment with percutaneous drainage of the cystic cavity is of limited value in patients with chronic pancreatitis and, at present, it is not utilized.

References

1. Sarles H, Sarles JC, Camatte R et al. Observations on 205 confirmed cases of acute pancreatitis, recurring pancreatitis, and chronic pancreatitis. Gut 1965; 6: 545–59.
2. Gullo L, Costa PL, Labò G. Chronic pancreatitis in Italy. Aetiological, clinical and histological observations based on 253 cases. Rendic Gastroenterol 1977; 9: 97–104.
3. Ammann RW, Akovbiantz A, Largiader F, Schueler G. Course and outcome of chronic pancreatitis. Longitudinal study of a mixed medical-surgical series of 245 patients. Gastroenterology 1984; 86: 820–8.

4. Bradley EL, Clements JL, Gonzalez AC. The natural history of pancreatitic pseudocysts: A unified concept of management. Am J Surg 1979; 137: 135–9.
5. Crass RA, Way LW. Acute and chronic pancreatic pseudocysts are different. Am J Surg 1981; 142: 660–3.
6. Van Sonnenberg E, Ferrucci J, Mueller P, Wittomberg J, Simeone J. Percutaneous drainage of abscesses and fluid collections: Technique, results and applications. Radiology 1982; 142: 1–10.
7. Sahel J, Bastid C, Pellat B, Schurgers P, Sarles H. Endoscopic cystoduodenostomy of cysts of chronic calcifying pancreatitis: A report of 20 cases. Pancreas 1987; 2: 447–53.
8. Cremer M, Deviere J, Engelholm L. Endoscopic management of cysts and pseudocysts in chronic pancreatitis: Long-term follow-up after 7 years of experience. Gastrointest Endosc 1989; 35: 1–9.
9. Grace PA, Williamson RCN. Modern management of pancreatic pseudocysts. Br J Surg 1993; 80: 573–81.
10. Sarles JC, Sahel J, Sarles H. Cysts and pseudocysts of the pancreas. In: Howat HT, Sarles H, eds. The Exocrine Pancreas. London: Saunders, 1979: 443–83.
11. Gullo L, Barbara L. Treatment of pancreatic pseudocysts with octreotide. Lancet 1991; 338: 540–1.
12. Creutzfeldt W, Lembcke B, Folsch UR, Schleser S. Effect of somatostatin analogue (SMS 201–995, Sandostatin) on pancreatic secretion in humans. Am J Med 1987; 82 (Suppl 5B): 49–54.
13. Williams ST, Woltering EA, O'Dorisio TM, Fletcher WS. Effect of octreotide acetate on pancreatic exocrine function. Am J Surg 1989; 157: 459–62.
14. Misumi A, Shiratori K, Lee KY, Barkin JS, Chey WY. Effects of SMS 201–995, a somatostatin analogue, on the exocrine pancreatic secretion and gut hormone release in dogs. Surgery 1988; 103: 450–5.
15. Gullo L, Biliotti G, Pezzilli R, Di Stefano M, Ancona D. Effect of octreotide (SMS 201–995) on meal-stimulated pancreatic secretion in three patients with external pancreatic fistula. Am J Gastroenterol 1991; 86: 892–4.
16. Gullo L, Pezzilli R, De Giorgio R. Effect of octreotide on pain in patients with chronic pancreatitis. Dig Surg 1996; 13: 465–8.
17. Sarles H, Adler G, Dani R et al. Classification of pancreatitis and definition of pancreatic diseases. Digestion 1989; 43: 234–6.
18. Ephgrane K, Hunt JL. Presentation of pancreatic pseudocysts: Implications for timing of surgical intervention. Am J Surg 1986, 151: 742–53.
19. Beebe DS, Bubrick MP, Onstad GR, Hitchcock CR. Management of pancreatic pseudocysts. Surg Gynecol Obstet 1984; 159: 562–4.
20. O'Malley VP, Cannon JP, Postier RG. Pancreatic pseudocysts. Cause, therapy, and results. Am J Surg 1985; 150: 680–2.
21. Yeo C, Bastidas JA, Lynch-Nyhan A, Fishman EK, Zinner MJ, Cameron JL. The natural history of pancreatic pseudocysts documented by computed tomography. Surg Gynecol Obstet 1990; 170: 411–7.
22. Karlson K, Martin EC, Fankuchen EI, Mattern RE, Schultz RW, Casarella WJ. Percutaneous drainage of pancreatic pseudocysts and abscesses. Radiology 1982; 142: 619–24.
23. Van Sonnenberg E, Wittich GR, Casola G et al. Percutaneous drainage of infected and noninfected pancreatic pseudocysts: experience in 101 case. Radiology 1989; 170: 757–61.
24. Gumaste UV, Dave PB. Editorial: pancreatic pseudocyst drainage – the needle or the scalpel? J Clin Gastroenterol 1991; 13: 500–5.
25. Di Candio G, Giulianotti P, Mosca F. Terapia delle pseudocisti pancreatiche: Indicazioni e risultati del trattamento mini-invasivo. In: Di Candio G, Giulianotti P, Mosca F, eds. Pancreas: Imaging diagnostico e interventistico. Poletto Editore, 1996: 227–60.

12.2 Endoscopic cyst drainage

R. Laugier

Introduction

During the course of chronic pancreatitis a cystic collection develops in one case out of five and usually in the relatively early stages of the disease. In only a minority of cases (7 to 8% of patients) those cysts resolve spontaneously [1]. All the other cysts will persist and are at risk of developing complications such as infection, compression of neighboring structures or organs hemorrhage, or rupture into anatomical cavities (pleural or peritoneal). Bradley et al. demonstrated long time ago that the rate of complications of those cysts increases with the duration of the observation time [2]. Thus among uncomplicated cysts which do not tend to resolve spontaneously, only small cysts in the head are not a mandatory indication for treatment. It should be pointed out that although they may be of small diameter, cysts in the tail of the pancreas are very often associated during their evolutive course with a thrombosis of the splenic vein.

The more serious complication of chronic pancreatitis cysts appears to be the hemorrhage which occurs in up to 10% of patients [3]. It's certainly not to be treated endoscopically. In fact, before having the temptation of treating endoscopically a cyst one has to check if signs of recent hemorrhage are present: acute abdominal pain with acute increase in cystic diameter, presence of a hyperechoic pattern of the cystic content or in some cases presence of pulsatility of the cystic wall. Those cases are to be treated either surgically or thanks to an endovascular approach (embolization): indeed the sudden decompression of the cystic content by a cystoenterostomy would enhance the bleeding phenomenon and thus enhance the morbidity and the risk of mortality, which is already very high in such condition.

In only some very special cases has it been possible to treat such an acute hemorrhage thanks to a combined angiographic and endoscopic method [4].

By contrast to hemorrhage, the other evolutive complications of the cysts are good indications for an endoscopic treatment. All sorts of compressions induced by the cystic development are fairly well treated thanks to endoscopy. This is the case for the main bile duct or the main pancreatic duct stenosis associated with the cyst as it is for some gastric antral compression or even some cases of recent portal segmental splenic hypertension. The spontaneous infection of the cystic content can be responsible for very serious generalized infection associated with a risk of septic shock. In those conditions, having to cope with very severely ill patients, the endoscopic drainage represents a very good alternative to surgical procedures.

The rupture within the digestive tract is in fact a way of spontaneous healing of some cysts. When the rupture develops into the pleural or the peritoneal cavity it is responsible for the development of a pleural or peritoneal collection with an amylase-, lipase-rich fluid content. For long time those complications have been considered as systematic surgical indications; now some cases have been reported to be treated successfully thanks to endoscopy [5, 6].

Technique of endoscopic procedures

The first endoscopic procedure which has been reported dealt in 1982 with the transgastric drainage of a cyst developed in the body of the pancreas [8]. This technique has later been described in more detail by Henkinbrand et al. [9], by Liguory et al. [10] in 1987 and Cremer et al. in 1989 [11]. A few years later the same technique initially described as a form of cystogastrostomy has been described for a duodenal approach [12, 13]. These procedures require a clear bulging of the cyst into the gastric or the duodenal cavity in order to ensure a very short distance between the digestive and the cystic walls. The endosonographic picture in those anatomical conditions clearly demonstrates that this distance is lower than 10 mm and it ensures safety of the procedure. In those conditions one understands very easily that cysts of the tail rarely give access to an endoscopic direct drainage! At the point of the maximal cyst bulging, the access to the cyst is obtained with the diathermy needle or some special device adapted to that specific purpose. We developed some years ago a special diathermy needle which allowed to remove the diathermic part of the device and to keep the catheter deep inside the cyst in such a way that after aspiration of some part of the cystic fluid (for biochemical and bacteriological analysis) cyst opacification becomes possible. Thereafter, another guide wire may be introduced within the catheter and thus within the cyst in order to perform a durable cystogastrostomy or duodenostomy. The "microknife" from Boston Scientific Company is perfectly adapted to this kind of procedure. Once the true communication between the cyst and the digestive tract has been created one used to introduce a papillotome in order to perform a relatively large cystoenterostomy. Obviously, the risk of such large communication was perforation and hemorrhage. This is because of those two risks that we now perform smaller cystoenterostomies using rather than a diathermic needle the dilation of the puncture thanks to a hydraulic inflatable balloon up to 6 or 8 mm in diameter. The risk of bleeding seems to be very much decreased in our experience by doing so.

Keeping the same guide-wire in position one introduces now one or two double pigtail plastic endoprosthesis of diameters ranging from 6 up to 12 French. In all publications the technical success rate appears better for the cystoduodenostomy than for the cystogastrostomy which is consequently associated with a higher complication rate [11–15]. The role of endosonography has been recently emphasized for minimizing as much as possible the risk of both perforation and hemorrhage [16–18]. In our experience endosonography was not only useful for predicting as best the risk of perforation but also for choosing the best point to be punctured and for extending indications of endoscopic puncture to some cysts which did not bulge into the duodenum although the distance between the walls was less than 5 mm [19]. This procedure has also been performed completely in one single step thanks to a large channel echoendoscope [21, 22]. Although this approach of direct cystoenterostomy seems to be easy (which is definitely not the case for the cystogastrostomy) it appears to be associated with some mortality due to the hemorrhagic risk [15, 24, 25]. One should note that reported cases of mortality are in the early experience of the technique. In all more recent reported series the mortality appears to be nil while morbidity ranges from 3 to 11% of patients [11–13, 25–27]. Cyst relapse seems to be lower than 20% for cystogastrostomy and less than 10% for cystoduodenostomy.

More recently, one has tried to reach the cystic cavity indirectly through the papilla and the ductal system [29–32]. A prerequisite of the technique is to demonstrate the patency of the cysto-ductal communication. This is easily documented by retrograde pancreatography when contrast medium leaves the pancreatic ductal system to fill the cyst cavity. Once such a communication has been documented one can introduce selectively a guide-wire into the main pancreatic duct to cannulate this communication with the tip of the guide-wire. Usually, a selective endoscopic pancreatic sphincterotomy may be required. The guide-wire having been introduced deeply into the cystic cavity, the communication has to be dilated using either the bougienage technique or rather a hydraulic inflatable balloon. At the end of the process, a double pig-tail endoprosthesis has to be introduced through the papilla into the cyst; its length between the 2 pig-tails has to be adapted to the distance between the cyst communication and the papilla. The role of this stent inserted after dilation of the communication is to keep this communication opened until the complete cyst healing. The duration of the stenting has thus to be adapted to the cyst diameter, its content and above all its evolution during drainage followed by ultrasonography or in some cases by computed tomography. This technique allows to drain all sorts of cysts whatever their size and their location (head, body or even tail) as long as communication with the ductal system may be documented. This elegant technique which does not require a diathermy knife has in our opinion to be attempted first before other approaches because it has a very low risk: no mortality so far has been reported [11–13, 26–32]. The morbidity is very low, usually reported between 2 and 7% and is mainly due to infection which in fact has to be treated eventually soon by a new procedure. Long-term results agree on a recurrence rate lower than 12% of all cases. In fact, the major problem of this technique is that it is not always feasible: stricture or stones between the papilla and cyst communication has to be first treated and above all, communication between the cyst and the ductal system is not always documented or in some cases documented but not catheterized by the guide-wire leading thus to a technical failure. It is very difficult to precisely appreciate the rate of unfeasibility of this technique in the literature: with growing experience it seems that the percentage of success rate is more than 3 cases out of 4. In the long-term prospect our opinion is that the late recurrence seems to be decreased by an association with a prolonged calibration of the main pancreatic duct with stents. So after the healing of the cyst we carry on with a complete clearance and treatment of main pancreatic duct stenosis downstream to the communication.

Conclusion

The endoscopic approach of cysts during chronic pancreatitis has to be attempted in all symptomatic cysts and in cysts located in the tail in the prevention of venous complications. The only definite contra-indication of the technique is the intra-cystic hemorrhage; all the other complications of cysts are good indications for endoscopic treatment. Although it has been described and generalized later, the first approach in our opinion is the indirect transpapillary cystoduodenostomy which is very often feasible and which appears to be particularly safe with very good short- and long-term results. If this approach is not anatomically possible one should attempt a direct approach either through the stomach or the duodenum according to the location and the size of the cystic cavity. Both those approaches give excellent results with a very low recurrence rate but in case of chronic pancreatitis it is generally considered that cystogastrostomy has slightly higher morbidity and mortality than cystoduodenostomy. One should always keep in mind that if those endoscopic techniques appear hazardous, if good anatomical conditions are not present or if there is contra-indication given by a preliminary endosonography it is better to refer the patients to a surgeon. This is also the case when we have to cope with an early recurrence of the cyst.

References

1. Bourliere M, Sarles H. Pancreatic cysts and pseudocysts associated with acute and chronic pancreatitis. Dig Dis Sci 1989; 34: 343–8.
2. Bradley EL III. Complications in chronic pancreatitis. Surg Clin North Am 1989; 481–97.
3. Gradacz TR, Trunkey D, Kiefer RF. Visceral vessel erosion associated with pancreatitis. Arch Surg 1978; 113: 1438–40.
4. Elton E, Howell DA, Amberson SM, Dykes TA. Combined angiograpyhic and endoscopic management of bleeding pancreatic pseudoaneurysms. Gastrointest Endosc 1997 Dec; 46 (6): 544–9.
5. Traverso LW, Kozarek RA. Interventional management of peripancreatic fluid collections. Surg Clin North Am 1999 Aug; 79 (4): 745–57.
6. Hastier P, Rouquier P, Buckley M, Simler JM, Dumas R, Delmont JP. Endoscopic treatment of wirsungo-cysto-pleural fistula. Eur J Gastroenterol Hepatol 1998 Jun; 10 (6): 527–9.
7. Nordback I, Sand J. The value of the endoscopic pancreatogram in peritoneal or pleural pancreatic fistula. Int Surg 1996 Apr–Jun; 81 (2): 184–6.
8. Bahari HM, Abdullah I. Endoscopic transgastric drainage of pseudopancreatic cyst. Med J Malaysia 1982 Dec; 37 (4): 316–7.
9. Henkinbrant A, Davaux A. Drainage of a pancreatic pseudocyst using endoscopic cystogastrostomy. Acta Gastroenterol Belg 1986 May–Jun; 49 (3): 341–7.
10. Liguory CL, Lefebvre JF, Dumont JL, Canard JM, Bonnel D. Dérivation kysto-digestive endoscopique. A propos de 10 cas. Chirurgie 1987; 113 (7–8): 726–32.
11. Cremer M, Deviere J, Engelholm L. Endoscopic management of cysts and pseudocysts in chronic pancreatitis: long-term follow-up after 7 years of experience. Gastrointest Endosc 1989 Jan–Feb; 35 (1): 1–9.
12. Sahel J. Endoscopic cysto-enterostomy of cysts of chronic calcifying pancreatitis. Z Gastroenterol 1990 Mar; 28 (3): 170–2.
13. Dohmoto M, Rupp KD. Endoscopic drainage of pancreatic pseudocysts. Surg Endosc 1992 May–Jun; 6 (3): 118–24.
14. Binmoeller KF, Seifert H, Soehendra N. Endoscopic pseudocyst drainage: a new instrument for simplified cystoenterostomy. Gastrointest Endosc 1994 Jan–Feb; 40 (1): 112.
15. Sahel J. Endoscopic drainage of pancreatic cysts. Endoscopy 1991 May; 23 (3): 181–4.
16. Grimm H, Binmoeller KF, Soehendra N. Endosonography – guided drainage of a pancreatic pseudocyst. Gastrointest Endosc 1992 Mar–Apr; 38 (2): 170–1.
17. Etzkorn KP, Deguzman LJ, Holderman WH, Abu-Hammour A, Schlesinger PK, Harig JM, Watkins JL. Endoscopic drainage of pancreatic pseudocysts: patient selection and evaluation of the outcome by endoscopic ultrasonography. Endoscopy 1995 May; 27 (4): 329–33.
18. Binmoeller KF, Soehendra N. Endoscopic ultrasonography in the diagnosis and treatment of pancreatic pseudocysts. Gastrointest Endosc Clin N Am 1995 Oct; 5 (4): 805–16.
19. Fockens P, Johnson TG, van Dullemen HM, Huibregtse K, Tytgat GN. Endosonographic imaging of pancreatic pseudocysts before endoscopic transmural drainage. Gastrointest Endosc 1997 Nov; 46 (5): 412–6.
20. Gerolami R, Giovanni M, Laugier R. Endoscopic drainage of pancreatic pseudocysts guided by endosonography. Endoscopy 1997 Feb; 29 (2): 106–8.
21. Giovannini M, Bernardini D, Seitz JF. Cystogastrostomy entirely performed under endosonography guidance for pancreatic pseudocyst: results in six patients. Gastrointest Endosc 1998 Aug; 48 (2): 200–3.

22. Pfaffenbach B, Langer M, Stabenow-Lohbauer U, Lux G. Endosonography controlled transgastric drainage of pancreatic pseudocysts. Dtsch Med Wochenschr 1998 Nov 27; 123 (48): 1439–42.
23. Seifert H, Dietrich C, Schmitt T, Caspary W, Wehrmann T. Endoscopic ultrasound-guided one-step transmural drainage of cystic abdominal lesions with a large channel echo endoscope. Endoscopy 2000 Mar; 32 (3): 255–9.
24. Donnelly PK, Lavelle J, Carr-Locke D. Massive haemorrhage following endoscopic transgastric drainage of pancreatic pseudocyst. BR J Surg 1990 Jul; 77 (7): 758–9.
25. Kozarek RA, Brayko CM, Harlan J, Sanowski RA, Cintora I, Kovac A. Endoscopic drainage of pancreatic pseudocysts. Gastrointest Endosc 1985 Oct; 31 (5): 322–7.
26. Huibregtse K, Schneider B, Vrij AA, Tytgat GNJ. Endoscopic pancreatic drainage in chronic pancreatitis. Gastrointest Endosc 1989; 34: 9–15.
27. Vitale GC, Lawhon JC, Larson GM, Harrell DJ, Reed Jr DN, Macleod S. Endoscopic drainage of the pancreatic pseudocyst. Surgery 1999 Oct; 126 (4): 616–21.
28. Froeschle G, Meyer-Pannwitt U, Brueckner M, Hennebruns D. A comparison between surgical, endoscopic and percutaneous management of pancreatic pseudocysts – long-term results. Acta Chir Belg 1993 May–Jun; 93 (3): 102–6.
29. Kozarek RA, Ball TJ, Patterson DJ, Freeny PC, Ryan JA, Traverso LW. Endoscopic transpapillary therapy for disrupted pancreatic duct and peripancreatic fluid collections. Gastroenterology 1991 May; 100 (5): 1362–70.
30. Barthet M, Bugallo M, Moreira LS, Bastid C, Sastre B, Sahel J. Management of cysts and pseudocysts complicating chronic pancreatitis. A retrospective study of 143 patients. Gastroenterol Clin Biol 1993; 17 (4): 270–6.
31. Pinkas H, Dolan RP, Brady PG. Successful endoscopic transpapillary drainage of an infected pancreatic pseudocyst. Gastrointest Endosc 1994 Jan–Feb; 40 (1): 97–9.
32. Figueira A, Colleoni Neto R, Jorge Jr ME, Caetano Jr EM, Ferraro JR, Trivino T. Transduodenal endoscopic drainage of pancreatic pseudocysts and peripancreatic collection. Rev Assoc Med Bras 1994 Jul–Sep; 40 (3): 202–6.

12.3 Endoscopic therapy: Common bile duct stenting

A. Eickhoff, J. F. Riemann

Abstract

Benign strictures of the bile ducts with their associated clinical signs of cholestasis, cholangitis and secondary biliary cirrhosis remain a challenging problem for gastroenterologists and surgeons. The overall incidence of common bile duct strictures due to chronic pancreatitis is reported to be approximately 10–30%. Higher incidences were demonstrated by adopting other criteria for diagnosis, such as laboratory or cholangiography findings. Most of the common bile duct strictures are not clinically manifest and therefore require no therapy. On the other hand, patients with persistent or recurrent jaundice and cholangitis are in danger of developing secondary biliary cirrhosis. This subgroup of patients need adequate treatment, either from surgery or endoscopy. The implantation of biliary plastic prostheses for other causes of benign bile strictures is well established. The exact role of *endoscopic stenting* of biliary strictures associated with chronic pancreatitis has not been clearly defined. There seems to be a therapeutic benefit for short-term treatment but medium-term and long-term outcome remains questionable. However, *endoscopic stenting* should be applied as initial therapy before surgery with its inherent higher morbidity and mortality. Additionally, it can be the definitive therapy for older and morbid patients or cases with complete stricture regression after stent removal. Results of metal prosthesis in this benign disease are limited and need further evaluation. Adequate management is therefore based more on a "team approach" combining treatment modalities from gastroenterology and surgery.

Introduction

The etiology of benign common bile duct stenosis is often associated with open or laparoscopic cholecystectomy, pancreatic diseases, sclerosing cholangitis or local infection [11]. Biliary strictures occur frequently in the natural course of chronic pancreatitis. However, they are clinically inapparent in most patients. The incidence has been described to be 10–30% of patients with chronic pancreatitis [7]. The great variability of incidence, between 3 and 45%, is due to the definition criteria adopted by different authors [10]. The pathogenesis of this type of stricture is frequently related to:

- compression by a pseudocyst,
- compression due to an edematous inflamed pancreatic head,
- periductal inflammation and subsequent fibrotic or scarred bile ducts.

Long-term complications may lead to recurrent chronic cholangitis in up to 9% and secondary biliary cirrhosis in about 7% of patients. Sepsis due to pyogenic liver abscess has also been described in a number of patients [10]. The indication for biliary drainage procedure, either by surgical or endoscopic approach, seems to be evident in symptomatic patients. Surgical drainage was the treatment of choice for biliary obstruction due to chronic pancreatitis for many years. However, surgical drainage has considerable mortality and morbidity rates, especially for patients with significant comorbidities like liver cirrhosis [13]. This led to the development of endoscopic drainage procedures at the beginning of the 1990s. Endoscopic biliary stenting is an alternative to the surgical approach, particularly for initial treatment of jaundice and cholangitis due to common bile duct stenosis. The outstanding position of endoscopic drainage is associated with its significantly lower mortality rate and its less invasive character. Therefore it is a desirable definitive treatment option for a subgroup of patients [1, 14]. However, endoscopic stent therapy has crucial limitations. Stent dysfunction and clogging with subsequent cholangitis occur frequently in the long-term follow-up. Elective or "programmed" stent exchange is necessary to prevent this complication. The beneficial effects of endoscopic drainage procedures and particularly their long-term outcome have been questioned. Today, the question of adequate management of *biliary stricture* due to chronic pancreatitis is still a point of discussion between surgeons and gastroenterologists [4, 7, 10].

Possible indications for biliary stenting

There is no question that endoscopic drainage is the treatment of choice for acute cholangitis. The aim of biliary stenting in patients with persistent or recurrent cholangitis is the prevention of secondary biliary cirrhosis. Additionally, patients with persistent obstructive jaundice are candidates for drainage procedures [9]. However, most patients with high-grade stricture of the common bile duct are asymptomatic only with moderate elevated cholestatic serum parameters. This group of patients do not need any invasive drainage, either by endoscopic or surgical approach. Most experts recommend drainage procedures only in symptomatic patients (acute cholangitis, persistent jaundice), regardless of the radiographic appearance of the bile ducts. A study by Stahl et al. approved this treatment plan; they found that most asymptomatic patients with verified common bile duct stricture due to chronic pancreatitis do quite well in the long-term outcome without any invasive drainage procedures [15].

In a time when new imaging techniques like magnetic resonance cholangiopancreatography belong to the diagnostic armamentarium of gastroenterologists, every indication of invasive diagnostic or therapeutic procedure has to be reconsidered regarding its pros and cons for the patients' outcome. Secondly, we should not forget that patients with chronic pancreatitis, although they usually present comorbidities, suffer from a potentially benign disease and should therefore not be treated in the same way as patients with malignant *biliary stricture* and its reduced prognosis. It is technically easy to implant an endoscopic stent in a *biliary stricture* for drainage. However, we should never forget the possible morbidity related to stent clogging, cholangitis and biliary sepsis. An adequate and individual indication is therefore strictly recommended for all patients [6, 7, 10].

Five indications for endoscopic biliary stenting are established worldwide:

1. to treat symptoms of cholestasis,
2. to drain infected bile,
3. to obtain time for regression of reversible inflammatory process or pseudocyst,
4. to prevent secondary biliary cirrhosis,
5. pain differentiation (due to biliary obstruction vs. pancreatitic pain).

Technique of biliary stenting

The first step in the diagnostic and therapeutic algorithm of biliary strictures after anamnesis and physical examination is percutaneous ultrasound. In case of biliary obstruction with a dilated common bile duct and obstructive jaundice, diagnostic ERCP is recommended. The aim of all diagnostic work-up is to clarify the etiology of the stenosis. It is important to distinguish benign biliary strictures from malignant strictures caused by a pancreatic carcinoma on top of chronic pancreatitis or a bile duct malignancy. The differential diagnosis may remain difficult even with modern imaging techniques; therefore a short-term surveillance program is strictly recommended for these patients. For management of patients with benign biliary strictures, standard selective deep cannulation of the bile duct is necessary. Usually, biliary sphincterotomy to facilitate repeated cannulations is unavoidable. Once the distal common bile duct is entered, traversing the stricture with a guide wire is necessary to insert either a plastic or metal transpapillary endoprosthesis. In very tight strictures, small 5–7 French prostheses may be the largest diameter that could be passed through the stenosis. Further dilatation to a size of 10 French or more with insertion of larger stents should be attained in the follow-up. Whether biliary stents should be changed regularly every 3 to 4 months or only "on demand" is a matter of debate [3, 6, 10]. We think that an elective exchange of biliary stents is connected with a significant lower rate of clogging, cholangitis and morbidity and therefore more appropriate for the patients. The role of metal mesh-stents for benign diseases in gastroenterology remains uncertain not only for this type of benign bile duct strictures but for others as well [2, 5]. Overall, endoscopic biliary stenting offers a convincing non-operative treatment with low morbidity and mortality and with excellent short-term results. As of now, there are seven published studies about *endoscopic stenting* of bile duct strictures due to chronic pancreatitis with plastic prosthesis, one abstract and one study addressing the use of *metal stents*. In our study, 38 patients had been treated with polyethylene stents and 5 patients with *metal stents*.

Use of polyethylene stents ("plastic")

As mentioned above, there are seven studies evaluating the effect of plastic prosthesis in biliary strictures caused by chronic pancreatitis [1, 3, 4, 6, 8, 14, 17]. The first paper was published by Deviere et al. in 1990. From 1982 to 1988 they investigated 25 patients with biliary stenosis and symptomatic cholestasis (obstructive jaundice, cholangitis, liver abscess). They used 10-French prosthesis and stent insertion was technically successful in all patients. Improvement of cholestasis was achieved shortly after stent implantation in all patients. Complete follow-up was possible in 19 patients; the median follow-up time was 14 months. Complications occurred in 8% of the patients, usually stent migration and stent clogging. The group preferred the stent exchange "on demand", this became necessary after a mean time of 6.5 months. Overall, only 3 patients remained asymptomatic after stent removal, so that the long-term success rate was 12%. Sixteen patients had to be treated with permanent biliary stenting and 6 of these patients underwent surgical therapy including biliodigestive bypass [3].

Four years later, Barthet et al. reported the outcome of 19 patients with symptomatic biliary obstruction and endoscopic therapy. This group favored elective stent exchange every 4 months and saw complications in two patients (stent migration, duodenal ulceration). Stent insertion was successful in all patients and was carried out over 10 (4–22) months. However, after follow-up of 18 months only 2 patients (10%) had complete clinical, biological and radiological recovery. Complete failure of the therapy occurred in 6 patients. The authors concluded that endoscopic stent therapy for bile duct strictures due to chronic pancreatitis is only a temporary approach although short-term results seem to be excellent [1]. The biggest study until now covered 58 patients and was published by Smits et al. in 1996. They adopted a multidisciplinary approach with subsequent endoscopic or surgical treatment after initial stent insertion. Stent placement was successful in all patients and was followed by rapid improvement of cholestatic symptoms. The complication rate was 9% and the median follow-up was 49 months. Regression of the stenosis was achieved in 16 patients after a median time of 10 months and the stents were permanently removed. In the follow-up of 46 months, no recurrent stenosis was noted in these 16 patients. Twenty-six of the patients had persistent stricture and required continued biliary stenting over 19 months. Improvement of cholestatic symptoms was achieved in all 26 patients. In the case of frequent stent-related complications, duodenal stenosis or chronic pancreatic pain, the indication for surgery was fulfilled. A surgical approach was necessary in 16 patients (28%) after a median time of stenting of 8.5 months. The remarkable early morbidity for these patients was 37.5%, but 15 of 16 patients experienced long-term improvement of their symptoms in the follow-up. The group summarized that although *endoscopic stenting* as a definitive approach was successful in more than one-quarter of their patients, it should be reserved only for temporary treatment or patients with contraindications for surgery [14]. Smaller studies published by Itani et al. and Kiehne et al. demonstrated similar results with long-term improvement rates from 10 to 25% [6, 8].

One study by Vitale et al. reported successful *endoscopic stenting* with regression of stenosis in 20 of their 25 patients. This remarkable outcome is probably due in part to the selection of patients with less severe chronic pancreatitis, different etiology of the disease and earlier stenting. In addition, this group actually presented medium-term (32 months) and not long-term results of endoscopic stent therapy [17]. A recently published paper by a German group revealed long-term success of *endoscopic stenting* of 32% in their 31 patients. After a median stenting-time of 10 months, there was a remarkable reduction in the bile duct diameter from 19.5 mm to 14.2 mm in 17 of 31 patients. Patients with complete regression of stenosis did not develop jaundice in a follow-up of 28 months. Overall, only 4 of the 31 patients (13%) presented complete regression in the

Table 12.3-1. Outcome of patients with polyethylene prostheses.

Author	n	Technical success	Long-term success	Complication rate	Follow-up (months)
Deviere 1990 [3]	25	100%	3 (12%)	8%	14
Barthet 1994 [1]	19	100%	2 (10%)	11%	18
Smits 1996 [14]	58	100%	16 (28%)	9%	46
Kiehne 2000 [8]	14	100%	2 (16%)	nm	52
Vitale 2000 [17]	25	100%	20 (80%)	20%	32
Farnbacher 2000 [4]	31	94%	10 (32%)	14%	28
Own data	38	95%	10 (26%)	18%	72

long run [4]. This stresses the argument that *endoscopic stenting* for biliary obstruction due to chronic pancreatitis should be performed only as a temporary treatment even if this therapy could be definitive with excellent long-term data in a subgroup of patients (Table 12.3-1).

Use of self-expandable metal stents ("Wallstents")

As mentioned previously, the use of biliary plastic prosthesis is an appropriate method for initial treatment of benign bile duct strictures with excellent short-term results. Additionally, it is a desirable alternative to surgery for poor operative candidates. However, stent clogging or stent migration and cholangitis are responsible for the significant morbidity leading to disappointing long-term results. Therefore, close monitoring with elective stent exchanges after biliary stenting is necessary to minimize complications. Moreover, the dilation effect of biliary plastic prosthesis is inadequate in many patients and responsible for the poor long-term outcome. Accordingly, to find an alternative with better long-term results, gastroenterologists developed treatment with self-expandable *metal stents* for these patients. Management with self-expandable *metal stents* has been well established in malignant bile duct strictures for years [10]. The occlusion rate is much lower than with *plastic stents* and elective stent exchanges are unnecessary also. However, the long-term results in tumor stenoses are affected by tumor overgrowth or ingrowth leading to unfavorable results in some cases. These tumor-related complications are not expected in biliary strictures due to chronic pancreatitis and that was the basis for their development in this benign disease. To the author's knowledge, there are only one published paper and one abstract concerning this form of therapy in a larger number of patients [2, 16]. Possible shortcomings of *metal stent* insertion in benign pancreatic or biliary diseases are epithelial hyperplasia with subsequent stent occlusion and possible malignant transformation by chronic irritation of the metal (Fig. 12.3-1A, B). In addition, *metal stents* are usually not removable either by endoscopy or surgery. Today, it remains

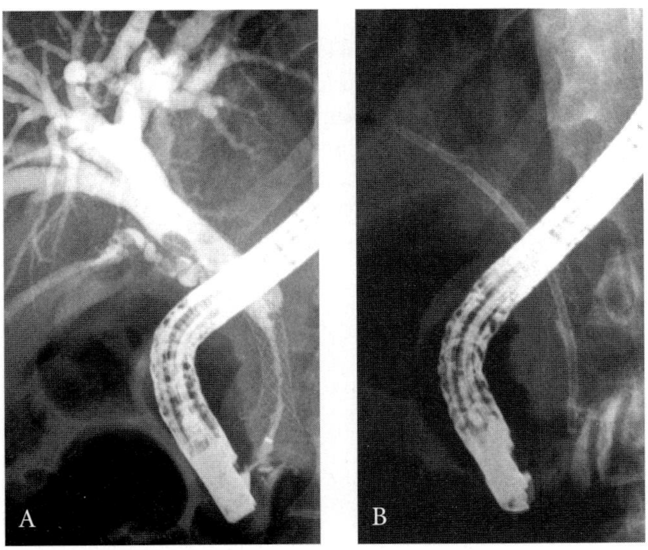

Figure 12.3-1A, B. Therapy with self-expandable Wallstent. **A:** Occlusion of Wallstent. **B:** Plastic stent in Wallstent.

questionable whether *metal stents* should be used in patients who are possible candidates for later biliodigestive bypass surgery or should better be reserved for patients not suitable for surgery.

In a prospective study Deviere et al. performed *endoscopic stenting* with self-expandable *metal stents* in 20 patients. Eleven of these cases had been treated with plastic prosthesis over a median time of 15 months previously. Endoscopic stent placement was successful in all patients. There were no problems of early clogging or stent migration. Symptoms of obstructive cholestasis improved quickly in all patients. After a mean follow-up of 33 months, success of stent therapy without any biliary problems was evaluated in 18 of the 20 patients (80%). All patients who were free of symptoms after six months remained asymptomatic in the further follow-up. Two patients developed epithelial hyperplasia in the stent lumen, leading to recurrent cholestasis and jaundice after three and six months. Second metal and *plastic stent* placement failed in one case and subsequent hepaticojejunostomy was inevitable. In order to guarantee technical success of hepaticojejunostomy or other drainage procedures, a short length of the stent (34 mm) with an internal diameter of 10 mm was chosen. Therefore, the proximal common bile duct remained free for future surgical approach. Despite excellent medium-term results with an success rate of 80%, the results of *metal stenting* in the long run remain uncertain [2]. Unfortunately, Deviere et al. published no further follow-up data on their patients; nevertheless long-term data is highly awaited to clarify the role of metal prosthesis in this benign disease.

A retrospective study by van Westerloo et al. was presented at the AGA Meeting this year. Self-expandable Wallstents were inserted in a subgroup of 15 patients, all had been treated by plastic prosthesis previously. Technical success was achieved in all cases. After a median follow-up of 14 months, the *metal stent* remained patent in 12 of 15 patients (80%). Failure of the stent therapy occurred in 3 patients after 1 week and 6 months leading to a stent-in-stent therapy first and subsequent hepaticojejunostomy finally [16]. Our experience with metal Wallstents is based on the results of 5 patients with benign biliary strictures due to chronic pancreatitis. Previous *plastic stenting* had been carried out in all cases over a median time of 14 months without clinical success. In a follow-up of 48 months, only 2 patients remained symptom-free and diagnostic ERCP demonstrated stent patency in these cases. Two patients received subsequent stent-in-stent therapy, and one patient underwent hepaticojejunostomy (Fig. 12.3-1A, B). These data stress the need for controlled clinical trials with longer follow-up in order to determine the exact role of *metal stent* therapy in the treatment of benign common bile duct stenoses. Overall, self-expandable *metal stents* seem to be desirable in a subgroup of patients with distal common bile duct stricture who are unfavorable candidates for surgical drainage (Table 12.3-2).

Table 12.3-2. Outcome of patients with metal prostheses.

Author	n	Technical success	Long-term success	Complication rate	Follow-up (months)
Deviere 1994 [2]	20	100%	18 (90%)	10%	33
Van Westerloo 2000 [16]	15	100%	12 (80%)	13%	14
Own data	5	100%	2 (40%)	40%	48

Discussion

Common bile duct stenosis caused by chronic pancreatitis represents a difficult clinical challenge for gastroenterologists. Approximately 10–30% of patients with chronic pancreatitis will develop such stenoses, which can result in cholestasis, cholangitis, jaundice and secondary biliary cirrhosis [6]. Biliary drainage procedures are indicated for symptomatic patients to prevent these complications in the follow-up [13]. However, many of these biliary stenoses present clinically asymptomatic with only temporary elevated cholestatic serum parameters. Usually, these asymptomatic strictures resolve spontaneously in the natural course of chronic pancreatitis. Conservative treatment is therefore recommended for those patients [12]. The optimal approach to the management of symptomatic biliary strictures in chronic pancreatitis has yet to be established.

Adequate management of the stricture is based on a "team approach" between endoscopists and surgeons. Dependant factors for the "team approach" are patients' age, comorbidities, course of chronic pancreatitis and the etiology of the stricture. *Plastic stents* offer satisfactory short-term and medium-term drainage but long-term follow-up data to clarify its role as definitive treatment is missing [4]. It can be used as a temporary treatment to relieve symptoms of cholestasis and to obtain time for regression of reversible inflammatory processes in the course of chronic pancreatitis. The endoscopic approach should therefore be the first-line therapy in symptomatic patients [10]. Immediate relief of symptoms is achieved in over 90% of cases but definitive improvement of the strictures is rarely seen in the follow-up. Endoscopic treatment offers low morbidity (0–9%) and mortality rates (0–4%) and especially the early complications are less frequent than in surgery [9] (Fig. 12.3-2A–C).

Adequate and definitive therapy for patients with recurrent cholestasis is provided by the surgical biliodigestive bypass procedure with either a pancreatic resection or drainage procedure. The surgical approach seems to be especially appropriate in young patients

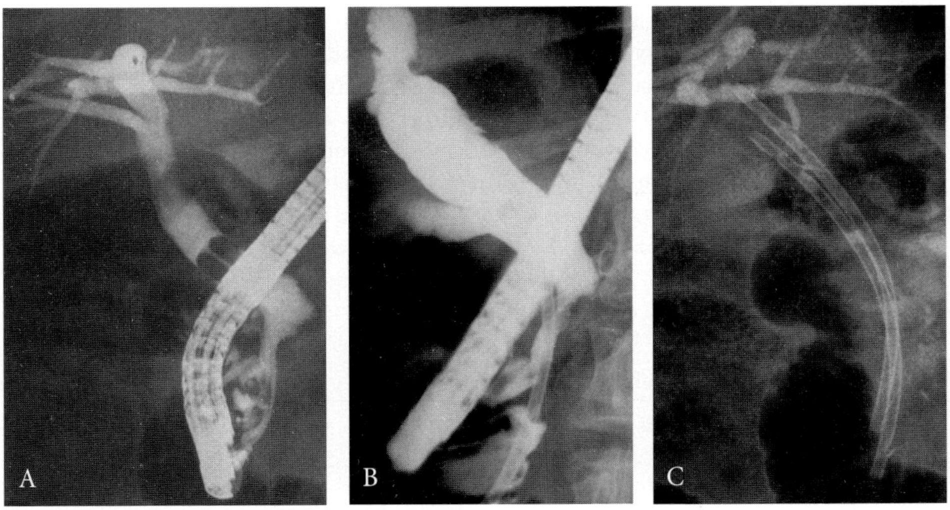

Figure 12.3-2A–C. Long-term stenting with polyethylene prostheses. **A:** Initial situation. **B:** Insertion of plastic stent. **C:** Adequate long-term drainage with 2 stents.

without any comorbidities. Endoscopic stent therapy could become the therapy of choice in poor surgical candidates or those who deny surgery [7]. As mentioned above, the long-term data revealed good clinical outcome with permanent normalization of the bile ducts only in a minority of patients. Major limitations such as stent clogging or migration and cholangitis frequently occurs in the follow-up [4, 10]. It is therefore recommended that the patients undergo elective stent exchange every 3–4 months to minimize the rate of complications. Self-expandable Wallstents could be an alternative for patients with frequent *plastic stent* occlusions [2, 5, 16]. *Metal stents* cannot migrate and offer a stent patency of over 80% in the follow-up. However, up to now there are only medium-term results of this approach with a re-occlusion rate of 20% due to epithelial hyperplasia [2]. As yet, no general recommendation for the use of metal prosthesis in patients with recurrent biliary stenoses can be given. Further studies determining the exact role of this approach are awaited.

Conclusions

The treatment of common bile duct stenoses in patients with chronic pancreatitis involves a "team approach" between endoscopists and surgeons. Endoscopic drainage should be performed as first line therapy to alleviate acute cholestasis before carrying out biliodigestive surgery. Obviously, there is a subgroup of patients that profits from *endoscopic stenting* with permanent regression of the stenosis after stent removal. The endoscopic approach is also the therapy of choice for unfavorable surgery candidates or patients who refuse surgery. The exact role of metal endoprosthesis and its cost-efficiency in this benign disease need to be defined in future studies.

References

1. Barthet M, Bernard JP, Duval JL, Affriat C, Sahel J. Biliary stenting in benign biliary stenosis complicating chronic calcifying pancreatitis. Endoscopy 1994; 26: 569–72.
2. Deviere J, Cremer M, Baize M, Love J, Sugai B, Vandermeeren A. Management of common bile duct stricture caused by chronic pancreatitis with metal mesh self-expandable stents. Gut 1994; 35: 122–6.
3. Deviere J, Devaere S, Baize M et al. Endoscopic biliary drainage in chronic pancreatitis. Gastrointest Endosc 1990; 36: 96–100.
4. Farnbacher MJ, Rabenstein T, Ell C, Hahn EG, Schneider HT. Is endoscopic drainage of common bile duct stenoses in chronic pancreatitis Up-to-Date? Am J Gastroenterol 2000; 95: 1466–71.
5. Hastier P, Buckley MJP, Peten EP, Dumas R, Delmont J. Long term treatment of biliary stricture due to chronic pancreatitis with a metallic stent. Am J Gastroenterol 1999; 94: 1947–8.
6. Itani KMF, Taylor TV. The challenge of therapy for pancreatitis-related common bile duct stricture. Am J Surg 1995; 170: 543–46.
7. Jakobs R, Riemann JF. The role of endoscopy in acute recurrent and chronic pancreatitis and pancreatic cancer. Gastroenterology Clinics of north America 1999; 28: 783–800.
8. Kiehne K, Fölsch UR, Nitsche R. High complication rate of bile duct stents in patients with chronic alcoholic pancreatitis due to noncompliance. Endoscopy 2000; 32: 377–80.
9. Löhr M, Schneider HT, Farnbacher M, Hahn EG, Fleig WE, Liebe S, Ell C. Endoskopisch interventionelle Therapie der chronischen Pancreatitis. Z Gastroenterol 1997; 35: 437–48.
10. Ng C, Huibregtse K. The role of endoscopic therapy in chronic pancreatitis-induced common bile duct strictures. Gastrointestinal Endoscopy Clinics of North America 1998; 8: 181–93.
11. Riemann JF, Maier M, Schilling D, Kohler B. Benigne Gallengangsstenosen – konservativ so lange wie möglich? Schweiz Rundschau Med Praxis 1994; 83: 883–5.

12. Schutz SM, Baillie J. Another treatment option for biliary strictures from chronic pancreatitis. Am J Gastroenterol 1995; 9(6): 1023–24.
13. Smith MT, Sherman S, Lehman GA. Endoscopic management of benign strictures of the biliary tree. Endoscopy 1995; 27: 253–66.
14. Smits ME, Rauws EAJ, van Gulik TM, Gouma DJ, Tytgat GNJ, Huibregtse K. Long-term results of endoscopic stenting and surgical drainage for biliary stricture due to chronic pancreatitis. British Journal of Surgery 1996; 83: 764–8.
15. Stahl TJ, Allen MO, Ansel HJ, Vennes JA. Partial biliary obstruction caused by chronic pancreatitis. An appraisal of indications for surgical biliary drainage. Ann Surg 1988; 207: 26–32.
16. Van Westerloo DJ, Bruno MJ, Bergman JJ, van de Heisteeg B, Rauws EA, Tytgat GN, Huibregtse K. Self-expandable wallstents for distal common bile duct strictures in chronic pancreatitis: Follow-up and clinical outcome of 15 patients. Gastroenterology 2000; A-913: 4693.
17. Vitale GC, Reed DN, Nguyen CT, Lawhon JC, Larson GM. Endoscopic treatment of distal bile duct stricture from chronic pancreatitis. Surg Endosc 2000; 14: 227–31.

12.4 Surgery versus endoscopic treatment in chronic pancreatitis

L. W. Traverso, R. A. Kozarek

Introduction

When conservative therapy of chronic pancreatitis is abandoned how can endoscopic therapy be helpful? Can endotherapy be used as primary treatment or is it just supportive therapy to allow safer surgery? This chapter will develop a schema that outlines criteria to implement treatment beyond medical therapy. Our algorithm utilizes endoscopic therapy (endotherapy) first, and if endotherapy fails, then surgical resection or drainage. The criteria for utilizing endotherapy and surgery are similar – a patient must have severe pancreatitis and be symptomatic with disabling abdominal pain. This chapter provides our definition of "severe" chronic pancreatitis and "disabling abdominal pain". In general endotherapy is indicated if the symptomatic patient has severe chronic pancreatitis that reaches the Cambridge Class V or "marked" stage of image severity (Table 12.4-1). If endotherapy fails then surgery is indicated. When patients require surgery they usually have pathological changes centered in the pancreatic head and a head resection is required. We then utilize a pylorus-preserving pancreaticoduodenectomy (PPW). Using this algorithm we found that virtually every resected patient received significant pain relief with an average follow-up after PPW of > 4 years.

All of our definitions are dependent on the pattern of anatomical changes that have occurred. We are therefore dependent on imaging studies to reflect the true anatomy. In a patient with disabling abdominal pain thought to be from chronic pancreatitis the

Cambridge Class[1]	Main PD	Abnormal Side Branches
I. NORMAL	Normal	None
II. EQUIVOCAL	Normal	< 3
III. MILD	Normal	≥ 3
IV. MODERATE	Abnormal	> 3
V. MARKED	Abnormal[2]	> 3

1 Roman numerals are assigned by the author and were not used in the original article

2 Marked abnormalities of main pancreatic duct are:

1. MPD terminates prematurely (abrupt, tapering, or irregular)
2. Multiple MPD strictures
3. MPD dilated > 10 mm
4. Ductal filling defects (stones)
5. "Cavities" intra- or extra-pancreatic
6. Contiguous organ involvement (CBD, duodenum, arterial venous fistula)

Table 12.4-1. Cambridge classification of "image severity".

clinician seeks evidence from imaging studies. Modern imaging is crucial for patient selection in order to make treatment decisions for chronic pancreatitis. Modern imaging allows the clinician to determine almost all of the anatomy before any treatment and then, using that anatomy, predict the likelihood for successful therapy. The pretreatment imaging studies include endoscopic retrograde cholangiopancreatography (ERCP), magnetic resonance cholangiopancreatography (MRCP), computer axial tomography directed at the pancreas (pancreas protocol CT), and endoscopic ultrasound (EUS). If surgery becomes necessary intraoperative imaging will include ultrasound (IUS), fluoroscopic pancreatography (IFP), and flexible pancreatoscopy. Postoperative imaging is just as important and includes the gross findings at the time of resection and those of the pathologist. We find it very informative to cut the specimen with the pathologist at the time of removal.

In general, in order for a patient to be a candidate for any type of interventional therapy directed at chronic pancreatitis, the patient must have specific anatomic changes and all forms of more conservative treatment must have failed. Endotherapy is the first interventional treatment. Surgery is the last resort, but when all forms of nonsurgical treatment have failed, *proper patient selection based on anatomy* will ensure that almost every one of these patients will receive considerable improvement.

Clinical presentation – must be "symptomatic" and have "severe chronic" pancreatitis

Disabling abdominal pain

Almost every patient that presents for medical treatment of chronic pancreatitis has abdominal pain. When the pain becomes disabling it is due to progressive disease that is documented by anatomical changes varying from ductal disruption, partial obstruction, or complete obstruction. Disabling abdominal pain is difficult to define but the patients will have a common pattern of chronic symptoms. In an earlier series we found that 94% of patients undergoing any form of surgical treatment for chronic pancreatitis had abdominal pain [1]. The pain had been present for an average of 5.6 years prior to surgery and was described as continuous in half the cases and intermittent chronic relapsing pancreatitis in the other 50%. The frequency of exacerbating episodes was every 5 months. The disabled patient has other patterns of clinical presentation – most of them are off alcohol (as it exacerbates symptoms) and all have at least oral narcotic requirements. Some are so disabled that they are dependent on total parenteral nutrition.

Once the physician has assessed that the patient has the above pattern of disabling abdominal pain, then the clinical diagnosis of "chronic pancreatitis" must be confirmed. The Marseilles classification of 1963 contains a preliminary definition of chronic pancreatitis, i.e., chronic pancreatitis represents "residual pancreatic damage either anatomical or functional that persists even if the primary cause or factors are eliminated". [2]. Once this general definition of the disease has been met then anatomic changes are assessed. Candidates for endotherapy or surgery must have the "marked" variety of anatomic changes according to the Cambridge Image Severity scale (Table 12.4-1) [3]. In the table, there are six items listed in the footnote that denote the "abnormal" findings associated with the "marked" stage on the scale. Any one of the six items will classify the patient into the Cambridge Class V or the "marked" stage of image severity.

The "composite pancreas"

Modern imaging information is derived from several types of imaging modalities. If the patient has surgery then observation of the gross specimen combined with the imaging data yields a *composite view* of the pancreatic parenchyma as well as the ductal system. The composite picture cannot be obtained utilizing just one imaging technique. Every patient undergoing endotherapy or surgery for chronic pancreatitis will have had at least a CT scan and ERCP. Many require visceral arteriography. Currently, the role of MRCP is still being evaluated. Intraoperatively, fluoroscopic pancreatography and ultrasound are frequently utilized. Even modern imaging is found to have limitations because gross specimen observations add more information.

This *"composite pancreas"* represents the anatomical picture that should be the baseline when selecting groups to compare outcomes of our procedures. An accurate composite pancreas compared to short- and long-term surgical outcomes has yielded reliable selection criteria [4].

What is endotherapy?

Endotherapy is an evolving concept that should only be utilized in pancreaticobiliary centers with extensive ERCP experience and where proficient management of complicated pancreatitis is already practiced. To expand on this statement, endotherapy must be practiced where a "multidisciplinary team" provides the additional modalities of interventional radiology, anesthesia in the fluoroscopy suite, extracorporeal shock wave lithotripsy (ESWL), and conventional surgery (resection and drainage). Endotherapy treatment decisions revolve around the status of the MPD, i.e., whether this duct is obstructed with stones and/or stricture or contains a ductal disruption. It must be emphasized that MPD obstruction is caused either by stones alone or, more commonly, by a stricture (with or without stones). Endotherapy can be definitive by itself. Alternatively, the use of endotherapy is complimentary to surgery allowing for resolution of inflammation or infection because of ductal decompression.

We found that 98% of patients who required surgery for chronic pancreatitis had a chief complaint of abdominal pain [4]. The pain of chronic pancreatitis has many potential causes. The pain can be due to ductal obstruction and ductal or parenchymal hypertension, pressure on contiguous organs, ductal disruption with activation of pancreatic enzymes, and, less commonly perineural inflammation and fibrosis. It is not surprising that the first criterion for endotherapy is almost always abdominal pain. In an asymptomatic patient there are essentially no indications for either interventional or surgical treatment, except the occasional patient that requires treatment for a persistent external pancreatic fistula.

Therefore, the sequence of therapy is to treat abdominal pain by addressing the anatomy that complicates the patient's case. Conservative medical therapy is essentially that as described by Ammann and colleagues – removal of the etiology, analgesics as necessary, and support of exocrine or endocrine insufficiency [5]. They had two groups of patients – those with and without exacerbation of chronic pain. In the group with exacerbation of chronic pain Ammann and coworkers found local complications, mainly ductal disruption anatomically expressed as a pseudocyst. For those Ammann patients without exacerbation of chronic pain we do not know their anatomy. Some of them may have had the "marked" variety of image severity and would have been considered for pain relief in our algorithm. In our experience an escalation of pain is invariably associated with anatomical changes such as development of a ductal disruption (pseudocyst), pancreatic duct stricture (with or without pancreatic duct stones), biliary stenosis, or duodenal stenosis.

Endotherapy is the first option with this escalation of pain. The consideration begins with mapping the MPD using MRCP or diagnostic ERCP. The anatomy of the MPD determines if endotherapy will be helpful. Patients may benefit from endotherapy if one of three potential anatomic findings is found – MPD stones (Fig. 12.4-1), MPD stricture (Fig. 12.4-2), and/or MPD disruption (leak, Fig. 12.4-3A and 3B) . In order to work endoscopically within the MPD a pancreatic sphincterotomy is required (Fig. 12.4-4). Since the sphincterotomy alone will result in transient edema and obstruction of the MPD, most patients will have a MPD stent left in place after sphincterotomy to insure adequate MPD decompression (Fig. 12.4-5). In the post-manipulation period the stent maintains MPD drainage and avoids post-procedure pancreatitis or ductal blowout that may occur due to transient edema in the sphincterotomy site. The transampullary MPD stent is temporary as a MPD stricture and more chronic pancreatitis can result if the stent is left in place longer than 4 to 6 weeks [6].

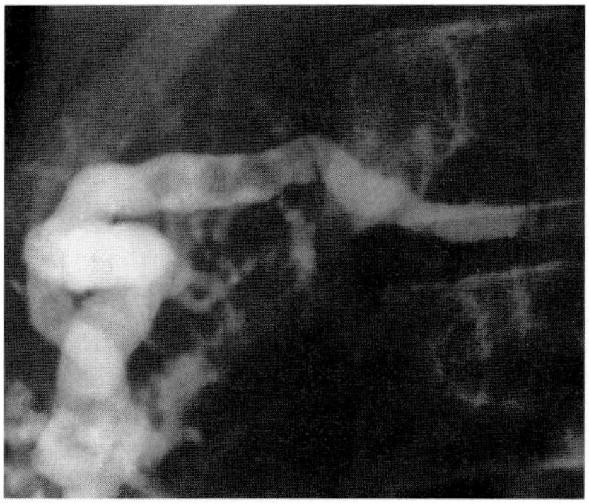

Figure 12.4-1. An ERCP shows a dilated main pancreatic duct (MPD) with multiple stones. The MPD does not have a stricture. Stones without a stricture in the MPD is an uncommon pattern.

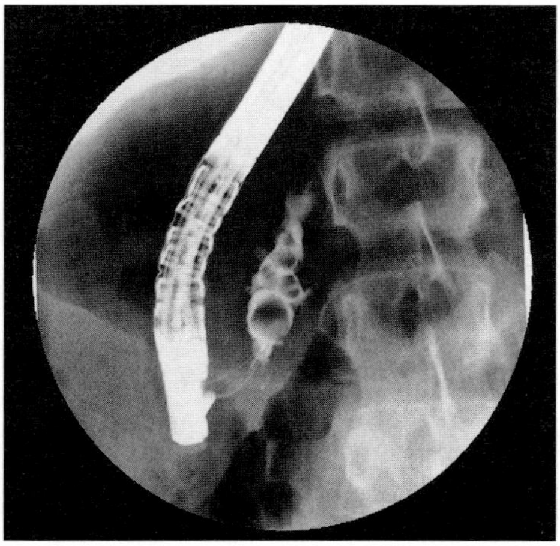

Figure 12.4-2. A main pancreatic duct (MPD) stricture is shown just inside the ampulla with multiple stones upstream.

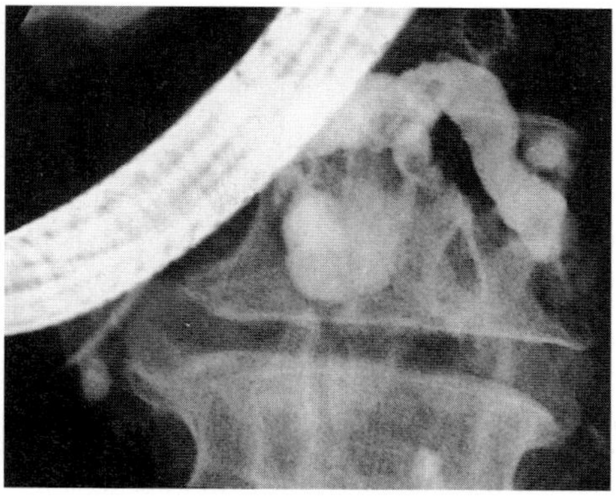

Figure 12.4-3A. A ductal disruption is shown inferior to the main pancreatic duct (center of photo) near the genu. Note that upstream from the disruption multiple small stones are seen in the MPD. Stones and stricture downstream (not shown) caused a disruption or blowout upstream.

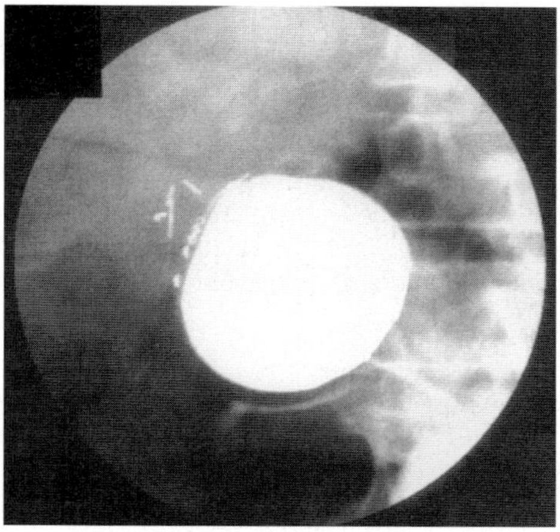

Figure 12.4-3B. An intraoperative pseudocystogram shows an intrapancreatic head cyst with injection of contrast (injection catheter at 4 o'clock to the cyst). Contrast from the cyst outlines the main pancreatic duct inferiorly (from 4 o'clock to 7 o'clock to the cyst) with a small amount of contrast seen emptying into the duodenum. This ductal disruption was probably caused by intrapancreatic necrosis eroding into the main pancreatic duct since the duct appears normal. Note that the cyst had previously eroded into the gastroduodenal artery in the form of a pseuodaneurysm that had to be embolized with coils seen at 10 o'clock to the cyst.

MPD strictures, stones, and leaks are common observations in many of these disabled patients with severe pancreatitis. It is interesting to compare endotherapy and ductal abnormalities between those patients with a more acute process, severe necrotizing pancreatitis, versus those with a very chronic process undergoing ESWL and then endotherapy (Table 12.4-2). Since ESWL is used to break stones all of these latter patients have stones. Approximately one third of chronic pancreatitis cases undergoing endotherapy will utilize ESWL. Endotherapy depends on ESWL to fracture and loosen impacted stones and then allow removal with the transampullary techniques of endotherapy. The table shows that MPD stones can be observed even in the more acute group. However both groups have MPD strictures observed frequently – from one third in the more acute group to one half in the more chronic forms of pancreatitis. Since 76% of patients with the more acute process have a ductal leak, endotherapy seems to have provided insight into the natural history of necrotizing pancreatitis, i.e., the frequent presence of pancreatic juice in the extrapancreatic space due to a pancreatic ductal disruption. We have found a strong correlation between necrosis and the presence of ductal disruption [7]. Both acute and chronic processes appear to benefit from endotherapy via decompression of the ductal system. The continued decompression of the ductal system with a temporary MPD stent can be definitive or it can allow the process to subside and facilitate surgery.

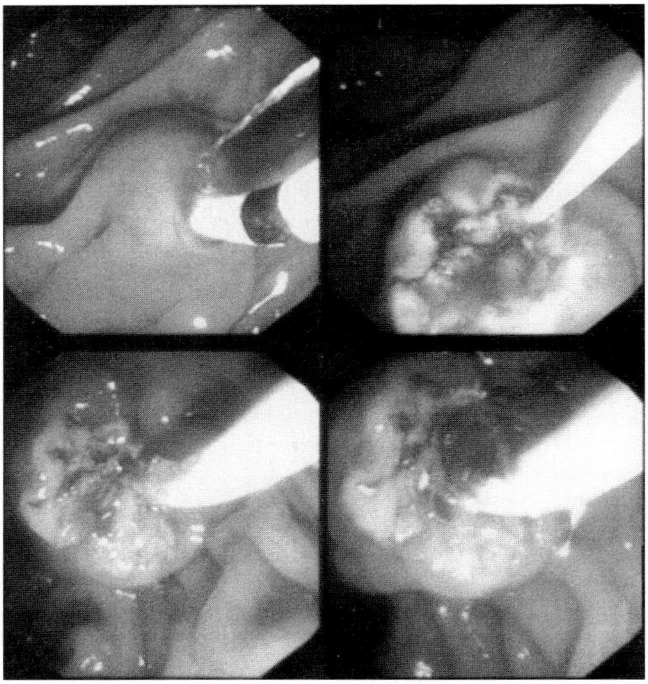

Figure 12.4-4. An endoscopic pancreatic sphincterotomy is being performed in the upper left corner. A wire is passed through the ampulla in the upper right hand corner photograph at the time of endotherapy. Subsequent balloon dilation of a MPD stricture is depicted in the lower two corners. A temporary transampullary stent was left in place (not shown).

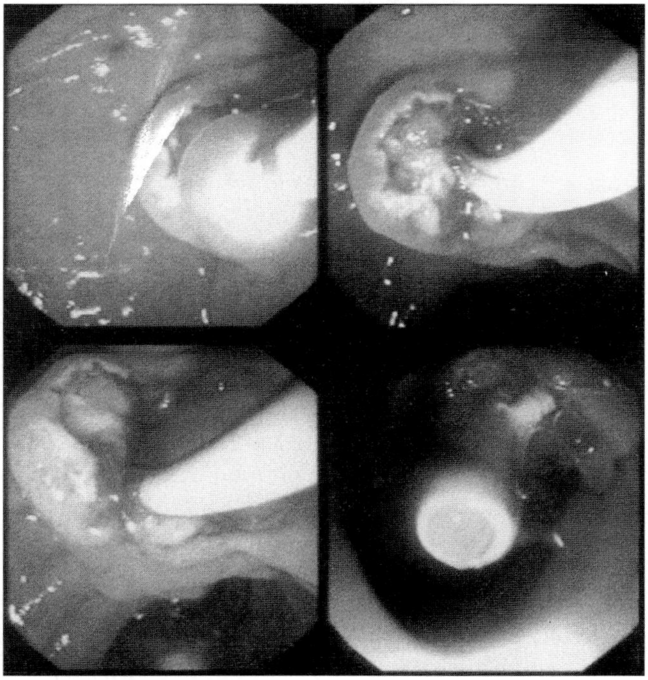

Figure 12.4-5. Multiple stone extractions were performed with a balloon (upper boxes). After clearance of stones and debris an endoscopic stent was left in place (temporarily) to avoid inflammatory edema that would transiently close the duct resulting in pain (right lower box).

Table 12.4-2. Ductal abnormalities in patients requiring endotherapy and ESWL for severe chronic pancreatitis versus those requiring endotherapy for severe necrotizing pancreatitis.

	Chronic pancreatitis, ESWL, endotherapy (n = 39)	**Severe necrotizing pancreatitis and endotherapy (n = 37)**
MPD Stricture	46%	35%
MPD Stones	100%	16%
MPD Leak	18%	76%

Unpublished results of patients treated since 1995

So how often does endotherapy fail and surgery is required? If surgery is required how do the patients respond? Does endotherapy make the chance of resolving the patient's symptoms with surgery more or less favorable? Teams that perform both endotherapy and surgery have not provided sufficient studies to answer these questions. However the acute and chronic extremes of pancreatitis used in Table 12.4-2 and 12.4-3 may provide some insight into the answer. The use of MPD stents is most prominent when there is either stricture and/or stones as they aid in ductal decompression. The stent also prevents more backpressure due to the inflammation from manipulation with wires and baskets. MPD sphincterotomy is almost always required to place stents and remove stones. Of most importance is that surgery appears to be avoided in the ESWL treated group in almost 80% of our cases with follow-up (mean 2.7 years). The ESWL patients had 48% complete pain relief while those that have gone on for a Whipple procedure would be expected to have 76% complete pain relief (see below). About half of the severe narcotizing pancreatitis cases avoided surgery – so it appears that endotherapy avoids surgery more often in the more chronic variety of severe pancreatitis (Table 12.4-3).

A decision tree based on ductal anatomy is provided in Table 12.4-4 and is modified or recreated from previous publications [8, 9]. In a symptomatic patient suppose the

Table 12.4-3. Results of endotherapy in patients with severe chronic pancreatitis that has endotherapy and ESWL versus those requiring endotherapy for severe necrotizing pancreatitis.

	Chronic pancreatitis, ESWL, endotherapy (n = 39)	**Necrotizing pancreatitis and endotherapy (n = 37)**
PD stents	82%	59%
PD Endoscopic sphincterotomy	90%	27%
Endoscopic cystogastrostomy or duodenostomy	0	13%
CT-guided drains	0	74%
Pain before treatment	92%	100%
Pain relief after treatment	85% some relief 48% complete at 2.7 yrs ± 0.6 yr	65%
Required surgery	18% (66% Whipple)	46% (66% debridement)

Unpublished results of patients treated since 1995

MPD in the pancreatic head does not have a stricture but is obstructed by stones (Fig. 12.4-1). There are no stones or stricture in the MPD of the body/tail but the duct in the body of the pancreas is "dilated" (> 5 mm as per the Cambridge classification). Look at the second row of Table 12.4-4 labeled "head MPD – no stricture but obstructed by stones" and under the "body/tail MPD dilated" column. This pattern is not as common as stones with strictures in the pancreatic head. As per Table 12.4-4, endotherapy is the first therapy and is therefore designated "A". Endotherapy first attempts to remove the stones using baskets and wires in a transampullary fashion. ESWL may be necessary to provide smaller stone fragments allowing their extraction. In this situation with short-term follow-up, we have found that about half of the patients will benefit; however, many go on to surgery [10]. In this patient without MPD stricture, if the process of endotherapy fails to break the chronic pancreatitis-associated pain cycle, then a Puestow procedure is indicated if the duct is dilated (designated "B" in Table 12.4-4). Failure of endotherapy is usually the result of further stone formation in the MPD after stent removal or repetitive clogging of the MPD stent. During a Puestow procedure the MPD is opened longitudinally in the neck of the gland extending into the pancreatic tail. If MPD stones deep in the head of the gland cannot be removed from the lateral pancreatic duct incision of the Puestow procedure, we will incorporate electrohydraulic lithotripsy (EHL) delivered through intraoperative pancreatoscopy. The goal is to ensure that the pancreatic duct is open into the duodenum. If this cannot be accomplished with EHL, then a ventral pan-

Table 12.4-4. Decision tree based on ductal anatomy in order of application, A to D. Modified after [8].

Status of main duct	Endo-therapy	Puestow ± EHL	Frey	PPW	Distal	No treatment
Head MPD – no obstruction						
Body/tail MPD:						
normal						A
dilated[1,2]		A				
stricture					B	A[2,3]
Head MPD – no stricture but obstructed by stones[1]						
Body/tail MPD:						
normal	A		B			
dilated[2]	A	B	C			
stricture	A					B[3]
Head MPD – obstructed by stricture ± stones						
Body/tail MPD:						
normal	A		B	C		
dilated[2]	A	B	C	D		
stricture[1]	A		C[4]	D[4]		B[3]

EHL = electrohydraulic lithotripsy
"A" is the first treatment consideration in each row, additional letters indicate the sequence if A fails.
[1] = uncommon anatomic pattern (< 10%)
[2] = MPD dilation defined by the Cambridge report is 6.5 mm in the head and 5.0 mm in body
[3] = consider current use of alcoholic beverages and, if so, any surgery is contraindicated
[4] = avoid total pancreatectomy and the 44% incidence of marginal ulceration, "Puestow" the duct through the stricture in the body or tail

creatic head resection (Frey) procedure may be utilized (designated "C" in row 2 of Table 12.4-4 where the body/tail MPD is dilated).

A more common anatomic pattern is MPD stricture (with stones) and the treatment used is depicted in the last row of Table 12.4-4. A short-term transampullary stent is utilized to provide ductal decompression upstream from the stricture. The endoscopist may be able to remove some or all of the stones through the stricture with or without ESWL. Balloon dilatation may be utilized. Operation is necessary if these endotherapy maneuvers followed by short term transampullary MPD stenting fail to break the pain cycle by relieving an inflammatory stricture in the MPD or if the appearance of the stricture suggests neoplasm. Head resection in the form of a pylorus-preserving Whipple procedure is then utilized.

Endotherapy is also applied to the ductal disruptions of chronic pancreatitis that result in pseudocysts, either intra-pancreatic or extra-pancreatic. These pseudocysts have been termed "cavities" in the Cambridge classification [3]. Endotherapy methods for treating ductal disruptions include transenteric or transampullary drainage of the pseudocyst with concomitant placement of double pigtail stents. The method is guided by the anatomy. This type of drainage procedure is only applicable to a pseudocyst and is *contraindicated* for a fluid collection that contains debris from peripancreatic necrosis. Note the infrequent use of endoscopic cystenterostomies in Table 12.4-3 when severe pancreatitis is associated with necrosis. Peripancreatic necrosis cavities will contain a significant amount of debris and are not amenable to drainage through the small diameter stents or drains that must be used with endotherapy. These smaller stents cannot be exchanged as readily as those percutaneous drains placed by interventional radiology. Because of clogged or small diameter stents or drains these cavities with debris will be inadequately drained by endotherapy. The result will be a peripancreatic abscess and the combination of transenteric drains and infected necrosis increases the possibility of drain erosion into a mesenteric artery (Fig. 12.4-6A and 12.4-6B). A true non-debris containing pseudocyst can be drained through a transgastric or transduodenal route. If the

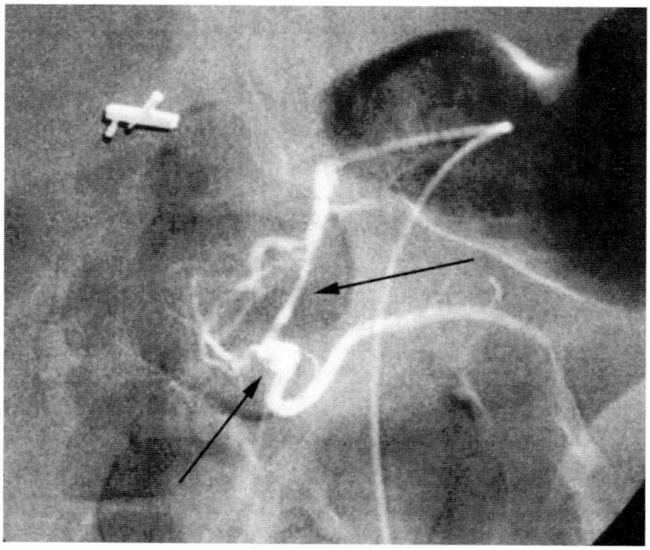

Figure 12.4-6A. A peripancreatic cavity filled with debris from necrosis was treated with placement of two transduodenal endoscopic stents at an outside institution. The stents became clogged and the cavity became infected. Gastrointestinal bleeding occurred from a bleeding gastroduodenal artery pseudoaneurysm (lower arrow) accompanied by spasm in the main vessel upstream (upper arrow).

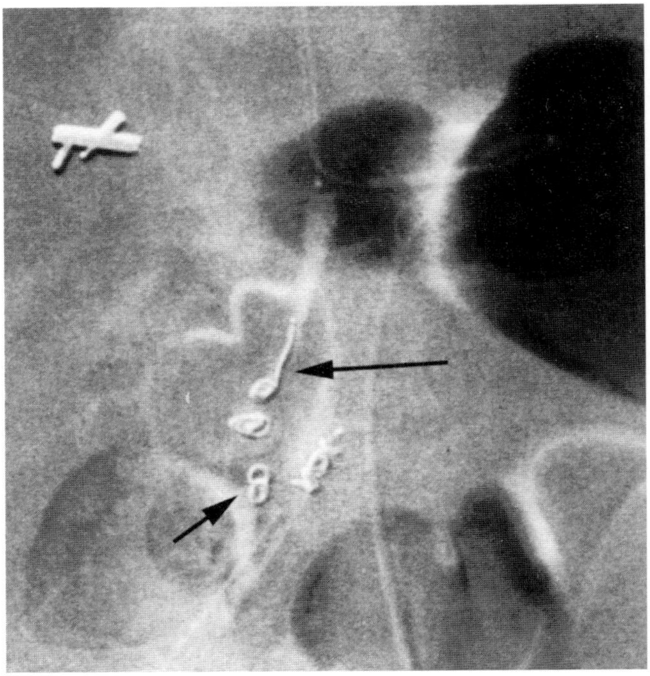

Figure 12.4-6B. The gastroduodenal artery was obliterated by coils, which included those placed in the main vessel (upper arrow) and over the pseudoaneurysm (lower arrow). This promptly stopped the bleeding and percutaneous drains were used to successfully decompress the abscess cavity.

ductal disruption at ERCP can be demonstrated to connect to the pseudocyst, then the cyst can be decompressed using a stent through the transampullary route through the MPD. In the latter case the stent is placed through the MPD obstruction into the cavity or beyond the cavity following the duct to bridge the disruption site and allow spontaneous resolution [11].

Surgical therapy for chronic pancreatitis

The foregoing discussion can be summarized. Resection or drainage procedures are reserved for patients who have all of the following criteria: presence of disabling pain, presence of chronic pancreatitis, presence of severe anatomical changes (Class V of the Cambridge Image Severity), endotherapy has failed, and lastly, but just as important, that the etiology for the chronic pancreatitis has been addressed (gallstones or alcohol). If all of these criteria are met then, in our experience, the majority of these patients require pancreaticoduodenectomy (60%) as the "pacemaker" for chronic pancreatitis appears to reside within the head of the pancreas. Outcome studies indicate that removing the head terminates the problem [4]. The remaining patients receive a drainage procedure like the Puestow (20%) or a distal pancreatectomy (20%).

Endotherapy may fail to be definitive in 20 to 50% of the cases as shown in Table 12.4-3. However, if surgery is required, the patient will have benefited during the endotherapy process as the surgery was facilitated in the following ways – pain was relieved by ductal or cyst decompression, portal venous congestion was decompressed with cyst decompression, time allowed nutrition to be optimized, biliary decompression allowed obstructive jaundice or cholangitis to be reversed, and peripancreatitis from ductal disruption was relieved. All of these benefits result in less morbidity during or after surgery such as less blood loss or wound infection. Note the frequent use of preoperative biliary or MPD stents in the following section.

Outcome analysis of PPW for chronic pancreatitis

If endotherapy fails does the delay lessen a patient's chance to obtain pain relief from surgery? The experience from our institution would suggest no. In 1997 [4], we summarized our results with 57 consecutive patients that had undergone pancreaticoduodenectomy for chronic pancreatitis. The indications for head resection in this group were as follows. All patients had intractable abdominal pain and chronic pancreatitis according to the Marseilles 1963 classification. All patients had the Cambridge Class V of "marked" image severity. To be more specific, 96% percent had MPD obstruction and the 4% without main pancreatic duct obstruction were patients with intrapancreatic "cavities" (or pseudocysts) in the head connected to the main pancreatic duct. In addition to MPD obstruction or pancreatic head pseudocyst, all patients had multiple other elements of the Cambridge Classification (Table 12.4-1) to support head resection. The patient characteristics were 63% male, 75% alcohol etiology, 56% pancreatic pseudocyst ("cavities") in the head, 23% with previous pancreatic operations such as pseudocyst or main ductal drainage procedures, and 33% were diabetic preoperative. All patients received ERCP and CT scans to develop a composite pancreas image and the surgeon dissected 100% of the gross specimens with the pathologist to draw the "composite pancreas".

The role of endotherapy is prominent in these patients because 65% had common bile duct obstruction and 47% had undergone preoperative common bile duct stenting. As listed previously, 96% had pancreatic duct obstruction while 39% had documented MPD disruption and 35% required MPD stenting. Percutaneous drainage was required in 19% for peripancreatic fluid collections.

Except for a minority, 97% of these patients were treated with PPW and the remaining 3% of patients, who had a previous antrectomy for peptic ulcer disease, could not be reconstructed with pylorus preservation (Kausch-Whipple procedure). Hospital and 30 day operative mortality was zero and 98% were available for follow-up after a mean of 42 months. The five-year actuarial survival rate was 93% and in the patients that were not diabetic preoperatively (n = 37), the actual five-year diabetic occurrence rate was 32%. This diabetes was not a consequence of the resection because no patient became diabetic sooner than 12 months after the surgery, indicating that the criteria for surgery had been accurate enough to ensure that nonfunctional pancreatic tissue had been excised. We did not see a predisposition for diabetes due to the pylorus-preserving Whipple procedure as has been suggested by others [12].

The patients with a follow-up of greater than 1 year (n = 43) had a mean follow-up time of 55 months. These patients were asked if they still had pain and if so was it still disabling. In the 96% of patients that had disabling pain as an indication for surgery, those patients asked in long-term follow-up about pain relief indicated a surprising finding. Every patient indicated that they had a "good" response to surgery and that their pain was no longer disabling. In addition, 76% of the patients indicated that their pain relief was "excellent" in as much as they were free of all pain. What about these 24% of patients who still had some residual discomfort (although no longer disabled)? Recall that the majority of these patients had alcohol-induced chronic pancreatitis. The psychological makeup of these patients became evident because the incidence of patients resuming alcohol was also 24%.

If endotherapy fails does the delay prevent patients from obtaining good results with surgery? The patients described above appeared to have obtained good pain relief with resection if they failed endotherapy. It is important to note that all patients with or without surgery were chosen with similar criteria for treatment as outlined in this chapter.

Summary

In order for a patient to be a candidate for any type of interventional therapy directed at chronic pancreatitis, the patient should have disabling abdominal pain, specific anatomic changes, and failed conservative treatment. Endotherapy is the first interventional treatment. Surgery is the last resort, but when endotherapy fails surgical resection will have been facilitated by endotherapy. If endotherapy and surgical resection are guided by *proper patient selection based on anatomy* then almost every one of these patients will receive considerable improvement after either endotherapy alone or failed endotherapy with added surgical resection.

References

1. Traverso LW, Tompkins RK, Urrea PT, Longmire WP. Surgical treatment of chronic pancreatitis – 22 years experience. Ann Surg 1979; 190: 312–9.
2. Sarles H. Proposal adopted unanimously by the participants of the symposium. In: Sarles H, ed. Pancreatitis. Symposium Marseilles April 25 and 26, 1963. Basel: S. Karger, 1963: VII–VIII.
3. Axon ATR, Classen M, Cotton PB et al. Pancreatography in chronic pancreatitis: international definitions. Gut 1984; 25: 1107–12.
4. Traverso LW, Kozarek RA. Pancreatoduodenectomy for chronic pancreatitis. Anatomic selection criteria and subsequent long-term outcome analysis. Ann Surg 1997; 226: 429–38.
5. Ammann RW, Muellhaupt B, Zurich Pancreatitis Study Group. Natural history of pain in alcoholic chronic pancreatitis. Gastroenterology 1999; 116: 1132–40.
6. Kozarek RA. Pancreatic stents can induce ductal changes consistent with chronic pancreatitis. Gastrointest Endosc 1990; 36: 93–5.
7. Lau ST, Simchuk EJ, Kozarek RA, Traverso LW. A pancreatic duct leak should be sought to direct treatment in patients with acute pancreatitis. Am J Surg 2001; 181: 411–5.
8. Traverso LW. The surgical management of chronic pancreatitis: the Whipple procedure. In: Cameron JL, ed. Advances in Surgery. St. Louis: Mosby, Inc., 1999, vol. 32: 23–39.
9. Traverso LW. Chronic pancreatitis – Endotherapy First Then Surgery. In : Kirby I, Bland MD, eds. The Practice of General Surgery. Philadelphia: WB Saunders Co., 2002: 743–49.
10. Mathews K, Correa RJ, Gibbons RP et al. Extracorporeal shock wave lithotripsy for obstructing pancreatic duct calculi. J Urol 1997; 158: 522–5.
11. Kozarek RA, Traverso LW. Pancreatic fistulas and ascites. In: Brandt LJ, ed. Clinical Practice of Gastroenterology. Philadelphia: Current Medicine, Inc., 1998: 17–23.
12. Büchler MW, Freiss H, Bittner R et al. Duodenum-preserving pancreatic head resection: long-term results. J Gastrointest Surg 1997; 1: 13–9.

13 Surgical treatment of chronic pancreatitis: Standard procedures

13.1 Drainage procedures for treatment of chronic pancreatitis

W. H. Nealon

Introduction

Although not proposed until the middle of the 20th century, drainage procedures in the treatment of certain patients with chronic pancreatitis would seem intuitively well conceived. Many, but not all, patients with chronic pancreatitis sustain structural derangements in the gland, which include dilatation of the main pancreatic duct and secondary ductular systems. Although there are often areas of narrowing and dilatation interspersed throughout the length of the main pancreatic duct (MPD), the dilatation almost always extends from one end of the gland to the other, and, therefore, suggests that there may be restriction to flow at the entry of the MPD into the duodenum. Although these abnormalities are easily defined preoperatively with our current imaging techniques, none of this information was obtainable before operation in the middle of the 20th century, and, therefore, strategies needed to be established at the time of operation. Perhaps this, combined with the fact that operative interventions in the pancreas were viewed as hazardous for most of the 20th century, explains why the earlier suggested techniques for drainage of the main pancreatic duct were minimalist in scope. Within close temporal proximity, the two earliest drainage procedures proposed were drainage at the ampulla, suggested by many but popularized by Doubilet [1], and resection of the small portion of the tail of the pancreas and drainage at the opposite end of the dilated main pancreatic duct, as suggested by Duval [2]. The physiologic basis for both of these operations was the supposition that all of the pain associated with chronic pancreatitis was related to restriction to flow out of the gland caused by the relative obstruction created by stenosis at the ampulla. Unfortunately, neither of these procedures resulted in significant relief of pain, and this fact remains one of the conundra associated with this disease. Why should relieving the restriction to flow of pancreatic juice in the head of the gland or in the tail of the gland not result in reduction in the amount of pressure within the pancreatic duct and, thereby, reduction in the pain associated with chronic pancreatitis? This historical surgical data may help predict that endoscopic drainage with plastic stents is unlikely to provide long-term relief of pain.

Structural abnormalities in chronic pancreatitis

It is well established that histologic examination of pancreatic tissue from patients with a diagnosis of chronic pancreatitis will characteristically show moderate to massive fibrosis. Interestingly, there appears to be preservation of islet tissue, although the fibrotic process appears to obliterate the communication between the islets and a complex portal venous system of interface between acinar tissue and islet tissue. Varying amounts of acinar tissue are destroyed or obliterated by the extensive fibrosis. There appears to be a specific clustering of inflammatory cells around nerves within the gland, and this fact has been proposed as one of the mechanisms for pain associated with this disease. Goecke, Friess and Büchler [3] have identified macrophages with chemokine receptor 5 (CCR5) as central to this process. Whether this fact plays a role in the success of drainage procedures for chronic pancreatitis is yet to be established. The role of inflammatory cells and of the products of these cells, including cytokines, is an active area of research. Because one of the earliest anatomic abnormalities seen in this disease is secondary ductular ectasia, there is general belief that this disease begins in the smaller ductules and that the process is initiated by deposition of proteins, which are poorly soluble, in the pancreatic juice. It is known from experimental models that obstruction of the ducts will result in this generalized fibrotic response. The disease will variably proceed to the main pancreatic duct, resulting in a variety of conformations. One of these, as previously described, is the classic "chain of lakes", in which there are areas of dilatation and narrowing throughout the main pancreatic duct. Pancreatic ductal stones which are composed of precipitated protein and calcium carbonate are variably seen within the gland and as stones within the main pancreatic duct or within the secondary ductules. A subset of patients will have generalized fibrosis but no dilatation of the duct. This is the so-called "small duct" variant of chronic pancreatitis. Additional features may be observed, including a mass effect, which is typically seen in the head of the pancreas. In certain geographic areas, this mass may reach a diameter as great as 15 cm. Cystic changes in the pancreas are well established, including what represent massively dilated ductules as well as the formation of pseudocysts. Each of these structural derangements may have implications for the operative procedure chosen. The clinical picture is not distinguishable among these varieties of anatomic derangements. In other words, patients with small duct chronic pancreatitis will not present in any different fashion than ones with a dilated duct or with cysts associated. Typically, the patient presents with a history of ethanol abuse and with a history of chronic pain with or without evidence of endocrine or exocrine insufficiency.

Strategies for operative intervention

There are a number of strategies that are routinely included by the pancreatic surgeon in approaching patients with chronic pancreatitis. Perhaps most significant is the concept of preservation of tissue. In view of the fact that this disease is so often associated with functional derangements, it would seem obvious that preservation of as much tissue as possible would be a goal. In this case, drainage procedures would appear to offer the best option, compared to alternatives which are based upon resectional therapy. In addition to preservation of function, one must keep in mind the relative risks of operation. In general, both the mortality and morbidity associated with drainage procedures has been lower than that associated with the more invasive resectional procedures [4–7]. Finally, there has, since the initiation of operations for chronic pancreatitis, been the hope that operative intervention would enhance the function of the pancreas after decompression. Again, one might intuitively believe that pancreatic juice which is unable to escape the obstructed pancreatic duct and therefore unable to participate in the digestive process may, upon release by a decompressive procedure, enhance exocrine function. In addition, many have suggested, and Reber et al. [8] has data to suggest, that pancreatic function is impacted by the high pressures within the main pancreatic duct. He has termed this condition "the pancreatic compartment syndrome". Thus, one might hope to see improved pancreatic endocrine and exocrine function after decompression. Although these goals have not routinely been met, these issues continue to be assessed in the operative management of this disease. More recently, attention has been directed towards the concept of preservation of function. We and others have evaluated the effect of decompressive procedures on the ongoing loss of function predictably seen in patients with chronic pancreatitis and have asked whether decompressive procedures may protect against further loss of function over time [4].

Operative options

Pancreatic duct sphincterotomy

As mentioned previously, the presumption was often drawn that stenosis at the sphincter for the main pancreatic duct in the major papilla was largely responsible for the diffuse dilatation of the pain pancreatic duct. For that reason, one of the earliest measures proposed for the operative management of this disease was a duodenotomy and operative sphincterotomy of the pancreatic duct. Doubilet [1] explored the usefulness of this procedure in the 1950s and early 1960s. Very little operative experience in pancreatic duct sphincterotomy has evolved since that time. The results obtained by these authors reflected a very high complication rate and a very low success rate for amelioration of pain.

Interestingly, there has been recent attention to attempting to enhance drainage of the main pancreatic duct by means of endoscopic sphincterotomy of the pancreatic duct sphincter with or without placement of a pancreatic duct stent. Unfortunately, enthusiasm for performing this procedure came well ahead of data to suggest that it had a therapeutic advantage. At present, there is little support for endoscopic pancreatic duct sphincterotomy in chronic pancreatitis.

Duval procedure

At almost the same time, and with a very similar strategy, Duval [2] proposed the procedure in which a small portion of the tail of the pancreas is resected and a loop of jejunum is anastomosed to the tail of the pancreas, facilitating drainage of the pancreatic duct through the tail. Unfortunately, this procedure also met with little success and was abandoned fairly promptly.

Longitudinal pancreaticojejunostomy

I believe it is pertinent to note that the original Puestow procedure was a modification of the Duval procedure. Puestow was the first to propose a longitudinal incision along the body of the pancreas with an anastomosis between a Roux-en-Y loop of jejunum and this longitudinal incision [9]. As a modification of the Duval procedure, Puestow suggested that the procedure include resection of the tail of the pancreas, followed by a longitudinal incision and an anastomosis. This procedure was recognized immediately as a safe and effective means of treating the pain associated with chronic pancreatitis. Partington and Rochelle [10] are credited with the procedure currently utilized exclusively as the technique for lateral pancreaticojejunostomy. The primary modification from the original description by Puestow [9] is the elimination of the resection of the tail of the pancreas. For this reason, many ascribe the eponym for this procedure to be the Partington-Rochelle procedure. It is my bias that Puestow was the originator of the concept of a longitudinal incision and I favor the terminology modified Puestow procedure. Many series have evolved to evaluate the success of the lateral pancreaticojejunostomy or modified Puestow procedure.

Important qualities inherent in this procedure include the fact that tissue is preserved. The avoidance of resection also greatly reduces both the mortality and the morbidity associated with this operation. Almost all large series have reported less than 1% mortality and morbidity less than 10% [5, 6, 11, 12]. More important is a consistent finding of long-term relief of pain in 85 to 95% of patients [4–6, 11, 12]. This procedure, when applied to appropriate patients, offers all of the best qualities sought in a procedure to treat the pain in this disease, no worsening of function and a very low mortality and morbidity.

The appropriate patient is one with chronic daily unrelenting abdominal pain, typically a patient dependent upon narcotics because of their pain and typically with considerable reduction in their quality of life, their ability to maintain employment, and their ability to meet the requirements of everyday life. These patients may or may not require frequent hospitalization [13]. Our data suggest that modified Puestow procedure successfully reduces the frequency of these acute exacerbations. It is clear that nutritional status is often affected by this disease, and data have been collected by our group and others to suggest that the drainage procedure results in uniform improvement in nutritional status, quality of life, and likelihood of employment [4].

Any study of outcomes of measures in chronic pancreatitis must be viewed with the perspective of many reports from Rudy Ammann [14, 15] in Zurich who has long examined the natural course and long-term follow-up of patients with chronic pancreatitis. Although his early studies focused on chronic pancreatitis managed medically, he has examined the effect of surgical intervention on this disease [15]. Many recognize these papers for having first proposed and repeatedly confirmed the process of "burnout" in this disease. Ammann proposes that over time the patient with chronic pancreatitis will have progressive loss of pancreatic endocrine and exocrine function, and that with this progressive loss of parenchyma, there is to be anticipated a diminution of pain to the point of achieving a status of "burnout" in which the patient has lost function but no longer is troubled by the pain of chronic pancreatitis. Naturally these data would argue that if surgery were simply delayed, then pain relief would be achieved without the expense, discomfort and risk of operative intervention. It is pertinent to note that in discussions undertaken by Dr. Ammann during this very symposium he pointed out an important distinction between his group and almost all other groups which have evaluated this disease. Dr. Ammann views narcotic dependence as a confounding variable and excludes all patients who require daily narcotics as a part of their disease. He only evaluates patients who are managed without narcotic analgesia. Degree of narcotics need is a standard, although subjective, measure of severity of CP for most authors. It is our belief that excluding patients with narcotic needs greatly reduces the severity of pain likely to be found in his population of patients. One might argue that his patients are more stoic, but a more reasonable speculation is that he has chosen patients whose pain is less severe. Thus, I would propose that his data are certainly valid, but apply to a subset of patients unlike the patients evaluated in most other large series. In general, most series include patients whose pain has been so severe that narcotic requirements is the rule.

There is a subset of patients who are ill-suited to the modified Puestow type drainage procedures. These include those patients who have the "small duct" variant of chronic pancreatitis. It would seem intuitive that patients without dilatation of the main pancreatic duct would gain little by decompression of this duct. Data have been collected to suggest that this is the case. Thus, in general, these patients are best suited to resectional therapy. In addition, patients with a dominant mass in the head of the pancreas are deemed poorly suited for a drainage procedure. The inflammatory mass (greater than 4.5 cm in diameter) may reach considerable size and is best suited to resection. Interestingly, a number of modifications of the standard lateral pancreaticojejunostomy have been proposed to address both of these issues. These modifications will be described subsequently, but briefly they include the duodenum-preserving pancreatic head resection created by Hans Beger [16] from Ulm, Germany, and excavation of the head of the pancreas in association with the longitudinal pancreaticojejunostomy as proposed by Frey [17]. Both of these procedures address the patients with the dominant mass in the head of the pancreas and a dilated duct. They may be viewed as combined resections and drainage procedures because they entail resecting a portion of the head of the pancreas. Finally, the so-called "V-shaped" excavation of the body of the pancreas along the main pancreatic duct followed by pancreaticojejunostomy has been proposed by Izbicki [12] and represents a variation on the standard drainage procedure, which may be better applied to patients with "small duct" variant of chronic pancreatitis.

Drainage procedures/impact upon function

Our group has long examined the impact on pancreatic endocrine and exocrine function that is seen after a variety of operative interventions in chronic pancreatitis [4, 13]. We have particularly focused on the modified Puestow procedure. Our method has been to evaluate all patients with chronic pancreatitis since 1985 that were seen in our clinic. A battery of structural and functional evaluations are performed, and we particularly focus upon endocrine function as measured by oral glucose tolerance test and pancreatic polypeptide release after a fatty meal. Exocrine function was analyzed by the bentiromide-PABA test and 72-hour fecal fat collection. Structural abnormalities were evaluated by ERCP and the Cambridge classification was utilized to grade patients as mild, moderate or severe changes, according to that formula. Using these five measures, two endocrine, two exocrine, and one anatomic, a grading system was created and baseline function was established for all patients. Patients were categorized as mild/moderate disease when their baseline analysis had 0, 1 or 2 of these 5 measures abnormal. Patients were categorized as severe when they had 3 to 5 of these risk factors abnormal (Table 13.1-1). We have

Table 13.1-1. Five-point system to grade severity of chronic pancreatitis.

Test	Threshold	Points assigned
ERCP	Cambridge "severe"	1
OGTT/Insulin	Abnormal hyperglycemia	1
Pancreatic polypeptide release after ingested fat	Flat response	1
72-hour fecal fat on 100 g Fat/24 hr	More than 7 gm in 24 hr	1
Bentiromide/PABA	Less than 50% absorption	1
		Total 5 points

Method for grading the severity of chronic pancreatitis

OGTT – oral glucose tolerance test

Patients with 0, 1 or 2 points were assigned a grade of "mild to moderate" chronic pancreatitis

Patients with 3, 4 or 5 points were categorized as severe chronic pancreatitis currently evaluated 223 patients with chronic pancreatitis. Seventy-six of these patients were categorized as severe chronic pancreatitis after initial evaluation. No patient with this level of disease had improvement of function over the period of analysis. A total of 104 patients have undergone modified Puestow procedure. We have had no deaths. The mean follow-up of patients in all categories after their initial evaluation is 76 months.

One hundred and forty-seven patients were categorized at baseline measures as mild to moderate chronic pancreatitis. Seventy-one of these patients have undergone modified Puestow procedure while 76 did not undergo a drainage procedure. The mean follow-up for the patients with mild to moderate chronic pancreatitis is 73 months. Among the mild to moderate patients, 52 of the 71 patients who underwent operation have remained mild to moderate chronic pancreatitis in follow-up. Nineteen operated patients have progressed to severe chronic pancreatitis with generalized loss of function. This contrasts with the data on patients who were originally categorized as mild to moderate pancreatitis who did not undergo operation. Among these 76 patients, only 29 (38%) were still categorized as mild to moderate disease in follow-up. Forty-seven patients or 62% had progressed to severe chronic pancreatitis during the follow-up period. Thus, 73% of patients operated had preservation of function compared to 38% who had preservation of function after no operation. It should be stressed that our finding is that loss of function is delayed. We do not claim to achieve improved function after decompression. Pain relief was achieved in 84% of patients, which is comparable to most reports in the literature. Success rates have varied from 75 to 92% for long-term relief of pain [4–7, 11, 12]. The data are remarkably consistent across a variety of series of patients who have undergone modified Puestow procedure to confirm these high rates of success for relief of pain. Our data were the first to suggest that an advantage may be appreciated beyond simple relief of pain. Our data suggest that the progressive loss of function, typically seen in chronic pancreatitis, may be delayed significantly by decompression of the main pancreatic duct. In separate studies, we have examined "small duct" chronic pancreatitis since most of our non-operated patients have this variant. Our data show that "small duct" disease has a more favorable outcome overall.

There have been observations made in other series of operative decompression of the main pancreatic duct suggesting similar outcomes. Beger et al. [18] have reported in their series of patients with limited resection and decompression in the so-called duodenum-preserving pancreatic head resection that both endocrine and exocrine function has improved dramatically in certain patients. In addition, a recent report from Sidhu et al. [19] reports remarkable improvement in endocrine function when patients with tropical chronic pancreatitis have been treated with the modified Puestow procedure. They compared 53 patients who underwent operation to 36 patients who did not. Four of the 11 patients who required insulin prior to operation were able to stop their insulin therapy entirely after decompression. The fasting and postprandial blood glucose levels and the overall insulin requirements decreased significantly. They found somewhat modest improvements in exocrine function as well.

Reber et al. [20] have produced scientific data to support these outcomes. By utilizing the model of partial obstruction of the pancreatic duct in cats, he is able to induce chronic pancreatitis. Reber has developed the "pancreatic compartment syndrome" theory. On the basis of this theory, the high intraductal and intraparenchymal pressures created by a partial obstruction of the main pancreatic duct results in a localized ischemia and a localized intracellular acidosis, which results in depression in functional measures in these cats. Reber [8] has further evaluated decompression by means of a Puestow type operation in the cats. In his studies, pancreatic exocrine and endocrine function improved considerably after decompression.

As mentioned briefly earlier in this manuscript, there are those who would suggest that the data from Ammann would dictate that simply waiting for "burnout" of the pancreas would achieve pain relief without intervention. I would again take note of the important distinction in Ammann's studies which came to light at this symposium, that his studies have excluded patients who are narcotic dependent. In addition, it is noteworthy that our data have failed to define a similar outcome in any of our patients followed for long-term. On the basis of our data and others, we advocate an aggressive attitude towards decompression of the main pancreatic duct in chronic pancreatitis. It is our belief that early decompression will result in prolonged preservation of pancreatic endocrine and exocrine function and possibly result in improved endocrine and exocrine function in individual patients.

Extended drainage procedures

Although discussed in some detail in other chapters in this book, I would like to make brief mention of extended drainage procedures, which have been evaluated as modifications of the simple longitudinal incision in the main pancreatic duct. Most significant of these and studied extensively is the duodenum-preserving pancreatic head resection, which was developed by Beger. Beger [16] and associates and subsequently studies by his protégée, Büchler, have consistently reported long-term pain relief in more than 90% of patients. In addition, as previously mentioned, their data suggest that a subset of patients have significant improvement in exocrine, and particularly endocrine, function after decompression. Many other sites have subsequently published data suggesting similar success rates for relief of pain using this operative procedure. It is the perceived advantage of this operative procedure that you have some preservation of pancreatic parenchyma and you have preservation of the gastroduodenal complex. Stenosis of the common bile duct may also be managed by simply unroofing the rigid wall of fibrosis that surrounds the common bile duct and thereby relieving any restriction to flow of bile caused by chronic pancreatitis. This negates the need for a separate choledochojejunostomy, which is, at times, indicated in patients undergoing modified Puestow procedure.

Subsequent to Beger's description of his operative procedure, Charles Frey [17] developed a procedure in which the body of the pancreas is not divided, as it is in the duodenum-preserving pancreatic head resection. He proposed a simple excavation of the head of the pancreas in combination with a longitudinal incision in the main pancreatic duct as one would do in a standard Puestow procedure. Both Beger [16] and Frey [17] target with their procedures the patients who have a dilated duct and a dominant mass in the head of the pancreas. The supposition is that the dominant mass will continue to cause pain unless some amount of this is resected. Frey believes that he preserves more parenchyma with his procedure than can be achieved with the duodenum-preserving pancreatic head resection. Frey has reported significant long-term pain relief with his operative procedure. He has made no analysis of the functional status of patients after his procedure.

Finally, in recent times, Izbicki [12] developed the "V-shaped excision" in association with a modified Puestow procedure. The target for this operation is patients with so-called "small duct" chronic pancreatitis. It is his belief that excising the tissue around the duct in combination with a drainage procedure may successfully ameliorate the pain associated with chronic pancreatitis in a subset of patients who otherwise would be managed with a more radical resection. His purpose, therefore, again is preservation of pancreatic parenchyma. He has an early series that presented promising data regarding early pain relief, and his subsequent report evaluated pain relief as well as endocrine insufficiency, exocrine insufficiency, and nutritional status. All of these measures were compared to more radical resections and he was able to confirm that his operation resulted in far less insufficiency and in improved nutritional status compared to the more radical resections.

References

1. Doubilet H. The physiologic basis of surgical treatment of acute and chronic pancreatitis. Sug Clin North Am 1958; 38: 505–11.
2. Duval MK, Jr, Enquist IF. The surgical treatment of chronic pancreatitis by pancreaticojejunostomy: an 8 year reappraisal. Surgery 1961; 50: 965–72.
3. Goecke H, Forssmann U, Uguccioni M, Friess H, Conejo-Garcia JR, Zimmermann A, Baggiolini M, Büchler MW. Macrophages infiltrating the tissue in chronic pancreatitis express the chemokine receptor CCR5. Surgery 2000; 128: 806–14.
4. Nealon WH, Thompson JC. Progressive loss of pancreatic function in chronic pancreatitis is delayed by main pancreatic duct decompression. A longitudinal prospective analysis of the modified Puestow procedure. Ann Surg 1993; 217: 458–68.
5. Proctor HJ, Mendes OC, Thomas CG, Jr, Herbst CA. Surgery for chronic pancreatitis. Drainage versus resection. Ann Surg 1979; 189: 664–71.
6. Prinz RA, Greenlee HB. Pancreatic duct drainage in 100 patients with chronic pancreatitis. Ann Surg 1981; 194: 313–20.
7. Sohn TA, Campbell KA, Pitt HA, Sauter PK, Coleman JA, Lillemo KD, Yeo CJ, Cameron JL. Quality of life and long-term survival after surgery for chronic pancreatitis. J Gastrointest Surg 2000; 4: 355–65.
8. Patel AG, Reber PU, Toyama MT, Ashley SW, Reber HA. Effect of pancreaticojejunostomy on fibrosis, pancreatic blood flow, and interstitial pH in chronic pancreatitis: a feline model. Ann Surg 1999; 230: 672–9.
9. Puestow CB, Gillesby WJ. Retrograde surgical drainage of pancreas for chronic relapsing pancreatitis. A. M. A. Arch Surg 1958; 76: 898–907.
10. Partington PF, Rochelle EL. Modified Puestow procedure for retrograde drainage of pancreatic duct. Ann Surg 1960; 152: 1037–943.
11. Evans JD, Wilson PG, Carver C, Bramhall SR, Buckels JA, Mayer AD, McMaster P, Neoptolemos JP. Outcome of surgery for chronic pancreatitis. Br J Surg 1997; 84: 624–9.
12. Izbicki JR, Bloechle C, Knoefel WT, Rogiers X, Kuechler T. Surgical treatment of chronic pancreatitis and quality of life after operation. Surg Clin North Am 1999; 79: 913–44.
13. Nealon WH, Matin S. Analysis of surgical success in preventing recurrent acute exacerbations in chronic pancreatitis. Ann Surg 2001; 233: 793–800.
14. Ammann RW, Muench R, Otto R, Buehler H, Freiburghaus AU, Siegenthaler W. Evolution and regression of pancreatic calcification in chronic pancreatitis. A prospective long-term study of 107 patients. Gastroenterology 1988; 95: 1018–28.
15. Ammann RW, Largiader F, Akovbiantz A. Pain relief by surgery in chronic pancreatitis? Relationship between pain relief, pancreatic dysfunction, and alcohol withdrawal. Scand J Gastroenterol 1979; 14: 209–15.
16. Beger HG, Schlosser W, Friess HM, Büchler MW. Duodenum-preserving head resection in chronic pancreatitis changes the natural course of the disease: a single-center 26-year experience. Ann Surg 1999; 230: 512–23.

17. Frey CF, Smith GJ. Description and rationale of a new operation for chronic pancreatitis. Pancreas 1987; 2: 701–7.
18. Bittner R, Butters M, Büchler M, Nagele S, Roscher R, Beger HG. Glucose homeostasis and endocrine pancreatic function in patients with chronic pancreatitis before and after surgical therapy. Pancreas 1994; 9: 47–53.
19. Sidhu SS, Nundy S, Tandon RK. The effect of the modified Puestow procedure on diabetes in patients with tropical chronic pancreatitis – a prospective study. Am J Gastroenterol 2001; 96: 107–11.
20. Reber HA, Karanjia ND, Alvarez C, Widdison AL, Leung FW, Ashley SW, Lutrin FJ. Pancreatic blood flow in cats with chronic pancreatitis. Gastroenterology 1992; 103: 652–9.

13.2 Duodenum-preserving pancreatic head resection changes the natural course of chronic pancreatitis

W. Schlosser, H. G. Beger

Natural course of alcoholic chronic pancreatitis

Chronic pancreatitis is a disease characterized by progressive inflammation of the endocrine and exocrine tissue which is mainly caused by chronic alcohol abuse in western countries. The morphological changes which occur during the disease can be best explained by the mechanism of alcohol-induced hypersecretion of acinar cells forming protein plugs, leading to periductal inflammation and fibrosis [8]. The pathomorphological result is a progressive destruction of acinar cells and an increase of extracellular matrix, which leads to deposition of fibrotic tissue. Besides this hypothesis the concept of recurrent attacks of acute pancreatitis causing acinar and fatty necrosis leading to perilobular fibrosis is more and more accepted [9]. According to this hypothesis, the periductal fibrosis causes ductal obstruction of the main duct and the side branches. After a period of more or less frequent pain attacks clinical signs of exocrine and endocrine pancreatic insufficiency appear in most of the patients. In around 30% of the patients with long lasting alcohol-induced chronic pancreatitis the development of an inflammatory mass in the head of the pancreas can be observed [3]. The clinical picture is dominated by nearly intractable upper abdominal pain in the majority of the patients. This pain syndrome may be caused by a chronic pancreatitis-associated neuritis, which is characterized by an enlargement of pancreatic sensory nerves in the area of the enlarged pancreatic head [1]. Pathomorphological characteristics of the inflammatory mass are focal necrosis, parenchymal calcifications, small cystic cavities and duct calculi deposition [10]. On the basis of a long-term follow-up observation the natural course of CP reveals a pain persistence in 55–85% of the patients 5 to 10 years after diagnosis [12]. Local complications like pseudocysts, common bile duct stenosis and compression of anatomical structures surrounding the pancreatic head are observed frequently. Long-term follow-up reveals that patients with CP have a 5-year survival of 67% and a 10-year survival of 43% [12, 13].

Pancreatic head: Pacemaker of chronic pancreatitis

In terms of CT scan for diagnosis of the pancreas, around 30% of all patients referred for surgical treatment reveal a pancreatic head enlargement, defined as a vertical pancreatic head diameter of 4 cm as borderline extension. In the normal pancreas, the pancreatic head including the neck of the pancreas covers approximately 45–55% of the pancreatic tissue. In terms of chronic inflammation characteristic pathomorphological changes can be found in the pancreatic head (Table 13.2-1). Furthermore the head of the pancreas covers two different embryological parts of the pancreas, the dorsal and the ventral pancreas, which might influence the pathomorphology of the chronic inflammation in the pancreatic head. The double duct system in the pancreatic head including the duct of Santorini and the duct of Wirsung is of clinical relevance for the pathomorphology of

Table 13.2-1. Pathomorphological changes in the pancreatic head with inflammatory mass (intraoperative findings in 504 patients*).

	Patients	
	n	%
Calcifications of the parenchyma	290	58
Pseudocystic small cavities (< 1 cm)	115	23
Large pseudocysts	46	9
Areas of focal necrosis (< 1 cm)	45	9
Pancreatic main duct stenosis	187	37
Common bile duct stenosis	217	43
Duct stones	148	29

* 11/1972–4/1982, Department of Surgery, Free University of Berlin, Germany
5/1982–12/1998, Department of General Surgery, University of Ulm, Germany

inflammation of the pancreas. The experience with recurrent pancreatitis in pancreas divisum and pancreatobiliary malfunction demonstrates that anomalies of the pancreatic duct system in the head of the pancreas sometimes lead to an inflammatory process in the head due to obstruction of the pancreatic juice flow and generation of local inflammatory process [11, 12].

Patients and methods

From 11/1972 to 12/1998, 504 patients underwent DPPHR for complicated chronic pancreatitis. 80% of the patients were male, 20% female, the mean age at the time of surgery was 44.4 years, the duration of pain was 3.6 years (median). 81% of the patients suffered from alcohol-induced CP and 19% of the patients had CP of unknown etiology, but 8% of them had an association with gallstones. Patients' data concerning etiology of the disease, medical history and pain had been documented prospectively. For preoperative diagnostic work-up sonography, computed tomography (CT) and endoscopic retrograde cholangio-pancreaticography (ERCP) were performed. Mesenterico-celiacography, hypotonic duodenography, endosonography, and magnetic resonance tomography (MRT) were used in some patients for special indications. For evaluation of endocrine function the oral glucose tolerance test (OGTT®) was performed in all patients except those suffering from manifest diabetes mellitus. A pancreolauryl test for evaluation of the exocrine pancreatic function was conducted in most patients. Preoperative morbidity and indications for surgery are listed in Tables 13.2-2 and 13.2-3. Follow-up investigations up to 26 years were evaluated to evaluate the early and late outcome of the patients with CP having undergone DPPHR. The results of these follow-up investigations were published in Surgery 1985 [4], Annals of Surgery 1989 [5], Journal of Gastrointestinal Surgery 1997 [6], and Annals of Surgery 1999 [7]. In the last follow-up investigation 388 patients operated on in the period from 5/1982 to 10/1996 were included. 310 (80%) of the patients were men and 78 (20%) were women; the mean age at the time of operation was 50.4 years (21–82 years). The in-hospital mortality was 1% (4 patients). The late mortality was 13% (49 pts.). 7 patients (2%) had to be reoperated for pain; 25 patients (6%) were lost for follow-up investigation. The late morbidity and quality of life after DPPHR was re-evaluated after 5.7 years in median (0–14.4 years) after surgical treatment. Most of the

		Patients n	%
Abdominal pain		**460**	**91**
	Occasional	53	12
	Frequent	196	43
	Daily	211	46
Pain treatment		3.6 years (median)	
Endocrine function (OGGT)	Normal range	246	49
	Latent	134	26
	IDDM	124	25
Exocrine function (PLT)	Reduced	284/329	86

* 11/1972–4/1982, Department of Surgery, Free University of Berlin, Germany
5/1982–12/1998, Department of General Surgery, University of Ulm, Germany

Table 13.2-2. Preoperative morbidity of patients with chronic pancreatitis and inflammatory mass in the head of the pancreas (IMH) (504 patients*).

	Patients n	%
Enlarged head (> 4 cm)	376	75
Pseudocystic lesion (> 1 cm)	46	9
Cholestasis	189	38
CBD-stenosis	232	46
PMD-stenosis	321	64
Duodenum stenosis	118	23
Vascular obstruction	80	16

* 11/1972–4/1982, Department of Surgery, Free University of Berlin, Germany
5/1982–12/1998, Department of General Surgery, University of Ulm, Germany

Table 13.2-3. Local complications of chronic pancreatitis with inflammatory mass in the head of the pancreas (504 patients*).

patients were reinvestigated in the outpatient department of the hospital. A proportion of the patients who were not able to join a hospital investigation program because of geographical or personal obstacles were reinvestigated by the family physician according to the protocol.

Preoperative morbidity of patients with chronic pancreatitis and IMH

Patients with chronic pancreatitis developing an inflammatory mass in the head of the pancreas are considered as a subgroup of about 30% of all patients with chronic pancreatitis [3]. The etiology is chronic alcohol overindulgence in more than 80%. The clinical picture is dominated by severe upper abdominal pain, often intractable by medical treatment. The patients have a history of a median pain treatment of 3.6 years. More than half of the patients present an impaired endocrine and exocrine function at the time of admission for surgery (Table 13.2-2). The average of the patients are male (70–90%) and the mean age is less than 40 years at the time of diagnosis. Due to involvement of the neighboring organ structures by the inflammatory mass, morphologic alterations like stenosis of the common bile duct, severe duodenum stenosis or compression of the portal vein occur in a remarkable number of the patients (Table 13.2-3).

Change in the natural course of chronic pancreatitis

504 patients with chronic pancreatitis and an inflammatory mass in the pancreatic head were treated with duodenum-preserving pancreatic head resection (DPPHR) between 11/1972 and 12/1998. Due to the limitation of the surgical procedure early postoperative morbidity and mortality were low. The hospital mortality was 0.8%, 5.6% of the patients had to be reoperated, postoperative hospitalization was in median 14.5 days. The most frequent indications for reoperations were bleeding from the pancreatic anastomosis, anastomotic leakage and intra-abdominal abscess. In addition to the standard reconstruction, a biliary anastomosis between common bile duct and excluded jejunal loop was necessary in 24% of the patients (Fig. 13.2-1). As a consequence of multiple stenosis of the pancreatic main duct a lateral pancreaticojejunostomy after longitudinal opening of the duct was performed in 9% of the patients (Fig. 13.2-2). The subtotal resection of the pancreatic head resulted in a decompression of the portal vein in 13%. Additional pseudocyst treatment was performed by anastomosis with the excluded jejunal loop in 7 patients. The intraoperatively observed macromorphological alterations in the pancreatic head are listed in Table 13.2-3. Subtotal resection of the pancreatic head resulted in an improved glucose metabolism of preoperatively latent or insulin-dependent diabetes

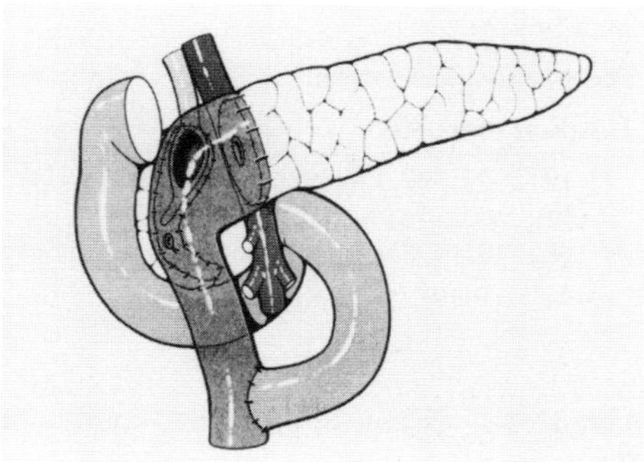

Figure 13.2-1. Duodenum-preserving pancreatic head resection combined with an internal biliary anastomosis.

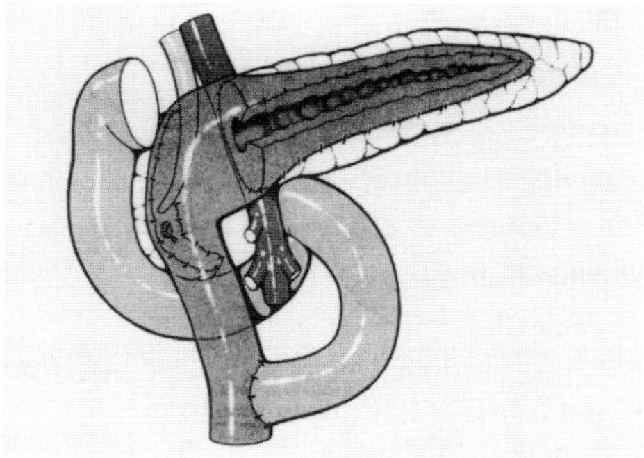

Figure 13.2-2. Duodenum-preserving pancreatic head resection combined with a lateral pancreaticojejunostomy.

in 9%; only 4% showed a deterioration with newly developed diabetes mellitus in the early postoperative period (Table 13.2-4).

During the follow-up period with a median of 5.7 years it has been demonstrated that late morbidity and mortality after DPPHR are surprisingly low (Table 13.2-5). Upper abdominal pain dropped from 93% preoperatively to 8.7% in the late follow-up. The average pain score of the patients still having pain after DPPHR was 4.8. The rate of patients who suffered from acute episodes of chronic pancreatitis fell from 69% to 12.5% postoperatively. 3.3% of the patients had to be reoperated due to pancreatitis-related complications. The late death rate was 13%. Concerning the endocrine function late after DPPHR 39% of the patients revealed normal glucose tolerance (Table 13.2-6). The number of patients with diabetes mellitus increased from 25% to 44%. However, 11% of the patients demonstrate an improved glucose metabolism compared to an impaired endocrine function preoperatively. The majority of the patients operated on with the DPPHR were reintegrated in their former profession or were working in a new profession (69%); 26% retired. In this respect, the Karnofsky index as an indicator of quality of life was 90–100 in 72% of the patients (Table 13.2-7).

Table 13.2-4. Early postoperative results after duodenum-preserving pancreatic head resection (504 patients*).

	Patients	
	n	%
Relaparotomy	28	5.6
Postop. deteriorated glucose metabolism	18	4
Postop. improved glucose metabolism	47	9
Postop. hospitalization	14.5 days (median)	
Hospital mortality	4	0.8

* 11/1972–4/1982, Department of Surgery, Free University of Berlin, Germany
5/1982–12/1998, Department of General Surgery, University of Ulm, Germany

Table 13.2-5. Change in the natural course of chronic pancreatitis (388 patients*; follow-up rate 94%).

	Preoperative 388 patients		Late postop., 5.7 yrs 303 patients	
	n	%	n	%
Abdominal pain	361	93[a)]	25	8.7[a)]
Acute episodes/hospitalization	268	69[b)]	38	12.5[b)]
Development of pancreatic cancer	22	5.6	2	0.7
Development of extrapancreatic cancer			4	1.3
Reoperation			10	1.3
Late death			49	13

* 5/1982–10/1996, Department of General Surgery, University of Ulm, Germany
a) $p > 0.0001$ (McNemar)
b) $p > 0.001$ (McNemar)

Table 13.2-6. Endocrine function after DPPHR.

	Preoperative 1972–1998 504 patients		Late postop. 1984 [4] 2.0 yrs[a)] 56 patients		Late postop. 1988 [5] 3.6 yrs[a)] 109 patients	Late postop. 1997 [7] 5.7 yrs[a)] 308 patients	
	n	%	n	%	%	n	%
OGTT normal	246	49	37	66	48	118	39
OGTT reduced	134	26			26	51	17
IDDM	124	25			26	134	44

OGTT = oral glucose tolerance test, IDDM = insulin-dependent diabetes mellitus
a) median years follow-up
[4] Beger, Surgery 1985; [5] Beger, Ann Surg 1989; [7] Beger, Ann Surg 1999

Table 13.2-7. DPPHR changes the natural course of the disease in chronic pancreatitis.

	1972–1983 [4] 58 patients 2.0 yrs[a)] 56 patients	1972–1987 [5] 128 patients 3.6 yrs[a)] 109 patients	1982–1996 [7] 388 patients 5.7 yrs[a)] 303 patients
Follow-up rate	100%	96%	94%
Pain free	92.8%	89%	91.3%
Pain	7.2%	11%	8.7%
Acute episodes	14%	11%	13%
Late death	3.6%	4.7%	13%
Endocrine function improved	15.8%	5.5%	11%
Professional rehabilitation	88.7%	67%	69%
Quality of life/Kanofsky Index > 80			82%

[4] Beger, Surgery 1985; [5] Beger, Ann Surg 1989; [7] Beger, Ann Surg 1999
a) median years follow-up

Discussion

The DPPHR results in a reduction or total absence of pain in the majority of the patients. The subtotal resection of the pancreatic head leads to relief of local complications such as stenosis of the pancreatic main duct, stenosis of the common bile duct, decompression of the duodenum and decompression of the portal and superior mesenteric vein. Compared to the Whipple operation which had been the standard procedure for a long time the DPPHR has the advantage of preserving the normal anatomical structures surrounding the pancreatic head combined with preservation of a maximum of pancreatic tissue. The superiority of the duodenum-preserving technique over pylorus-preserving resection could be shown in prospective studies [16, 58]. Concerning the pain status after DPPHR the results of 4 reevaluations in a period of 26 years show a cumulative pain-free status in 88–92.8% of the patients. In the natural course of pancreatitis without surgical intervention, the rate of patients suffering from pain decreases to 85% after 5 years. However, the majority of the patients (53%) still has pain after more than 10 years [11, 12]. In this series 91% of the patients were pain-free in an observation period of up to 14 years after DPPHR. During the observation period only 9% of the patients suffered from further acute episodes with the need of hospitalization due to pancreatitis.

Compared to the Whipple procedure and its modification, the pylorus-preserving modification, the DPPHR offers the major advantage of preserving the duodenum. Mainly due to the preserved physiologic gastrointestinal passage the endocrine function of the pancreas is preserved at least early postoperatively [4, 5]. It could be shown that the improvement of the endocrine function in 5–15% after DPPHR is the result of reduced levels of the anti-insulinary hormones glucagon and somatostatin [2]. Nevertheless, in the long-term follow-up 21% of the patients developed new incidence of diabetes mellitus. Compared to the natural course of chronic pancreatitis with 17% normal glucose metabolism [12], patients following DPPHR reveal preserved endocrine function in 39%. In terms of quality of life after DPPHR 69% of the patients were professionally rehabilitated, 26% retired, and only 5% of the patients were still in the status of disease. Using the Karnofsky-Index scoring system, 72% of the patients were scored within the normal range after DPPHR. After DPPHR the death rate was 8.9 and 13% in two groups with a median observation time of more than 5 years (Table 13.2-7). In studies with a comparable observation time the reported death rate was 20.8 to 35% [12, 14, 15]. The lower late mortality after DPPHR compares favorably with the late mortality after Whipple procedure [16, 17]. In the series between 1982 and 1996 6.3% of the patients developed a ductal pancreatic carcinoma in the pancreatic head after a long period of clinical treatment for chronic pancreatitis. This emphasizes the increased risk of developing pancreatic cancer in patients suffering from chronic pancreatitis with an inflammatory mass in the head.

Conclusion

Obviously DPPHR leads to an interruption of the inflammatory process in the left pancreas, sparing the patients further hospitalizations and pain attacks. The surgical excision of the main inflammatory process in the head of the pancreas promotes the transformation of clinically manifest chronic pancreatitis into a silent status of the disease in most patients. With regard to pain status, frequency of acute episodes of chronic pancreatitis, the need for further hospitalization, the low early and late mortality and the restoration of quality of life, DPPHR results in a change in the natural course of the disease.

References

1. Bockman DE, Büchler MW, Malfertheiner P, Beger HG. Analysis of nerves in chronic pancreatitis. Gastroenterology 1988; 94: 1459–69.
2. Bittner R, Butters M, Büchler MW, Nägele S, Roscher R, Beger HG. Glucose hemostasis and endocrine pancreatic function in patients with chronic pancreatitis before and after surgical therapy. Pancreas 1994; 9: 47–53.
3. Beger HG, Büchler MW. Duodenum-preserving resection of the head of the pancreas in chronic pancreatitis with inflammatory mass in the head. World J Surg 1990; 14: 83–7.
4. Beger HG, Krautzberger W, Bittner R. Duodenum-preserving resection of the head of the pancreas in patients with severe chronic pancreatitis. Surgery 1985; 97: 467–73.
5. Beger HG, Büchler MW, Bittner R, Öttinger W, Roscher R. Duodenum-preserving resection of the head of the pancreas in severe chronic pancreatitis. Ann Surg 1989; 209(3): 273–9.

6. Büchler MW, Friess H, Bittner R, Roscher R, Krautzberger W, Müller MW, Malfertheiner P, Beger HG. Duodenum-preserving pancreatic head resection: Long-term results. J Gastrointest Surg 1997; 1: 13–9.
7. Beger HG, Schlosser W, Friess H, Büchler MW. Duodenum-preserving head resection in chronic pancreatitis changes the normal course of the disease: a single-center 26-year experience. Ann Surg 1999; 230(4): 512–9.
8. Sarles H, Dagorn JC, Giorgi D, Bernard JP. Remaining pancreatic stone protein as "lithostatin". Gastroenterology 1990; 99: 900–5.
9. Klöppel G, Maillet B. Pseudocysts in chronic pancreatitis: a morphological analysis of 57 resection specimens and 9 autopsy pancreata. Pancreas 1991; 6: 266–74.
10. Beger HG, Witte C, Kraas E. Erfahrungen mit einer das Duodenum erhaltenden Pankreaskopfresektion bei chronischer Pankreatitis. Chirurg 1980; 51: 303–9.
11. Widmaier U, Schmidt A, Schlosser W, Beger HG. Die duodenumerhaltende Pankreaskopfresektion in der Therapie des Pancreas divisum. Chirurg 1997; 68: 180–6.
12. Lankisch PG, Löhr-Happe A, Otto J, Creutzfeld W. Natural course in chronic pancreatitis. Pain, exocrine and endocrine pancreatic insufficiency and prognosis of the disease. Digestion 1993; 54: 148–55.
13. Lankisch PG, Izbicki JR, Binmoeller KF, Soehendra N, eds. Chronic Pancreatitis. Berlin, New York: Walter de Gruyter & Co., 1997; Natural course of chronic pancreatitis. 1–14.
14. Ammann R, Akovbiantz A, Largiader F, Schueler G. Course and outcome of chronic pancreatitis. Longitudinal study of a mixed medical-surgical series of 245 patients. Gastroenterology 1984; 86: 820–8.
15. Miyake H, Harada H, Kunichika K, Ochi K, Kimura I. Clinical course and prognosis of chronic pancreatitis. Pancreas 1987; 2: 378–85.
16. Howard JM. Howard JM, Jordan GL, Reber HA, eds. Surgical Disease of the Pancreas. Philadelphia: Lea & Febiger; 1987; Surgical treatment of chronic pancreatitis. 496–521.
17. Christiansen J, Olsen JH, Worning H. The pancreatic function following subtotal pancreatectomy for cancer. Scand J Gastroenterol 1971; 6(Suppl): 189–93.

13.3 Modifications of the duodenum-preserving pancreatic head resection

T. Strate, C. Busch, C. Bloechle, W. T. Knoefel, J. R. Izbicki

Summary

Surgery for chronic pancreatitis has gained wide acceptance because of excellent results regarding pain alleviation and control of complications arising from adjacent organs. After the introduction of the duodenum-preserving pancreatic head resection by Beger almost three decades ago, many modifications have been proposed, evaluated and compared. This article reviews the variety of operations, the reported results and potential advantages.

The indications for surgical intervention are intractable pain, complications related to adjacent organs, endoscopically not permanently controlled pancreatic pseudocysts in conjunction with ductal pathology, and conservatively intractable internal pancreatic fistula [1]. Occasionally the inability to exclude pancreatic cancer despite broad diagnostic work-up also requires surgery [2]. The ideal surgical approach should address all these problems.

Pain is the crucial symptom in severe chronic pancreatitis. Reflecting experimental evidence and clinical experience, ductal and parenchymatous hypertension and neural alterations in combination with extensive fibrosis have been developed as basic hypotheses on the pathogenesis of pain in chronic pancreatitis [3, 4].

Referring to these different ideas of pain origin, drainage and resection have emerged as the main principles of surgery in chronic pancreatitis. Exclusively draining or resective operations [5, 6] have failed to meet all the aims of an ideal surgical treatment for chronic pancreatitis.

Surgical methods

Duodenum-preserving resection of the head of the pancreas (DPRHP) according to Beger [7, 8]

Beger devised this operation in the early 70s and reported his results some years later [7].

After ventral dissection and dorsal mobilization of the head of the pancreas, frozen sections are sampled. The gland is tunneled above the portomesenteric vein, where it is divided. Hemostasis of the left resection margin is achieved by transfixing stitches. The resection is carried out towards the papilla of Vater. The pancreatic head is resected almost completely leaving only a small margin of pancreatic tissue between the duodenum and the common bile duct. Towards the vena cava a small rim of pancreatic tissue is preserved, too. The bile duct is freed from scarring tissue to ensure sufficient bile flow. Preservation of the gastroduodenal artery is not mandatory. While resecting the uncinate process, care should be applied to spare the meso-duodenal vessels. A pancreaticojejunostomy and pancreatojejunostomy is performed using a Roux-en-Y loop of proximal jejunum. If the common bile duct cannot be decompressed, a choledochotomy proximal to the papilla should be performed fixating the margins to the dorsal pancreatic plate, so bile can drain into the resection cavity.

Warren's modification [9]

Four years after Beger's report on duodenum-preserving pancreatic head resection, Warren et al. suggested a modification of this procedure. After performing the pancreatic head resection much in the way Beger described it, the body and tail of the pancreas are denervated by ligating and dividing the splenic vein at its junction with the superior mesenteric vein. The splenic artery is divided as it approaches the pancreas from the celiac axis. Viability of the spleen is ensured through its extensive arterial and venous collateral circulation, principally the gastroepiploic and short gastric systems. The entire flap (pancreas, splenic artery and vein and associated nerve fibers) is freed from all tissue until the pancreas is attached only to the vessels at the hilus of the spleen. This maneuver supposedly severs all somatic and autonomic nerve fibers. Finally a Roux-en-Y loop of jejunum is prepared and the pancreatic duct anastomosed with a small mucosal opening.

The longitudinal pancreaticojejunostomy combined with local pancreatic head excision (LPJ-LPHE) according to Frey [10]

Frey and co-workers reported on a modification of the DPRHP [7, 10]. The operative difference between the two methods is a more radical resection of the pancreatic head in the Beger procedure. Frey's technique combines a modified longitudinal pancreaticojejunostomy according to Partingtom-Rochelle with limited excision of the pancreatic head.

After a Kocher maneuver and identification of the superior mesenteric and portal vein, the pancreatic duct is opened longitudinally, proximally and distally. Absorbable sutures are placed parallel to, and not less than 3–4 mm from, the duodenum along the inner aspect of the duodenum for hemostasis. The head of the pancreas is cored out leaving a cuff of pancreas along the inner aspect of the duodenum. Care should be taken not to interrupt the gastroduodenal artery and the anterior pancreaticoduodenal arcade on the same patient. Medially, a margin of at least 4–5 mm of pancreatic head is left right to the portal vein to avoid dividing the pancreas. Posteriorly, a shell of pancreas remains between the cored out head, the uncinate process and the inferior vena cava. A Roux-en-Y double layer pancreaticojejunostomy is performed.

Takada's modification [11]

In 1993 Takada et al. proposed a variation of a duodenum-preserving pancreatic head resection [11]. The mobilization is similar to the Beger procedure, but a Kocher maneuver is not performed. After transection of the pancreatic gland over the portal vein, a polyvinyl tube is inserted into the pancreatic duct and a suture is placed to fix the tube. The anterior superior pancreatoduodenal artery is divided and the pancreatic head is resected towards the duodenum. The pancreatic duct is divided at its junction with the bile duct. After complete resection of the pancreatic head, the remaining pancreatic duct is anastomosed to the duodenum. The posterior cut edge of the pancreas is sutured to the duodenal wall. A small incision is made into the duodenum opposite to the remaining pancreatic duct and the pancreatic duct tube is introduced into the duodenum and brought out of the intestinal tract through the anterior wall of the middle third of the stomach. The pancreaticoduodenal anastomosis is performed. Then the duodenum is sutured to the anterior cut edge of the pancreas.

Kimura's and Sapy's modifications [12–14]

Kimura et al. suggested a different modification of a duodenum-preserving pancreatic head resection with detailed description of how to preserve the duodenal blood supply.

After a complete Kocher maneuver is performed, the pancreas is cut above the portal vein and removed from the third portion of the duodenum. Then the posterior surface of the pancreatic head is removed from the connective tissue membrane, which should be left intact in order to ensure blood flow to the duodenum. The main pancreatic duct is cut at its junction with the terminal portion of the bile duct. The pancreas is cut in the line of the anterior superior pancreaticoduodenal artery (running along the right side of the common bile duct and supplying the papilla of Vater with blood). In essence the pancreatic tissue between the duodenum and the common bile duct is left intact so as to preserve sufficient blood flow to the papilla. After careful suturing of the cut surface of the pancreas with nylon mono-filament strings, the remaining body of the pancreas is anastomosed in the posterior wall of the stomach. A very similar technique using a pancreatogastrostomy for reconstruction of the alimentary tract was described by Sapy et al. a few years later [14]. He did not indicate how much pancreatic tissue was left at the duodenal wall and to what extend the common bile duct was freed from pancreatic and connective tissue.

Nakao's modification [15]

Nakao described a pancreatic head resection with segmental duodenectomy including minor and major papilla in 1998.

After cholecystectomy, the pancreas is divided above the portal vein. The extra-pancreatic nerve plexus between the uncinate process and the superior mesenteric artery is preserved, so the inferior pancreatoduodenal artery is preserved. The posterior inferior pancreatoduodenal artery is ligated and divided. The anterior inferior pancreatoduodenal artery is divided near the major papilla. The common bile duct is divided at the upper border of the pancreas. Two to three centimeters of ischemic area of the duodenum is observed including the major and minor papilla. The oral side of the duodenum is divided at 5 to 7 cm from the pyloric ring. The distal part of the duodenum is divided at the margin of the anterior inferior pancreatoduodenal artery ligation. The gastroduodenal artery is completely spared. The length of the resected duodenum ranges from 3 to 5 cm. The reconstruction of the alimentary tract is performed with pancreatogastrostomy, duodenoduodenostomy, and choledochoduodenostomy.

The V-shaped excision [16]

Most recently, another "extended" drainage procedure has been described addressing the rare entity of sclerosing ductal pancreatitis referred to as "small duct disease" with maximal Wirsungian duct diameter of less than 3 mm [16]. This operation features a longitudinal V-shaped excision of the ventral aspect of the pancreas combined with a longitudinal pancreatojejunostomy sewn to the edge of the organ.

After performing an extensive Kocher maneuver, a metal probe is placed into the common bile duct through a proximal choledochotomy to identify the intrapancreatic course of the distal common bile duct. Starting from the upper and lower edges of the gland, the ventral pancreatic aspect is longitudinally excised, with the tip of the excised wedge being located deep in the dorsal part of the pancreas. A longitudinal triangular cavity results to ensure adequate drainage of secondary and tertiary ductal branches. In case of common bile duct stenosis, the intrapancreatic course of the choledochal duct is freed from fibrotic tissue. Finally, a Roux-en-Y pancreatojejunostomy is performed using a single layer monofilament running suture. A T-tube is placed into the common bile duct.

Results of the surgical intervention

The duodenum-preserving resection of the head of the pancreas (DPRHP) according to Beger [8] and the longitudinal pancreaticojejunostomy combined with local pancreatic head excision (LPJ-LPHE) according to Frey [10]

Duodenum-preserving pancreatic head resection as introduced by Beger has been shown to offer both reliable pain relief and the advantage of low mortality and acceptable morbidity with preservation of endocrine and exocrine function [17].

Of the first 57 patients reported by Beger, 86% were completely rehabilitated and only 5.4% developed diabetes mellitus after surgery [8]. Compared to the pylorus-preserving Whipple procedure, patients undergoing a duodenum-preserving pancreatic head resection according to Beger have less pain, greater weight gain, a better glucose tolerance and a higher insulin secretion capacity at comparable morbidity rates (15% vs. 20%) and 0% mortality [18].

The finding that patients undergoing the DPRHP procedure suffer from less pain, however, is somewhat puzzling, as the extent of resection in both operations is rather similar. Thus, it is difficult to understand why the preservation of the gastroduodenal passage and common bile duct continuity should cause better pain relief.

Another randomized controlled trial comparing the duodenum-preserving pancreatic head resection according to Beger with the classical Whipple procedure showed advantages regarding preservation of the pancreatic function and occupational rehabilitation for the DPRHP procedure [19].

The experience with LPJ-LPHE has so far been limited to the reports of the institution, the procedure originated from [10, 20] and the Hamburg experience [17, 21, 22].

Both the DPRHP and LPJ-LPHE have been found to effectively control pain with 0% procedure related mortality in a randomized controlled trial [17]. Effective control of complications of adjacent organs was achieved in 90% (Beger) vs. 100% (Frey). Both groups displayed an improvement in quality of life index of 67%. Neither procedure led to further deterioration of endocrine or exocrine pancreatic function. But in this trial morbidity was 20% in the DPRHP group compared to 9% in the LPJ-LPHE group. The resection of the head of the pancreas is not as radical as in the DPRHP procedure, which makes the LPJ-LPHE technically less demanding. This fact could be an explanation for the observed lower morbidity.

As depicted from data reported in the literature and recently shown by a prospective randomized trial, the results of the "extended" drainage operation (LPJ-LPHE) in terms of pain relief and management of pancreatitis-associated complications of adjacent organs match the outcome achieved by resections, such as the partial pancreatoduodenectomy (PD) according to Whipple [2], the pylorus-preserving pancreatoduodenectomy (PPPD) according to Longmire-Traverso [18], and DPRHP [17]. Within an intermediate follow-up period, preservation of pancreatic function and social and occupational rehabilitation were also shown to be comparable after LPJ-LPHE and DPRHP [17, 21]. As mortality of resectional procedures like PD [2], PPPD [18] or DPRHP [17] has dropped to nearly nil in experienced centers, the argument of increased mortality cannot be used any longer in favor of drainage operations. However, significantly lower peri- and postoperative morbidity still favors draining procedures. Moreover, with regard to development of endocrine and exocrine pancreatic insufficiency a definitive advantage can be shown for the "extended" drainage operation LPJ-LPHE as well as for DPRHP [17] as compared to PD [2] or PPPD [18]. Preservation of the gastroduodenal passage and of the continuity of the common bile duct seems to be of utmost importance for regulation of the exocrine secretory capacity and glucose metabolism [23]. Results of a prospective randomized trial comparing LPJ-LPHE with PPPD confirmed these findings [22].

Warren's modification [9]

Two patients were treated according to the Warren modification [9] and both were pain-free after the operation (the observation period is not mentioned). Interestingly the flap survived in both patients. It is very likely, that pain control was achieved because the pancreatic head had been resected, since it is most likely that this part is the "motor" of the disease [24]. The number of patients investigated does not allow any conclusions about the efficacy of this procedure.

Takada's modification [11]

Takada's technique [11] offers "physiologic" restoration of the alimentary tract, since no Roux-en-Y reconstruction is needed. However, despite its technical feasibility, its results have never been evaluated in comparison to other pancreatic head resection methods (Whipple, PPPD, DPRHP, LPJ-LPHE), so an improvement regarding pain-control, preservation of exocrine and endocrine function, postoperative gastrointestinal function and mobility, mortality and morbidity can only be hypothesized. Moreover Takada reported on a series of 11 patients that 3 patients developed duodenal necrosis, of whom 1 patient died. In all three cases the gastroduodenal artery was divided. Therefore this routine was changed to preservation of the posterior superior gastroduodenal artery, and duodenal necrosis did not occur any more [11]. But whether or not the duodenal necrosis was induced through the anastomosis or through the division of the gastroduodenal artery remains speculative. This is even more so as Beger states in his report on the first cases of duodenum-preserving pancreatic head resection that preservation of the gastroduodenal artery is not crucial to maintaining sufficient blood-flow to the duodenum [8].

Kimura's and Sapy's modifications [12–14]

Sapy's report included 14 patients [14]. Morbidity was 28,5% with 0% mortality. Complete pain relief was achieved in 80% of patients. Body weight was unchanged in 50%, decreased in 15% and gained in 35% of patients. Progression of endocrine dysfunction was observed in 2 patients (average follow-up of 2 years).

Unfortunately, Kimura et al. only reported on one patient suffering from mucin-producing carcinoma undergoing this procedure. The postoperative course was uneventful except for a "slight deformity" in the distal common bile duct. So on the one hand the procedure with its two main alterations, i.e. drainage of the remaining pancreas into the stomach and leaving substantial pancreatic tissue between the duodenum and the common bile duct, has to be shown to be safe and effective in chronic pancreatitis in a bigger group of patients. On the other hand, the reported "slight deformity" in the distal common bile duct can be caused by leaving a pancreatic rim in the vicinity of the duct. Since common bile duct stenosis is a common complication in chronic pancreatitis [18], this procedure could potentially leave the narrowing part around the duct leading to persistent stenosis, therefore making this operation unsuitable for selected patients. Also it is not obvious why the pancreatic rim needs to be left in place, since the common bile duct is freed completely from the surrounding pancreatic and connective tissue in the Beger procedure and reports on papillar or duodenal necrosis are missing.

Nakao's modification [15]

In 14 cases (including mucin-producing cystic tumor (n = 9), annular pancreas (n = 1), anomalous arrangement of the pancreaticobiliary ductal system (n = 1), carcinoma of the duodenum (n = 1), carcinoma of the papilla (n = 1) and distal common bile duct cancer (n = 1), mortality was 0% [15]. Minor leakage from the duodenoduodenostomy and choledochoduodenostomy was observed in 3 cases and 1 case respectively. All responded to conservative treatment. During a follow-up period of 3 months to 6 years, one patient died due to liver metastasis (distal bile duct carcinoma). All other patients are still alive.

The proposed advantage of this procedure is that the risk of duodenal necrosis close to the papilla due to accidental division of the posterior superior pancreatoduodenal artery is nil, since this portion of the duodenum is resected anyway. This way a more radical pancreatic head resection can be performed. If the risk of inducing duodenal necrosis justifies an a priori segmental duodenal resection with the additional risk of duodenoduodenostomy leakage remains to be seen. Also, if a more radical pancreatic head resection is wanted e.g. in cases of malignancies, two well established methods (Whipple or pylorus-preserving Whipple) can be considered the gold standard. Nakao did not report about the possible advantages of segmental duodenectomy in comparison with the standard procedures (improved exocrine or endocrine pancreatic function, etc.).

The V-shaped excision [16]

Mortality was nil with a morbidity of 15,4% in a series of 13 patients [16]. During a median follow-up of 30 months, complete relief of symptoms was observed in 92% of patients. Exocrine and endocrine pancreatic function was well preserved and quality of life increased significantly postoperatively.

With this new procedure, the role of distal pancreatectomy, which has until now been indicated only in sclerosing chronic pancreatitis limited to the pancreatic body and tail [25], will further be diminished. This procedure effectively drains secondary and tertiary pancreatic ducts in small duct disease. For small duct disease, a rare form of chronic pancreatitis, this organ sparing operation seems to be a valuable alternative to resectional procedures.

Conclusion

Of the duodenum-preserving pancreatic head resections, two methods can be considered standard procedures in chronic pancreatitis: the LPJ-LPHE and DPRHP. Both procedures can be performed in a "custom-made" fashion to fit the individual situation. Crucial is the resection of peri-papillary pancreatic tissue in chronic pancreatitis, since neglecting this area leads to higher recurrences.

Only the operations outlined above have undergone a critical evaluation in multiple trials, confirming their superiority as surgical procedures for chronic pancreatitis.

All other modifications outlined above have so far not been compared to LPJ-LPHE and DPRHP in terms of mortality, morbidity, functional status etc. Still, some technical aspects like the potential benefit of different reconstruction methods (pancreaticoduodenostomy, pancreaticogastrostomy or pancreaticojejunostomy) are probably worth evaluating.

References

1. Warshaw AL. Pain in chronic pancreatitis – patients, patience, and the impatient surgeon. Gastroenterology 1984; 86: 987–9.
2. Saeger HD, Schwall G, Trede M. Standard Whipple in chronic pancreatitis. In: Beger HG, Büchler MW, Malfertheimer P, eds. Standards in pancreatic surgery. Berlin: Springer, 1993: 385–91.
3. Ebbehoj N, Svendsen LB, Madsen P. Pancreatic tissue pressure in chronic obstructive pancreatitis. Scand J Gastroenterol 1984; 19: 1066–8.
4. Bockmann DE, Büchler MW, Malfertheimer P, Beger HG. Analysis of nerves in chronic pancreatitis. Gastroenterology 1988; 94: 1459–69.
5. Greenlee HB, Prinz RA, Aranha GV. Long-term results of side-to-side pancreaticojejunostomy. World J Surg 1990; 14: 70–6.
6. Frey CF, Child CG, Fry W. Pancreatectomy for chronic pancreatitis. Ann Surg 1976; 184: 403–13.
7. Beger HG, Witte C, Krautzberger W, Bittner R. [Experiences with duodenum-sparing pancreas head resection in chronic pancreatitis]. Chirurg 1980; 51: 303–7.
8. Beger HG, Krautzberger W, Bittner R, Büchler MW, Limmer J. Duodenum-preserving resection of the head of the pancreas in patients with severe chronic pancreatitis. Surgery 1985; 97: 467–73.
9. Warren D, Millikan WJ, Henderson JM, Hersh T. A denervated pancreatic flap for control of chronic pain in pancreatitis. Surg Gynecol Obstet 1984; 159: 581–3.
10. Frey CF, Smith GJ. Description and rationale of a new operation for chronic pancreatitis. Pancreas 1987; 2: 701–7.
11. Takada T, Yasuda H, Uchiyama K, Hasegawa H. Duodenum-Preserving Pancreatoduodenostomy. A New Technique for Complete Excision of the Head of the Pancreas with Preservation of the Biliary and Alimentary Integrity. Hepatogastroenterology 1993; 40: 356–9.
12. Kimura W, Muto T, Makuuchi M, Nagai H. Subtotal Resection of the Head of the Pancreas Preserving Duodenum and Vessels of the Pancreatic Arcade. Hepatogastroenterology 1996; 43: 1438–41.
13. Kimura W, Morikane K, Futakawa N et al. A New Method of Duodenum-Preserving Subtotal Resection of the Head of the Pancreas based on the Surgical Anatomy. Hepatogastroenterology 1996; 43: 463–72.
14. Sapy P, Arkosy P, Szappanos M. Simple Reconstructive Method in Cases of Duodenum-Preserving Subtotal Resection of the Head of the Pancreas. Hepatogastroenterology 1998; 45: 1870–3.
15. Nakao A. Pancreatic Head Resection with Segmental Duodenectomy and Preservation of the Gastroduodenal Artery. Hepatogastroenterology 1998; 45: 533–5.
16. Izbicki JR, Bloechle C, Broering DC, Kuechler T, Broelsch CE. Longitudinal V-shaped excision of the ventral pancreas for small duct disease in severe chronic pancreatitis. Ann Surg 1998; 227: 213–9.
17. Izbicki JR, Bloechle C, Knoefel WT, Kuechler T, Binmoeller KF, Broelsch CE. Duodenum-preserving resections of the head of the pancreas in chronic pancreatitis – A prospective randomized trial. Ann Surg 1995; 221: 350–8.
18. Büchler MW, Friess H, Mueller MW, Wheatley AM, Beger HG. Randomized trial of duodenum-preserving pancreatic head resection versus pylorus-preserving Whipple in chronic pancreatitis. Am J Surg 1995; 169: 65–70.

19. Klempa I, Spatny M, Menzel J et al. Pankreasfunktion und Lebensqualität nach Pankreaskopfresektion bei der chronischen Pankreatitis. Chirurg 1995; 66: 350–9.
20. Frey CF, Amikura K. Local resection of the head of the pancreas combined with longitudinal pancreaticojejunostomy in the management of patients with chronic pancreatitis. Ann Surg 1994; 220: 492–507.
21. Izbicki JR, Bloechle C, Knoefel WT, Binmoeller KF, Soehendra N, Broelsch CE. Drainage versus Resektion in der chirurgischen Therapie der chronischen Kopfpankreatitis: eine randomisierte Studie. Chirurg 1997; 68: 369–77.
22. Izbicki JR, Bloechle C, Broering DC, Knoefel WT, Kuechler T, Broelsch CE. Extended drainage versus resection in surgery for chronic pancreatitis – Prospective randomized trial comparing the longitudinal pancreaticojejunostomy combined with local pancreatic head excision with the pylorus-preserving pancreatoduodenectomy. Ann Surg 1998; 228: 771–9.
23. Bittner R, Butters M, Büchler MW, Naegele S, Roscher R, Beger HG. Glucose homeostasis and endocrine pancreatic function in patients with chronic pancreatitis before and after surgical therapy. Pancreas 1994; 9: 47–53.
24. Büchler MW, Friess H, Bittner R et al. Duodenum-preserving pancreatic head resection: Long-term results. J Gastrointest Surg 1997; 1: 13–9.
25. Sawyer R, Frey CF. Is there still a role for distal pancreatectomy in surgery for chronic pancreatitis? Am J Surg 1994; 168: 6–9.

13.4 The Whipple resection for chronic pancreatitis

H. A. Reber

Abstract

Pancreaticoduodenectomy remains the gold standard for the various resection operations that are used to treat pain in chronic pancreatitis. It is used most commonly when 1) the pancreatic duct is normal in diameter, 2) the head of the pancreas is enlarged, often containing calcifications and cysts, 3) a previous drainage procedure was ineffective, and 4) even in the absence of pain, when there is concern about the presence of a pancreatic neoplasm in the head of the gland. The operative mortality rate is < 5%, and about 80% of patients experience long-term pain relief. Increasing experience with several newer operations (Beger, Frey) that resect some of the head of the pancreas while preserving the duodenum, suggests that they may prove to be attractive alternatives to the Whipple procedure.

Introduction

The most common indication for operation in chronic pancreatitis is intractable pain. The design of an operative strategy to treat the pain is complicated by the subjective nature of that symptom as well as a limited understanding of its causes. Although pancreatic duct hypertension [1], perineural inflammation and loss of the protective perineural barrier [2], and pancreatic ischemia [3] have all been implicated, probably none of these mechanisms explains the pain in all patients. In some, complications like pseudocysts, infection, and biliary or duodenal obstruction may also play a role. As a result, a variety of operations, including pancreatic denervation, several forms of pancreatic ductal drainage, and different types of pancreatic resection, have been used with varying success.

Whipple first performed pancreaticoduodenectomy for chronic pancreatitis , and in 1946 he described the results of a two-stage operation in three patients [4]. Seven years later, Cattell and Warren reported their experience with a one-stage operation in 11 patients with the disease [5]. The results from the perspective of pain relief were judged to be good in eight, fair in two, and poor in one. The authors went on to comment that "although (the Whipple operation) has not been effective in every case, it has given the best results, and we consider it the current method of choice when obstruction of the duct of Wirsung can be demonstrated ... In electing this choice, it should be remembered that (it) is a procedure of considerable magnitude ... in which the hazards and technical requirements are even greater than they are in resection of malignant lesions ... The physician should likewise be mindful of the fact that the disease is benign, and that alternative methods of surgical therapy are available ..."

Although it was soon recognized by others as well that pain relief was usually excellent following the Whipple operation, the operative morbidity and mortality rates were high [6] so surgeons sought simpler and safer approaches. However, today the mortality rates for pancreaticoduodenectomy are less than 5% and long-term morbidity is lower as well, so objections to the performance of the Whipple procedure for both benign and malignant diseases are less than ever before.

Goals of operation and indications for resection

The goals of any operation for chronic pancreatitis are to relieve the symptoms, to minimize side effects like diabetes and malabsorption, and to accomplish this with the lowest operative morbidity and mortality rates.

Pain is the most common symptom that leads to a consideration for surgical treatment in all reported series, and it is the most frequent indication for pancreatoduodenectomy as well. It is present in about 90% of cases. Resection is preferred by most surgeons if the pancreatic duct is not dilated (i.e. > 6–7 mm in diameter measured in the body of the gland).

The Whipple resection may also be indicated even when the pancreatic duct *is* dilated, if the head of the pancreas is enlarged. The anterior-posterior diameter of the head on CT scan can measure 5–6 cm or more, and multiple calcifications and parenchymal cysts may be seen. The rest of the gland often appears less involved. With such extensive disease in the head, duodenal and/or common bile duct obstruction also may be present. In a minority of cases, superior mesenteric-portal vein compression also occurs.

In some patients with chronic pancreatitis, usually those with a mass in the head of the gland, the clinician may be concerned about the possibility of malignancy. This can occur when the patient is jaundiced and there is little or no pain, when there is a short and asymmetric bile duct stricture, or when the serum CA19-9 level is elevated. Although this is a less common indication today than in earlier years when preoperative diagnostic techniques were less sophisticated, it probably still is the principal indication for operation in up to 10% of cases [7]. In Trede's recent review of 100 Whipple resections performed for what was presumed preoperatively to be chronic pancreatitis, 15 patients (15%) were found also to have pancreatic carcinoma [8]. Of 311 patients who underwent resection with the preoperative diagnosis of pancreatic carcinoma, 43 (14%) were found to have only chronic pancreatitis. These authors felt that the high frequency of misdiagnoses in their review was because some of their patients were treated before techniques like CT scans and fine needle aspiration were available. Nevertheless, all pancreatic surgeons agree that the distinction between benign and malignant disease remains an unsolved dilemma in some patients.

Pancreaticoduodenectomy also should be considered in patients who have undergone pancreaticojejunostomy, in whom pain relief was inadequate or, after a period of satisfactory relief, the pain has recurred [9, 10]. Such recurrence has been reported in up to 50% of these cases. Although rare patients may benefit from revision of a strictured pancreaticojejunal anastomosis as confirmed by ERCP [11], most will do better with a resection. Markowitz and associates [12] performed pancreaticoduodenectomies in 11 patients after failed previous drainage procedures. There was significant pain relief in seven (64%).

Another factor in the decision to perform pancreatoduodenectomy is the bias of the individual surgeon involved. Since it is generally accepted that the likelihood of permanent pain relief is higher with a Whipple resection than with a drainage procedure, many surgeons prefer to resect even in patients with dilated ducts. This is particularly true since the risks of resection are quite low. One clue to surgeon bias in the operative procedure chosen to treat chronic pancreatitis is the frequency of specific indications for resection, which varies widely in different series. For example, at UCLA 77% of Whipple resections done for patients who ultimately were found to have only chronic pancreatitis, were done because the surgeon suspected pancreatic cancer (unpublished). Corresponding frequencies were Mayo Clinic (64%) [13], Johns Hopkins ((30%) [14, 15], and Mannheim, Germany (34%) [8, 16]. The inference is that UCLA and Mayo Clinic surgeons are more inclined to treat patients with chronic pancreatitis with operations other than pancreaticoduodenectomy. Surgeons at Hopkins and Mannheim are more likely to resect for chronic pancreatitis even when the diagnostic possibility of pancreatic cancer is low.

Etiology of chronic pancreatitis

The cause of the pancreatitis differs considerably in various reported series. For example, ethanol, which is the most common cause of chronic pancreatitis around the world, was the etiologic agent in 70% of the patients who underwent pancreatoduodenectomy in the series from Birmingham in the United Kingdom [17]. It was the cause in 55% of the Mayo Clinic patients [13], 43% of the Johns Hopkins patients [14], but only 27% of the patients from the Massachusetts General Hospital [18]. Indeed, another 27% of the MGH patients were felt to have developed pancreatitis on the basis of pancreas divisum. This reflects the interest of the MGH surgeons, but the high frequency of this entity in their series is unlikely to be duplicated elsewhere. These observations are important because they point out the difficulty in comparing the results of any form of treatment of chronic pancreatitis from different centers with such disparate causes of the disease, since the natural history is likely to differ according to etiology.

Whipple resection in patients with pancreatitis

Over the last decade, there has been an increase in the willingness of most surgeons to consider performing pancreaticoduodenectomy for both benign and malignant disease. In patients with pancreatic cancer, several major centers have reported large series with operative mortality rates less than 5% and morbidities in an equally acceptable range [19–21]. Anecdotal data suggest that a Whipple resection done for chronic pancreatitis may be more difficult than the same operation done for pancreatic cancer. Adhesions and inflammation in the area of the superior mesenteric and portal veins may account for a somewhat greater operative blood loss and operative time. Nevertheless, in patients with either chronic pancreatitis or pancreatic cancer, published series give similar results [22, 23]. In part, this is due to the performance of these operations at specialized centers by surgeons with considerable experience. Improvements in perioperative care also probably play a role. Closed suction drainage and parenteral nutrition have considerably simplified the management of leaks from the pancreaticojejunal anastomosis, the single leading cause of morbidity in earlier series. Several prospective randomized studies suggest that the incidence of pancreatic fistula also may be reduced with the use of the drug octreotide. Of course, the likelihood of a fistula complicating a Whipple resection in patients with chronic pancreatitis has always been lower than in cases where the operation is done for cancer. In the latter case, the pancreas is usually softer and sutures are more likely to tear through the pancreatic tissue.

Several newer operations have been described which are being used increasingly as alternatives to the standard Whipple resection in patients with chronic pancreatitis. Beger et al. have considerable experience with a duodenal preserving resection of the head of the pancreas combined with a pancreaticojejunostomy [24]. Frey has performed a pancreaticojejunostomy which is combined with a "coring" out of much of the tissue in the head of the pancreas; this approach is less extensive than the Beger operation [25]. The results of both of these procedures suggest that they are safe and that they relieve pain effectively in most patients. Indeed, they may eventually be proven to be excellent alternatives to the Whipple operation in certain situations.

Results

In the absence of any randomized, controlled trials, the results of pancreaticoduodenectomy as well as all of the other operations for chronic pancreatitis are difficult to assess. Despite efforts to standardize reporting, pain relief remains difficult to evaluate objectively. Many patients are addicted to narcotics, so the possibility of secondary gain always must be considered. Nevertheless, most series suggest that the results after pancreaticoduodenectomy are better than those that follow distal resections or drainage procedures, averaging more than 85% good or fair pain relief at 5 year follow-up [9]. Exocrine insufficiency develops in approximately 70% of patients and the incidence of diabetes is more than 50% [9]. Neither of these appear to be the result of the operation, but occur over the long term as pancreatic exocrine and endocrine function continue to deteriorate [26].

Conclusions

The choice among operative procedures for chronic pancreatitis depends on the operative indications and the surgeon's prejudices and expertise. With experience that goes back 50 years, the Whipple pancreaticoduodenectomy remains the "gold standard" of all of the resection operations currently performed for pain relief in patients with chronic pancreatitis. The newer operations that resect some of the head of the pancreas while preserving the duodenum appear to be attractive alternatives to the Whipple procedure. Nevertheless, proof that the results are as good or better than the Whipple will require experience from a larger number of centers and longer follow-up.

Indications for the Whipple resection include those patients with a small pancreatic duct, a particularly diseased and often enlarged pancreatic head, situations where there is an inability to rule out malignancy, and patients who have failed a previous pancreaticojejunostomy.

The Whipple resection can be performed with an acceptably low operative mortality rate ($< 5\%$) and low long-term morbidity. The likelihood of permanent pain relief is probably about 85%, which is higher than after a drainage operation.

References

1. Ebbehoj N, Borly L, Bulow J, Rasmussen SG, Madsen P, Matzen P, Owre A. Pancreatic tissue fluid pressure in chronic pancreatitis relation to pain, morphology, and function. Scand J Gastroenterol 1990; 25: 1046–51.

2. Bockman DE, Büchler MW, Malfertheiner P, Beger HG. Anatomy of nerves in chronic pancreatitis. Gastroenterology 1988; 90: 1459–69.
3. Patel AG, Toyama MT, Alvarez C, Nguyen TN, Ashley SW, Reber HA. Pancreatic interstitial pH in human and feline chronic pancreatitis. Gastroenterology 1995; 109: 1639–45.
4. Whipple AO. Radical surgery for certain cases of pancreatitis associated with calcareous deposits. Ann Surg 1946; 124: 991–1008.
5. Cattell RB, Warren KW, eds. Surgery of the Pancreas. Philadelphia: W. B. Saunders 1953: 125–7.
6. Rhoads JE, Folin LS. History of surgery of the pancreas. In: Howard JM, Jordan GL, Jr, Reber HA, eds. Surgical Diseases of the Pancreas. Philadelphia: Lea & Febiger, 1987: 3–11.
7. Ashley SW, Reber HA. Surgical management of exocrine pancreatic cancer. In: Go VLM et al., eds. The Exocrine Pancreas: Biology, Pathobiology, and Diseases. Second Edition. New York: Raven Press, 1993: 913–29.
8. Saeger HD, Schwall G, Trede M. Standard Whipple in chronic pancreatitis. In: Beger HG, Büchler M, Malfertheiner P. Standards in pancreatic surgery. Berlin: Springer Verlag, 1993.
9. Frey CF. Surgical treatment of chronic pancreatitis. In: Go VLW et al., eds. The Pancreas: Biology, Pathobiology, and Disease. Second Edition. New York: Raven Press, 1993: 707–40.
10. Greenlee HB, Prinz RA, Aranha GV. Long-term results of side-to-side pancreaticojejunostomy. World J Surg 1990; 14: 70–6.
11. Prinz RA, Aranha GV, Greenlee HB. Redrainage of the pancreatic duct in chronic pancreatitis. Am J Surg 1986; 151: 150–6.
12. Markowitz JS, Rattner DW, Warshaw AL. Failure of symptomatic relief after pancreaticojejunal decompression for chronic pancreatitis. Arch Surg 1994; 129: 374–80.
13. Sakorafas GH, Farnell MB, Nagorney DM, Sarr MG, Rowland CM. Pancreatoduodenectomy for chronic pancreatitis. Arch Surg 2000;135: 517–24.
14. Barnes SA, Lillemoe KD, Kaufman HS, Sauter PK, Yeo CJ, Talamini MA, Pitt HA, Cameron JL. Pancreaticoduodenectomy for benign disease. Am J Surg 1996; 171: 131–5.
15. Sohn TA, Campbell KA, Pitt HA, Sauter PK, Coleman J, Lillemoe KD, Yeo CJ, Cameron JL. Quality of life and long-term survival after surgery for chronic pancreatitis. J Gastrointest Surg 2000; 4: 355–65.
16. Rumstadt B, Forssmann K, Singer MV, Trede M. The Whipple partial duodenopancreatectomy for the treatment of chronic pancreatitis. Hepatogastroenterology 1997; 44: 1554–9.
17. Evans JD, Wilson PG, Carver C, Bramhall SR, Buckels JAC, Mayer AD, McMaster P, Neoptolemos JP. Outcome of surgery for chronic pancreatitis. British J Surgery 1997; 84: 624–9.
18. Jimenez RE, Fernandez-del Castillo C, Rattner DW, Chang Y, Warshaw AL. Outcome of pancreatoduodenectomy with pylorus preservation or with antrectomy in the treatment of chronic pancreatitis. Ann Surg 2000; 231: 293–300.
19. Trede M, Schwall G, Saeger H. Survival after pancreaticoduodenectomy. Ann Surg 1990; 211: 447–58.
20. Grace PA, Pitt HA, Tompkins RK. Decreased morbidity and mortality after pancreaticoduodenectomy. Am J Surg 1986; 151: 141–9.
21. Crist DW, Sitzmann JV, Cameron JL. Improved hospital morbidity, mortality, and survival after the Whipple procedure. Ann Surg 1987; 206: 358–65.
22. Rossi RL, Rothschild J, Braasch JW, Munson JL, ReMine SG. Pancreaticoduodenectomy in the management of chronic pancreatitis. Arch Surg 1987; 122: 416–21.
23. Stone WM, Sarr MG, Nagorney DM, McIlrath DC. Chronic pancreatitis. Results of Whipple's resection and total pancreatectomy. Arch Surg 1988; 123: 815–9.
24. Beger HG, Büchler HG. Duodenum-preserving resection of the head of the pancreas in chronic pancreatitis with inflammatory mass in the head. World J Surg 1990; 14: 83–7.
25. Frey CF, Smith GJ. Description and rationale for a new operation for chronic pancreatitis. Pancreas 1987; 2: 701–4.
26. Traverso LW, Kozarek RA. Pancreatoduodenectomy for chronic pancreatitis. Ann Surg 1997; 226: 429–38.

13.5 Pancreatic left resection in chronic pancreatitis – indications and limitations

A. Bauer, W. Uhl, O. Tcholakov, M. Wagner, H. Friess, M. W. Büchler

Summary

Many different surgical procedures have been proposed to relieve pain and reduce the incidence of complications associated with chronic pancreatitis. An important question is whether pancreatic left resection is an adequate surgical treatment of chronic pancreatitis, as the pancreatic head has turned out to be the pacemaker in chronic pancreatitis. A careful preoperative work-up is mandatory to exclude further complications not caused by the inflamed body or tail of the pancreas and to select the very small number of patients who may benefit from pancreatic left resection.

Of the total number of 171 patients who underwent surgery for chronic pancreatitis between 11/1993 and 7/1999, only 12 patients (7%) had a pancreatic left resection. Inflammatory complications, recurrent acute pancreatitis or the suspicion of a neoplasm were in most cases the indication for pancreatic left resection. Concerning the surgical approach, no differences between the technique of suturing the pancreatic stump or creating a Roux-en-Y pancreaticojejunostomy were observed. Preservation of the spleen should be desirable in patients undergoing pancreatic left resection if there is no clear indication for splenectomy such as perisplenic pseudocyst or inflammatory or fibrotic encasement of the splenic vessels. Postoperative outcome was without any major complication. The risk of surgery-induced endocrine and exocrine pancreatic insufficiency is not increased in a 40–60% pancreatic left resection.

Although the pancreatic head is the pacemaker in the disease progression of chronic pancreatitis and therefore most patients undergo a duodenum-preserving pancreatic head resection, pancreatic left resection is a beneficial surgical treatment for a small and carefully selected group of patients.

Introduction

The history of pancreatic left resection dates back to 1884, when Billroth reported a distal resection in a patient with malignant pancreatic tumor. Case reports by Finney at Hopkins and Mayo in Rochester followed in the early beginning of the 20th century, describing surgical technique and short-term outcome in patients undergoing distal pancreatectomy [21]. In 1957 Barret and Bowers described a distal pancreatectomy, resecting 95% of the pancreatic gland in patients with chronic pancreatitis (CP) [24]. Significant increase in pancreatic exocrine and endocrine insufficiency led to a less radical distal resection, performed by Fry and Child in 1980 [17, 24].

The principal indication for surgery in patients with CP is intractable pain, followed by inflammation-related complications such as pancreatic pseudocysts [13]. The pathogenesis of pain in chronic pancreatitis is incompletely understood. Inflammation, fibrosis and varying degrees of duct obstruction are morphologic hallmarks of the disease.

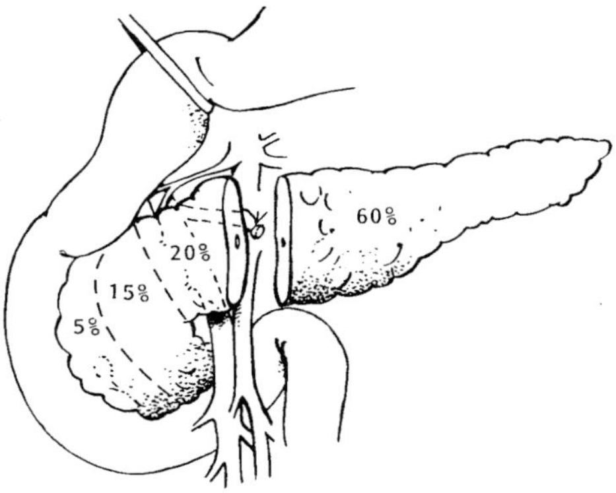

Figure 13.5-1. Extent of pancreatic left resection in chronic pancreatitis (Note: Recommendation of 40–60% distal resection to avoid insulin-dependent diabetes mellitus; from [12]).

Neuropathic mechanisms are also said to play an important role as ductal drainage procedures provide pain relief in only 60–80% of patients suffering from chronic pancreatitis [4, 6, 7, 16, 23]. Introduction of new surgical techniques as described by Beger or Frey seemed to supersede the Whipple procedures and distal pancreatectomy in patients with chronic pancreatitis, and especially in patients with an inflammatory mass in the pancreatic head [2, 3, 8, 9, 10, 15, 24].

Modern imaging techniques such as CT scan, ERCP or all-in-one MRI may allow us to select a special group of patients who will benefit most from pancreatic left resection, such as patients with severe pain, small-duct-disease and a lesion limited to the body or the tail of the pancreas with no other complications of chronic pancreatitis [24]. Distal subtotal resection proved effective in reducing pain, but increased the incidence of endocrine and exocrine insufficiency [23]. A 40–60% resection of distal pancreatic tissue as recommended by Eggink et al. turned out to give adequate relief of pain in patients with chronic pancreatitis (Fig. 13.5-1) [12]. The risk of diabetes or steatorrhea is not increased, so that distal pancreatectomy should be carried out as organ-preserving procedure whenever possible [12].

Herein we describe a retrospective analysis of patients who underwent pancreatic left resection for chronic pancreatitis between November 1993 and July 1999, as well as the indications leading to left resection and the pre-operative work-up with special reference to the literature. This review additionally compares different surgical approaches, e.g. splenectomy versus spleen-preserving operation, and whether drainage of the pancreatic duct should be recommended.

Methods

From November 1993 to July 1999 the total number of patients who underwent pancreatic resection for chronic pancreatitis at the Inselspital Bern, Switzerland, was 171. However, out of this patient population only 12 patients (7%) had a pancreatic left resection.

The data concerning age, etiology, history of chronic pancreatitis, indication for operation as well as post-operative hospital stay and complications were assessed retrospectively by reviewing patients' records. Due to the very small group of patients (n = 12) data were evaluated only qualitatively and not statistically analyzed.

Results

Patients

During the time of observation, the total number of patients who were operated on for chronic pancreatitis was 171 (Fig. 13.5-2). Of these, 12 patients, 9 male and 3 female, underwent distal pancreatectomy for chronic pancreatitis (Table 13.5-1). The mean age was 47.5 years (range 20–60 years). Analyzing the patients' history, 4 of them had a documented history of severe acute pancreatitis, and the histological examination showed peripancreatic necrosis and in the body and tail of the pancreas chronic inflammation. Seven patients were suffering from alcoholic pancreatitis. One patient had a history of gallstone disease and therefore a biliary etiology of chronic pancreatitis. The etiology was unknown in 2 of the other 4 patients and not clearly defined in the other 2. The history of recurrent pain from chronic pancreatitis had a duration from 6 months in 2 patients up to more than 2 years. In 5 patients the history of chronic pancreatitis could not be evaluated.

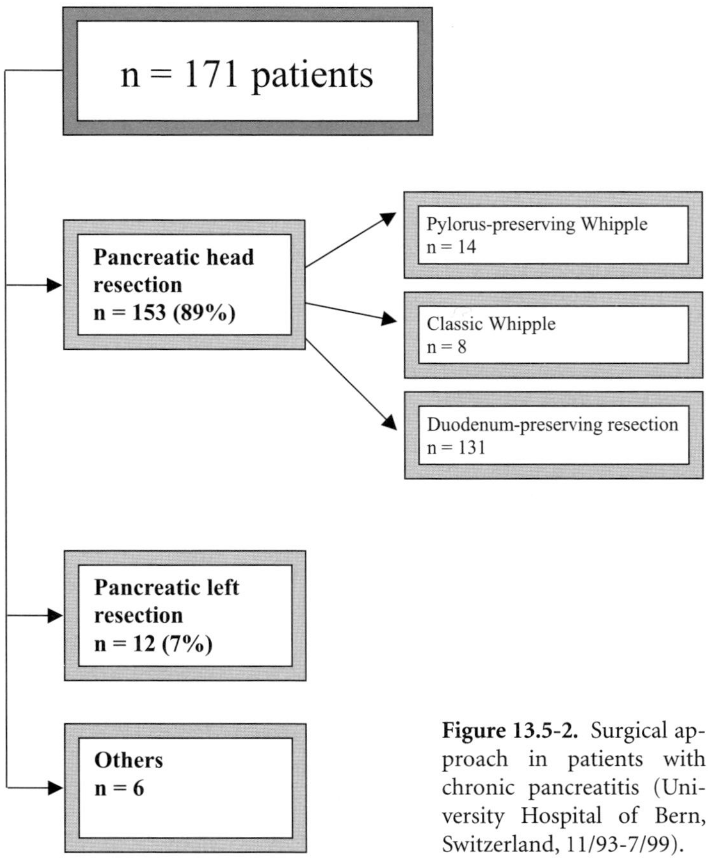

Figure 13.5-2. Surgical approach in patients with chronic pancreatitis (University Hospital of Bern, Switzerland, 11/93-7/99).

	n = 12	
Gender	Male	9
	Female	3
Age	20–29 years	–
	30–39 years	3
	40–49 years	5
	50–60 years	3
	> 60 years	1
Etiology	Alcoholic	7
	Biliary	1
	Other	2
	Unknown	2
History of pain	< 1/2 year	2
	1/2–2 years	–
	1–2 years	2
	> 2 years	3
	Unknown	5

Table 13.5-1. Characterization of patients with pancreatic left resection for chronic pancreatitis (University Hospital of Bern, Switzerland, 11/93–7/99).

Surgical indications, preoperative work-up

Inflammatory complications were the leading indication for distal pancreatectomy, as most of the patients showed one or more inflammation-related complications of chronic pancreatitis. Two of the patients had a history of recurrent acute pancreatitis. Four patients suffering from chronic pancreatitis underwent diagnostic laparotomy, as the suspicion of possible malignancy could not be excluded. One patient had a history of traumatic rupture of the spleen that needed surgical intervention, so the chronically inflamed pancreas was also removed during this laparotomy session (Table 13.5-2).

Leading diagnostic technique among these patients was the CT scan, and all-in-one MRI (including MRCP) was performed in 6 patients. Five patients had an ERCP preoperatively, which turned out to show false-negative results in 2 patients.

Table 13.5-2. Indication for pancreatic surgery and preoperatively performed work-up (University Hospital of Bern, Switzerland, 11/93–7/99).

		n = 12	
Indication for operation	Inflammatory complications	Pseudocyst	2
		Fistula	2
		Pancreatic main duct stenosis	4
	Suspicious of neoplasm		4
	Recurrent acute pancreatitis		2
	Other	Trauma	1
		Autoimmune reaction	1

Surgical technique performed

Distal pancreatectomy was performed conservatively, combined with splenectomy in 8 out of 12 patients. In 4 patients a spleen-preserving operation was chosen. Indication for splenectomy was an undefined intraoperative situation such as suspected malignancy. Three of the patients had inflammatory complications such as pancreatic fistula or

Table 13.5-3. Surgical management in pancreatic left resection for chronic pancreatitis (University Hospital of Bern, Switzerland, 11/93–7/99).

	n = 12	
Surgical approach	Distal pancreatectomy + splenectomy	8
	Distal pancreatectomy + spleen preservation	3
	Other technique used	1
Management of pancreatic stump	Roux-en-Y drainage	7
	Other drainage mechanism	1
	Stump oversewing	4

perisplenic pseudocyst so that the spleen had to be removed. Traumatic rupture of the spleen was the indication for distal pancreatectomy and splenectomy in one patient. One patient with biliary chronic pancreatitis underwent a segmental resection of the distal pancreas and a concrement in the pancreatic duct was removed.

Concerning the distal pancreatic stump, 7 patients had a Roux-en-Y drainage operation, while 4 patients were left with the oversewn pancreatic stump. One patient had a duodenum-preserving pancreatic head resection and a re-laparotomy with an extended pancreatic resection 2 and 1 years before he underwent spleen-conserving pancreatic left resection. During this procedure a revision of the anastomosis was also necessary. Table 13.5-3 shows the surgical technique performed and the management of the pancreatic stump.

Complications

Preoperatively, diabetes mellitus due to chronic pancreatitis was known in 3 patients. Other common complications were pancreatic fistula or thrombosis of the splenic vein, occurring in 2 patients. One patient had had 2 previous abdominal operations and one had had a traumatic rupture of the spleen. Alterations of hepatic or cardiac function were detected in 1 patient, and one had neurological problems due to persistent diabetic polyneuropathia.

Table 13.5-4 shows the postoperative complications found in patients who underwent pancreatic left resection. The postoperative course was without any major surgical or medical complications and all patients could be discharged within the range of 8–19 days (mean 12.4 days) (Table 13.5-4).

Table 13.5-4. Postoperative complications and hospital stay in 12 patients undergoing pancreatic left resection for chronic pancreatitis (University Hospital of Bern, Switzerland, 11/93–7/99).

	n = 12	
Postoperative complications	Nausea and vomiting	2
	Post-splenectomy thrombocytosis	1
	New incidence of hyperglucosemia	2
	Need of anti-diabetic treatment	1
	Substitution of pancreatic enzymes	7
Postoperative hospital stay	Mean	12.4 days
	Range	8–19 days

Minor postoperative complications observed were nausea and vomiting after start of oral intake in two patients and transient thrombocytosis due to splenectomy in one patient. Postoperative incidence of pathological hyperglucosemia occurred in two patients and led to oral antidiabetic medication in one patient. Medication was not yet necessary in the other, but regular controls of glucose level were recommended.

Pancreatic enzyme substitution was necessary in seven patients.

Discussion

Many different surgical procedures have been proposed to relieve pain and reduce the incidence of complications associated with chronic pancreatitis. The most important question is whether pancreatic left resection is an adequate treatment of chronic pancreatitis and which form of distal pancreatectomy is superior to the other.

While some authors recommend pancreatic left resection for its tissue-conserving benefit in patients with chronic pancreatitis, others criticize that it is rarely effective in the reduction and relief of pain, as a high incidence of persistent pain in patients after distal pancreatectomy is reported [13, 14, 21, 23, 25].

The pacemaker in the European form of chronic pancreatitis seems to be the pancreatic head. In around 30% of patients with chronic pancreatitis an inflammatory mass in the head of the pancreas develops, leading frequently to an enlargement of this part of the pancreas [2, 3, 4, 8, 9, 10]. The total proportion of patients who undergo a duodenum-preserving pancreatic head resection or a Whipple procedure for chronic pancreatitis is about 80%.

Criteria for performing a distal pancreatectomy were recently defined by Sawyer et al. [24]. Patients with severe pain, small ducts and a disease process limited to the body and/or tail of the pancreas benefit most from a 40–60% distal resection [24]. Our own data presenting 12 patients who underwent distal pancreatectomy show that distal pancreatectomy is a rarely performed procedure and should be restricted to a very selected number of patients. Between 5 and 15% of all patients who have surgical intervention for chronic pancreatitis seem to benefit from distal pancreatectomy [24]. Therefore, a careful preoperative work-up is mandatory to exclude further complications of chronic pancreatitis not caused by the inflamed body or tail of the pancreas. That distal pancreatectomy turned out to be unsuccessful mostly in the past, might have been due to a poorly performed pre-operative selection of patients.

But even when the anatomic evidence suggested that chronic pancreatitis primarily involved the tail, or a stricture of the mid-pancreatic duct was believed to cause the symptoms, a distal resection seldom provided sustained pain relief [23]. Furthermore, preoperatively diagnostic findings did not always predict the parenchymal changes observed at laparotomy [23]. Of the patients analyzed, 5 had an ERCP preoperatively, and it showed positive diagnostic findings in 3 patients. During laparotomy the other two ERCP results turned out to be false-negative. So preoperatively performed diagnostic procedures are not always reliable in patients with chronic pancreatitis.

Alcohol abuse is in most cases the main etiology for chronic pancreatitis and this alcohol-related form of pancreatitis is characterized by a diffuse disease process that is seldom limited to the body or tail of the pancreas [19, 23]. Another explanation for the worse outcome could be ongoing alcohol abuse in patients with alcohol-related chronic pancreatitis after surgical intervention. So the prediction whether a distal pancreatectomy can be successfully performed is difficult, especially in patients with chronic alcohol abuse or idiopathic chronic pancreatitis.

An often discussed disadvantage in pancreatic left resection is the high incidence of insulin-dependent diabetes mellitus (IDDM) occurring after surgical intervention [2, 3, 9, 10, 13]. The reason is the preponderance of islet cells in the pancreatic body and tail. The data published by Evans et al. in 1997 showed an increase in the incidence of IDDM in all patients who underwent surgery. No significant differences between the various surgical procedures were shown [13]. In pancreatic left resection development of IDDM seems to be a long-term complication. After 24 months, the incidence of IDDM rose up to 30%, continuing to nearly 40% after 36 months [13]. Among our patients the incidence of postoperatively occurring IDDM was not increased; 2 patients had an IDDM that was already known pre-operatively. Analyzing long-term results after distal pancreatectomy, it seems to be difficult to tell operation-related pancreatic endocrine insufficiency from the late deterioration in pancreatic function due to the progressive disease process [25]. The development of IDDM is also determined by the natural course of chronic pancreatitis [25].

Trying to define standards for pancreatic resection, Fernandez-del Castillo et al. reported that growing experience in pancreatic surgery led to a lower incidence of complications and a minimal mortality rate [14]. Their conclusion was that in a high-volume setting, pancreatic resection could be carried out with a mortality and morbidity rate that is comparable to that of other types of gastrointestinal surgery [14]. So the best treatment of this very selected group of patients being operated on for chronic pancreatitis should be carried out in pancreatico-biliary units, providing interdisciplinary care [13]. Good indications for pancreatic left resection in chronic pancreatitis are pancreatic duct stenosis and therefore obstructive disease due to trauma, history after acute necrotizing pancreatitis and chronic pancreatitis with pseudocysts in the tail of the pancreas [27].

If pancreatic left resection is indicated, the next question is whether it should be performed with or without splenectomy. The intimate relationship between splenic artery and vein to the body of the pancreas is the reason that in the past splenectomy has been included as an expedient component routinely performed during left resection [1, 20, 27]. The recognition of postsplenectomy sepsis as an unwanted added risk and the importance of the spleen for the host defense system has changed the routine indication for splenectomy and made conservation of the spleen desirable [1, 27].

The French surgeon Mallet-Guy first described the technique of spleen-preserving pancreatic left resection in the 1940s for patients with chronic pancreatitis [1]. During the following years three different means of spleen preservation in distal pancreatectomy were established [20]. The first technique is a distal pancreatectomy without preserving the splenic artery and vein, so the short gastric and gastroepiploic arteries are the only blood supply to the spleen [27]. Splenomegaly is a contraindication for this means of spleen conservation because the increased mass is insufficiently nourished by the short gastric vessels. Using another technique, the splenic, short gastric and gastroepiploic arteries and veins can be sacrificed. This procedure is only rarely if ever performed, because the blood supply to the spleen is uncertain. Distal pancreatectomy can also be performed in the third technique, preserving the splenic artery and vein as described by Kimura et al. [20]: In this way the blood supply to the spleen is well maintained and the danger of splenic necrosis and abscess formation is reduced [20]. On the other hand distal pancreatectomy with conservation of the splenic artery and vein is both time- and labor-consuming. Dissecting the splenic vessels from the pancreas could probably induce or facilitate the development of pancreatitis and is very difficult to perform in an inflamed or fibrotic pancreas [27]. To exclude the bias of various pancreatic diseases that might effect the outcome after distal pancreatectomy with or without splenectomy, Benoist et al. analyzed 40 patients undergoing distal pancreatectomy for other indications than chronic pancreatitis [5] (Table 13.5-5). Fifteen patients underwent distal pancreatectomy with spleen conservation, 25 had a splenectomy. Pancreatic left resection with splenectomy turned out to have a lower morbidity rate, as pancreatic complications such as fistula or

Table 13.5-5. Literature research 2000.

Author	Pancreatic left resection	±Splenectomy Management of the pancreatic stump	Morbidity Mortality Reoperation
Shankar et al. (1990)	n = 113	Stump suture: n = 67 (59%) Roux-en-Y drainage: n = 46 (41%)	*Complications:* Suture: n = 29 (43%) Drainage: n = 21 (46%) *Morbidity:* Suture: n= 19 (28%) Drainage: n =21 (45%) *Mortality:* n = 4 (3.5%)
Fernandez-del Castillo et al. (1995)	n = 71	Spleen preservation in n = 14 (20%)	*Reoperation:* n = 1 (1.4%)
Rattner et al. (1996)	n = 20	Spleen preservation in n = 4 patients (20%)	Good results: n = 11 (55%) Poor results: n = 9 (45%)
Evans et al. (1997)	n = 13	Spleen preservation in n = 4 patients (31%)	Complications: n = 3 Increase in IDDM and exocrine pancreatic insufficiency
Benoist et al. (1998)	n = 40	Spleen preservation: n = 15 (37.5%) Splenectomy: n = 25 (62.5%)	*Splenectomy:* Morbidity: 20% *Spleen preservation:* Morbidity: 40% *Reoperation:* 6%
Lillemoe et al. (1999)	n = 235	Splenectomy: n = 198 (84%) Spleen preservation: n = 37 (16%)	*Splenectomy:* Morbidity: 30% Mortality: 1% *Spleen preservation:* Morbidity: 29% Mortality 0% *Reoperation:* 14%
Schoenberg et al. (1999)	n = 74	Spleen preservation in n = 25 patients (34%)	Relaparotomy: n = 3 (4%)
Govil et al. (1999)	n = 38	Spleen preservation in n = 22 patients (57.9%)	Mortality: n = 4 (10.5%) Morbidity: n = 8 (21%) Post-op. IDDM: n = 12 (31.6%)

subphrenic abscess occurred more frequently in patients after spleen-conserving surgery [5]. The incidence of post-splenectomy sepsis is about 0.28–1.9% with a mortality rate of 2.2%, which means that complications due to splenectomy do not occur frequently. Data after immunization against Pneumococci and Haemophilus influenzae are lacking: maybe the risk is lowered to 0%. A increased risk, however, is observed in children below the age of 15 years or patients with malignant hematological disorders [5].

Splenic complications in chronic pancreatitis leading to splenectomy are favored by splenic vein occlusion and pseudocyst or necrosis of the pancreatic tail [22].They may even represent the first manifestation of chronic pancreatitis [22]. Among our 12 patients who underwent distal pancreatectomy only 3 had a spleen-conserving distal pancreatic left resection, and one had a spleen-preserving pancreatic segmental resection with interposition of a jejunal loop. Splenectomy was necessary in 8 patients because of complications such as pancreatic fistula (n = 2), perisplenic pseudocyst (n = 2), suspicion of a neoplasm (n = 4) or a traumatic splenic rupture (n = 1). The final standard, whether distal pancreatectomy should be performed with or without splenectomy, is not yet clear. As Table 13.5-5 shows, most studies indicate that pancreatic left resection can be performed without sacrificing the spleen in various pancreatic conditions, including chronic pancreatitis [1]. In severe chronic pancreatitis followed by gross pancreatic calcification, marked edema and fibrosis that also encases the splenic vessels, the conventional distal pancreatectomy with splenectomy remains the appropriate procedure [1]. In the present study, pancreatic left resection combined with splenectomy was performed in 8 cases and all patients were immunized on the 10th postoperative day against Pneumococci and Haemophilus influenzae. In 4 patients spleen preservation was possible (Table 13.5-4). In the postoperative outcome, spleen preservation did not influence the mean duration of hospital stay after surgery. The mean of postoperative time in hospital for patients with splenectomy was 12.5 days, while patients who had a spleen-preserving pancreatic resection stay 12.2 days in the mean.

Splenic autotransplantation, as suggested by some surgeons is no substitute for splenic preservation as the risk of overwhelming sepsis still exists [19]. In cases where splenectomy is unavoidable, autotransplantation is reported to restore a degree of immune function and red cell scavenging capacity, and should therefore be recommended [19]. At least the incidence of post-operative IDDM seems to be less in patients who underwent spleen-preserving distal pancreatectomy.

Different opinions exist concerning the remaining pancreatic stump after distal pancreatectomy. The surgical objective of draining the pancreatic cut surface is to avoid the effects of a leak from the pancreatic stump and to achieve better drainage. As the anastomosis is often found to be occluded, this frequently occurring stenosis rate may be reflected in failure to provide long-term relief after pancreaticojejunostomy [26]. Shankar et al. analyzed 113 patients after distal pancreatectomy. The pancreatic stump was sutured in 67 patients without any drainage procedure; 46 patients had a Roux-en-Y loop of the jejunum after pancreatic resection (Table 13.5-5). As the postoperative outcome was similar in both groups, caudal pancreatic drainage seems to confer no benefit [26]. Therefore, their suggestion was that the distal pancreatic stump should be closed without drainage [26]. Anastomosis should be reserved for patients with a dilated duct or a stricture in the pancreatic head [1].

Four of the patients analyzed were left without any drainage system and the pancreatic stump was oversewn. In the seven patients who had a pancreaticojejunostomy, drainage was considered necessary as they had complications such as stenosis, pseudoysts or duct irregularities. A special drainage technique was used in a patient who underwent 2 laparotomies before distal pancreatectomy, so anastomosis was indicated to optimize the post-operative outcome. According to the data published by Shankar et al. no difference in the outcome, complication rate or duration of hospital stay could be found [26].

Finally, we conclude that distal pancreatectomy is a beneficial surgical treatment for a small selected group of patients with chronic pancreatitis caused by trauma with obstructive chronic pancreatitis due to stenosis or occlusion of the pancreatic main duct or a history after severe acute pancreatitis with so-called persisting necrotizing pancreatitis. Whenever distal pancreatectomy is performed for chronic pancreatitis it should be carried out as tissue preserving as possible. Spleen preservation is desirable if there is no clear indication for splenectomy such as perisplenic pseudocyst, inflammatory and fibrotic encasement of the splenic vessels or suspicion of malignancy. Inflammatory complications such as stenosis or pseudocyst may be an indication for a pancreatic drainage procedure; in other cases the stump can be carefully oversewn. In the future pancreatic left resection might also be performed laparoscopically, as initial data published by Cuschieri et al. and Gagner et al. show good results [11, 18].

References

1. Aldridge MC, Williamson RCN. Distal pancreatectomy with and without splenectomy. Br J Surg 1991; 78: 976–9 (E).
2. Beger HG, Krautzberger W, Bittner R, Büchler MW, Limmer J. Duodenum-preserving resection of the head of the pancreas in patients with severe chronic pancreatitis. Surgery 1985; 97: 467–73.
3. Beger HG, Schlosser W, Friess H, Büchler MW. Duodenum-preserving head resection in chronic pancreatitis changes the natural course of the disease: a single-center 26-year experience. Ann Surg 1999; 230: 512–9.
4. Beger HG, Schlosser W, Siech M, Poch B. The surgical management of chronic pancreatitis: Duodenum-preserving pancreatectomy. Advances in Surgery 1999; 32: 87–105.
5. Benoist S, Dugué L, Sauvanet A, Valverde A, Mauvais F, Paye F, Farges O, Belghiti J. Is there a role of preservation of the spleen in distal pancreatectomy? J Am Coll. Surg 1999; 188: 255–60 (G).
6. Bockmann DE, Büchler MW, Malfertheiner P, Beger HG. Analysis of nerves in chronic pancreatitis. Gastroenterol 1988; 94: 1459–69.
7. Büchler MW, Weihe E, Friess H, Malfertheiner P, Bockmann E, Müller S, Nohr D, Beger HG. Changes in peptidergic innervation in chronic pancreatitis. Pancreas 1992; 7: 183–92.
8. Büchler MW, Friess H, Mueller MW, Wheatley AM, Beger HG. Randomized trial of duodenum-preserving pancreatic head resection versus pylorus-preserving Whipple in chronic pancreatitis. Am J Surg 1995; 169: 65–70.
9. Büchler MW, Friess H, Baer HU, Neoptolemos JP. Surgical treatment of chronic pancreatitis: new standards. Dig Surg 1996; 13: 66.
10. Büchler MW, Friess H, Bittner R. Duodenum-preserving pancreatic head resection: Long-term results. J Gastroint Surg 1997; 1: 13–9.
11. Cuschieri A, Jakimowicz JJ, van Spreeuwel J. Laparoscopic distal 70% pancreatectomy and splenectomy for chronic pancreatitis. Ann Surg 1996; 223: 280–5 (F1).
12. Eggink WF, Bauer FLR, Schattenkerk Effetinck M, Obertop H, Bruining HA, Jeekel J, Van Houten H. Surgical treatment of chronic pancreatitis by distal pancretectomy. Neth J Surg 1983; 35: 184–7 (2).
13. Evans JD, Wilson PG, Carver C, Bramhall SR, Buckels JAC, Mayer AD, McMaster P, Neoptolemos JP. Outcome of surgery for chronic pancreatitis. Br J Surg 1997; 84: 624–9 (4).

14. Fernandez-del Castillo C, Rattner DW, Warshaw L. Standards for pancreatic resection in the 1990s. Arch Surg 1995; 130: 295–300 (B).
15. Frey CF, Smith CJ. Description and rationale of a new operation for chronic pancreatitis. Pancreas 1987; 2: 701–7.
16. Friess H, Büchler MW, Mueller C, Malfertheiner P. Immunopathogenesis of chronic pancreatitis. Gastroenterol 1998; 115: 1018–22.
17. Fry WJ, Child CG. Ninety-five per cent distal pancreatectomy for chronic pancreatitis. Ann Surg 1965; 162: 543–9.
18. Gagner M, Pomp A. Laparoscopic pancreatic resection: Is it worthwhile? J Gastrointest Surg 1997, 1: 20–6 (F2).
19. Govil S, Imrie CW. Value of splenic preservation during distal pancreatectomy for chronic pancreatitis. Br J Surg 1999; 86: 894–8 (D).
20. Kimura W, Inoue T, Futakawa N, Shinkai H, Han I, Muto T. Spleen-preserving distal pancreatectomy with conservation of the splenic artery and vein. Surgery 1996; 120: 885–90 (H).
21. Lillemoe KD, Kaushal S, Cameron JL, Sohn TA, Pitt HA, Yeo CJ. Distal pancreatectomy: indications and outcomes in 235 patients. Ann Surg 1998; 229: 693–700 (1).
22. Malka D, Hammel P, Lévy P, Sauvanet A, Ruszniewski P, Belghiti J, Bernades P. Splenic complications in chronic pancreatitis: prevalence and risk factors in a medical-surgical series of 500 patients. Br J Surg 1998; 85: 1645–9 (C).
23. Rattner DW, Fernadez-del Castillo C, Warshaw AL. Pitfalls of distal pancreatectomy for relief of pain in chronic pancreatitis. Am J Surg 1996; 171: 142–6 (5).
24. Sawyer R, Frey CF. Is there still a role for distal pancreatectomy in surgery for chronic pancreatitis? Am J Surg 1994; 168: 6–9 (3).
25. Schoenberg MJ, Schlosser W, Rück W, Beger HG. Distal pancreatectomy in chronic pancreatitis. Dig Surg 1999; 16: 130–6 (A).
26. Shankar S, Theis B, Russell RCG. Management of the stump of the pancreas after distal pancreatic resection. Br J Surg 1990; 77: 541–4 (S1).
27. Warshaw AL. Conservation of the spleen with distal pancreatectomy. Arch Surg 1988; 123: 550–3 (F).

13.6 Laparoscopic pancreatic surgery in patients with chronic pancreatitis

L. Fernández-Cruz, A. Sáenz, J. P. Pantoja, E. Astudillo, S. Navarro

Introduction

Laparoscopy was initially introduced in the field of pancreatic surgery for staging pancreatic cancer. In 1911, Bernheim reported the use of diagnostic laparoscopy in a patient with a pancreatic mass, declaring that the presence of liver metastases precluded the possibility of any curative surgical attempt [1]. Cushieri in 1978, and Warshaw in 1986, also performed laparoscopic staging for the detection of metastases and tumor ingrowth [2, 3].

In recent years, technological advances and the experience accumulated with laparoscopic procedures for upper gastrointestinal tract and biliary tree diseases have made it possible to attempt with success the laparoscopic approach in pancreatic surgery.

The aim of this article is to analyze the recent advances in laparoscopic pancreatic surgery in the management of patients with chronic pancreatitis. This approach has been performed with clinical success in the management of patients with distal chronic pancreatitis and patients with chronic pancreatic pseudocysts.

Indications and technique of laparoscopic surgery in patients with chronic pancreatitis

Sawyer and Frey have stated that the ideal operation for patients with chronic pancreatitis should offer a low operative mortality, induce permanent pain relief, not exacerbate pancreatic exocrine and endocrine insufficiency, be easy to perform and not increase susceptibility to infection [4].

Distal pancreatectomy has been considered to have a limited role in the management of pain secondary to chronic pancreatitis. However, in 5 to 15% of patients with chronic pancreatitis, the disease is mainly located in the body and tail of the pancreas [4].

The analysis of the literature suggests the following factors that could select those patients who could benefit from distal pancreatectomy. 1) Patients with obstructive pancreatitis fulfilling the criteria defined and described in the 1994 Marseilles Classification of pancreatitis: Dominant stricture in the main pancreatic duct, normal main pancreatic duct and side branches proximal to the stricture on ERCP and normal pancreatic parenchyma on CT scan and at surgery, and no history of alcohol abuse. 2) Patients with a pseudocyst in the tail of the pancreas. 3) Patients with alcoholic chronic pancreatitis, with disease limited to the body and tail of the pancreas and minimally dilated duct (< 5 mm) according to CT scans and ERCP studies. 4) Patients with an inflammatory tumor suspected of being malignant.

Sawyer and Frey reported the results of a group of 17 patients who underwent distal pancreatectomy for chronic pancreatitis [4]. Of 10 patients with disease limited to the body and tail of the pancreas, 9 had no pain or mild pain postoperatively. Of 7 patients with diffuse disease or disease localized to the head of the pancreas, 6 required further hospitalization and surgery for severe persistent pain.

Rattner et al. reported the results of surgery for relief of pain in 20 patients, who underwent distal pancreatic resection for chronic pancreatitis. Alcohol abuse was the only etiology for chronic pancreatitis in 5 patients. Postoperative mortality was 5%, and 35% of the patients had a significant morbidity (2 abscesses, 2 intraoperative hemorrhages, 1 pancreatic fistula, 1 splenic infarction and 1 episode of delayed gastric emptying). Eleven patients (55%) had good results, 3 (15%) fair results and 6 (30%) poor results. The presence of a pseudocyst in the tail of the pancreas was associated with a good result. In this series, 3 of the 20 patients (15%) had unsuspected carcinoma of the pancreas [5].

Sakarofas et al. from the Mayo Clinic have reported the early and late morbidity and mortality in a group of 484 patients undergoing surgery for chronic pancreatitis. In this study 135 patients (28%) underwent distal pancreatectomy including splenectomy except in 11 (8%) of the patients in whom splenic salvage was achieved. Hospital mortality and morbidity after distal pancreatectomy was 1% and 20% respectively. The mean hospital stay in this group of patients after left resection was 13 days. Pain relief was achieved in 80% of patients after distal pancreatectomy. These excellent results may be due to a careful patient selection [6].

Govil and Imrie have recently reported good results after distal pancreatectomy in 23 of 36 patients with chronic pancreatitis. In this report, of the group of 21 patients in whom alcohol abuse was the etiology only 11 had good results but 10 had fair or poor results. However all 11 patients with obstructive pancreatitis had good results. In this series, the presence of pseudocysts was not invariably associated with a good outcome after distal pancreatectomy [7].

In the series of Shoenberg et al. 72% of the patients were pain-free after distal pancreatectomy during a median observation period of 58 months [8].

This analysis of the literature suggests that distal pancreatectomy, when indicated in the selected group of patients produces excellent results. However, morbidity is not infrequent in this limited pancreatic resection with a prolonged hospital stay.

Distal pancreatectomy is usually performed with *en bloc* resection with the spleen. The rationale of this approach is accepted for malignant disease of the pancreas but is questioned in patients with benign pancreatic disease [9]. Two studies have compared patients undergoing distal pancreatectomy with and without splenectomy, reporting no postoperative deaths in either one and similar complication rates. However overwhelming sepsis after distal pancreatectomy and splenectomy has been reported [4, 7, 8].

The *en bloc* distal pancreatic and spleen resection is performed, most of the time, for technical reasons, to make the operation short and easy but without any beneficial effect for the patient. Spleen preserving distal pancreatectomy is technically demanding and a more time-consuming procedure.

Splenic preservation is sometimes not possible in patients undergoing distal pancreatectomy for chronic pancreatitis in whom the pancreatic tissue is firmly and densely adherent to the splenic vessels. However, when the spleen preservation was attempted, the spleen was successfully salvaged in 25 out of 74 patients (34%) by Shoenberg et al. and 22 out of 26 patients (85%) by Govil and Imrie [7, 8]. These results compare favorably with 8% and 20% splenic preservation by Sakarofas et al. and Rattner et al. respectively [5, 6].

As an alternative, Warshaw has reported distal pancreatectomy and conservation of the spleen by dividing the splenic artery and vein but preserving the short gastric vessels [10]. However, the long-term function of the spleen for immunological defense is unknown.

More than a decade ago Pacher et al. [11] and Fitzgibbons et al. [12] managed the transected pancreas following distal pancreatectomy using the stapling device. Since then mechanical staplers have offered a quick and simple method for pancreatic transection. This technology as well as vascular staplers allowed Soper et al. to establish the safety and efficacy of laparoscopic distal pancreatectomy using an animal model without evidence of pancreatic leak or fistulae [13].

The first attempt to apply laparoscopic surgery in the surgical management of chronic pancreatitis was performed by Gagner and Pomp in 1994 [14]. Pylorus-preserving pancreaticoduodenectomy was successfully performed in a 30-year-old woman with chronic pancreatitis. Delayed gastric emptying complicated the postoperative course requiring nasogastric tube drainage for 20 days. The patient was discharged in good condition on the 30th postoperative day. This procedure proved to be time-consuming with an operative time of 10 hours. The authors concluded that, although technically feasible, the laparoscopic Whipple procedure may not improve the postoperative outcome or shorten the postoperative period. Cushieri has emphasized that the likely benefit of laparoscopic surgery over conventional open surgery is dependent on the ratio of access to procedural trauma [15]. In pancreaticoduodenectomy, the access trauma forms only a small component of the total operative insult to the patient. Therefore, this operation through the laparoscopic approach could be applied only when the postoperative course of the patient promised a better outcome than with the current open approach. At present, there is no place for laparoscopic pancreaticoduodenectomy in patients with chronic pancreatitis and a mass in the head of the pancreas.

However, Cushieri et al. in 1996 described the technique of laparoscopic distal 70 to 80% pancreatectomy with *en bloc* splenectomy performed in a group of 7 patients with intractable pain due to chronic pancreatitis [16]. The patients were placed in a supine position and five access ports were used, one at the umbilical area and two on each side at the subcostal region. The splenic artery is ligated first close to its origin from the celiac axis to minimize the risk of major bleeding during the subsequent dissection and to reduce the size of the spleen. The splenic vein is ligated at the confluence with the portal vein. The authors demonstrated that this operation using the laparoscopic technique can be performed within an acceptable operating time and without major complications. Also this technique achieved sustained pain relief in all patients.

Laparoscopic distal pancreatectomy has been performed also with clinical success by several surgeons in the management of benign tumors of the pancreas, including insulinoma [17–24].

From February 1998 to October 2000 we used the laparoscopic approach in 5 consecutive patients (3 male and 2 female) with distal chronic pancreatitis, median age 39.5 years ranging from 23 to 52 years. The etiology was obstructive pancreatitis. Abdominal pain for at least 6 months was the main complaint in all patients, partially alleviated with the use of non-opiate analgesics. Hospitalization due to exacerbation of the abdominal pain with increased serum amylase over 1000 IU/L (Normal value 10–400) was necessary in 4 patients. CT scan only showed an enlargement of the body and tail of the pancreas in 2 patients and a pseudocyst of 5 cm in size in one patient in the tail of the pancreas. ERCP showed a complete stop in the Wirsung duct in one patient and in 4 patients a stricture in the pancreatic duct in the body-tail of the pancreas. A normal size (3–4 mm) of the Wirsung duct was observed in all patients.

In our approach the patient is placed in half-lateral position with the left side up and reverse Trendelenburg. The surgeon and assistant stand on the left of the patient, whereas the camera person and the scrub nurse stand on the opposite side. Four 10–12-mm trocars are inserted in the abdominal wall: 3–4 cm above the umbilicus, on the xiphoid area, subcostal on the mid-axillary line, subcostal on the mid-clavicular line. The first step of the surgery is to start with dissection of the lieno-renal ligament and subjacent fascia, lateral to the spleen. The spleno-colic ligament is divided using laparoscopic coagulating shears (harmonic scalpel, Ethicon ultracision or USSC ultrasonics). The splenic flexure of the colon is mobilized downwards. The tail of the pancreas is then visualized, the gastrocolic omentum is widely open up to the level of the mesenteric vessels. Exposure of the anterior aspect of the pancreas is performed by dividing the adhesions between the posterior surface of the stomach and the pancreas. Care must be taken to preserve the short gastric vessels. At this point a clear demarcation between normal and abnormal pancreas is obtained. The limit of the resection was determined by the extent of the disease. It included 40 to 70% of the gland. The planning of the operation was to preserve the splenic vessels and in all 5 cases a spleen preserving distal pancreatectomy was performed. The inferior border of the pancreas is dissected and a complete detachment of the body and tail of the pancreas from the retroperitoneum is performed. This mobilization of the left pancreas allows visualization of the posterior wall of the gland where the splenic vein is easily identified. With gentle blunt dissection, the splenic vein is pushed away from the posterior pancreatic wall (Fig. 13.6-1). Visual magnification through the laparoscope permits excellent control of the small pancreatic veins that are coagulated using a Ligasure (USSC) device. We try to avoid whenever possible the use of hemostatic clips. A tunnel is created between the splenic vein and the pancreas. Through this space the splenic artery is identified by using blunt careful dissection with a curve dissector (Fig. 13.6-2). In some cases because of the fibrosis it took some time to surpass the superior border of the pancreas above the splenic artery. The pancreas is then transected with an endoscopic linear

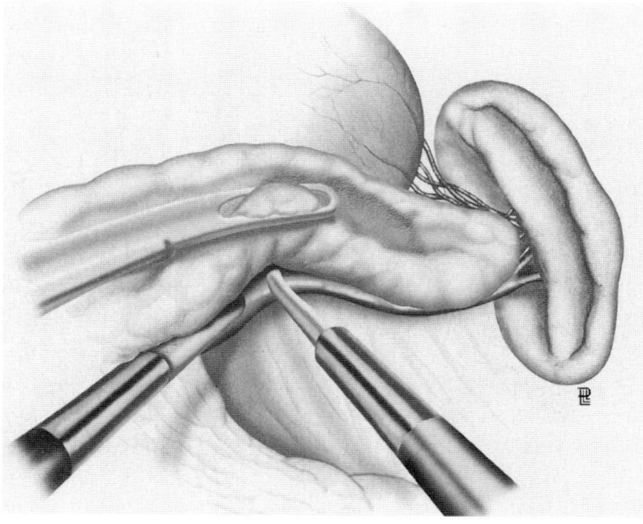

Figure 13.6-1. Gentle separation of the splenic vein from the posterior aspect of the pancreas.

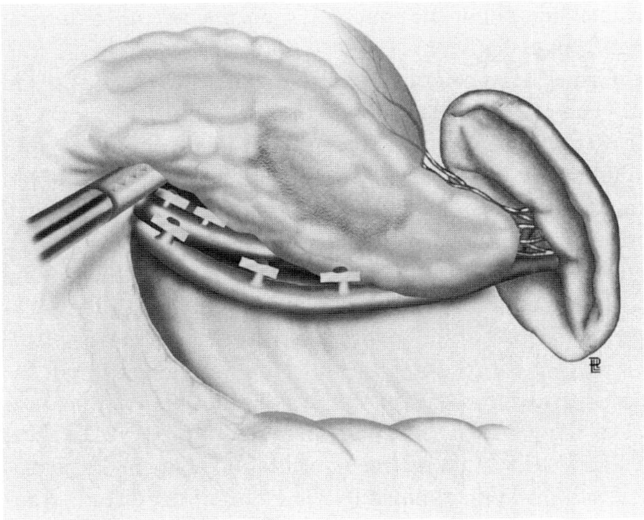

Figure 13.6-2. Creation of a tunnel between the splenic vessels and the body of the pancreas.

stapler. Usually two stapler applications are necessary. The mid-body of the pancreas is then grasped and retracted anteriorly with a 5-mm forceps and traction is applied to expose the small branches of the splenic artery and vein that are coagulated using a Ligasure (USSC) device (Fig. 13.6-3). The dissection is continued laterally to the splenic hilium. The specimen is then extracted using a non-permeable nylon bag through an enlarged trocar incision. A sylastic drain is placed in the pancreatic bed near the pancreatic stump.

The mean operative time was 4 hours ranging from 3 to 5 hours. The mean blood loss was 450 ml ranging from 300 to 800 ml. One patient was re-operated on 4 days after surgery for perforation of a duodenal ulcer; through mid-line incision a simple closure of the duodenal ulcer was performed. The mean hospital stay was 6 days ranging from 5 to 14 days. In these patients the mean time to resume daily activities was 3.8 weeks ranging

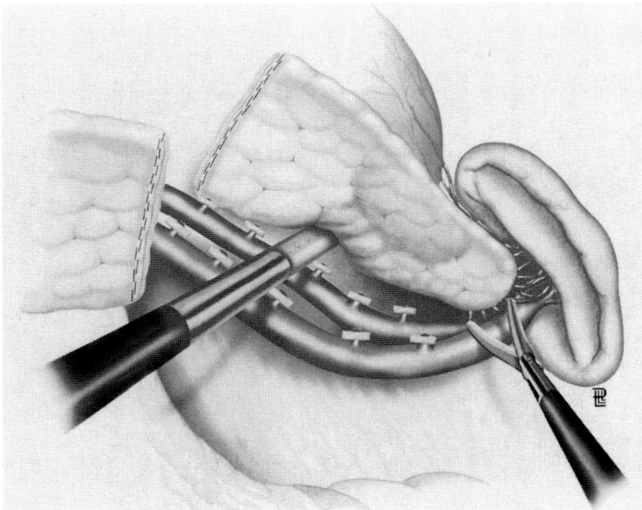

Figure 13.6-3. Dissection of the resected gland from the splenic vessels laterally to the splenic hilium.

from 3 to 4 weeks. All patients are pain-free with a mean follow up of 7 months ranging between 2 months and 2 years.

In summary, laparoscopic surgery in patients with chronic pancreatitis may offer the advantage of a minimally invasive approach in terms of cosmetic results, hospital stay and postoperative recovery.

The clinical experience with the laparoscopic approach is rather limited but with the excellent results achieved with this procedure, we believe, laparoscopic pancreatic surgery will soon become the standard treatment for benign pancreatic disease.

Indications and techniques of laparoscopic surgery in patients with chronic pancreatic pseudocysts.

Pancreatic pseudocysts are frequent complications of severe acute pancreatitis and are defined as fluid collections arising in or adjacent to the pancreas but lacking an epithelial lining. Surgery is infrequently indicated. However, pseudocysts in chronic pancreatitis have a mature capsule and rarely resolve spontaneously. Therapeutical intervention is indicated in symptomatic pseudocysts and when the size is over 6 cm in diameter. Bradley et al. found that complications occurred in 41% of patients with pseudocysts over 6 cm [25]. However, Vitas and Sarr have reported that observation was successful in three patients with pseudocysts over 10 cm [26]. It seems that in selected patients observation may be a good alternative.

The management of pancreatic pseudocysts includes percutaneous drainage, surgical decompression by external or internal drainage (into the stomach or jejunum) and pancreatic resection. More recently, endoscopic drainage and laparoscopic drainage have been proposed as minimally invasive procedures. The success or failure of each one of these therapeutical options is sometimes difficult to interpret in the current literature, especially when it is not clear whether the pseudocysts were the result of acute or chronic pancreatitis and whether there is a communication between the pseudocysts and the Wirsung duct. This communication occurs in 20% of pseudocysts in acute pancreatitis and in 49% of pseudocysts in chronic pancreatitis [27].

Percutaneous drainage has demonstrated in several studies long duration of catheter drainage and hospital stay, increased pseudocyst persistence and complications. In a recent study percutaneous drainage was successful only in 42% of patients [28].

Surgical treatment has included internal drainage into the stomach, duodenum, or jejunum, external drainage or resection. The mortality rate ranged from 0 to 10% with a complication rate of 25% and recurrence rates from 0 to 17% [29–33]. Recurrence is not infrequent in patients with chronic pancreatitis and persistent alcohol abuse due to stenosis of pancreatic duct or pancreatic duct stones.

Computed tomography scans allow identification of pancreatic pseudocysts bulging into the stomach or duodenum lumen suitable for minimally invasive methods. Endoscopic drainage can be performed using transpapillary cyst drainage or transmural techniques (endoscopic cystogastrostomy and endoscopic cystoduodenostomy). Transpapillary cyst drainage is technically demanding but in selected cases successful drainage was achieved in 84% with 9% recurrence rate over a mean follow-up of 2 years [34]. The stent is left *in situ* for 4 to 16 weeks and removed when the pseudocyst has resolved but carries the risk of stent-induced duct damage. Transmural pseudocyst drainage mimics the technique used in open surgery to drain the pseudocyst into the stomach or duodenum.

A side-viewing endoscope localizes the most prominent side of pseudocyst and a papillotome is used to make a diathermy incision to enter the pseudocyst. Usually, a stent is left within the cyst cavity to maintain patency for 2 to 4 months or until ultrasonographic confirmation of cyst resolution. Endoscopic cystogastrostomy and endoscopic cystoduodenostomy in the collective series achieved successful drainage in 82% and 89% and a recurrent rate of 18% and 6% respectively [34]. Perforation occurred less commonly with endoscopic cystoduodenostomy (4%) than with endoscopic cystogastrostomy (18%). Bleeding requiring surgery due to opening into a large vessel occurred in 7% of patients after endoscopic cystogastrostomy and 3% after cystoduodenostomy. Sahel et al. have reported 65% successful cystoduodenostomy drainage in 20 patients with chronic calcifying pancreatitis [35]. Recently, Beckingham et al. have reported the long-term outcome of endoscopic drainage of pancreatic pseudocyst from 34 patients selected for this method [36]. The etiologies were chronic pancreatitis in 20 patients, acute pancreatitis in 4 patients and trauma in 10 patients. Pseudocysts associated with chronic pancreatitis were successful drained in 75% of cases with no recurrences at 4 years median follow-up. Thick walled pseudocysts (> 1 cm) and location in the tail of the pancreas were factors associated with technical failures. Applying these criteria endoscopic transmural drainage is safely recommended in less than 50% of pancreatic pseudocysts.

The principles of both open and endoscopic drainage have been adopted by laparoscopic surgeons in the management of pancreatic pseudocysts. Since the first reports in 1994 different techniques have been described for laparoscopic pseudocyst drainage:

1. Laparoscopic intraluminal cystogastrostomy was introduced by Gagner and Way et al. [37, 38]. In this technique, radially expanding dilator 5 mm are inserted into the stomach, allowing the introduction into the stomach of a 5-mm laparoscope and instruments. A cystogastrostomy is created by using electrocautery. The holes in the stomach are closed with intracorporeal sutures. Trias et al. used the same intraluminal approached but inserting 12 mm cannulas with a balloon allowing the introduction of the endostapler device creating a wide cystogastrostomy [39]. After removing the cannulas, both gastric holes were closed by application of staples. 2. Laparoscopic anterior cystogastrostomy was described by Meltzer and Amaral [40] and published by Holeczy and Danis [41] and more recently by Smadja et al. [42]. An anterior gastrostomy is performed allowing easy access to the posterior wall of the stomach. Upon location of the cystogastric interface the pseudocyst cavity is penetrated using electrocautery. Both cystogastrostomy and anterior gastric wall closure are performed using an endoscopic linear stapling device. 3. Laparoscopic posterior cystogastrostomy was described by Morino [43] and recently published by Park et al. [44]. This technique uses the lesser sac approach; the anastomosis is performed between the cystostomy and posterior wall gastrostomy using an endoscopic linear stapling device.

Before deciding to choose one of the techniques described above, ERCP should be used to get information on the anatomy of the main pancreatic duct. A pseudocyst communication with the Wirsung duct was found in 44% to 68% in some series [45]. Pancreatic duct strictures and calculi are not infrequent findings in patients with chronic pancreatitis. Also, endoscopic ultrasound is a valuable adjunctive imaging technique in the management of pancreatic pseudocyst allowing identification of the area pseudocyst-gastric or duodenum apposition, exclusion of the presence of pseudoaneurysms and differentiation of pseudocysts from cystic neoplasms with increased accuracy.

We believe that pseudocysts, independent of the size, when associated with an inflammatory mass in the head of the pancreas or big duct in the head of the gland with calculi should be treated with pancreatic head resection. Also, patients with ductal strictures in the body of the pancreas and a distal pancreatic pseudocysts are best treated by a distal pancreatectomy. The laparoscopic approach using internal drainage of the pseudocyst should be reserved for pseudocysts larger than 5–6 cm located in the head or body of the pancreas. The communication with the main pancreatic duct does not exclude laparoscopic internal drainage except in patients with obvious multiple pancreatic duct strictures. Nevertheless, patients with chronic pancreatitis and continued alcohol abuse because of persistent changes may develop pancreatic inflammation, mass lesions or duct dilatation indicative of obstruction. In these patients, laparoscopic internal drainage may not be a definitive treatment and a more radical surgery may be needed in the course of the disease.

From October 1998 to October 2000, we used the laparoscopic approach in 6 patients (4 male and 2 female) with pancreatic pseudocysts. Median age 42 years ranging from 38 to 63 years. The etiology of the pseudocysts was chronic pancreatitis, alcoholic in 4 and idiopathic in 2. An inflammatory mass in the pancreas or pancreatic calculi was not observed by CT scans. ERCP failed to show a communication between the pancreatic duct and the pseudocysts. The pseudocysts were located 2 in the head and 4 in the body of the gland. The median size was 8 cm, ranging between 7 and 10 cm. Abdominal pain with a feeling of fullness after food intake was the main complaint in all patients for at least 3 months.

Patients were placed supine with general endotracheal anesthesia. A 10-mm trocar was introduced at the umbilicus. A 0° angle laparoscope was used. Two 10 to 12-mm trocars were placed, one under the xiphoid process and another under the left costal margin. Another 10 to 12-mm trocar was inserted under the right costal margin when necessary. In all cases the pancreatic pseudocysts were located using intraoperative ultrasound allowing identification of the most appropriate pseudocyst gastric apposition. In addition, in two patients the confirmation of the pseudocyst's position was done by puncture of the pseudocysts with a Verres needle. This maneuver allows aspiration of pseudocyst fluid for culture and cytological analysis. The injection of radio-opaque contrast under fluoroscopic control allows identification of the site for enteric drainage. In two patients with pseudocyst in the head of the pancreas laparoscopic intraluminal cystogastrostomy was performed. Under laparoscopic guidance two balloon-tipped trocars were placed in the anterior wall of the stomach through gastrostomies (Fig. 13.6-4). Once the balloons were inflated inside the gastric lumen, low pressure insuflation was applied to one of the tro-

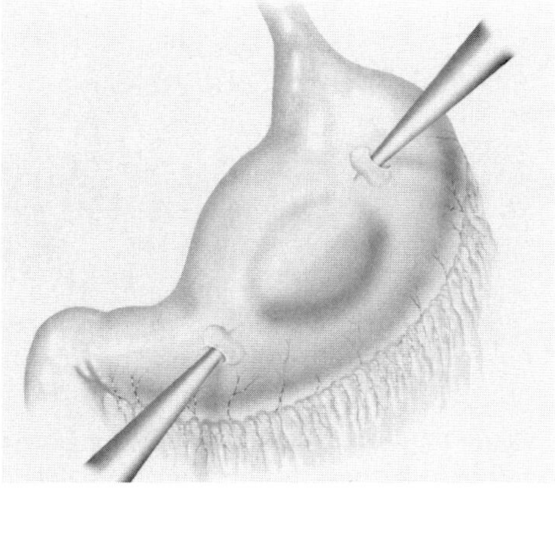

Figure 13.6-4. Placement of the trocars in the gastric lumen.

cars. A 0° laparoscope and the use of laparoscopic ultrasound identified the position of the pseudocyst (Fig. 13.6-5). The pseudocysts were penetrated using electrocautery. The insertion of the gastroscope into the cyst allows loculations to be lysed and the area for pancreatic pseudocyst biopsy to be identified. The cystogastrostomy was performed by using an endoscopic linear stapler device. The operative time was 120 and 150 minutes respectively. Patients were discharged 4 days after surgery. In four patients with pancreatic pseudocyst in the body of the pancreas, cystogastrostomy was performed through a laparoscopic anterior gastrostomy. In this approach the anterior wall of the stomach was opened 3.5 cm in length using the Harmonic Scalpel with direct access to the posterior gastric wall (Fig. 13.6-6). The use of electrocautery communicates the pseudocyst cavity with the stomach, confirmed by a rapid fluid loss through the entry site. The opening is enlarged using a harmonic scalpel. A cystogastrostomy anastomosis was performed with an endoGIA lineal stapler 3 cm in length (Fig. 13.6-7). The anterior gastric wall was closed with an endoGIA stapler (Fig. 13.6-8). The mean operative time was 100 minutes ranging from 60 to 120 minutes. The mean hospital stay was 4.5 days, ranging from 3 to 5 days. All patients resumed their daily activities within 2 weeks after laparoscopic surgery and are free of symptoms. The mean follow-up is 8 months ranging from 2 months to 2 years.

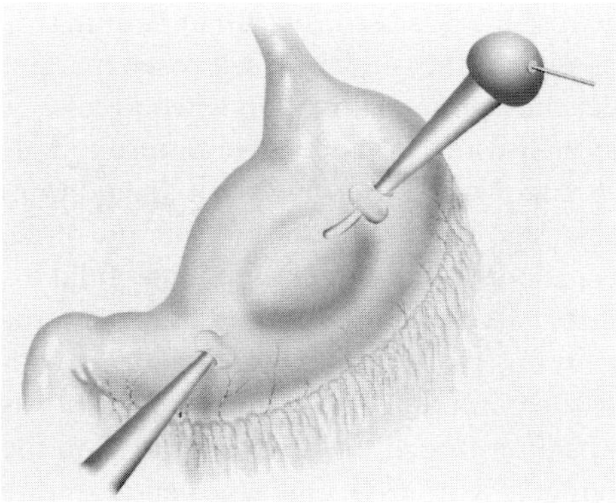

Figure 13.6-5. Use of laparoscopic ultrasound for the location of the pseudocyst.

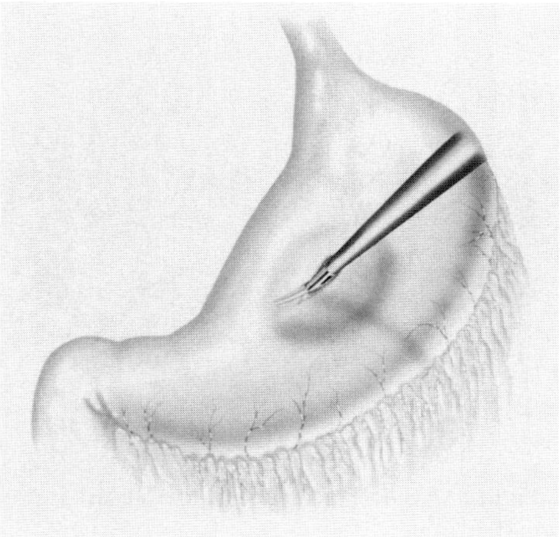

Figure 13.6-6. Incision of the anterior gastric wall with electrocautery or harmonic scalpel.

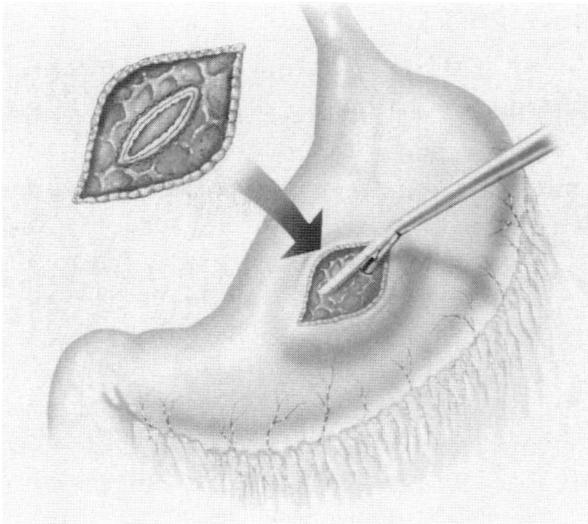

Figure 13.6-7. Creation of the cystogastrostomy with the use of a endoscopic linear stapling device.

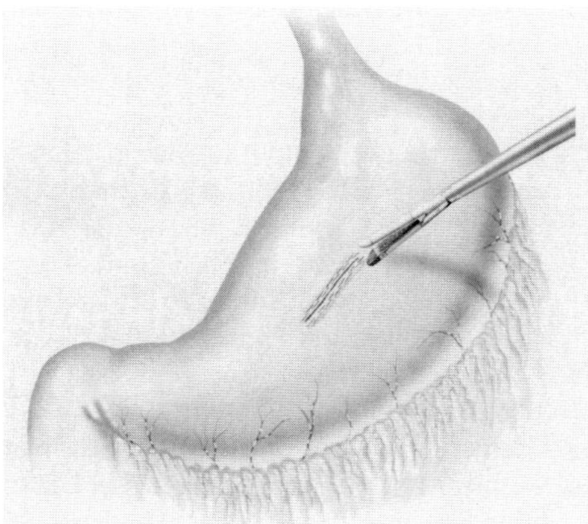

Figure 13.6-8. Closure of the anterior gastric wall with an endoscopic linear stapling device.

In summary, both laparoscopic intraluminal cystogastrostomy and laparoscopic anterior cystogastrostomy are safe and effective methods to treat symptomatic large pseudocysts of the pancreas. The benefit of a minimally invasive method using the laparoscopic approach may be in the good visualization of the structures, avoiding complications such as bleeding and perforation not infrequently found in the endoscopic management of pancreatic pseudocysts using transmural endoscopic drainage. Furthermore, the use of a stapling device to make the cystogastrostomy anastomosis not only prevents hemorrhage from the anastomosis site but provides a wide opening to prevent recurrence of the pseudocysts. The benefit may also be in the relatively short operative time and short hospital stay. The mean hospital stay of 4.5 days compares favorably with the mean hospital stay of 17.2 days recently published in a group of 58 pancreatic pseudocyst patients managed surgically with success [28]. Based on the prompt recovery and early period to resume daily activities patients appear to benefit from the laparoscopic approach. In the future prospective studies comparing endoscopic management with the laparoscopic approach will define the most appropriate patient who could benefit from one of these minimally invasive methods of treating pancreatic pseudocysts. The cost-benefit issue will also play a role in the decision-making.

References

1. Bernheim BM. Organoscopy: cystoscopy of the abdominal cavity. Ann Surg 1911; 53: 764–7.
2. Cushieri A, Hall AW, Clark J. Value of laparoscopy in the diagnosis and management of pancreatic cancer. Gut 1978; 19: 672–7.
3. Warshaw AL, Tepper JE, Shipley WU. Laparoscopy in the staging and planning of therapy for pancreatic cancer. Am J Surg 1986; 151: 76–80.
4. Sawyer R, Frey CF. Is there still a role for distal pancreatectomy in surgery for chronic pancreatitis? Am J Surg 1994; 168: 6–9.
5. Rattner DW, Férnandez del Castillo C, Warshaw AL. Pitfalls of distal pancreatectomy for relief of pain in chronic pancreatitis. Am J Surg 1996; 171: 142–6.
6. Sakarofas GH, Farnell MB, Farley DR, Rowland CM, Sarr MG. Long-term results after surgery for chronic pancreatitis. Int J Pancreat 2000; 27: 131–42.
7. Govil S, Imrie CW. Value of splenic preservation during distal pancreatectomy for chronic pancreatitis. Br J Surg 1999; 86: 895–8.
8. Shoenberg MH, Schlosser W, Rück W, Beger HG. Distal pancreatectomy in chronic pancreatitis. Dig Surg 1999; 16: 130–6.
9. Cooper MJ, Williamson RCN. Splenectomy: indications, hazards and alternatives. Br J Surg 1984; 71: 173–80.
10. Warshaw AL. Conservation of the spleen with distal pancreatectomy. Arch Surg 1988; 123: 550–3.
11. Pacher HL, Pennington R, Chassin J, Spencer FC. Simplified distal pancreatectomy with the auto suture stapler: preliminary clinical observations. Surgery 1979; 85: 166–70.
12. Fitzgibbons TJ, Yellin AE, Maruyama MM, Donovan AJ. Management of the transected pancreas following distal pancreatectomy. Surg Gynecol Obstet 1982; 154: 225–31.
13. Soper NJ, Brunt LM, Dunnegan DL, Meininger TA. Laparoscopic distal pancreatectomy in the porcine model. Surg Endosc 1994; 8: 57–61.
14. Gagner M, Pomp A. Laparoscopic pylorus-preserving pancreaticoduodenectomy. Surg Endosc 1994; 8: 408–10.
15. Cushieri A. Laparoscopic surgery of the pancreas. J R Coll Surg Edinb 1994; 39: 184–7.
16. Cushieri A, Jakimowicz JJ, Spreeuwel J. Laparoscopic distal 70 % pancreatectomy and splenectomy for chronic pancreatitis. Ann Surg 1996; 223: 280–5.
17. Gagner M, Pomp A, Herrera MF. Early experience with laparoscopic resections of islet cell tumors. Surgery 1996; 120: 1051–4.
18. Sussman LA, Christie R, Whittle DE. Laparoscopic excision of distal pancreas including insulinoma. Aust N Z J Surg 1996; 66: 414–6.
19. Cushieri A, Jakimowicz JJ. Laparoscopic pancreatic resections. Semin Laparosc Surg 1998; 5: 168–79.
20. Burpee S, Jossart G, Gagner M. The laparoscopic approach to gastropancreatic tumors. Acta Chir Austriaca 1999; 31: 207–13.
21. Vezakis A, Davides D, Larvin M, McMahon MJ. Laparoscopic surgery combined with preservation of the spleen for distal pancreatic tumors. Surg Endosc 1999; 13: 26–9.
22. Matsumoto T, Kitano S, Yoshida T, Bandoh T, Kakisako K, Nonomiya K, Tsuboi S, Baatar D. Laparoscopic resection of a pancreatic mucinous cystadenoma using laparoscopic coagulation shears. Surg Endosc 1999; 13: 172–2.
23. Tihany TF, Morvay K, Nehez L, Winternitz T, Rusz Z, Flautner LE. Laparoscopic distal resection of the pancreas with the preservation of the spleen. Acta Chir Hung 1997; 36: 359–61.
24. Klingler PJ, Hinder RA, Menke DM, Smith SL. Hand-assisted laparoscopic distal pancreatectomy for pancreatic cystadenoma. Surg Laparosc Endosc 1998; 8: 180–4.
25. Bradley E, Clements J, Gonzalez A. The natural history of pancreatic pseudocysts: a unified concept of management. Am J Surg 1979; 137: 135–41.
26. Vitas GJ, Sarr MG. Selected management of pancreatic pseudocysts: operative versus expectant management. Surgery 1992; 111: 123–30.

27. Barthet M, Sahel J, Bodiou-Bertei C, Bernard JP. Endoscopic transpapillary drainage of pancreatic pseudocysts. Gastrointest Endosc 1995; 42: 208–13.
28. Heider R, Meyer AA, Galanko JA, Behrns KE. Percutaneous drainage of pancreatic pseudocysts is associated with a higher failure rate than surgical treatment in unselected patients. Ann Surg 1999; 229: 781–9.
29. Gumaste UV, Dave PB. Pancreatic pseudocyst drainage – the needle or the scalpel? J Clin Gastroenterol 1991; 13: 500–5.
30. Newell KA, Liu T, Aranha GV, Prinz RA. Are cystgastrostomy and cystjejunostomy equivalent operations for pancreatic pseudocysts? Surgery 1990: 108: 635–40.
31. Schattenkerk ME, De Vries JE, Bruining HA, Eggink WF, Obertop H. Surgical treatment of pancreatic pseudocysts. Br J Surg 1982; 69: 593–4.
32. Frey CF. Pancreatic pseudocyst – operative strategy. Ann Surg 1978; 188: 652–62.
33. Kohler H, Schafmayer A, Ludtke PE, Lepsien G, Peiper HJ. Surgical treatment of pancreatic pseudocysts. Br J Surg 1987; 74: 813–5.
34. Beckingham IJ, Krige JEJ, Bornman PC, Terblanche J. Endoscopic management of pancreatic pseudocysts. Br J Surg 1997; 84: 1638–45.
35. Sahel J, Bastid C, Pellat P, Schurgers P, Sarles H. Endoscopic cystoduodenostomy of cysts of chronic calcifying pancreatitis: a report of 20 cases. Pancreas 1987; 2: 447–53.
36. Beckingham IJ, Krige JEJ, Bornman PC, Terblanche J. Long term outcome of endoscopic drainage of pancreatic pseudocysts. Am J Gastroenerol 1999; 94: 71–4.
37. Gagner M. Laparoscopic transgastric cystogastrostomy for pancreatic pseudocyst. Surg Endosc 1994; 8: 235.
38. Way LW, Legha P, Mori T. Laparoscopic pancreatic cystogastrostomy: the first operation in the new field of intraluminal laparoscopic surgery. Surg Endosc 1994; 8: 235.
39. Trias M, Targarona EM, Balagué C, Cifuentes A, Taurá P. Intraluminal stapled laparoscopic cystogastrostomy for treatment of pancreatic pseudocyst. Br J Surg 1995; 82: 403.
40. Meltzer RC, Amaral JF. Laparoscopic pancreatic cystogastrostomy. Minimally Invasive Ther 1994; 3: 289–94.
41. Holeczy P, Danis J. Laparoscopic transgastric pancreatic pseudocystogastrostomy – first experience with extraluminal approach. Hepatogastroenterology 1998; 45: 2215–8.
42. Smadja C, Badaway A, Vons C, Giraud V, Franco D. Laparoscopic cystogastrostomy for pancreatic pseudocyst is safe and effective. J Laparoendosc Adv Surg Tech 1999; 9: 401–3.
43. Morino M, Garrone C, Locatelli L, Cavuoti G, Miglietta C. Laparoscopic management of benign pancreatic cystic lesions. Surg Endosc 1995; 9: 625.
44. Park A, Schwartz R, Tandan V, Anvari M. Laparoscopic pancreatic surgery. Am J Surg 1999; 177: 158–63.
45. Vitale GC, Lawhon JC, Larson GM, Harrel DJ, Reed DN, Macleod S. Endoscopic drainage of the pancreatic pseudocyst. Surgery 1999; 126: 616–23.

13.7 Complications in pancreatic surgery: Prevention and treatment

K. Z'graggen, B. M. Schmied, M. W. Büchler

Introduction

Pancreatic surgery has evolved over the last three decades and is safe in experienced hands. The current management allows a mortality below 5% and a morbidity of 20–40%. The most commonly performed pancreatic operation is a pancreatic head resection, which includes the classic pancreatoduodenectomy (Whipple-Kausch operation), the pylorus-preserving pancreatoduodenectomy (Longmire-Traverso procedure) and for patients with chronic pancreatitis, the duodenum-preserving pancreatic head resection (Beger operation). Safe pancreatic surgery includes a careful preoperative assessment of the patients' risk factors and access to specialized endoscopy (ERCP) and diagnostic radiology (CT and MR tomography) [1]. Curative surgery in pancreatic cancer patients may be limited because of tumor size and extension but pancreatic resection in chronic pancreatitis can be challenging because of inflammatory changes and portal/ mesenteric hypertension.

Complications of pancreatic surgery can be prevented by different strategies, including prophylactic administration of octreotide [2] and a meticulous surgical technique during resection and reconstruction. From November 1993 to August 2000 547 patients underwent pancreatic resections at our institution, of whom the majority (76%) underwent pancreatic head resection. The following overview focuses on the prevention and treatment of pancreatic complications and discusses the results of pancreatic surgery with special reference to pancreatic head resection and chronic pancreatitis.

Preventive strategies in pancreatic surgery

The formation of *specialized centers* in pancreatic surgery allowed the improvement of operative and postoperative results in the past. Quality and efficiency in the surgical treatment of pancreatic diseases depend on the volume of patients treated. Recent publications analyzed the relation between patient volume and outcome [3, 4]. A correlation between the number of pancreatic resections, morbidity and in-hospital mortality has repeatedly been shown and a recent publication also demonstrated that high-volume centers have lower cost [5–7]. Although these data confirm the volume-outcome relationship in other areas of interest, including colorectal and liver surgery [6], hospital experience is particularly important with pancreaticoduodenectomy. The evidence that patients considering this procedure should be given the option of care at a high-volume referral center is rather solid [5, 8]. The specialized care includes not only the technical expertise of the procedure but also the postoperative care and in particular the management of associated complications. However, the patient with suspected pancreatic cancer or severe chronic pancreatitis usually presents to a physician or institution that does not focus on pancreatic diseases. At present, more than half of these patients are treated at low-volume institutions performing two or less pancreatoduodenectomies per year [9,10].

The *routine administration of octreotide* intra- and postoperatively (3 × 100–200 mcg/d subcutaneously) has been established as a concept to prevent surgical morbidity through randomized controlled trials [11–14]. Octreotide is a somatostatin analogon that reduces exocrine pancreatic function and splanchnic blood flow [15]. Although two studies from centers in the United States did not demonstrate a benefit of perioperative routine application of octreotide with regard to pancreatic fistula and morbidity [16, 17], the concept was demonstrated to be cost effective in elective pancreatic surgery, including pancreatic resections in chronic pancreatitis [2,12]. The controversy over the use of routine octreotide in pancreatic resections has been difficult to resolve. Reasons for the ongoing dispute may be decisive differences in surgical management and technique that may render interinstitutional comparisons inconclusive.

A meticulous and standardized *surgical technique* is the cornerstone of successful pancreatic surgery. The pancreatic anastomosis is the crucial step during reconstruction of gastrointestinal continuity after pancreatic head resection. Leakage of the pancreatic anastomosis has been associated with complications and mortality [18–21]. Several techniques and modifications have been proposed during the last decades, but regardless of the technique used, many large studies describe pancreatic fistula rates of more than 10% [19, 22–24]. Pancreatogastrostomy has also been proposed as an alternative to the more commonly used pancreaticojejunostomy, but anastomotic bleeding has been demonstrated to be a postoperative problem that disfavors its routine application [25]. Several steps, such as duct-to-mucosa adaptation and temporary ductal stenting, are thought to be important for a safe pancreatic anastomosis, but their technical quality is notoriously difficult to assess.

Complications after pancreatic surgery

Pancreas-specific complications are pancreatic fistula and delayed gastric emptying. The prevalence of pancreatic fistula is reported as 2–16% in major series, the prevalence of delayed gastric emptying 20–40%, and there has been considerable controversy concerning the optimal treatment of these complications. We have recently reported a pancreatic fistula rate of 2.1% in 331 patients undergoing pancreatic head resection [26]. The mortality in the series was 2.1%, the total morbidity 38%, including a local morbidity of 28% (Table 13.7-1) and a reoperation rate of 3.9%. The low mortality reported by many cen-

Local complication	%
Delayed gastric emptying	16.3
Wound sepsis	3.9
Intra-abdominal abscess	1.2
Bleeding	3.6
Cholangitis	2.1
Pancreatic fistula	2.1
Biliary fistula	0.9
Colonic fistula	0.9

Table 13.7-1. Local complications in 331 patients after pancreatic head resection (from [26]).

ters should not detract from the fact that morbidity after pancreatic resections remains rather high. The majority of local complications can be managed conservatively but intra-abdominal complications require experienced interventional radiologists who are able to treat abscesses and fluid collections and prevent reoperation under such circumstances.

Pancreatic fistula

The breakdown of a pancreatic anastomosis with development of a pancreatic fistula is a complication that can lead to further septic complications, bleeding and reoperation. A pancreatic fistula is typically defined as 30 ml or more secretion of amylase-rich drain fluid (≥5000 IU) per day for more than 10 days after the operation. Pancreatic fistula was associated with mortality in many reports and completion pancreatectomy has been considered to be the treatment in this situation until recently [27]. Pancreatic fistula can be categorized into low output (> 200 ml/d) and high output fistula for practical purposes. All patients with pancreatic fistula in our series were treated conservatively or interventionally and none of them died [26]. However, all had low output fistula without clinical signs of sepsis. We therefore think that a completion pancreatectomy for a pancreatic fistula should be a rare exception after pancreatic head resection. Although these results contradict recommendations from other groups, many centers report a higher prevalence of fistula and intra-abdominal sepsis [28–30].

The pancreatic anastomosis in patients with chronic pancreatitis is usually considered to have a much lower risk for a pancreatic fistula than in patients with periampullary tumors, in particular benign tumors or tumors of the common bile duct [31]. In our experience, the prevalence of pancreatic fistula was equal in patients with chronic pancreatitis (2.4%) and others (2.0), which included the patients with benign and ampullary tumors that had a soft pancreatic parenchyma. The prevalence of pancreatic fistulae was also similar whether a Whipple procedure, a pylorus-preserving pancreatoduodenectomy or a duodenum-preserving pancreatic head resection was performed [26]. The conclusion from this series with regard to pancreatic fistula was that although it is technically more difficult to do an anastomosis to a soft pancreas the consistency of the pancreatic remnant is certainly not the only, maybe not even the main risk factor for a pancreatic fistula. Strict adherence to a meticulous technique may be more important than pancreatic texture and consistency.

Delayed gastric emptying

The most frequent complication after pancreatic head resection is delayed gastric emptying and it occurs in 20–40% of patients. In our own series the prevalence of delayed gastric emptying is 33% after a classic Whipple procedure and 20% after a pylorus-preserving pancreatoduodenectomy. The definitions used vary from one report to another and sometimes explain the difference from one group to another. Most commonly delayed gastric emptying is defined as the need for a nasogastric tube for more than 10 days postoperatively. The median hospital stay after pancreatoduodenectomy is approaching 10 days in centers specialized in pancreatic diseases. Therefore, this definition is clinically relevant in patients that are well postoperatively and ready to leave hospital.

Many factors have been associated with delayed gastric emptying including intra-abdominal complications [18] and the technique of reconstructing the gastrointestinal continuity [32, 33]. Treatment options, however, are limited and there is only one randomized controlled trial that examined the effect of erythromycin on delayed gastric emptying. Erythromycin increases the interdigestive gastric motility and has been demonstrated to be beneficial in diabetic gastroparesis [34]. Yeo and colleagues demonstrated that erythromycin reduced the prevalence of delayed gastric emptying from 30% in the control group to 19% in the treatment group [35]. Despite the availability of many prokinetic drugs, delayed gastric emptying remains a significant clinical problem after pancreatic resections and other drugs with prokinetic activity on the stomach are currently being evaluated.

In patients with chronic pancreatitis delayed gastric emptying can be avoided altogether by performing a duodenum-preserving pancreatic head resection. In our series of more than 130 Beger operations, delayed gastric emptying did not occur. Therefore, the maintenance of the duodenal passage does facilitate the postoperative course for a significant proportion of patients with chronic pancreatitis undergoing surgery [26].

Surgery in chronic pancreatitis: the Bern experience

From November 1993 to August 2000 40% (217/547) of patients undergoing pancreatic resection were operated on for chronic pancreatitis (Table 13.7-2). The Beger operation was used as the standard procedure in 61% of our patients and a pancreatoduodenectomy was only performed if cancer in the head of the pancreas was suspected preoperatively or could not be ruled out during the procedure.

Table 13.7-2. Surgery in chronic pancreatitis: The Bern Experience 11/1993–08/2000 (n = 217).

Operation	No. of patients	%
DPPHR (Beger operation)	132	61
Pancreatoduodenectomy	22	11
Pancreatic left resection	12	6
Others	4	2
Non-resective procedures	47	22

The morbidity and mortality of the 132 patients with duodenum-preserving pancreatic head resection were 23% and 0.8% respectively. Systemic morbidity was 8% and local morbidity 15%. This was significantly lower than after pancreatoduodenectomy, mainly because delayed gastric emptying does not occur after a duodenum-preserving resection of the head of the pancreas. The fistula rate was 4.5%, including biliary, colonic and pancreatic (3%) fistula.

Conclusions

Many factors impact on the quality of pancreatic surgery. The current literature supports the view that the formation of specialized units, through an increased case load and readily available expertise in the management of patients with pancreatic diseases, including chronic pancreatitis, contributed significantly to the process. Centralization may be the most important determinator for the prevention of complications and for the improvement in results seen after pancreatic surgery over the last three decades. A further reduction of complications specific to pancreatic surgery (pancreatic fistula, delayed gastric emptying) can be expected from using already established strategies (octreotide), and from research into and development of new therapeutic drugs for delayed gastric emptying, which is the biggest contributor to morbidity after pancreatoduodenectomy.

References

1. Schmied BM, Z'graggen K, Redaelli CA, Büchler MW. Problems in staging of pancreatic and hepatobiliary tumours. Ann Oncol 2000; 11 (Suppl 3): 161–4.
2. Rosenberg L, MacNeil P, Turnacioglu K. Economic evaluation of the use of octreotide for prevention of complications following pancreatic resection. J Gastrointest Surg 1999; 3: 225–32.
3. Elixhauser A, Halpern MT. Economic evaluations of gastric and pancreatic cancer. Hepatogastroenterology 1999; 46: 1206–13.
4. Z'graggen K, Schmied BM, Büchler MW. Cost effective strategies in staging and imaging of pancreatic cancer. In: Arnold R, Galmiche JP, eds. Barret's esophagus, colon cancer and tumor imaging. Update Gastroenterology 2000.
5. Begg CB, Cramer LD, Hoskins WJ, Brennan MF. Impact of hospital volume on operative mortality for major cancer surgery. JAMA 1998; 280: 1747–51.
6. Choti MA, Bowman HM, Pitt HA, Sosa JA, Sitzmann JV, Cameron JL, Gordon TA. Should hepatic resections be performed at high-volume referral centers? J Gastrointest Surg 1998; 2: 11–20.
7. Birkmeyer JD, Finlayson SR, Tosteson AN, Sharp SM, Warshaw AL, Fisher ES. Effect of hospital volume on in-hospital mortality with pancreaticoduodenectomy. Surgery 1999; 125: 250–6.
8. Kingsnorth AN. Major HPB procedures must be undertaken in high-volume quaternary centres? HPB Surg 2000; 11: 359–61.
9. Gordon TA, Bowman HM, Tielsch JM, Bass EB, Burleyson GP, Cameron JL. Statewide regionalization of pancreaticoduodenectomy and its effect on in-hospital mortality. Ann Surg 1998; 228: 71–8.
10. Neoptolemos JP, Russell RC, Bramhall S, Theis B. Low mortality following resection for pancreatic and periampullary tumours in 1026 patients: UK survey of specialist pancreatic units. UK Pancreatic Cancer Group. Br J Surg 1997; 84: 1370–6.
11. Büchler MW, Friess H, Klempa I, Hermanek P, Sulkowski U, Becker H et al. Role of octreotide in the prevention of postoperative complications following pancreatic resection. Am J Surg 1992; 163: 125–30.
12. Friess H, Beger HG, Sulkowski U, Becker H, Hofbauer B, Dennler HJ, Büchler MW. Randomized controlled multicentre study of the prevention of complications by octreotide in patients undergoing surgery for chronic pancreatitis. Br J Surg 1995; 82: 1270–3.
13. Pederzoli P, Bassi C, Falconi M, Camboni MG. Efficacy of octreotide in the prevention of complications of elective pancreatic surgery. Italian Study Group. Br J Surg 1994; 81: 265–9.
14. Montorsi M, Zago M, Mosca F, Capussotti L, Zotti E, Ribotta G et al. Efficacy of octreotide in the prevention of pancreatic fistula after elective pancreatic resections: a prospective, controlled, randomized clinical trial. Surgery 1995; 117: 26–31.
15. Escorsell A, Bandi JC, Andreu V, Moitinho E, Garcia-Pagan JC, Bosch J, Rodes J. Desensitization to the effects of intravenous octreotide in cirrhotic patients with portal hypertension. Gastroenterology 2001; 120: 161–9.
16. Lowy AM, Lee JE, Pisters PW, Davidson BS, Fenoglio CJ, Stanford P, Jinnah R, Evans DB. Prospective, randomized trial of octreotide to prevent pancreatic fistula after pancreaticoduodenectomy for malignant disease. Ann Surg 1997; 226: 632–41.
17. Yeo CJ, Cameron JL, Lillemoe KD, Sauter PK, Coleman J, Sohn TA, Campbell KA, Choti MA. Does prophylactic octreotide decrease the rates of pancreatic fistula and other complications after pancreaticoduodenectomy? Results of a prospective randomized placebo-controlled trial. Ann Surg 2000; 232: 419–29.

18. Van Berge-Henegouwen MI, de Wit LT, van Gulik TM, Obertop H, Gouma DJ. Incidence, risk factors, and treatment of pancreatic leakage after pancreaticoduodenectomy: drainage versus resection of the pancreatic remnant. J Am Coll Surg 1997; 185: 18–24.
19. Yeo CJ, Cameron JL, Sohn TA, Lillemoe KD, Pitt HA, Talamini MA et al. Six hundred fifty consecutive pancreaticoduodenectomies in the 1990s: pathology, complications, and outcomes. Ann Surg 1997; 226: 248–57.
20. Trede M, Saeger HD, Schwall G, Rumstadt B. Resection of pancreatic cancer – surgical achievements. Langenbecks Arch Surg 1998; 383: 121–8.
21. Obertop H. Improving the technique of performing a pancreaticoenterostomy and pancreatoduodenectomy. J Am Coll Surg 1996; 182: 557–8.
22. DiCarlo V, Balzano G, Zerbi A, Villa E. Pancreatic cancer resection in elderly patients. Br J Surg 1998; 85: 607–10.
23. Cullen JJ, Sarr MG, Ilstrup DM. Pancreatic anastomotic leak after pancreaticoduodenectomy: incidence, significance, and management. Am J Surg 1994; 168: 295–8.
24. Marcus SG, Cohen H, Ranson JH. Optimal management of the pancreatic remnant after pancreaticoduodenectomy. Ann Surg 1995; 221: 635–45.
25. Yeo CJ, Cameron JL, Maher MM, Sauter PK, Zahurak ML, Talamini MA, Lillemoe KD, Pitt HA. A prospective randomized trial of pancreaticogastrostomy versus pancreaticojejunostomy after pancreaticoduodenectomy. Ann Surg 1995; 222: 580–8.
26. Büchler MW, Friess H, Wagner M, Kulli C, Wagener V, Z'graggen K. Pancreatic fistula after pancreatic head resection. Br J Surg 2000; 87: 883–9.
27. Van Berge-Henegouwen MI, de Wit LT, van Gulik TM, Obertop H, Gouma DJ. Incidence, risk factors, and treatment of pancreatic leakage after pancreaticoduodenectomy: drainage versus resection of the pancreatic remnant. J Am Coll Surg 1997; 185: 18–24.
28. Smith CD, Sarr MG, van Heerden JA. Completion pancreatectomy following pancreaticoduodenectomy: clinical experience. World J Surg 1992; 16: 521–4.
29. Cullen JJ, Sarr MG, Ilstrup DM. Pancreatic anastomotic leak after pancreaticoduodenectomy: incidence, significance, and management. Am J Surg 1994; 168: 295–8.
30. Farley DR, Schwall G, Trede M. Completion pancreatectomy for surgical complications after pancreaticoduodenectomy. Br J Surg 1996; 83: 176–9.
31. Barens SA, Lillemoe KD, Kaufman HS, Sauter PK, Yeo CJ, Talamini MA, Pitt HA, Cameron JL. Pancreaticoduodenectomy for benign disease. Am J Surg 1996; 171: 131–4.
32. Kingsnorth AN, Berg JD, Gray MR. A novel reconstructive technique for pylorus-preserving pancreaticoduodenectomy: avoidance of early postoperative gastric stasis. Ann R Coll Surg Engl 1993; 75: 38–42.
33. Muller MW, Friess H, Beger HG, Kleeff J, Lauterburg B, Glasbrenner B, Riepl RL, Büchler MW. Gastric emptying following pylorus-preserving Whipple and duodenum-preserving pancreatic head resection in patients with chronic pancreatitis. Am J Surg 1997; 173: 257–63.
34. Tack J, Janssens J, Vantrappen G, Peeters T, Annese V, Depoortere I, Muls E, Bouillon R. Effect of erythromycin on gastric motility in controls and in diabetic gastroparesis. Gastroenterology 1992; 103: 72–9.
35. Yeo CJ, Barry MK, Sauter PK, Sostre S, Lillemoe KD, Pitt HA, Cameron JL. Erythromycin accelerates gastric emptying after pancreaticoduodenectomy. A prospective, randomized, placebo-controlled trial. Ann Surg 1993; 218: 229–37.

14 Surgical treatment of chronic pancreatitis: Long-term results

14.1 Current surgical trends in Japan for managing chronic pancreatitis

T. Takada, Y. Takada, K. Takada

Summary

The main purpose of surgery for chronic pancreatitis is to relieve patient's persistent pain and preserve pancreatic exocrine/endocrine function. In this study, we analyzed the details of 2,936 patients with chronic pancreatitis who underwent surgery and who were listed in the 1985 National Statistics Registry, Japan, and afterward, we reviewed the literatures concerning the current surgical trends in Japan. We reached the following conclusions: 1) A side-to-side pancreaticojejunostomy or Frey's operation is frequently performed for patients showing a uniform dilatation of the main pancreatic duct from the pancreatic head to the tail. 2) A pancreatic resection is indicated in patients showing a marked inflammatory lesion in the pancreatic parenchyma. For a proximal pancreatic resection, a pylorus-preserving pancreatico-duodenostomy was the most favored technique. However, recently a duodenum-preserving pancreatic head resection is increasingly being performed. This latter technique is attracting more attention as it allows the excision of the inflamed pancreatic head while preserving the integrity of the biliary and alimentary tracts. 3) There is also a hypothesis that the pancreatic head acts as a so-called "pacemaker" in chronic pancreatitis.

Introduction

The main purpose of surgery is to relieve intractable patient's pain, which is characterized by persistent abdominal/and or back pain, while preserving pancreatic exocrine or endocrine functions or both. A side-to side pancreaticojejunostomy is performed for patients showing a marked dilatation of the main pancreatic duct; Partington's or Puestow's operation, or Frey's operation. Whereas pancreatic resection is the surgical choice for patients presenting mass-producing pancreatitis; Whipple, PPPD (pylorus-preserving pancreaticoduodenectomy), or DPPHR (duodenum-preserving pancreatic head resection). Especially, DPPHR showed significant results in relieving pain while still preserving pancreatic exocrine function. At a few institutions, pancreatic denervation is performed. These listed operative procedures would be discussed by an advocator or by doctors currently supporting each surgical technique [1]. We analyzed the details of 2,936 patients with chronic pancreatitis who underwent surgery and who were listed in the 1985 National Statistics Registry, Japan , and afterward, we also reviewed the literatures concerning the current surgical trends in Japan.

Pancreatic ductal drainage

Since Coffey's first report on pancreatic drainage in 1909 and Link's report of an external pancreatic drainage resulting in a marked recovery of the patient's condition [2, 3], reports on pancreatic drainage have been notable.

Mainly, there are three kinds of pancreatic ductal drainage procedure: Sphinctero-plasty or sphincterotomy, caudal pancreaticojejunostomy, and side-to-side pancreaticoje-junostomy. Based on the National Statistics Registry, pancreatic drainage procedures were performed in about 60% of the surgically treated patients in Japan in 1985.

Transduodenal sphincteroplasty/sphincterotomy

Dubilet and Mylholland first reported transduodenal sphincteroplast in 1948 [4], and in 1956 they reported on 190 cases through follow-up research, where 88% had relief of pain [5], and Bartlett followed this operation and reported a pancreatic orifice plasty in 1959 [6]. Nardi reported that over 50% of his patients experienced relief of pain after trans-duodenal sphincteroplasty with pancreatic orifice plasty [7, 8]. However, in most clinics, due to the ambiguity of the report, this operative procedure is not commonly conducted.

According to the 1985 National Statistics for Japan, either a sphincteroplasty or sphincterotomy was performed for 99 patients. However, these procedures are not currently conducted in Japan because they are ineffective for pain relief.

Caudal pancreaticojejunostomy

DuVal and Zollinger reported on caudal pancreaticojejunostomy in 1954 [9, 10]. However, this operative technique is not effective when there are multiple pancreatic stenoses, and currently this is not commonly conducted in Japan.

Side-to-side pancreaticojejunostomy

Puestow reported a side-to-side pancreaticojejunostomy following longitudinal excision of the pancreatic duct after distal pancreatectomy and splenectomy in 1956 [11]. Partington and Rochelle reported modified Puestow's procedure (longitudinal side-to-side pancreaticojejunostmy without removal of the distal pancreatectomy and splenectomy) in 1960 [12]. Further, A. P. Thal reported a modified Partington's procedure for those cases without dilatation of the pancreatic duct (< 5 mm) [13].

According to the 1985 National Statistics for Japan, a side-to-side pancreaticojejunostomy had been performed in about 30% of the 2,936 registered patients. Particularly,

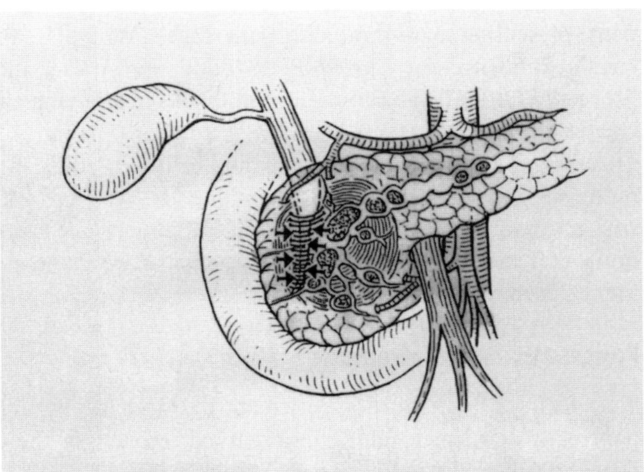

Figure 14.1-1. The cause of failure of a side-to-side pancreaticojejunostomy. Matsuno indicated that the failure of Puestow's/Partington's operation was due to inadequate drainage caused by the presence of pancreatic stones and/or ductal stenosis in the secondary branches of the main pancreatic duct.

T. Sato of Tohoku University advocated this surgery in Japan. Dr. Sato analyzed 134 chronic pancreatitis patients and reported that 97% of the patients who underwent side-to-side pancreaticojejunostomy showed pain relief [14]. On the other hand, Matsuno (a successor of Sato at the Tohoku University School of Medicine) indicated the failure of side-to-side pancreaticojejunostomy due to inadequate drainage caused by the presence of pancreatic stones and/or ductal stenosis in the secondary branches of the main pancreatic duct (Fig. 14.1-1) [15].

Frey's operation

In the 1985 National Statistics in Japan, there were no reports of Frey's Operation being performed. Afterwards, Matsuno of Tohoku University [15] and Fujimaki of Toyama Medical and Pharmaceutical University [16] reported their experiences using Frey's operation. Matsuno preferred Frey's operation to either Partington's or Puestow's operation, or resectional surgery, and they also concluded that Frey's operation was superior to Partington's side-to-side pancreaticojejunostomy [17].

Frey's operation is composed of two steps; coring-out the head of the pancreas and making the longitudinal pancreatic ductal incision, and side-to-side pancreaticojejunostomy (Fig. 14.1-2) [18, 19].

Pancreatic resection

Pancreatic resection includes total pancreatectomy, proximal pancreatic head resection (Whipple, PPPD, DPPHR), distal pancreatectomy, and middle pancreatectomy (or medial pancreatectomy).

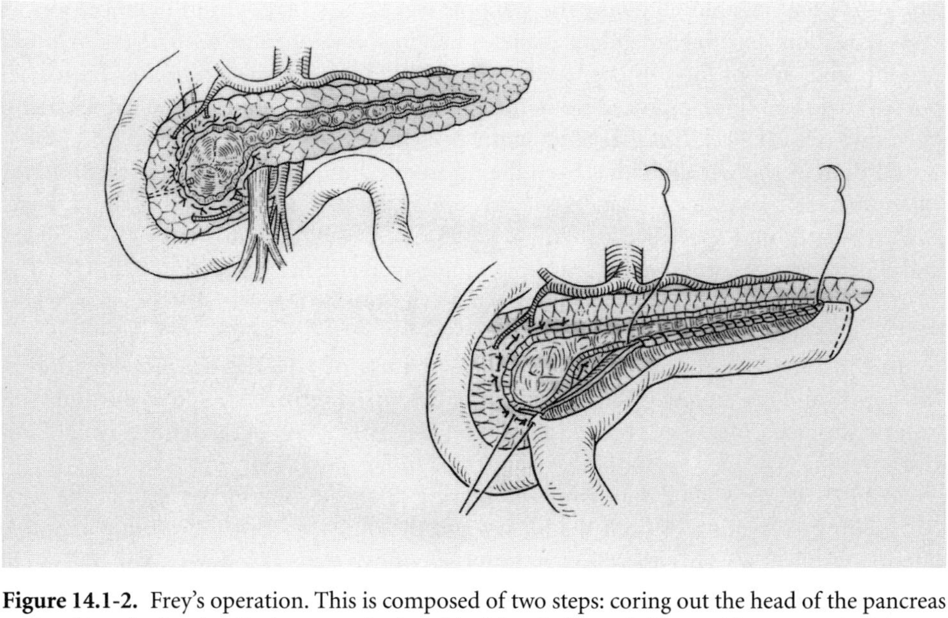

Figure 14.1-2. Frey's operation. This is composed of two steps: coring out the head of the pancreas and making the longitudinal pancreatic ductal incision (left), and side-to-side pancreaticojejunostomy (right).

Total pancreatectomy

Of the 2,936 surgically treated patients reported in the 1985 National Statistics for Japan, 36 underwent total pancreatectomy. At present, total pancreatectomy is not actively performed in Japan because of the resulting difficulties in controlling diabetes mellitus in the apancreatic state or difficulties in the management of impaired digestion and absorption or both.

The mainstream procedure used in pancreatic resection is either a pylorus-preserving pancreaticoduodenectomy (PPPD) or a duodenum-preserving pancreatic head resection (DPPHR).

Proximal pancreatic head resection

Proximal pancreatectomy has been preferred for removal of the "inflamed pacemaker" in the major portion of the diseased gland, in the pancreatic head [20], while preserving a sufficient segment of the body and tail of the gland to prevent the onset of diabetes.

Whipple procedure. 161 out of 1,936 surgically treated patients underwent the Whipple procedure. Later, Hanyu reported that their experience with 81 Whipple procedure patients showed feasible results [21]. Later, Imaizumi & Hanyu analyzed operative techniques in view of their effect on pain relief and preferred a proximal pancreatectomy such as pancreaticoduodenectomy or duodenum-preserving pancreatic head resection to a drainage operation [22] .

PPPD. The Whipple procedure had been used for all of the pancreaticoduodenectomies. However, since the report by Traverso and Longmire in 1978 [23], a pylorus-preserving pancreaticoduodenectomy, PPPD, has become the favored operative procedure for cases of chronic pancreatitis. Rossi reported that 66% of the patients who underwent Whipple procedure suffered from postoperative diabetes mellitus and 75% of the patients required pancreatic supplement [24]. Further, Traverso reported that the overall reduction of abdominal pain following the Whipple was 78%, whereas in PPPD there was an 85% reduction. Insulin-dependent diabetes mellitus developed in 47% of the Whipple patients and 26% of the PPPD patients, where PPPD was considered useful. Takada reported that the Whipple procedure induces postgastrectomy sequelae and sacrifices gut hormone-releasing cells that are abundantly present in the resected regions [25].

DPPHR. Although PPPD has been the favored technique for proximal resection, the extent of resection is very large despite the size of the lesion. On the other hand, Beger et al. reported on a specialized proximal pancreatic resection that preserved the biliary and digestive tracts, the duodenum-preserving pancreatic head resection, DPPHR (Fig. 14.1-3) [26, 27]. Beger recently reported wonderful results for 504 DPPHR cases, where 91.3% of patients were pain-free [28].

In the 1985 National Statistics for Japan, the use of DPPHR was not mentioned. Mizumoto and his successor Kawarada of Mie University were the first to report on their experiences using Beger's operation in Japan [29]. After 1990, many reports of DPPHR and a modified Beger's operation have appeared in Japan [30–34].

In 1993, we reported a duodenum-preserving total resection of the head of the pancreas with preservation of both the biliary and the digestive tract following pancreatoduodenostomy [34]. This operation is composed of two steps as follows: total excision of the head of the pancreas while preserving the integrity of the digestive and biliary tract, and reconstruction through pancreatoduodenostomy (Fig. 14.1-4). This procedure allows complete resection of the inflammatory mass in the pancreatic head. This approach also

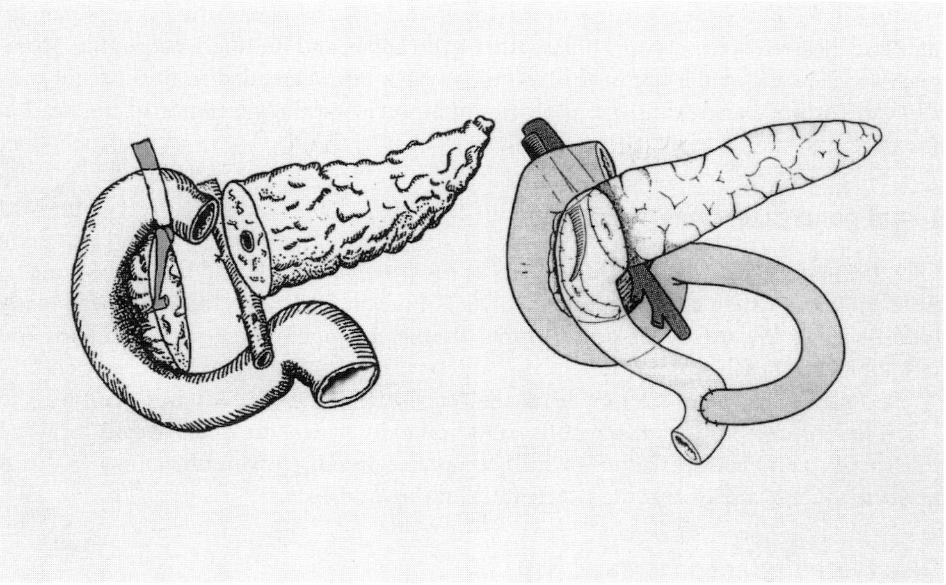

Figure 14.1-3. Beger's operation. This is composed of two steps: first, a partial resection of the head of the pancreas is performed while preserving biliary and digestive tracts (left). Then the reconstruction is performed with Roux-en Y pancreaticojejunostomy (right).

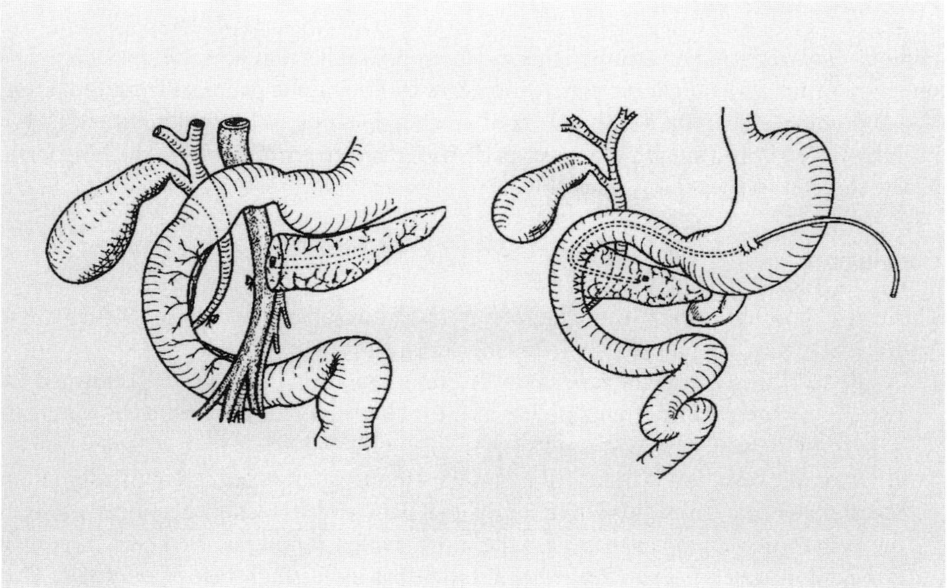

Figure 14.1-4. Takada's operation. This procedure is composed of two steps: a total excision of the head of the pancreas while preserving both the biliary tract and alimentary tract (left). In this operation, maintenance of the duodenal blood supply is required, so for this purpose it is very important to preserve the posterior arcade of pancreaticoduodenal artery without performance of Kocher's maneuver.

maintains the physiologic process of mixing food, bile, and pancreatic juice, as pancreatoduodenostomy preserves the biliary tract, gallbladder, and the duodenal papilla. Moreover, indications for the use of this technique have been extended to include not only cases of chronic pancreatitis but also cases of a mucin-producing tumor of the head of the pancreas.

Distal pancreatectomy

Of 2,936 patients, 197 underwent removal of the pancreatic body and tail, and 48 underwent removal of the pancreatic tail only. The 95% distal pancreatectomy has been rarely used in Japan because of the postoperative problems; impaired digestive functions and development of diabetes mellitus.

Recently, segmental resection or medial pancreatectomy [35, 36] was attempted in Japan for treating chronic pancreatitis complicated by pancreatic duct stenosis localized in the pancreatic body. In addition, a spleen-preserving distal pancreatectomy [37] was performed for a case of chronic pancreatitis on the caudal side.

Denervated splenopancreatic flap

Warren reported denervated splenopancreatic flap in 1984 [38]. In Japan, H. Kato developed a modified operation which combined Beger's operation with a denervated pancreatic flap described by Warren et al. [39].

Pancreatic denervation

Hiraoka et al. reported on two patients in whom pain relief was achieved by a complete resection of the postganglionic pancreatic nerve by freeing the pancreas from the posterior abdominal wall [40]. Takahashi reported thoracoscopic splanchnicectomy in 1996 [41]. However, only a small number of patients remain free from pain in the long term, so few surgeons perform this operation.

Conclusion

Through a thorough review of the literatures and a careful analysis of the 1985 Japanese National Statistics, we came to the following conclusions:

1. A side-to-side pancreaticojejunostomy or Frey's operation is frequently performed for patients showing a uniform dilatation of the main pancreatic duct from the pancreatic head to the tail.
2. A pancreatic resection is indicated in patients showing a marked inflammatory lesion in the pancreatic parenchyma. For a proximal pancreatic resection, a pylorus-preserving pancreatico-duodenostomy was the most favored technique. However, recently a duodenum-preserving pancreatic head resection is increasingly being performed. This latter technique is attracting more attention as it allows the excision of the inflamed pancreatic head while still preserving the integrity of the biliary and alimentary tracts.
3. There may be validity to the hypothesis that the pancreatic head acts as a so-called "pacemaker" in chronic pancreatitis.

References

1. Takada T, Yasuda H, Amano H et al. Current surgical trends in Japan for managing chronic pancreatitis. Pancreas 1998; 16: 337–42.
2. Coffey RC. Pancreaticoenterostomy and pancreatectomy. Ann Surg 1909; 50: 1238–64.
3. Link G. Treatment of chronic pancreatitis by pancreatotomy. Ann Surg 1911; 53: 768–82.
4. Doubilet H, Mulholland JH. Recurrent acute pancreatitis. Observation on etiology and surgical treatment. Ann Surg 1948; 128: 768–82.
5. Doubilet H, Mulholland JH. Eight-year study of pancreatitis and sphincteroplasty. JAMA 1956; 160: 521–8.
6. Bartlett MK, McDermott WV. Exploration of the pancreatic duct for pancreatitis. Surg Gynecol Obstet 1957; 104: 377–9.
7. Nardi GL. Papillotis and stenosis of the sphincter of Oddi. Surg Clin North Amer 1973; 53: 1149–60.
8. Nardi GL, Michaelassi F, Zannini P et al. Transduodenal sphincteroplasty. 5–25 year follow-up of 89 patients. Ann Surg 1983; 198: 435–61.
9. Duval MK Jr. Caudal pancreaticojejunostomy for chronic relapsing pancreatitis. Ann Surg 1954; 140: 775–85.
10. Zollinger RM, Keith LM, Ellison EH et al. Pancreatitis. N Engl J Med 1954; 251: 521–8.
11. Puestow CB, Gillesby WL. Retrograde surgical drainage of the pancreas for chronic relapsing pancreatitis. Arch Surg 1956; 76: 898–907.
12. Partington CB, Rochelle RL. Modified Puestow procedure for retrograde drainage of the pancreatic duct. Ann Surg 1960; 152: 1037–43.
13. Thal AP. A technical for drainage of the obstructed pancreatic duct. Surgery 1962; 51: 313–9.
14. Sato T, Miyashita E, Yamauchi H et al. The role of surgical treatment for chronic pancreatitis. Ann Surg 1986; 203: 766–71.
15. Egawa S, Takeda K, Matsuno S et al. Frey's operation for chronic pancreatitis. Tan to Sui 1998; 19: 1115–21.
16. Neto FC, Fujimaki M,Shizukuda M et al. Frey's operation for chronic pancreatitis. Shujutu 1995; 49: 495–502.
17. Akimura K, Matsuno S, Arai K et al. Surgery for chronic pancreatitis – extended pancreaticojejunostomy. Hepato Gastroenterology 1997; 44: 1547–53.
18. Frey CF, Amikura K. Local resection of the head of the pancreas combined with longitudinal pancreaticojejunostomy in the management of patients with chronic pancreatitis. Ann Surg 1994; 220: 492–507.
19. Frey CF, Suzuki M, Isaji S et al. Pancreatic resection for chronic pancreatitis. Surg Clin North Amer 1989; 69: 499–528.
20. Longmire WP. The surgical treatment of pancreatic disease. Jpn J Surg 1978; 4: 249–60.
21. Hanyu F, Suzuki M, Imaizumi T. Surgical management in chronic pancreatitis. Geka-Chiryo 1990; 62: 515–20.
22. Iamizumi T, Suzuki M, Hanyu F et al. Surgical treatment and results of chronic pancreatitis. Clinical Gastroenterology 1995; 10: 1093–1101.
23. Traverso LW, Longmire WP. Preservation of the pylorus in pancreatoduodenectomy. Surg Gynecol Obstet 1978; 146: 959–62.
24. Rossi RL, Rothschild J, Braasch JW et al. Pancreatoduodenectomy in the management of chronic pancreatitis. Arch Surg 1987; 122: 416–20.
25. Takada T, Yasuda H, Shikata J et al. Postprandial plasma gastrin and secretin concentrations after a pancreatoduodenectomy: a comparison between a pylorus-preserving pancreatoduodenectomy and the Whipple procedure. Ann Surg 1989; 210: 47–51.
26. Beger HG, Witte CH, Krantzberger W. Erfahrung mit einer das Duodenum erhaltenden Pankreaskopfresektion bei chronischer Pankreatitis. Chirurg 1980; 51: 303–9.
27. Beger HG, Krantzberger W, Wittner R et al. Duodenum-preserving resection of the head of the pancreas in patients with severe chronic pancreatitis. Surgery 1985; 97: 467–73.

28. Beger HG, Schlosser W, Friess HM et al. Duodenum-preserving head resection in chronic pancreatitis changes the natural course of the disease. A single-center 26 year experience. Ann Surg 1999; 230: 512–23.
29. Mizumoto R, Kawaharada Y. Surgical treatment of chronic pancreatitis. Geka-Chiryo 1982; 47: 501–9.
30. Yasuda H, Takada T, Uchiyma K et al. Resection of the head of the pancreas with preservation of biliary tract and duodenum. Tan to Sui 1990; 11: 967–73.
31. Takada T, Yasuda H, Uchiyama K et al. Duodenum-preserving pancreatoduodenostomy: a new technique for complete excision of the head of the pancreas with preservation of biliary and alimentary integrity. Hepato Gastroenterology 1993; 40: 356–9.
32. Imaizumi T, Hanyu F, Suzuki M et al. Clinical experience with duodenum-preserving total resection of the head of the pancreas with a pancreatico-choledocho-duodenostomy. J Hepatobiliary Pancreat Surg 1995; 2: 38–44.
33. Kimura W, Nagai H. Study of surgical anatomy for duodenum-preserving total resection of the head of the pancreas. Ann Surg 1995; 221: 359–63.
34. Takada T, Yasuda H, Uchiyama K et al. Complete duodenum-preserving resection of the head of the pancreas with preservation of the biliary and alimentary tract. J Hepatobiliary Pancreat Surg 1995; 2: 32–7.
35. Takada T, Yasuda H, Uchiyama K et al. A proposed new pancreatic classification system according to segments; operative procedure for a medial pancreatic segmentectomy. J Hepatobiliary Pancreat Surg 1994; 1: 322–5.
36. Ikeda S, Matsumoto S, Maeshiro K et al. Segmental pancreatectomy for the diagnosis and treatment of small lesions in the neck or body of the pancreas. Hepato Gastroenterology 1995; 42: 730–3.
37. Kimura W, Inoue T, Futagawa N et al. Spleen-preserving distal pancreatectomy with conservation of the splenic artery and vein. Surgery 1996; 120: 885–90.
38. Warren WD, Millikan WJ Jr, Henderson JM et al. A denerved pancreatic flap for control of chronic pain in pancreatitis. Surg Gynecol Obstet 1984; 159: 581–3.
39. Kato H, Abe I, Shimozawa E et al. New surgical procedure for chronic pancreatitis: partial resection of the head of the pancreas and complete isolation of the body and tail of the pancreas. Geka-Chiryo 1985; 53: 331–6.
40. Hiraoka T, Watanabe E, Kato T et al. A new surgical approach for control of pain in chronic pancreatitic. Am J Surg 1986; 152: 550–3.
41. Takahashi T, Kakita A, Izumika H et al. Thoracoscopic splanchnicectomy for the relief of intractable abdominal pain. Surg Endosc 1996; 10: 65–8.

14.2 Surgery of chronic pancreatitis: The Massachusetts General Hospital experience

C. Fernández-del Castillo, D. W. Rattner, A. L. Warshaw

Introduction

Chronic pancreatitis is a relentlessly progressive disease, and no treatment – medical, surgical, or endoscopic –, can reverse its course or provide an expectation for improvement in pancreatic function once the disease is established. Thus, treatment has been aimed at the control of symptoms, and pain is by far the most common and recalcitrant complaint of these patients.

In North America, efforts to treat the pain of chronic pancreatitis by surgical means began in the mid-twentieth century, with transduodenal sphincteroplasty and with caudal pancreatojejunostomy (DuVal procedure), both of which gave variable and usually poor results [1, 2]. A more extensive drainage procedure, lateral pancreatojejunostomy, was described by Puestow and Gillesby in 1958 [3] and subsequently modified by Partington and Rochelle [4]. This became the first surgical treatment widely considered to be effective for pain in this disease. However, at that time its application was hampered because there was no way to determine preoperatively if a patient with chronic pancreatitis had the dilated ducts required for the procedure, since ERCP and CT were not available until the 1970s. Thus, at the time of exploration the surgeon would perform an intraoperative pancreatogram to determine if the patient would be a candidate for a lateral pancreatojejunostomy. In those patients without dilated pancreatic ducts, the remaining options were to perform a sphincteroplasty (which was largely abandoned because of its failure) or to do nothing further. In the 1960s surgeons began performing pancreatic resections for chronic pancreatitis, initially distal pancreatectomies (with poor results) and later distal subtotal (95%) resections, which were more effective for pain but rendered most patients diabetic [5]. Proximal resections of the head of the pancreas (i.e Whipple-type procedures) were not widely applied until the 1980s, when the associated operative morbidity and mortality fell quite substantially [6–9].

At the Massachusetts General Hospital, surgical interventions for chronic pancreatitis have been done for over 40 years [10–12]. More than 90% of patients are referred to surgery because of chronic incapacitating pain that has failed to respond to medical treatment. Other indications are related to complications of chronic pancreatitis, such as biliary and duodenal obstruction, pseudocysts, pancreatic fistula or ascites, portal hypertension, as well as inability to exclude cancer.

In this chapter, we present a recent 8-year experience with surgical procedures for the management of pain in 134 patients with chronic pancreatitis. At the MGH, the preferred approach for this problem is a lateral pancreatojejunostomy because it is a safe operation, with good results, that does not compromise further pancreatic exocrine or endocrine function. Although it has been claimed that the Puestow procedure may retard pancreatic insufficiency [13], that has not been our experience [11], and this is not a reason for our preference. To determine if a patient is a candidate for this procedure, we obtain pre-

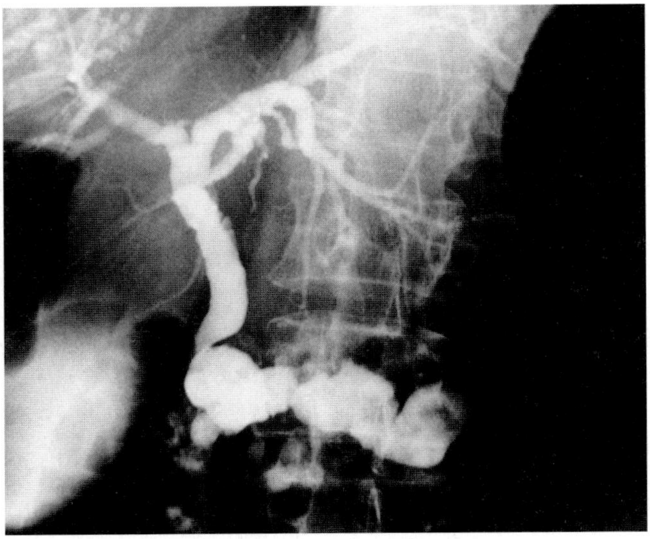

Figure 14.2-1. ERCP showing a dilated pancreatic ductal system as well as a bile duct stricture.

operatively a CT and an ERCP or an MRCP (except when the pancreatic duct is clearly and sufficiently dilated by CT examination and when further morphologic delineation is not considered necessary). Our cutoff to select a drainage procedure is a pancreatic duct diameter of 7 mm or more (Fig. 14.2-1), since smaller ducts are invariably associated with poor results if a drainage operation is performed. If the ducts are not dilated, we choose a Whipple procedure, unless the imaging studies clearly indicate that the disease is localized to the distal pancreas (dominant mid-duct stricture or pseudocyst), in which case we perform a distal pancreatectomy.

At our institution, the current proportion of patients with chronic pancreatitis undergoing surgery that have dilated ducts is 29%, with the rest of the patients being treated by resection (Fig. 14.2-2). For comparison, a recently published experience from the Mayo Clinic reports that 35% of patients with chronic pancreatitis undergoing surgery had a Puestow-type procedure [14], and in another series from Johns Hopkins the proportion is 19% [15].

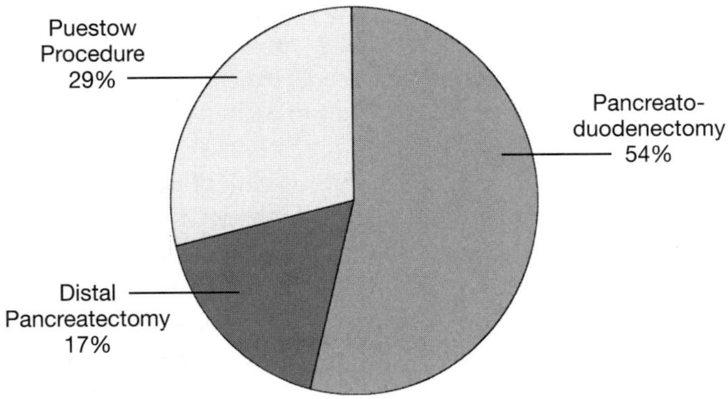

Figure 14.2-2. Surgery for pain in chronic pancreatitis. Massachusetts General Hospital (MGH), 1991 to 1997 (n = 134).

Pancreatoduodenectomy

From 1991 to 1997, we performed 72 pancreatoduodenectomies in patients with chronic pancreatitis and pain. The clinical characteristics and operative outcomes are summarized in Table 14.2-1. The series is unusual in that the most common etiology was obstructive chronic pancreatitis from ampullary stenosis or pancreas divisum (35%), reflecting a long-standing interest of our Institution in this problem. The second most common indication was alcohol abuse in 25%.

Table 14.2-1. Clinical characteristics and operative outcomes.

	(n)	(%)	Age	Duration of CP (years)	Alcohol abuse (%)	Post-op. length of stay	Operative mortality (%)
Pancreatoduodenectomy	72	50	47.2	5.3	28	15.6	1.3
Distal pancreatectomy	23	43	42.6	3.5	30	8.2	0
Puestow procedure	39	43	48.0	8.3	51	10.1	0
All procedures	134	47	46.6	5.8	35	12.7	0.7

There was a single perioperative death (mortality of 1.4%). The most common postoperative complication was delayed gastric emptying, occurring in 24%, followed by pancreatic fistula in 8%. Three patients required reoperation (4%).

Complete follow-up was available for 90% of patients, with an average follow-up of 41 months (Table 14.2-2). The success rate of pancreaticoduodenectomy in either eliminating or greatly reducing the pain and narcotic use associated with chronic pancreatitis was 65%. Poor results, indicated by lack of improvement of pain, occurred in 23 patients, six of whom underwent completion pancreatectomy within a year of surgery.

Table 14.2-2. Long-term follow-up.

	Follow-up (n)	(%)	Mean length of follow-up (months)	Good results (%)	Fair results (%)	Poor results (%)	Late death (%)
Pancreatoduodenectomy	72	90	41	46	19	35	7
Distal pancreatectomy	23	79	24	42	32	26	0
Puestow procedure	39	87	54	50	24	26	11

Five patients died during follow-up. Three of these resulted from malnutrition and failure to thrive as a consequence of progressive chronic pancreatitis (at 19, 60, and 77 months) and the other 2 were unrelated. There were no deaths related to cancer, in the pancreas or elsewhere in the GI tract.

In a recent study we compared the outcome of the 39 patients within this group who had the pylorus-preserving variant of pancreatoduodenectomy (PPPD) with that of the 33 patients who underwent the conventional pancreatoduodenectomy with antrectomy [16]. There was no difference in the preoperative characteristics of the patients. A significantly higher incidence of delayed gastric emptying was seen in the PPPD (33% vs. 12%), which resulted in a mean postoperative hospital stay that was on average three days longer (14.2 vs. 17.2). In the long term, there was no difference in postoperative nutritional indices at six months (PPPD and PD with antrectomy patients had body mass indexes > 20 in 73% and 78% of cases, respectively), need for pancreatic enzyme replacement (63% and 77%), new onset of diabetes (10% and 12%) or pain relief. There was a higher, although not statistically significant, incidence of peptic ulcer and gastrointestinal bleeding in the PPPD patients and one instance each of dumping and biliary gastritis in the PD with antrectomy group. Currently, we perform pancreatoduodenectomy with antrectomy almost exclusively, and consider the pylorus-preserving variant only for the patient who is severely malnourished (although our data do not support the theoretical rationale of this procedure).

Distal pancreatectomy

In the same time period, 23 patients with chronic pancreatitis were selected for distal pancreatectomy for the purpose of pain relief. All of them had CT, ERCP or intraoperative findings that suggested that inflammation was largely confined to the tail of the pancreas and had a pancreatic duct size of less than 7mm. These patients frequently had a mid-duct stricture or a pseudocyst in the tail. Their clinical characteristics and operative outcomes are shown in Table 14.2-1, and the long-term results in Table 14.2-2. The prevalence of alcohol abuse was similar to those patients who underwent Whipple procedures (22%) but pancreas divisum or ampullary stenosis was not an etiologic factor in this group. Trauma or previous episodes of biliary pancreatitis resulting in stricture of the pancreatic duct was the cause in 35% of patients, and in the remaining it was unknown.

17 patients (74%) had either good or fair results, and the remaining had no improvement in pain. In a previous study we evaluated the factors associated with good results in distal pancreatectomy for chronic pancreatitis, and found that the presence of a pseudocyst or a complete occlusion of the midpancreatic duct can predict a good outcome in terms of pain relief [17].

Lateral pancreatojejunostomy

Thirty-nine patients underwent a Puestow-type procedure. 51% of them had alcohol abuse as an etiologic factor, and 30% and 15%, respectively, were idiopathic or related to pancreas divisum. Their clinical characteristics are shown in Table 14.2-1. The average duration of chronic pancreatitis prior to surgery was 8.3 years. Concomitant surgical procedures included a biliary bypass in 10 patients, pseudocyst drainage in 3, resection of the pancreatic tail in 3, and one each gastrojejunostomy and right colectomy (for a villous adenoma). There were no operative deaths and the average length of hospital stay was 10 days.

Follow-up was available in 34 patients (87%), with an average duration of 54 months. 50% of them were judged to have good results, 24% of them fair, and 26% poor. Three patients who initially did well had recurrent pain 2, 6 and 7 years after surgery. The first subsequently underwent a thoracoscopic splanchnicectomy with good results, and the others are being managed medically. An ERCP confirmed a patent anastomosis in the patient who developed recurrent pain 7 years following the Puestow procedure.

Of the 9 patients with poor results, three underwent a subsequent Whipple procedure 4, 9 and 15 months later. One was found to have pancreatic cancer (misdiagnosed as chronic pancreatitis initially), and died 10 months later; the other two had fair results. We previously reported on 14 patients with failed Puestow procedures who underwent subsequent Whipple-type resection of the pancreatic head, with fair or good results in 10 of them (71%) [18].

Four patients died during the follow-up period. One was the patient with the failed Puestow who underwent a Whipple and was found to have pancreatic cancer. While it is likely that she had pancreatic cancer at the time of the initial surgery, it is of note that she had had symptoms of chronic pancreatitis for 17 years. Two other patients died of pancreatic cancer, one 2.5 years after surgery (with an 18-year history of chronic pancreatitis) and the other 7 years following the Puestow. The last patient died of peritonitis of uncertain origin 14 months after the surgical procedure.

Difficulty in the differential diagnosis between chronic pancreatitis and cancer is also underscored by seven additional patients who underwent pancreatic resection (4 distal and 3 proximal) for presumed chronic pancreatitis in the same time period, and who were found to have a malignant tumor. However, none of these patients had had symptoms for more than one year. In choosing between drainage and resection, this uncertainty can be weighed in the decision.

Future directions

Our group has begun to develop experience with thoracoscopic splanchnicectomy for the management of pain in chronic pancreatitis. Our preliminary results are encouraging. If long-lasting pain relief is obtained, as reported by others [19], this may well replace pancreatoduodenectomy in the treatment algorithm of some patients, particularly those who do not have significant symptoms of nausea and vomiting, which are unlikely to be affected by the neurectomy.

References

1. DuVal MK. Caudal pancreaticojejunostomy for chronic relapsing pancreatitis. Ann Surg 1954; 140: 775–85.
2. Jones SA, Smith LL, Gregory G. Sphincteroplasty for recurrent pancreatitis. Ann Surg 1958; 147: 180–90.
3. Puestow CB, Gillesby WJ. Retrograde surgical drainage of pancreas for chronic relapsing pancreatitis. Arch Surg 1958; 76: 898–906.
4. Partington PF, Rochelle RE. Modified Puestow procedure for retrograde drainage of the pancreatic duct. Ann Surg 1960; 152: 1037–43.
5. Frey CF, Child CG, Fry W. Pancreatectomy for chronic pancreatitis. Ann Surg 1976; 184: 403–14.
6. Grace PA, Pitt HA, Tompkins RK, DenBesten L, Longmire WP. Decreased morbidity and mortality after pancreatoduodenectomy. Am J Surg 1986; 151: 141–8.
7. Pellegrini CA, Heck CF, Raper S, Way LW. An analysis of the reduced morbidity and mortality rates after pancreaticoduodenectomy. Arch Surg 1989; 124: 778–81.
8. Crist DW, Sitzmann JV, Cameron JL. Improved hospital morbidity, mortality, and survival after the Whipple procedure. Ann Surg 1987; 206: 358–65.
9. Fernández-del Castillo C, Rattner DW, Warshaw AL. Standards for pancreatic resection in the 1990's. Arch Surg 1995; 130: 295–300.

10. Nardi GL, Acosta JM. Papillitis as a cause of pancreatitis and abdominal pain: role of evocative test, operative pancreatography, and histologic evaluation. Ann Surg 1966; 164: 611–21.
11. Warshaw AL, Popp JW, Schapiro RH. Long-term patency, pancreatic function, and pain relief after lateral pancreaticojejunostomy for chronic pancreatitis. Gastroenterology 1980; 79: 289–93.
12. Warshaw AL. Conservation of pancreatic tissue by combined gastric, biliary, and pancreatic duct drainage for pain from chronic pancreatitis. Am J Surg 1985; 149: 563–9.
13. Nealon WH, Thompson JC. Progressive loss of pancreatic function in chronic pancreatitis is delayed by main pancreatic duct decompression. Ann Surg 1993; 217: 458–68.
14. Sakorafas GH, Farnell MB, Farley DR, Rowland CM, Sarr MG. Long-term results after surgery for chronic pancreatitis. Int J Pancreatol 2000; 27: 131–42.
15. Sohn TA, Campbell KA, Pitt HA et al. Quality of life and long-term survival after surgery for chronic pancreatitis. J Gastrointest Surg 2000; 4: 355–65.
16. Jimenez RE, Fernández-del Castillo C, Rattner DW, Chang Y, Warshaw AL. Outcome of panreaticoduodenectomy with pylorus-preservation or with antrectomy in the treatment of chronic pancreatitis. Ann Surg 2000; 231: 293–300.
17. Rattner DW, Fernández-del Castillo C, Warshaw AL. Pitfalls of distal pancreatectomy for relief of pain in chronic pancreatitis. Am J Surg 1996; 171: 142–6.
18. Markowitz JS, Rattner DW, Warshaw AL. Failure of symptomatic relief after pancreaticojejunal decompression for chronic pancreatitis. Arch Surg 1994; 129: 374–80.
19. Menezes N, Carter CR, Imrie CW. Minimally invasive thoracoscopic splanchnicectomy (MITS) in the management of chronic pancreatitis. Int J Pancreatol 2000 (in press).

14.3 Surgical treatment of chronic pancreatitis: The Hungarian experience

T. F. Tihanyi, L. E. Flautner, A. Magyar, I. Pulay

Abstract

Systematic surgical therapy for chronic pancreatitis began with the advent of ERCP, introduced in Hungary towards the end of the 1960s. In the earlier periods cyst drainage operations were performed, or occasionally pancreatoduodenectomies for suspicion of pancreatic cancer. With the help of ERCP the imaging of ductal morphology gave impetus to the development of different surgical treatment modalities for chronic pancreatitis and its complications. Between 1972 and 1998 3468 operations were performed for the treatment of chronic pancreatitis. 1920, 713 and 835 of these were cyst drainage, resections and decompressions respectively. The overall mortality rate was 2.6%. The choice of the procedure was based on ductal morphology and the localization of the disease within the gland. Thus a policy of differential patient and treatment selection was adopted. To decrease the high morbidity and mortality rates associated with the traditional Kausch-Whipple pancreatoduodenectomy the pylorus-preserving procedure – reintroduced by Traverso and Longmire – in combination with pancreatogastrostomy was applied from 1978. Due to its favorable results it very soon spread in Hungary and became the method of choice in pancreatic head resections. The organ preservation tendency brought about by the duodenum-preserving technique of Beger and the limited head resection proposed by Frey stimulated further changes in the surgical approach to chronic pancreatitis. Combined drainage procedures were developed to improve long-term results, resections are becoming more limited and the technique of local head resection with extended distal drainage is becoming more popular in our institutional experience.

Chronic pancreatitis is a confronting disease. Although it is not a surgical one *"per se"*, many patients undergo surgery most frequently because of intractable pain and/or different complications arising during the clinical course of chronic pancreatitis. In spite of the numerous types of surgical procedures developed over the years surgical treatment of chronic pancreatitis is still a great challenge. Many centers dealing with chronic pancreatitis apply either resection or decompression based on theoretical principles [1, 2], while others use a more selective approach [3]. Many new techniques like endoscopic drainage or stone clearance were introduced recently to avoid surgery [4, 5]. None of the options has proved its superiority over the others in the long run.

In Hungary the number of operations rapidly increased during the 1970s and 1980s. This tendency can still be observed, indicating a continuously increasing incidence of pancreatic diseases, both chronic pancreatitis and pancreatic cancer (Fig. 14.3-1). A plausible explanation for this can be given from the etiologic point of view. The most frequent etiologic factor in Hungary is chronic alcohol consumption. According to statistical data the annual pure alcohol consumption is quite high: during the last three decades with 12–14 liters per person Hungary has stood sixth among high-rate consumers in Europe

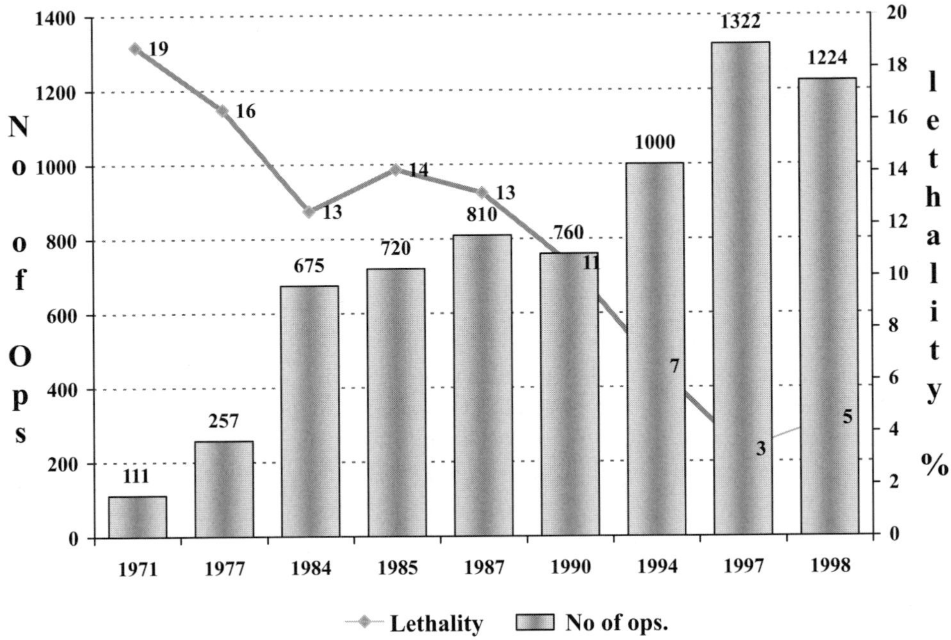

Figure 14.3-1. Number of surgical procedures performed on the pancreas in Hungary from 1971 to 1998. Data collected by the National Institute of Surgery.

(Table 14.3-1). Another important factor is the type of drinks consumed. Hungary was previously a "wine drinking" country but drinking habits have changed substantially. Spirits consumption accounts for 48% of the total and with this Hungary precedes all other European countries except Poland, Russia and Rumania (Table 14.3-2) [6–8].

It is not surprising therefore that alcohol-related diseases like liver cirrhosis and pancreatitis are frequent in Hungary, where mortality from alcoholic liver diseases and pancreatitis was 60 and 4/100,000 inhabitants respectively in 1999 [9, 10]. The incidence of chronic pancreatitis falls between 12 and 18 cases per 100,000 inhabitants yearly.

Till the end of the 1960s, although sporadic cases of chronic pancreatitis were recognized and operated on, pancreatic resections were performed mostly with the suspicion of tumor. The most frequent operation in chronic pancreatitis was drainage of pseudocysts complicating the disease. The greatest impact on the diagnosis of the different ductal alterations in chronic pancreatitis came from the introduction of ERCP. The technique was introduced in Hungary at the end of the 60s [11]. Different drainage procedures based on ductal morphology were introduced at the 1st Department of Surgery of Semmelweis University in Budapest, and very soon this institute became the largest referral center in Hungary for pancreatic diseases [12].

Institutional experience

Between 1972 and 1998 3468 operations were performed for the treatment of chronic pancreatitis at the 1st Department of Surgery, Faculty of Medicine of Semmelweis University Budapest. The overall postoperative mortality was 2.6% (90 patients). The distri-

Table 14.3-1. Total annual consumption of alcohol in Hungary in comparison with other European countries.

Country	Liters per person older than 15 [8] 1975	1980	1986	1990	1995
Luxembourg	13.09	13.46	14.36	14.75	14.24
Slovenia			15.46	12.85	13.88
France	20.94	18.98	16.69	15.64	13.76
Portugal	18.36	14.85	14.57	12.69	13.56
Germany					13.00
Hungary	**12.68**	**15.11**	**14.49**	**14.42**	**12.54**
Czech Republic			11.32	11.33	12.21
Denmark	11.77	11.5	12.21	11.69	12.14
Belgium	12.98	13.55	12.62	12.09	12.10
Ireland	11.22	10.50	9.43	10.46	12.06
Austria	14.47	13.84	12.19	12.59	11.75
Switzerland	13.53	13.45	13.31	13.03	11.29
Romania	10.17	10.91	10.31	9.55	11.11
Spain	19.58	18.34	14.96	13.45	11.09
Slovakia			13.21	12.44	10.64
Greece		13.21	9.18	10.66	10.40
Netherlands	11.65	11.33	10.62		9.92
Bulgaria	10.51	11.17	11.75	11.69	9.45
United Kingdom	8.87	9.26	9.14	9.51	9.42
Italy	16.86	16.66	12.30	10.90	9.27
Russia		13.40	6.74	7.14	9.20
Finland	8.08	7.91	8.56	9.54	8.26
Poland	9.59	11.49	9.69	8.28	7.97
Sweden	7.98	7.09	6.71	6.70	6.04
Norway	5.64	5.91	5.23	5.06	5.10

bution of the different types of procedures is shown on Table 14.3-3. In comparison to the Hungarian performance the data of the year 1997 indicate that 40% of the operations performed for chronic pancreatitis are done in this institute (Table 14.3-4) [13].

The evolution of the surgical attitude to the management of chronic pancreatitis becomes quite apparent if one analyzes the patients' data in two consecutive periods, taking the last ten years' data separately. Tables 14.3-5 and 14.3-6 clearly show a substantial increase in the number of operations with stable distribution of the main type of procedures in both periods. Overall mortality is significantly reduced. During the period between 1972 and 1988 the double choledocho-Wirsungoplasty and Wirsungojejunostomy was a preferred type among the decompressions. The classical Kausch-Whipple pancreatoduodenectomies carried quite a high mortality rate (Tables 14.3-7 and 14.3-8). Analyzing results at that time, it was found that in the early follow-up period around 70% of the patients were free of symptoms after either resections, decompressions or cyst drainage, but in the long term this rate decreased to 50–60% (Table 14.3-9). During this period the rate of subsequent operations performed for recurrent symptoms after resec-

Country	1975	1980	1985	1992	1995	1997
	Liters pro year per capita [8]					
Russia				3.8	7.0	5.5
Romania	1.9	0.92	2.0	3.5	3.96	4.49
Poland	4.6	6	4.6	3.5	3.5	3.4
Hungary	**3.61**	**4.75**	**5.4**	**3.4**	**3.42**	**3.25**
Bulgaria	2.91	3.15	3.21	2.81	2.75	2.46
Spain	2.7	3.2	2.8	2.7	2.5	2.6
France	2.42	2.52	2.33	2.63	2.48	2.43
Finland	3.01	2.98	3.01	2.25	1.95	2.07
Netherlands	3.44	2.72	2.24	1.9	1.73	1.72
Ireland	2.03	2.04	1.8	1.6	1.7	1.7
Luxembourg	1.74	1.69	1.62	1.6	1.6	1.6
Austria	1.65	1.59	1.46	1.26	1.5	1.5
Switzerland	1.94	2.05	2.18	1.61	1.49	1.47
Iceland	2.4	2.25	2.26	1.87	1.46	1.22
United Kingdom	1.47	1.78	1.72	1.48	1.35	1.37
Sweden	2.97	2.74	2.06	1.6	1.33	1.09
Belgium	1.99	2.37	2.12	1.2	1.1	1.0
Denmark	1.74	1.52	1.64	1.19	1.07	1.11
Norway	1.84	1.91	1.41	0.81	0.81	0.87
Portugal	0.9	0.9	0.8	0.8	0.8	0.8
Italy	1.8	1.9	1.3	1	0.7	0.7
Turkey	0.5	0.44	0.3	0.4	0.4	0.4

Table 14.3-2. Annual consumption of spirits in Hungary in relation to other European countries.

Types of operations	No.	Lethality (%)
Resection	704 (20%)	32 (4.5%)
Decompression	821 (24%)	9 (1.1%)
Cyst drainage	1943 (56%)	49 (2.5%)
Total	**3468**	**90 (2.6%)**

Table 14.3-3. Distribution and lethality of the different types of surgical procedures for chronic pancreatitis at the 1st Dept. of Surgery, Medical Faculty of Semmelweis University Budapest between 1972 and 1998.

tions, decompressions and cyst drainage was 11–21–18% respectively. In the next period – between 1989 and 1998 – the type of the most frequently applied operation changed markedly. Among the resections the pylorus-preservation with pancreatogastrostomy was favored, becoming the standard for pancreatic head resection (Table 14.3-10). Double-plasty has rarely been performed. Combined cyst-duct decompression was introduced, and among the distal decompressions the Wirsungo-gastric anastomosis were preferred (Table 14.3-11). Late results clearly show that the 30.5% subsequent operation rate after the double-plasty could be reduced to 10% after the combined drainage procedures.

Table 14.3-4. Pancreatic operations performed for chronic pancreatitis in Hungary in the year 1997.

	Hungary		1st Dept. of Surgery Semmelweis University		Percent of 1stDept of Hungary
	No.	Lethality (%)	No.	Lethalithy (%)	
Decompression total	**132**	**0**	**47**	**0**	**35.61**
Double plasty	11		2		18.18
C-W-G	27		18		66.67
W-G	73		24		32.88
C-W-J	7		2		28.57
W-J	14		1		7.14
Resection total	**135**	**0**	**58**	**0**	**42.96**
PD total	9		3		33.33
PD partialis	75		28		37.33
Distal resection	51		27		52.94
Pseudocyst drainage total	**540**	**3 (0.56)**	**218**	**2 (0.92)**	**40.37**
Total	**807**	**3 (0.37)**	**323**	**2 (0.62)**	**40.02**

PD = pancreatoduodenectomy, CWG = cysto-Wirsungo-gastrostomy, WG = Wirsungo-gastrostomy, CWJ = cysto-Wirsungo-jejunostomy, WJ = Wirsungo-jejunostomy

Table 14.3-5. Types of operations performed for chronic pancreatitis between 1972 and 1988.

Types of operations	No.	Lethality
Resection	300 (20%)	20 (6.7%)
Decompression	295 (24%)	6 (2.0%)
Cyst drainage	681 (56%)	26 (3.8%)
Total	**1276**	**52 (4.1%)**

Table 14.3-6. Types of operations performed for chronic pancreatitis between 1989 and 1998.

Types of operations	No.	Lethality
Resection	404 (18.4%)	12 (3.0%)
Decompression	526 (24%)	3 (0.6%)
Cyst drainage	1262 (57.6%)	23 (1.6%)
Total	**2192**	**38 (1.73%)**

Table 14.3-7. Decompressions performed for chronic pancreatitis during the period between 1972 and 1988.

Types of operations	No.		Lethality (%)
Double plasty		138	4 (2.9%)
Distal decompression		157	2 (1.3%)
– Wirsungo-jejunost	83		
– Wirsungo-gastrost	23		
– cysto-Wirsungo-gastrostomy	51		
Total		**295**	**6 (2.0%)**

Types of operations		No.	Lethality (%)
Pancreatoduodenectomy		173	18 (10.4)
– Total	30		6 (20%)
– Whipple	58		8 (13.8%)
– pylorus-preservation	85		4 (4.7%)
Duodenum-preserving		6	0
Distal resection		121	2 (1.6%)
Total		**300**	**20 (6.7%)**

Table 14.3-8. Types of resections performed for chronic pancreatitis during the period between 1972 and 1988.

Types of operations	"Good" results	
	After 1 year	After 5 years
Decompression	69.8%	57.2%
Resection	67.1%	52.4%
Cyst drainage	72.2%	63.5%

Table 14.3-9. Long-term results of the different operations in chronic pancreatitis.

Types of operations		No.	Lethality (%)
Pancreatoduodenectomy		226 (56%)	10 (4.4)
– Total	17		2 (11.7%)
– Whipple	42		3 (7.1%)
– pylorus-preservation	167		5 (3.0%)
Duodenum-preserving		40 (9.9%)	1 (2.5%)
Distal resection		138 (34.1%)	1 (0.7%)
Total		**404**	**12 (3.0%)**

Table 14.3-10. Resections performed for chronic pancreatitis during the period between 1989 and 1998.

Types of operations		No.	Lethality (%)
Pancreatoduodenectomy		226 (56%)	10 (4.4)
Double plasty		52 (9.9%)	1 (1.9%)
Distal decompression		474 (90.1%)	2 (0.4%)
– Wirsungo-jejunost	27		
– Wirsungo-gastrost	260		
– cysto-Wirsungo-gastrostomy	187		
Total		**526**	**3 (0.6%)**

Table 14.3-11. Decompressions performed for chronic pancreatitis during the period between 1989 and 1998.

Discussion

Pain has been the main indication for surgical treatment over the years. Many theories were tried as to the origin of pain in chronic pancreatitis. Obstruction theory was justified by the clinical experience that ductal decompression relieved pain. It was demonstrated later by Bradley, Madsen and Ebbehoy that there is increased ductal and tissue pressure associated with dilatation. Decompressive procedures causing pain relief were associated with decreased intraductal and tissue pressures [14]. Reber experimentally proved that ductal obstruction and increased tissue pressure leads to decreased tissue per-

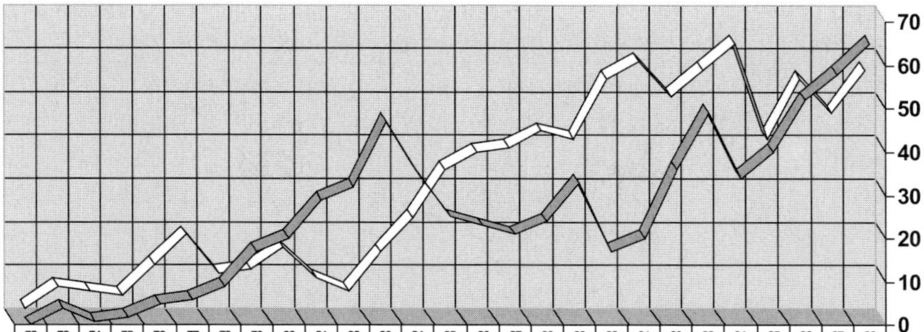

	72	73	74	75	76	77	78	79	80	81	82	83	84	85	86	87	88	89	90	91	92	93	94	95	96	97	98
■ Resection	0	4	1	2	5	6	9	17	20	29	32	47	35	25	23	21	24	33	17	20	36	49	34	40	52	58	65
□ Decompr.	2	7	6	5	12	19	10	11	16	9	6	15	23	34	38	39	43	41	55	59	51	57	63	41	55	47	57

Figure 14.3-2. Changing trends in the rate of resections and decompressions performed between 1972 and 1998 at the 1st Department of Surgery, Faculty of Medicine, Semmelweis University, Budapest.

fusion. As a consequence the lowered tissue pH may add to the mechanism of pain [15]. Recently this microcirculatory disturbance was demonstrated in human chronic pancreatitis, too [16]. On the other hand Bockmann demonstrated neural inflammatory lesions that are also responsible for causing pain [17]. The rationales of the different surgical procedures are based on these hypotheses of pathogenesis of pain.

Basically two main types of operations – namely resection and decompression – were adopted in our Institute with changing frequency (Fig. 14.3-2). The interlacing curves clearly show the changes in institutional preferences over the years. During the first period mostly decompressions like double-plasty or distal pancreatojejunostomy were performed because the traditional Kausch-Whipple resection carried high morbidity and mortality. Szécsény introduced the technique of the transduodenal choledocho-Wirsungoplasty in Hungary in 1972 [18]. This aimed to provide drainage of the pancreatic duct in cases of periampullary obstruction (Fig. 14.3-3). But as it turned out, long-term results

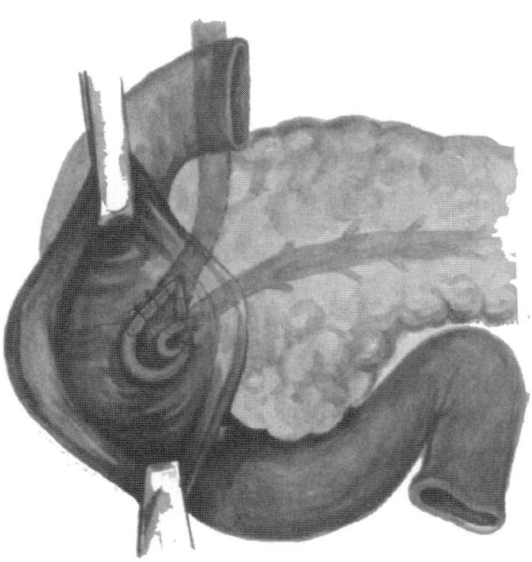

Figure 14.3-3. Transduodenal choledocho- and Wirsungo-plasty.

Table 14.3-12. Mortality of 368 partial pancreatoduodenectomies from 1983 to 1998 in relation to the type of procedure, etiology and management of the pancreatic remnant.

	Pancreato-jejunostomy			**Pancreato-gastrostomy**			**Total**
	Whipple	PPPD	Subtot	Whipple	PPPD	**Subtot**	
Malignant	13	5	18	10	117	127	145
Lethal	1	1	2 (11.1%)	2	10	12 (9.4%)	14 (9.6%)
Benign	29	6	35	13	175	188	223
Lethal	2	–	2 (5.7%)	1	5	6 (3.2%)	8 (3.6%)
Total	**42**	**11**	**53**	**23**	**292**	**315**	**368**
Lethal	3	1	4 (7.5%)	3	15	18 (5.7%)	22 (5.9%)

of these drainage procedures were disappointing. At an average of 1.5 years 30% of these patients required subsequent surgery, in most cases resection, because of recurrent symptoms. So our attention turned back to pancreatoduodenectomy. A major impact on our attitude was made by the adoption of the pylorus-preserving technique of Traverso and Longmire [19]. With a new type of pancreatic reconstruction – pancreatogastrostomy – the results of pancreatoduodenectomy improved substantially [20]. Operative mortality and morbidity requiring reoperations was lowered, the rate of postoperative pancreatic fistula decreased. These differences in the rate of pancreatic leaks were more marked in patients with malignant disease then in chronic pancreatitis. The fistula occurrence was more likely with a soft pancreas (Tables 14.3-12, 14.3-13 and 14.3-14). Many authors described delayed gastric emptying as the most frequent complication following pylorus-preserving pancreatoduodenectomy [21–23]. In our experience this did not present real concern. Delayed emptying occurred in less then 10% of the cases, all resolving spontaneously. Gastric emptying studies with isotopic labeled standard food showed gastric emptying profiles similar to those of normal subjects (Fig. 14.3-4). In our practice care is taken to preserve the right gastric artery and its supraduodenal branch. The stomach is not mobilized to avoid denervation of the antrum and pylorus. On the other hand, pancreatogastric anastomosis was associated with a somewhat higher rate of postoperative bleeding originating from the surface of the resected pancreas. Only 7 of the 15 cases required reoperation while the others were managed endoscopically. Survival data were similar to those of drainage procedures and significantly better then the traditional Kausch-Whipple procedure (Fig. 14.3-5).

Table 14.3-13. Morbidity and mortality of pancreato-jejunal anastomosis following pancreatoduodenectomy (1983–1998).

Type of lesion	No.	Reoperation	P-j leak	Lethality
Malignant	18	3 (16.7%)	2 (11.1%)	2 (11.1%)
Benign	35	6 (17.1%)	2 (5.7%)	2 (5.7%)
Total	**53**	**9 (16.9%)**	**4 (7.5%)**	**4 (7.5%)**

Table 14.3-14. Morbidity and mortality of pancreato-gastric anastomosis following Pancreatoduodenectomy (1983–1998).

Type of lesion	No.	Reoperation	P-j leak	Lethality
Malignant	127	28 (22.0%)	8 (6.3%)	12 (9.4%)
Benign	188	15 (8.0%)	8 (4.2%)	6 (3.2%)
Total	**315**	**43 (13.6%)**	**16 (5.0%)**	**18 (5.7%)**

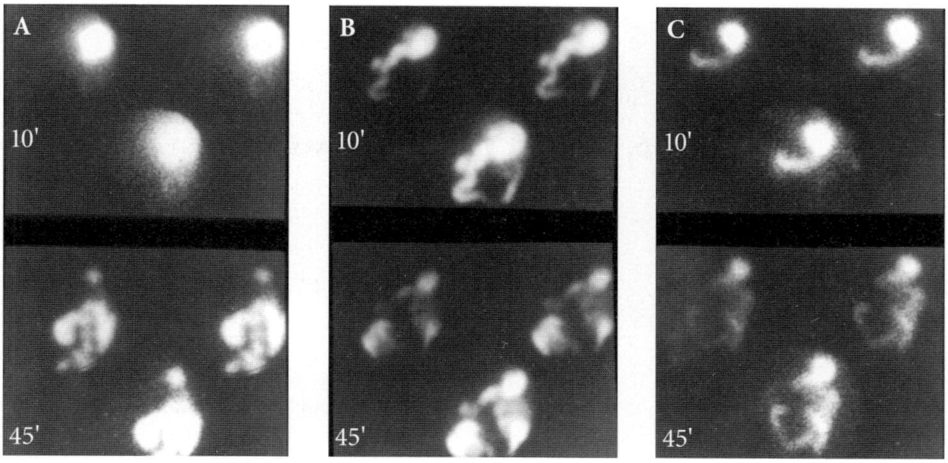

Figure 14.3-4A–C. A: Gastric emptying after standard Kausch-Whipple, **B:** pylorus-preserving pancreatoduodenectomy with pancreatogastric anastomosis, and **C:** normal subjects. Scintigraphy with Tc99-labeled standard food, 4 weeks postoperatively.

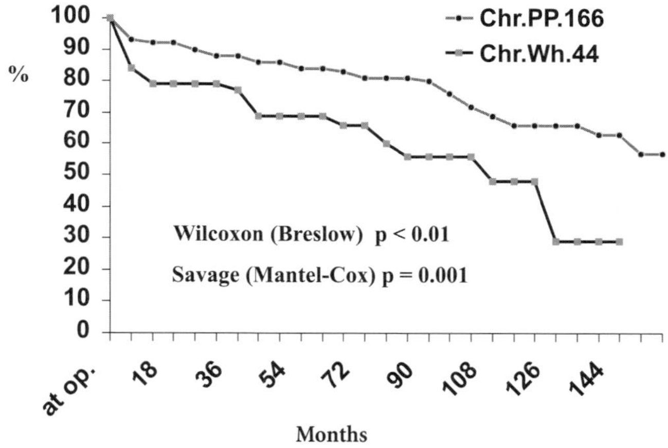

Figure 14.3-5. Cumulative survival after standard Kausch-Whipple and pylorus-preserving pancreatoduodenectomy of patients with chronic pancreatitis. PP = pylorus-preserving, Wh = Whipple type of resection, Chr = chronic pancreatitis

We analyzed the causes of failure of drainage operations. Early recurrences occurring within 18 months were mostly the consequence of such multiple morphologic alterations of the pancreas that were not recognized at the time of the initial procedure. These might be multiple strictures of the duct, pseudocysts or sometimes multiple necrotic cavities in the head. Simple drainage of either the pseudocyst or the pancreatic duct alone would not provide lasting pain relief. Combined drainage procedures like cysto-Wirsungo-jejunostomy and cysto-Wirsungo-gastrostomy were developed. This latter became the preferred anastomosis type, being technically less demanding, less time consuming and giving results equal to or even superior to the jejunal anastomosis [24] (Fig. 14.3-6). Another observation on follow-up of the drainage procedures was the influence of the length of the disease period before surgery upon survival. Patients with a length of symptoms less then 18 months had a more favorable outcome then those with a longer period (Fig. 14.3-7).

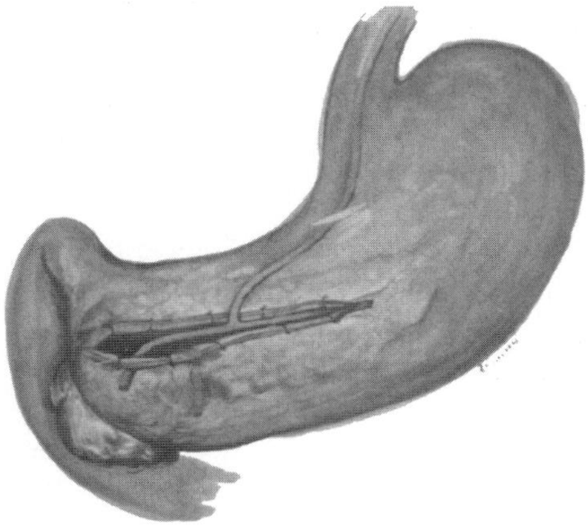

Figure 14.3-6. Combined drainage procedure; cysto-Wirsungo-gastrostomy.

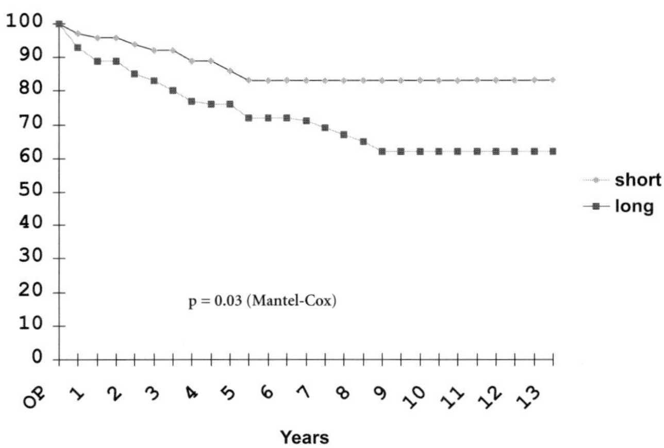

Figure 14.3-7. Cumulative survival after decompressions in chronic pancreatitis. The effect of the length of symptoms (short = < 18 months, long = > 18 months).

This seems to confirm the observations of Nealon, who found that early decompression of the ductal system could prevent the progressive functional loss of the pancreas [25].

In the 1980s a new tendency of application of organ-preserving techniques was seen. These procedures addressed both the problem of the inflammatory head-mass and the necessity of adequate ductal drainage. With different extent of local resection of the pancreatic head the duodenum and the continuity of the common bile duct is preserved [26, 27]. Randomized clinical trials comparing Whipple, pylorus-preserving and duodenum-preserving techniques proved the superiority of this latter [28–30], while the duodenum-preserving Beger procedure and the extended drainage procedure of Frey provide similar results in respect of pain relief, functional restoration and quality of life [31]. Both the Beger and the Frey procedure were adopted in Hungary with several modifications [32, 33]. In our experience total excision of the pancreatic head was performed with an attempt to preserve the duodenal blood supply from the inferior arcade of the pancreaticoduodenal artery. The pancreatic remnant was managed by the traditional pancreatogastric anastomosis. Results of the 21 duodenum-preserving procedures show that complications like duodenal and biliary fistula were related to local circulatory problems (Table 14.3-15). From 1998 the extended drainage was adopted instead of the total head excision. The low rate of major complications, no mortality (Table 14.3-16) and very good responses to quality of life measurements further promote its clinical application.

Table 14.3-15. Results of duodenum-preserving total excision of the head of the pancreas with pancreatogastric reconstruction (n = 21, 1988–1998).

Complication	No.	Reoperation	Lethality
Duodenum necrosis	2	2	1
Biliary fistula	2	2	–
Late biliary stenosis	1	1	–
Total	5 (24%)	5	1 (4.7%)

Table 14.3-16. Results of extended drainage with local excision of the head of the pancreas (Frey procedure, n = 19).

Complication	No.	Reoperation	Lethality
Delayed gastric emptying	1	–	–
Abdominal abscess	1	3 times	–
Recurrent attack	1	–	–
Total	3 (15.8%)		–

Comments

There were significant changes in the surgical treatment of chronic pancreatitis during the last 30 years. The experiences drawn can be summarized as follows:

Morbidity and mortality of the pancreatoduodenectomies have decreased to an acceptable level.

Combined drainage procedures like cysto-Wirsungo-gastrostomy decreased the incidence of subsequent operations following simple decompressions. Results indicate that the combined drainage can provide prolonged pain relief with low morbidity and mortality.

Application of extended drainage procedures with local resection of the head of the pancreas such as the Beger and the Frey procedures preserve the duodenum and the common bile duct, thus maintaining the continuity of the gastrointestinal and biliary tract. The complication rate was very low and rehabilitation quicker than after pancreatoduodenectomies.

The responses of patients to quality of life measurements were seemingly better after the extended drainage procedures. In our experience, similarly to international data, these procedures further decreased morbidity and improved long-term functional results following the surgical treatment of chronic pancreatitis.

References

1. White T, MJ. H. Pancreaticojejunostomy versus resection in the treatment of chronic pancreatitis. Am. J. Surg. 1979; 138: 129–134.
2. Prinz RA, Greenlee HB. Pancreatic duct drainage in chronic pancreatitis. Hepatogastroenterology 1990; 37: 295–300.

3. Falconi M, Valerio A, Caldiron E, et al. Changes in pancreatic resection for chronic pancreatitis over 28 years in a single institution. Br J Surg 2000; 87: 428–33.
4. Binmoeller KF, Jue P, Seifert H, Nam WC, Izbicki J, Soehendra N. Endoscopic pancreatic stent drainage in chronic pancreatitis and a dominant stricture: long-term results. Endoscopy 1995; 27: 638–44.
5. Delhaye M, Vandermeeren A, Baize M, Cremer M. Extracorporeal shock-wave lithotripsy of pancreatic calculi. Gastroenterology 1992; 102: 610–20.
6. Harkin A, Anderson P, Goos C. Smoking, drinking and drug-taking in Europe. . Copenhagen, Denmark: Alcohol, drug and tobacco programme WHO Regional Office for Europe, 1997: 72–97.
7. Olah A, Belágyi T, Wellner I, Varga G. Trends and consequences of alcohol consumption and pancreatitis in Hungary. Magy. Seb. 2000; 53: 3–6.
8. European Public Health Information for Eastern Europe: WHO Euphin-East Network, 1999.
9. Yearbook of health statistics 1998. Budapest: Hungarian Central Statistical Office, 1999.
10. Demographic Yearbook 1999. Budapest: Hungarian Central Statistical Office, 2000.
11. Papp J. Significance of ERCP in the diagnosis of pancreatic diseases. Thesis I.Dept. Internal Medicine Semmelweis University. Budapest, 1978.
12. Szécsény A. Surgery of the pancreas. Magy. Seb. 1979; 32: 81–96.
13. Magyar A, Flautner L, Forgács A. New trends in pancreatic surgery. Magy.Seb 1998; 51: 331–336.
14. Ebbehoj N, Borly L, Bulow J, Rasmussen SG, Madsen P. Evaluation of pancreatic tissue fluid pressure and pain in chronic pancreatitis. A longitudinal study. Scand J Gastroenterol 1990; 25: 462–6.
15. Reber PU, Patel AG, Toyama MT, Ashley SW, Reber HA. Feline model of chronic obstructive pancreatitis: effects of acute pancreatic duct decompression on blood flow and interstitial pH. Scand J Gastroenterol 1999; 34: 439–44.
16. Schilling MK, Redaelli C, Reber PU, et al. Microcirculation in chronic alcoholic pancreatitis: a laser Doppler flow study. Pancreas 1999; 19: 21–5.
17. Bockmann DE. BM, Malfertheiner P., Beger HG.,. Analysis of nerves in chronic pancreatitis. Gastroenterology 1988; 94: 1459–1469.
18. Szécsény A, Flautner, L.,Bock, Gy., Tihanyi, T., Unsere Ergebnisse in der chirurgischen Behandlung der chronischen Pankreatitis. Acta Chir. Austr. 1982; 43: 32.
19. Traverso LW, Longmire WPJ. Preservation of the pylorus in pancreaticoduodenectomy. Surgery, Gynecology and Obstetrics 1978; 146: 959–62.
20. Flautner L, Tihanyi T, Szécsény A. Pancreatogastrostomy; An ideal complement to pancreatoduodenectomy. Am. J. Surg. 1985; 150: 608–611.
21. Olah A, Bogdan-Rajcs S, Pardavi G, Matrai T. [Delayed gastric emptying as a frequent complication of pylorus-preserving pancreatoduodenectomy]. Orvosi Hetilap 1993; 134: 1857–60.
22. Yeo CJ, Cameron JL, Sohn TA, et al. Six hundred and fifty consecutive pancreaticoduodenectomies in the 1990s: pathology, complications, and outcomes. Ann Surg 1997; 226: 248–57; discussion 257–60.
23. Vickers SM, Chan C, Heslin MJ, Bartolucci A, Aldrete JS. The role of pancreaticoduodenectomy in the treatment of severe chronic pancreatitis. Am Surg 1999; 65: 1108–11; discussion 1111–2.
24. Tihanyi T, Flautner, L, Szécsény, A. Simultaneous treatment of pancreatic pseudocyst and chronic pancreatitis by cysto-Wirsungo-enteral anastomosis. Magy. Seb. 1989; 42: 145–150.
25. Nealon WH, Thompson JC. Progressive loss of pancreatic function in chronic pancreatitis is delayed by main pancreatic duct decompression. A longitudinal prospective analysis of the modified Puestow procedure. Ann Surg 1993; 217: 458–66; discussion 466–8.
26. Beger H, Krautzberger W, Bittner R, Buechler M, J. L. Duodenum-preserving resection of the head of the pancreas in patients with severe chronic pancreatitis. Surgery 1985; 97: 467–473.
27. Frey C, Smith G. Description and rationale of a new operation for chronic pancreatitis. Pancreas 1987; 2: 701–707.
28. Klempa I, Spatny M, Menzel J, et al. [Pancreatic function and quality of life after resection of the head of the pancreas in chronic pancreatitis. A prospective, randomized comparative study

after duodenum-preserving resection of the head of the pancreas versus Whipple's operation]. Chirurg 1995; 66: 350–9.
29. Büchler MW, Friess H, Muller MW, Wheatley AM, Beger HG. Randomized trial of duodenum-preserving pancreatic head resection versus pylorus-preserving Whipple in chronic pancreatitis. Am J Surg 1995; 169: 65–9; discussion 69–70.
30. Büchler MW, Friess H, Muller MW, Beger HG. [Duodenum-preserving resection of the head of the pancreas: a new standard operation in chronic pancreatitis]. Langenbecks Arch Chir Suppl Kongressbd 1997; 114: 1081–3.
31. Izbicki JR, Bloechle C, Knoefel WT, et al. [Drainage versus resection in surgical therapy of chronic pancreatitis of the head of the pancreas: a randomized study]. Chirurg 1997; 68: 369–77.
32. Sapy P, Arkosy P, Szappanos M. Simple reconstructive method in cases of duodenum-preserving subtotal resection of the head of pancreas. Hepatogastroenterology 1998; 45: 1870–3.
33. Kelemen D, Endredi J, Horvath OP. [Comparative study of pancreatic head resection in chronic pancreatitis]. Orv Hetil 1999; 140: 2101–5.

14.4 Surgery for chronic pancreatitis: The Amsterdam experience

D. Boerma, H. Obertop, D. J. Gouma

Chronic pancreatitis is a multidimensional disease that causes symptoms directly related to the chronic inflammation and destruction of the gland, such as upper abdominal pain and (later) exocrine and endocrine insufficiency. Symptoms may also be caused by the development of complications of the disease, such as pseudocysts, bile duct stenosis, duodenal or portal vein compression, or pseudoaneurysms. Pain, jaundice, duodenal obstruction, portal hypertension or even hemorrhagic shock due to acute bleeding into a pseudocyst may be the result. Chronic pancreatitis mainly affects males around 40 years of age and the predominant cause of the disease is excessive use of alcohol (40 to 50% of all patients), whereas in 40% of the patients the cause remains unknown [1].

During the past decades research in the field of chronic pancreatitis and its clinical presentation has led to clearly distinguished morphological characteristics of this disease and indications for treatment, in particular surgical treatment, are well defined. It is generally agreed upon that patients with asymptomatic chronic pancreatitis may be managed expectantly. Symptoms due to complications of the disease usually require early intervention, whereas symptoms due to gland destruction can be treated longer by non-surgical means. Intractable abdominal pain due to chronic inflammation and/or ductal hypertension and the suspicion of cancer are then the indications for intervention. Eventually, the majority of patients undergo surgery during the course of their disease [1]. Despite these well-defined morphologic characteristics and indications for surgery, treatment strategies may differ between countries.

Treatment of abdominal pain and/or symptoms due to complications of the disease greatly depends on the clinical presentation. The treatment of a bleeding pseudoaneurysm is often surgical, but more recently interventional radiology has shown to be beneficial. The treatment of pain depends on its presumed origin, and the treatment of a symptomatic pseudocyst depends on its morphological relation to surrounding structures, such as the pancreatic duct, but also adjacent intestines. Two concepts of treatment of abdominal pain exist: drainage (of the pancreatic duct, choledochal duct or pseudocysts) or resection (of the diseased parenchyma), both of which have been subject of discussion and amendments during the past decades.

The beneficial effect of drainage of the pancreatic duct in terms of pain relief underscores the hypothesis that one of the mediators of pain in chronic pancreatitis is increased pressure in the pancreatic duct [2, 3]. Ductal dilatation and parenchymal hypertension were proven to cause pain. Thus, in these patients drainage of the duct seems the treatment of choice. In other patients, however, partial resection of the pancreas has proven beneficial, supposedly because in these patients perineural inflammation as demonstrated by Bockmann et al. in 1988 is the cause of the pain [4]. Others have suggested that the pacemaker of the disease is located in the head of the gland and head resection should be the treatment of choice [5]. This was recommended for many years even when no abnormalities were visible in the pancreatic head. Thus, a symptomatic patient with a dilated pancreatic duct should be treated by drainage of the duct and a patient who presents with an inflammatory mass in the pancreas by resection. In patients who have a combination of an inflammatory mass in the pancreatic head and concomitantly a dilated pancreatic duct, drainage and resection should be combined in one operative procedure. Finally, the suspicion of cancer is without doubt a clear indication for resection.

For many years drainage of the pancreatic duct was performed according to the Puestow procedure [6], but mostly the modification by Partington and Rochelle is used and a side-to-side anastomosis of the duct with a jejunal loop is performed [7]. When applied to selected patients this "modified Puestow" procedure results in long-term pain relief in 65 to 90% of the patients, with acceptable postoperative morbidity of 5 to 15% and almost no mortality [3, 8, 9]. In the 1980s Frey suggested that lateral drainage of the pancreatic duct should be accompanied by partial resection of the pancreatic head and the duodenum-preserving resection of the pancreatic head as introduced by Beger was increasingly carried out [10, 11]. Another concept was introduced by Izbicki et al. in 1998, consisting of a V-shaped excision of the ventral pancreas and subsequent drainage of the pancreas in a jejunal loop, resulting in drainage of the main duct but also of the secondary and tertiary ductuli, that could also be used in patients with "small duct" chronic pancreatitis [12].

In the Academic Medical Center (AMC) patients who are candidates for surgery undergo standard preoperative work-up to evaluate the presence of an inflammatory mass, the size of the pancreatic duct and the integrity of the biliary ductal system, the duodenum and surrounding vascular structures. Previously the methods used were ultrasonography (with or without Doppler signaling) to determine the relation to surrounding structures, and early ERCP to visualize the pancreatic and biliary ductal systems. More recently standard work-up includes spiral CT scanning and MRCP. In a minority of patients angiography is performed.

It is a result of the referral pattern that two groups of patients can be distinguished in the AMC. Most patients who are referred directly to the surgical department require the differential diagnosis of chronic pancreatitis and pancreatic cancer, and often undergo resection of a suspicious pancreatic head. Patients who are considered candidates for drainage (i.e. who have a dilated pancreatic duct or a pseudocyst) are mostly primarily referred to the gastroenterologist for endoscopic drainage of the duct or cyst. And almost no patients are referred to the surgeon for the resection of an inflammatory mass in the pancreatic head. This is reflected in the procedures performed in our hospital (Table 14.4-1): the majority of patients underwent a drainage procedure (72%), and only 4% of patients required a concomitant head resection. An Italian series reports the same percentages, with anastomotic procedures being performed in 80% of their patients versus 20% resections. Also these authors rarely perform a duodenum-preserving head

Table 14.4-1. Discrepancy in type of surgical procedures performed for chronic pancreatitis in two referral centres for pancreatic surgery (Ulm, Germany, and Amsterdam, the Netherlands).

	Ulm [14] n = 750 (%)	**Amsterdam** n = 243 (%)
Drainage procedures	102 (14)	175 (72)
Left resection	81 (11)	25 (10)
DPPHR	448 (60)	10 (4)
(PP)PD	69 (9)	33 (14)
Others	50 (7)	–

resection for chronic pancreatitis since an inflammatory mass of substantial diameter in the head is in their practice an uncommon finding [13]. In a large series published by Beger's group, of the 750 patients operated for chronic pancreatitis 14% underwent a drainage procedure and 60% underwent drainage of the pancreatic duct combined with a duodenum-preserving head resection [14] (Table 14.4-1).

Again only the different referral pattern and treatment philosophy can explain these differences in treatment. It is clear that patients in whom pancreatic cancer can not be ruled out on the basis of clinical history and radiological imaging, invariably primarily require resection of the diseased parenchyma. Between 1983 and 1999 463 patients underwent pancreaticoduodenectomy because of suspected pancreatic carcinoma or doubtful differentiation between (focal) chronic pancreatitis and carcinoma [15]. Whereas in earlier years the classical Whipple's resection was routinely performed, by now almost all patients undergo pylorus-preserving pancreaticoduodenectomy (Table 14.4-2). Postoperative mortality has decreased to 1% and hospital stay is relatively short (15 days). The number of patients who were operated upon for suspected carcinoma, but who appeared to have chronic pancreatitis, has increased from 3.7% to 12.6%. The increase in pancreatitis patients undergoing head resections reflects a change in treatment philosophy since in a follow-up study of patients who were initially treated for chronic pancreatitis 22 patients finally appeared to have pancreatic cancer [16]; 11 of these patients appeared to have cancer within 9 months after the diagnosis of chronic pancreatitis (Fig. 14.4-1). It may very well be that these patients suffered from cancer at the time of diagnosis of chronic pancreatitis. This remarkable finding together with the decreased morbidity and mortality after pancreaticoduodenectomy has prompted us to be more liberal in per-

	1983–1992 n = 163	1993–1996 n = 149	1997–1999 n = 151
PD	163 (100)	41 (28)	12 (8)
PPPD	0	108 (72)	139 (92)
Mortality	4.9%	1.3%	0.7%
Hospital stay (days)	24	18	15
Pancreatitis	6 (3.7)	14 (9.4)	19 (12.)

Table 14.4-2. Type of pancreatic head resection performed in 463 patients between 1983 and 1999, operated upon because of suspicion of pancreatic cancer [15]. Percentages in parentheses.

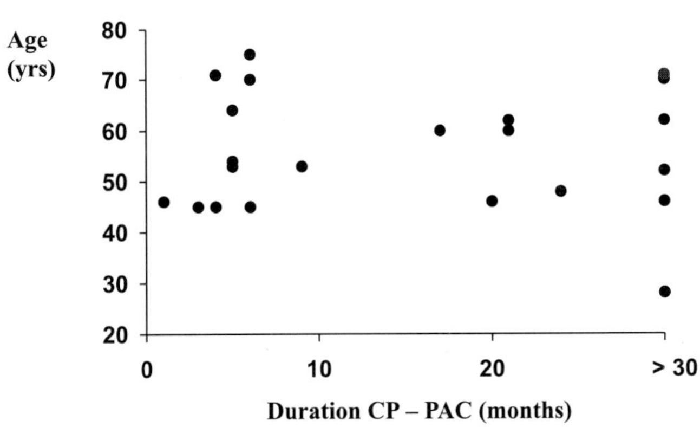

Figure 14.4-1. Time until diagnosed with pancreatic carcinoma (PAC) in 22 patients who were initially treated for chronic pancreatitis (CP). With permission from Van Gulik et al. [16].

forming a resection in case of pancreatic head abnormalities, offering the definite differential diagnosis between focal pancreatitis and pancreatic cancer.

Thus, the indication in our center for a more extensive procedure today is almost exclusively the inability to otherwise rule out pancreatic carcinoma. In case of "clear" chronic pancreatitis without suspicion of cancer, resectional procedures are seldom performed and when these are thought to be indicated an organ-sparing resection such as a Beger's or Frey's procedure is preferred. This change in number and type of resections for chronic pancreatitis has been recognized in other series as well [13, 17]. Falconi reported that the indication for pancreatic head resection was less often pain than in earlier years (40% versus 62%), whereas pancreatic carcinoma was suspected in 25% of their recently operated patients versus 4% in earlier years [13]. Pancreatic tail resection is infrequently carried out in our hospital (n = 25 between 1985 and 1999) and mainly for recurrent pseudocysts in the tail area, massive pancreatic stone disease or in case of doubt about the benign origin of any lesion in the area. The mortality of this procedure was zero and the most important complication was the development of a pancreatic fistula, which was effectively treated by early ERP and stent placement [18]. In a large series of 235 patients who underwent distal pancreatectomy (30% for chronic pancreatitis) Lillemoe et al. showed that this procedure is associated with low mortality and an acceptable morbidity rate of 31% [19]. Total pancreatectomy is no longer performed, since it bears the risk of late mortality due to brittle diabetes. In the Italian series all patients submitted to total pancreatectomy (n = 5) died as a result of decompensated glucose metabolism disorders [13].

When drainage is indicated, endoscopic and surgical treatment are both applied frequently in our center. As a less invasive procedure with high rates of immediate pain relief and short hospitalization endoscopic drainage has been suggested to be a useful alternative for surgical drainage and gained ground in the Netherlands. Many reports have been published reporting immediate pain relief to be as high as 90 to 100%, with a low complication rate [20–23]. But after stent removal only 15 to 20% of the patients maintain their pain relief, leading to repetitive stent exchanges or delayed surgery in most of the patients [21, 23, 24]. In a Belgian series of 75 patients ductal strictures had disappeared in only 7 patients after 13 months of stenting and 35 patients still underwent repetitive stent exchanges (after a mean follow-up of 37 months). At the time of follow-up 33 patients were candidates for pancreaticojejunostomy [21]. In a previous study from our center that included 49 patients with stents 3 patients had undergone pancreaticojejunostomy because of failure of stent-therapy [22]. Up to now, after 7 years of follow-up a total of 10 patients of that study group (20%) have undergone surgical drainage.

Of the patients who underwent lateral pancreaticojejunostomy between 1991 and 1997 in the AMC (n = 71) 81% had undergone some sort of endoscopic treatment prior to surgery. Postoperative morbidity and mortality were low (16% and 0 respectively) and median hospital stay was relatively short (11 days). A major concern of endoscopic pancreatic duct drainage as primary treatment for patients with chronic pancreatitis is the potential of pancreatic stents to cause damage to the pancreatic duct or to introduce infection. It is unknown whether prior endotherapy jeopardizes the outcome of subsequent surgery in terms of septic complications or recurrence of pain. Therefore the outcome of pancreaticojejunostomy in this endoscopic era was evaluated. In an attempt to homogenize the study population patients who had undergone a concomitant partial resection of the pancreas were excluded from the analysis. Thus, 50 patients who had undergone a lateral pancreaticojejunostomy according to Partington and Rochelle were studied. Of

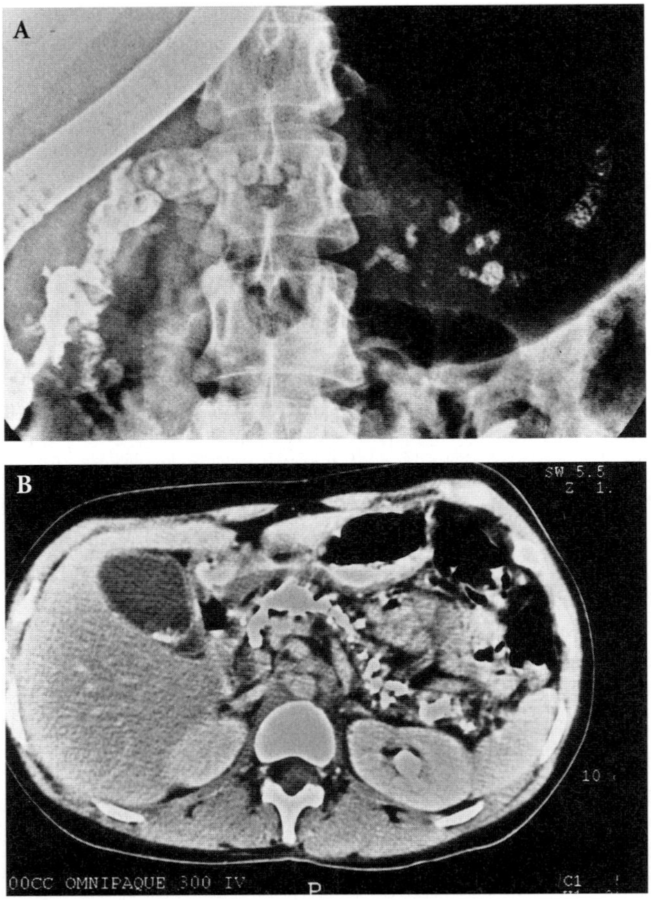

Figure 14.4-2A, B.
A 34-year-old female patient with pancreas divisum and chronic pancreatitis was primarily treated by endoscopic drainage of the pancreatic duct. After 8 stent exchanges (via the minor papilla) within two years, she was referred for surgical treatment by the gastroenterologist, because the multiple stones in the pancreatic duct inhibited adequate drainage (**A**). A CT scan was performed to determine the operative strategy and since no inflammatory mass was seen in the pancreatic head (**B**) a lateral pancreaticojejunostomy was constructed after removal of all stones (**C** and **D**, see p. 593). She was discharged 7 days later and is currently pain-free.

these 50 patients 50% had undergone endoscopic stenting of the pancreatic duct. Patients who initially had undergone endoscopic duct drainage were evaluated separately from those who had not. Although the groups represent a different patient population preoperatively, no difference in postoperative complications was found (12% versus 8%), mortality was zero and median hospital stay was 9 days in both groups. Recurrence of pain during the long-term follow-up was the same in both groups (20%). But patients who had undergone prior stenting of the pancreatic duct were operated on 60 months after their first symptoms, whereas patients who had not been treated endoscopically underwent pancreaticojejunostomy within 17 months after the onset of symptoms. Patients received their first endoprosthesis after 36 months of symptoms and underwent pancreaticojejunostomy 24 months later, after a median of 2 stents per patient (range 1 to 8 stents). In a series of Falconi et al. surgery was performed after 4.1 years (SD 3.8) of the onset of disease. They found that patients underwent surgery at an older age as compared to earlier years (51 versus 54 years) [13].

Pseudocysts were until the wide application of endoscopic and radiological techniques drained by surgical anastomosis with an adjacent intestine. Nowadays only patients with a pseudocyst not amenable to non-surgical drainage are considered candidates

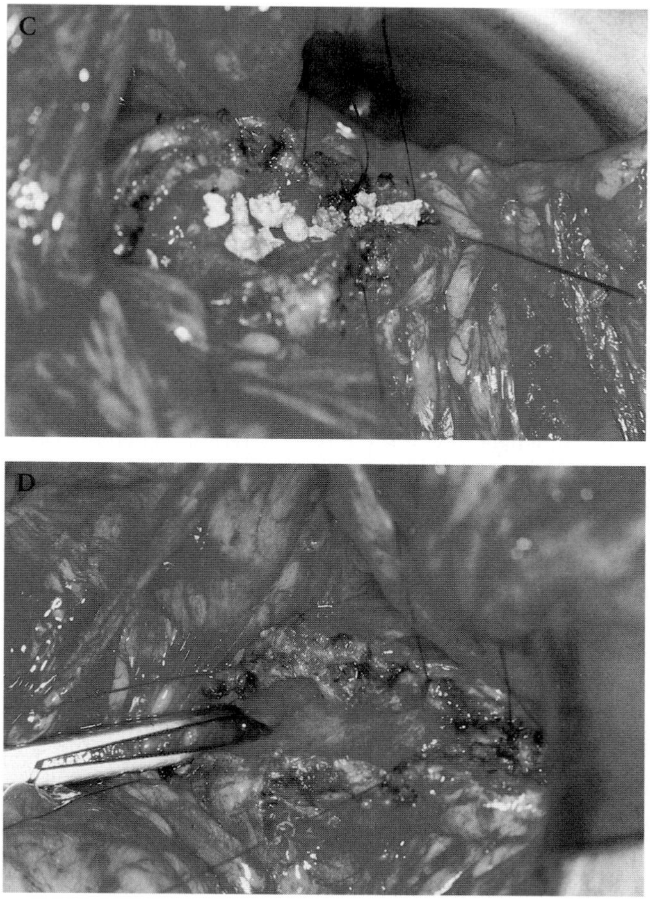

Figure 14.4-2C, D.

for surgery. Whether interventional or surgical drainage is indicated depends on multiple factors such as localization, size, multiplicity, maturity and recurrence of the cyst. When these criteria are meticulously applied results of interventional drainage are highly favorable, with a resolution rate around 90% and few short-term recurrences [24–28]. On the other hand surgical drainage still is a safe and very effective treatment method for symptomatic pseudocyst: in 43 patients who underwent cystoenterostomy between 1984 and 1994 morbidity was 14% and there was no mortality. During a follow-up period of 7 years only 3 pseudocysts recurred (8%) [29]. In a recent large British series comparable good results were shown, urging the authors to state that the introduction of newer techniques will have to withstand comparison to this traditional approach [30]. Even when interventional drainage leads to complications such as secondary infection (9% risk of infection after endoscopic procedures [32]) internal drainage of a pseudocyst is safe [32].

Among gastroenterologists in the Netherlands it is widely accepted that endoscopic therapy should be the first line of treatment for chronic pancreatitis when drainage is indicated. Most patients are referred for pancreaticojejunostomy or surgical cystoenterostomy after prior endoscopic attempts to minimize symptoms. Surgeons are confronted with patients in a later phase of their disease still awaiting a more definitive therapy (Fig. 14.4-2).

It could be hypothesized that due to the development of endoscopic stenting only the patients that are difficult to treat are referred to the surgeon. These patients did not respond to endotherapy or required (semi-)acute surgery because of an endoscopic complication. If that were true a risk factor for postoperative complications or poor outcome in terms of pain relief would be endoscopic treatment prior to surgery. In our series of 50 patients who underwent lateral pancreaticojejunostomy risk factors were calculated. Regression analysis showed that the outcome of pancreaticojejunostomy was less favorable in patients with a history of alcohol abuse, as was also found in earlier studies [5]. But most importantly prior stenting was not found to be a risk factor for recurrent pain after pancreaticojejunostomy. Therefore it seems that therapeutic endoscopy, albeit often not a definitive solution, can be safely applied as initial treatment of patients with chronic pancreatitis to achieve relief of symptoms. On the other hand surgery may be avoided in 15 to 20% of patients but is only postponed in the majority of patients, who require repetitive stent exchanges and need surgery after all. Whether patients with recurrent symptoms after one episode of stenting are best treated by continued stent exchanges or early pancreaticojejunostomy remains to be determined by prospective comparative studies.

The difference in implementation of the newer treatment concepts has resulted in much discrepancy between numbers of resection and type of drainage procedures among published series, despite the well-defined indications for either treatment concept. Whether drainage is always performed surgically or may be performed endoscopically seems to depend on regional (national) habits, as does the question whether resection stands for partial pancreaticoduodenectomy or duodenum-preserving pancreatic head resection. In our practice virtually no patients are referred for treatment because of chronic pancreatitis with an inflammatory mass in the pancreatic head, although these patients should exist in the Netherlands just as well as in Germany. It would be most likely that physicians simply do not refer these patients for surgical treatment, possibly due to a more conservative attitude of physicians in the Netherlands, believing that the disease will be self-limiting and eventually "burn out" [5]. Referral policy is directly related to local expertise, which may play an important role in this discrepancy. There is no center in the Netherlands with extensive experience (> 50) with Beger's procedures. Since the AMC is known for its expertise in pancreatic resections for cancer, patients are mainly referred for pancreatic head resection because of a suspicious lesion in the pancreatic head and more often turn out to have benign disease. This is also shown in other series from departments with extensive experience with surgery for pancreatic carcinoma [33]. A large center with extensive experience in resectional surgery for chronic pancreatitis will probably attract more patients with parenchymal abnormalities amenable for resection [14]. And in a medical center with a large gastroenterology department with pancreatobiliary interest, for instance in Brussels, patients may be referred primarily for pancreatic stenting [21]. The latter also accounts for the gastroenterology department of our hospital [20]. Consequently, a relatively large number of patients referred to us are candidates for drainage of the pancreatic duct or pseudocyst. Whether this sequence of treatment is beneficial, and at what point endotherapy should be considered to have failed and surgery to be indicated, is unknown. Future prospective randomized studies, although logistically extremely difficult, are necessary to answer this question.

In our series of 71 patients undergoing lateral pancreaticojejunostomy 3 patients (4%) underwent partial resection of the pancreatic head during follow-up (2 Frey's and 1 Beger's procedure). At the time of lateral pancreaticojejunostomy the presence of an inflammatory mass had been excluded, but 20 to 30% of all patients are claimed to develop an inflammatory mass in the pancreatic head [14]. Possibly secondary surgery would not have been necessary in these patients if these patients had undergone concomitant partial head resection at the time of the initial pancreaticojejunostomy. Should we do a standard partial head resection only in patients with an inflammatory head mass of more than 4 cm or should we even consider extension of the drainage procedures in other patients? Considering the 3 failures in our series we should probably perform more resections. The results of (lateral) drainage combined with a partial pancreatic head resection, as in the Beger's or Frey's procedure, are very promising so far, although follow-up is relatively short [34–36]. No evidence has been presented that these procedures are superior to the modified Puestow procedure in patients with a dilated duct and without a pancreatic head mass or one of 1–2 cm. It would be extremely interesting to compare details of the European data in an attempt to analyze the different treatment strategies and indications for different surgical procedures.

References

1. Ammann RW, Muellhaupt B. The natural history of pain in alcoholic chronic pancreatitis. Gastroenterology 1999; 116: 1132–40.
2. Bradley EL III. Pancreatic duct pressure in chronic pancreatitis. Am J Surg 1982; 144: 313–6.
3. Bradley EL III. Long-term results of pancreaticojejunostomy in patients with chronic pancreatitis. Am J Surg 1987; 153: 207–13.
4. Bockmann DE, Büchler MW, Malfertheiner P, Beger HG. Analysis of nerves in chronic pancreatitis. Gastroenterology 1988; 94: 1459–69.
5. Ammann RW, Akovbiantz A, Lagarder F, Schueler G. Course and outcome of chronic pancreatitis. Longitudinal study of a mixed medical-surgical series of 245 patients. Gastroenterology 1984; 82: 820–8.
6. Puestow CB, Gillesby WJ. Retrograde surgical drainage of the pancreas for chronic relapsing pancreatitis. Arch Surg 1958; 76: 898–904.
7. Partington PF, Rochelle REL. Modified Puestow procedure for retrograde drainage of the pancreatic duct. Ann Surg 1960; 152: 1037.
8. Greenlee HB, Prinz RA, Aranha GV. Long-term results of side-to-side pancreaticojejunostomy. World J Surg 1990; 14: 70–6.
9. Sielezneff I, Malouf A, Salle E, Brunet C, Thirion X, Sastre B. Long-term results of lateral pancreaticojejunostomy for chronic alcoholic pancreatitis. Eur J Surg 2000; 166: 58–64.
10. Frey CF, Smith GJ. Description and rationale of a new operation for chronic pancreatitis. Pancreas 1987; 2: 701–7.
11. Beger HG, Büchler MW, Bittner RR, Oettinger W, Roscher R. Duodenum-preserving resection of the head of the pancreas in severe chronic pancreatitis. Early and late results. Ann Surg 1989; 209: 273–8.
12. Izbicki JR, Bloechle C, Broering DC, Kuechler T, Broelsch CE. Longitudinal V-shaped excision of the ventral pancreas for small duct disease in severe chronic pancreatitis: prospective evaluation of a new surgical procedure. Ann Surg 1998; 227: 213–9.
13. Falconi M, Valerio A, Caldiron E, Salvia R, Sartori N, Talamini G, Bassi C, Pederzoli P. Changes in pancreatic resection for chronic pancreatitis over 28 years in a single institution. Br J Surg 2000; 87: 428–33.
14. Schlosser W, Beger HG. Organ-preserving surgery in chronic pancreatitis: the duodenum-preserving pancreatic head resection. Ann Ital Chir 2000; 71: 65–70.
15. Gouma DJ, van Geenen RCI, van Gulik TM, de Haan RJ, de With LT, Busch ORC, Obertop H. Morbidity and mortality after pancreaticoduodenectomy. Risk factors and the impact of hospital volume. Ann Surg 2000; 232(6).

16. Van Gulik TM, Moojen TM, van Geenen R, Rauws EAJ, Obertop H, Gouma DJ. Differential diagnosis of focal pancreatitis and pancreatic cancer. Ann Oncol 1999; 10 (Suppl 4): 85–8.
17. Traverso LW, Kozarek RA. Pancreatoduodenectomy for chronic pancreatitis. Ann Surg 1997; 226: 429–38.
18. Boerma D, Rauws EAJ, van Gulik TM, Huibregtse K, Obertop H, Gouma DJ. Endoscopic stent placement for pancreaticocutaneous fistula after drainage of the pancreas. Br J Surg 2000; 87: 1506–9.
19. Lillemoe KD, Kaushal S, Cameron JL, Sohn TA, Pitt HA, Yeo CJ. Distal pancreatectomy: indications and outcomes in 235 patients. Ann Surg 1999; 229: 698–700.
20. Huibregtse K, Schneider B, Vrij AA, Tytgat GNJ. Endoscopic pancreatic drainage in chronic pancreatitis. Gastrointest Endosc 1988; 34: 9–15.
21. Cremer M, Deviere J, Delhaye M, Baize M, Vandermeeren A. Stenting in severe chronic pancreatitis: results of medium-term follow-up in seventy-six patients. Endoscopy 1991; 23: 171–6.
22. Smits ME, Badiga SM, Rauws EAJ, Tytgat GNJ, Huibregtse K. Long-term results of pancreatic stents in chronic pancreatitis. Gastrointest Endosc 1995; 42: 461–7.
23. Binmoeller KF, Jue P, Seifert H, Nam WC, Izbicki JR, Soehendra N. Endoscopic pancreatic stent drainage in chronic pancreatitis and a dominant stricture: long-term results. Endoscopy 1995; 27: 638–44.
24. Cremer M, Deviere J, Engelholm L. Endoscopic management in cysts and pseudocysts in chronic pancreatitis: long-term follow-up after 7 years of experience. Gastrointest Endosc 1989; 35: 1–9.
25. Van Sonnenberg E, Wittich GR, Casola G et al. Percutaneous drainage of infected and noninfected pancreatic pseudocysts: experience in 101 cases. Radiology 1989: 170: 757–61.
26. Freeny PC. Percutaneous management of pancreatic fluid collections. Baill Clin Gastroenterol 1992; 6: 259–72.
27. Smits ME, Rauws EAJ, Tytgat GNJ et al. The efficacy of endoscopic treatment of pancreatic pseudocysts. Gastrointest Endosc 1995; 42: 202–7.
28. Beckingham IJ, Krige JE, Bornman PC et al. Long-term outcome of endoscopic drainage of pancreatic pseudocysts. Am J Gastroenterol 1999; 94: 71–4.
29. Boerma D, van Gulik TM, de Wit LT, Obertop H, Gouma DJ. Long-term results of surgical drainage of pancreatic pseudocysts. In: Cavallari A, Mazziotti A, Principe A, eds. Proceedings of the Second World Congress of the IHPBA, Bologna (Italy). Monduzzi Editore 1996; 1069–73.
30. Usatoff V, Brancatisano R, Williamson RCN. Operative treatment of pseudocysts in patients with chronic pancreatitis. Br J Surg 2000; 87: 1494–9.
31. Bilbao MK, Dotter CT, Lee TG, Katon RM. Complications of endoscopic retrograde cholangiopancreatography (ERCP). A study of 10 000 cases. Gastroenterology 1976; 70: 314–20.
32. Boerma D, van Gulik TM, Obertop H, Gouma DJ. Internal drainage of infected pancreatic pseudocyst: safe or sorry? Dig Surg 1999; 16: 501–5.
33. Yeo CHJ, Cameron JL, Sohn TA et al. Six hundred and fifty consecutive pancreaticoduoenectomies in the 1990s. Ann Surg 1997; 226: 248–60.
34. Izbicki JR, Bloechle C, Knoeffel WT, Kuechler T, Binmoeller KF, Broelsch CE. Duodenum-preserving resection of the head of the pancreas in chronic pancreatitis. A prospective, randomized trial. Ann Surg 1995; 221: 350–8.
35. Bloechle C, Izbicki JR, Knoeffel WT, Kuechler T, Broelsch CE. Quality of life in chronic pancreatitis – results after duodenum-preserving resection of the head of the pancreas. Pancreas 1995; 11: 77–85.
36. Beger HG, Schlosser W, Friess HM, Büchler MW. Duodenum-preserving head resection in chronic pancreatitis changes the natural course of the disease: a single-center 26-year experience. Ann Surg 1999; 230: 512–9.

14.5 Evidence-based surgery in chronic pancreatitis

K. Z'graggen, W. Uhl, H. Friess, M. W. Büchler

Introduction

Evidence-based medicine (EBM) is the implementation of the currently best available treatment according to scientific studies. The term EBM was proposed by Sackett and colleagues [1] and EBM aims to integrate scientific knowledge according to its level of evidence into medical routine. In analogy, to perform evidence-based surgery should be the primary and daily goal in treating our patients. However, surprisingly few treatment strategies are supported by randomized controlled trials, which represent the gold standard in evidence-based medicine.

Surgeons have been accused of basing their treatment strategies on personal opinion rather than on systematic studies [2] and may at times be particularly reluctant to incorporate external evidence (gathered by a different group) into their "surgical philosophy". This seems particularly important in the surgical treatment of chronic pancreatitis since the two main treatment strategies consist of drainage operations, type Partington-Rochelle, and pancreatic head resection, and arguments for or against different types of operations are often influenced by personal preference (drainists versus resectionists). In the light of the recent emergence of evidence-based medicine, we discuss the available randomized controlled trials in the surgical treatment of patients with chronic pancreatitis and define areas with a need for carefully designed studies in the future.

What is evidence-based surgery?

Evidence-based surgery is defined as the application of the currently best scientific evidence/knowledge in the treatment of an individual patient [3]. To apply the best available evidence in the diagnosis and treatment of surgical patients is a complex process [1]. The availability of scientific information has greatly improved through the use of electronic media, but only the critical analysis and timely implementation of new evidence into daily practice will result in improved patient care. Evidence-based medicine therefore is an instrument to integrate science and clinical expertise. The Cochrane Collaboration, organized in different centers throughout the world, is at present the most prominent proponent of evidence-based medicine [4]. Its aim is "to help people make well-informed decisions about healthcare by preparing, maintaining and promoting the accessibility of systematic reviews of the effects of healthcare interventions" (mission statement of the Cochrane Collaboration).

According to Table 14.5-1, evidence can be classified into different levels. Randomized controlled trials and a meta-analysis of randomized controlled trials are the gold standards of evidence-based medicine and surgery [5]. While level-I evidence can be compared to a soccer game in the European Champions League, personal opinions of even re-

I a	Meta-analysis of randomized controlled trials (> 1)
I b	Randomized controlled trials
II a	Well designed controlled trials
II b	Well designed cohort/case control studies
II c	Uncontrolled studies (dramatic results)
III	Opinions of respected authorities

Table 14.5-1. Classification of evidence according to Ellis [5].

spected authorities (level III) may only reach the level of a decent game of amateurs or sometimes street soccer when it comes to decision-making according to evidence-based surgery. More than 80% of published results in surgery is not level-I evidence and among publications in prominent surgical journals, only 2.8% were randomized controlled trials [3]. The situation in the literature on chronic pancreatitis is similar. A literature search on chronic pancreatitis and surgery with the most commonly used database "pubmed" (www.ncbi.nlm.nih.gov/entrez) revealed approximately 100 prospective studies among 1800 articles on chronic pancreatitis and surgery but only seven of these papers reported on randomized controlled trials in chronic pancreatitis.

Evidence-based surgery in chronic pancreatitis

The discussion of optimal surgical treatment in chronic pancreatitis is usually based on level-II and level-III evidence. Seven randomized controlled trials in the surgical treatment of chronic pancreatitis were identified (Table 14.5-2). Four studies compared surgical techniques [6–9], while the remaining three trials examined individual aspects of surgical treatment such as gastric emptying delay [10–12], the use of octreotide to prevent complications after surgery and venous splanchnic blood flow after drainage versus resection procedures. Despite the fact that the classic drainage procedure (pancreaticojejunostomy type Partington-Rochelle) have not been examined in randomized controlled

Table 14.5-2. Randomized controlled trials in chronic pancreatitis.

	First author	Journal	Comparison of	Patients
1	**Büchler MW et al. 1995**	Am J Surg (Ref. 6)	**Beger vs. PPPD**	**40**
2	**Klempa I et a. 1995**	Chirurg (Ref. 7)	**Beger vs. Whipple**	**43**
3	**Izbicki JR et al. 1995**	Ann Surg (Ref. 8)	**Beger vs. Frey**	**42**
4	**Izbicki JR et al. 1998**	Ann Surg (Ref. 9)	**PPPD vs. Frey**	**61**
5	**Friess H et al. 1995**	Br J Surg (Ref. 10)	**octreotide vs. placebo surgery and complications**	**247**
6	**Müller MW et al. 1997**	Am J Surg (Ref. 11)	**PPPD vs. DPPHR gastric emptying delay**	**20**
7	**Bloechle et al. 1997**	Br J Surg (Ref. 12)	**resection vs. drainage venous splanchnic blood flow**	**14**

trials, a recent AGA Technical Review on "treatment of pain in chronic pancreatitis" concluded that "current consensus among surgeons is, that drainage operations are safest and most likely to be effective" [13]. The lack of randomized controlled trials does not exclude the possibility that pure drainage by pancreaticojejunostomy is less effective than resection in the majority of patients with chronic pancreatitis. However, the current trend towards various types of resectional procedures, such as the Beger operation (duodenum-preserving pancreatic head resection) [14], the Frey procedure (limited pancreatic head resection in combination with longitudinal pancreaticojejunostomy) [15], a recently described modification of the Beger and Frey procedure [16], and pylorus-preserving and classic pancreaticoduodenectomies [17–19], is indicated by the recent literature and the availability of level-I evidence evaluating safety and outcome of some of the duodenum-preserving procedures.

The four randomized controlled trials on surgical treatment in chronic pancreatitis (Table 14.5-2, trials 1–4) indicate that the Beger and Frey operation have advantages compared with pancreatoduodenectomies. Büchler and colleagues (trial 1) demonstrated that while the Beger operation and a pylorus-preserving pancreatoduodenectomy were both safe, the duodenum-preserving pancreatic head resection resulted in a significant improvement with regard to pain, weight gain and glucose tolerance [6]. They concluded that the Beger operation should be considered an alternative procedure in the surgical treatment of chronic pancreatitis. The favorable results in the postoperative course of the Beger operation compared with a classical pancreatoduodenectomy were confirmed by Klempa and colleagues in trial 2. They observed a quicker recovery and a significant benefit with regard to postoperative hormonal status in patients undergoing a Beger operation [7]. Izbicki and colleagues (trial 3) reported very similar results with regard to pain reduction, pancreatic endocrine and exocrine function, and quality of life after the Beger and Frey procedures [8]. Finally, trial 4 by Izbicki and colleagues, comparing the Frey procedure to a pylorus-preserving pancreatoduodenectomy, demonstrated that the more limited resection of the pancreatic head resulted in equally effective pain relief compared with a pancreatoduodenectomy but provided a better quality of life [9]. The four randomized controlled trials all demonstrate a benefit for patients who undergo a resection of the pancreatic head with preservation of the duodenum, and the advantages are significant in trials of relatively limited size.

Despite the available level-I evidence many surgeons and centers of excellence continue to use the original drainage operation (side-to-side pancreaticojejunostomy) and the pancreatoduodenectomy as their primary approach in the surgical treatment of patients with chronic pancreatitis. The arguments for continuing these strategies may be valid, but will in the future have to be tested in randomized controlled trials. Future studies may be facilitated by standardization of surgical procedures and possibly an improvement in the classification of chronic pancreatitis.

Conclusions and outlook

The application of the principles of evidence-based medicine and surgery will improve the surgical treatment of patients with chronic pancreatitis. The classification of studies into their respective levels of evidence will facilitate the implementation of published evidence in routine treatment strategies. However, the review of the literature demonstrates a considerable lack of evidence from randomized controlled trials in chronic pancreatitis and in particular in the surgical treatment of chronic pancreatitis. Current level-I evidence demonstrates that results after duodenum-preserving pancreatic head resections compare favorably with pancreatoduodenectomy in patients with chronic pancreatitis. Future trials will have to compare drainage procedures with different types of resection and help define specific indications for the various surgical procedures. With evolving new technologies future randomized controlled trials will also compare interventional endoscopic or radiologic treatment with surgery and possibly medical strategies with surgical concepts.

References

1. Sackett DL, Rosenberg WM, Gray JA, Haynes RB, Richardson WS. Evidence-based medicine: what it is and what it isn't. BMJ 1996; 312(7023): 71–2.
2. Horton R. Surgical research or comic opera: questions but few answers. Lancet 1996; 347: 984–5.
3. Uhl W, Wente MN, Büchler MW. Surgical clinical studies and their practical realization. Chirurg 2000; 71: 615–25.
4. Altman DG, Burton MJ. The Cochrane Collaboration. Langenbecks Arch Surg 1999; 384: 432–6.
5. Ellis J, Mulligan I, Rowe J, Sackett DL. Inpatient general medicine is evidence-based. A-Team, Nuffield Department of Clinical Medicine. Lancet. 1995; 346: 407–10.
6. Büchler MW, Friess H, Muller MW, Wheatley AM, Beger HG. Randomized trial of duodenum-preserving pancreatic head resection versus pylorus-preserving Whipple in chronic pancreatitis. Am J Surg. 1995; 169: 65–9.
7. Klempa I, Spatny M, Menzel J, Baca I, Nustede R, Stockmann F, Arnold W. Pancreatic function and quality of life after resection of the head of the pancreas in chronic pancreatitis. A prospective, randomized comparative study after duodenum-preserving resection of the head of the pancreas versus Whipple's operation. Chirurg 1995; 66: 350–9.
8. Izbicki JR, Bloechle C, Knoefel WT, Kuechler T, Binmoeller KF, Broelsch CE. Duodenum-preserving resection of the head of the pancreas in chronic pancreatitis. A prospective, randomized trial. Ann Surg 1995; 221: 350–8.
9. Izbicki JR, Bloechle C, Broering DC, Knoefel WT, Kuechler T, Broelsch CE. Extended drainage versus resection in surgery for chronic pancreatitis: a prospective randomized trial comparing the longitudinal pancreaticojejunostomy combined with local pancreatic head excision with the pylorus-preserving pancreatoduodenectomy. Ann Surg 1998; 228: 771–9.
10. Friess H, Beger HG, Sulkowski U, Becker H, Hofbauer B, Dennler HJ, Büchler MW. Randomized controlled multicentre study of the prevention of complications by octreotide in patients undergoing surgery for chronic pancreatitis. Br J Surg 1995; 82: 1270–3.
11. Muller MW, Friess H, Beger HG, Kleeff J, Lauterburg B, Glasbrenner B, Riepl RL, Büchler MW. Gastric emptying following pylorus-preserving Whipple and duodenum-preserving pancreatic head resection in patients with chronic pancreatitis. Am J Surg 1997; 173: 257–63.
12. Bloechle C, Busch C, Tesch C, Nicolas V, Binmoeller KF, Soehendra N, Izbicki JR. Prospective randomized study of drainage and resection on non-occlusive segmental portal hypertension in chronic pancreatitis. Br J Surg 1997; 84: 477–82.
13. Warshaw AL, Banks PA, Fernandez-Del Castillo C. AGA technical review: treatment of pain in chronic pancreatitis. Gastroenterology 1998; 115: 765–76.
14. Beger HG, Krautzberger W, Bittner R, Büchler MW, Limmer J. Duodenum-preserving resection of the head of the pancreas in patients with severe chronic pancreatitis. Surgery 1985; 97: 467–73.
15. Frey CF, Smith GJ. Description and rationale of a new operation for chronic pancreatitis. Pancreas 1987; 2: 701–7.

16. Gloor B, Friess H, Uhl W, Büchler MW. A modified technique of the Beger and Frey procedure in patients with chronic pancreatitis. Dig Surg 2001; 18: 21–5.
17. Traverso LW, Kozarek RA. Pancreatoduodenectomy for chronic pancreatitis: anatomic selection criteria and subsequent long-term outcome analysis. Ann Surg. 1997; 226: 429–35.
18. Sakorafas GH, Farnell MB, Nagorney DM, Sarr MG, Rowland CM. Pancreatoduodenectomy for chronic pancreatitis: long-term results in 105 patients. Arch Surg 2000; 135: 517–23.
19. Jimenez RE, Fernandez-del Castillo C, Rattner DW, Chang Y, Warshaw AL. Outcome of pancreaticoduodenectomy with pylorus preservation or with antrectomy in the treatment of chronic pancreatitis. Ann Surg 2000; 231: 293–300.

14.6 Quality of life in chronic pancreatitis

C. D. Johnson, D. Fitzsimmons

Chronic pancreatitis is a progressive incurable condition which can severely disrupt a patient's life as a result of severe symptoms or complications. Medical and surgical treatments are designed to ameliorate the severity of symptoms and to deal with complications which may be life-threatening. However the disease process continues unabated and so all treatments for the condition must be regarded as palliative.

Some treatments for chronic pancreatitis have significant adverse affects on the quality of life of the patient. For example major surgery requires a period of convalescence that may last several months. Medical treatment may be burdensome, requiring consumption of numerous capsules or frequent injections, and it may be ineffective, for example when pain is poorly controlled.

For all of these reasons, the quality of life of patients is now recognized as an important outcome measure for the success or otherwise of medical or surgical treatment. Treatment designed to relieve a particular symptom, even if effective, may have little effect on the overall quality of life because of adverse effects of the treatment.

The major difficulty in the measurement of quality of life is the lack of appropriate assessment instruments. Many quality of life questionnaires exist, designed for different purposes. For example the Nottingham Health Profile and the Short Form 36 are designed to detect changes in the quality of life of generally healthy populations [1, 2]. Such questionnaires are unsuitable for patients with severe symptoms because their focus is on the identification of minor symptoms [3, 4].

System-based questionnaires, such as the Gastrointestinal Quality of Life Index (GIQLI) [5] have not been validated in patients with chronic pancreatitis. However they do contain a very wide range of questions dealing with all aspects of gastrointestinal disease, and although they are sensitive to changes in a disease population the large proportion of irrelevant material (in the context of chronic pancreatitis) makes them cumbersome to use.

Pancreas-specific assessment

We have developed a quality of life assessment tool in association with the EORTC for use in patients with pancreatic cancer. This consists of a core module (EORTC QLQ-C30) and a pancreas specific module (EORTC QLQ-PAN26) which when used together cover all of the quality of life issues of relevance to patients with pancreatic cancer [6].

Some of the similarities between chronic pancreatitis and pancreatic cancer have been noted above. Table 14.6-1 shows the extensive overlap in symptoms, signs and prognosis between chronic pancreatitis and pancreatic cancer. These similarities led us to the hypothesis that the C30/PAN26 system could be a useful instrument for the assessment of quality of life in patients with chronic pancreatitis.

Table 14.6-1. Similarities between the clinical presentation and progression of chronic pancreatitis and pancreatic cancer.

	Chronic pancreatitis	Pancreatic cancer
Symptoms		
Pain		
Constant	✓	✓
Radiates to back	✓	✓
Needs opiates	✓	✓
Jaundice	Sometimes	Often
Vomiting	✓	✓
Anorexia	✓	✓
Steatorrhea	Late	Rare unless jaundiced
Signs		
Mass	Rare	Rare
Weight loss	✓	✓
Cachexia	Late	Often
Diabetes	✓	✓
Prognosis		
Relentless and progressive	✓	✓
Duration	Years	Months

In order to test this hypothesis we studied a sample of fifty-three patients, drawn from three clinics in different countries [7]. This sample was chosen to allow testing of the C30/PAN26 in different languages and different cultures. Two clinics were heavily surgically oriented and one clinic provided medical patients only (Table 14.6-2). Each patient completed the questionnaires and then provided information in a structured debriefing interview to indicate the appropriateness of each item and to raise any other issues not included in the questionnaire that had a significant effect on their quality of life. The responses were analyzed for content validity (was the meaning clear? and were the questions relevant to the patient?); reliability (was there good correlation between related items?), and discriminant validity (was a clinically significant difference in symptoms or treatment related to differences in quality of life?). These analyses were conducted using the methods required by EORTC for validation of their questionnaires in cancer patients [8]. The C30/PAN26 had already been through this process for assessment of quality of life in patients with pancreatic cancer.

Table 14.6-2. Characteristics of patients in validation study.

	Cape Town n = 16	Southampton n = 13	Magdeburg n = 25
Age (yrs)	47 (36–54)	40 (28–60)	48 (31–66)
M/F	16/0	9/4	21/4
Duration of disease (yr)	8 (3–17)	6 (2–13)	2 (1–13)
Alcohol/other cause	16/0	10/3	24/1
Treatment, medical/surgical	1/15	2/11	25/0
Opioids	16	4	21

Content validity

All but three of the fifty-four patients were able to complete the questionnaire unaided in a median time of nine minutes (range 6–20). There was missing data in 4% of responses, related to the patient's ability to care for his or herself, and to sexuality. All other items were answered by all patients. No patient found the questionnaire difficult to answer and in the debriefing interview no additional items or issues were identified that ought to have been included.

Reliability

Correlations between linked items in the various scales within the questionnaires were all satisfactory (Cronbach's alpha > 0.7), with the sole exception of jaundice (Table 14.6-3). This anomaly had been noted also in the responses from pancreatic cancer patients but it had been felt desirable to include jaundice in the questionnaire. The inconsistencies arose from the fact that many patients had not experienced jaundice in the preceding week prior to completing the questionnaire. However in those patients who were jaundiced this had a substantial impact on their quality of life.

C30	PAN26
Physical functioning	Pancreatic pain
Role functioning	Digestive function
Emotional functioning	Bowel habit
Cognitive functioning	Body image
Pain	Satisfaction with care
Fatigue	Sexuality
Nausea & vomiting	

Table 14.6-3. Scales showing adequate reliability (Cronbach's alpha > 0.7).

Discriminant validity

This was tested by dividing the patients into two groups for analysis and comparing the values obtained on each scale between the two groups. Three separate analyses were performed, for patients who required or did not require opiate analgesia, patients with good or poor performance status, and the prior use or not of surgical treatment. The effect of gender was also analyzed as a negative control.

Previous surgical treatment had no effect on quality of life, except for significant differences in cognitive functioning and the presence of nausea and vomiting. There were no differences between men and women.

Good performance status was significantly associated with better quality of life in almost every domain of the questionnaires, whereas the consumption of opiate analgesia was associated with differences in the responses in about half of the scales on the questionnaire (Table 14.6-4).

These findings suggest that the discriminant validity of the questionnaires is high. Patients with good performance status scored generally higher in almost all areas of quality of life, as would be expected, whereas the consumption of opiate analgesia had more selective effects, consistent with the known side effects of opiates.

Table 14.6-4. Differences in values of scales in patients requiring or not requiring opiate treatment.

Significant difference	No difference
Cognitive function	Physical function
Emotional function	Role function
Fatigue	Body image
Nausea and vomiting	Digestive function
Pain/Pancreatic pain	Satisfaction with care
Social function	Sexuality
Jaundice	
Overall quality of life	

Application of the QLQ-C30 and QLQ-PAN26 in chronic pancreatitis

We conclude from these observations that the combination of the QLQ-C30 and the QLQ-PAN26 is a suitable system for assessing quality of life in patients with chronic pancreatitis. Furthermore it is clear that patients who have had surgical treatment have no overall difference in quality of life when compared with patients who have had medical treatment only.

Two preliminary reports confirm that these questionnaires are suitable for assessing quality of life in patients with chronic pancreatitis who have had either medical or surgical treatment [9, 10]. In patients with alcoholic chronic pancreatitis, medical treatment reduced pain, and there were significant improvements in pain scales and function scales in quality of life assessment after starting medical treatment [9]. Endocrine and exocrine insufficiency was associated with impaired physical functioning, role functioning and emotional and cognitive function.

In patients who had undergone surgery, decompression procedures were associated with more rapid recovery of nutritional status and with better quality of life scores related to fatigue, sleeping and appetite [10]. Duodenum preserving techniques were associated with better emotional and cognitive functioning and better scores in the pain and diet scales. The authors suggest that there is a significant association between preservation of other organs and good quality of life after pancreatic surgery.

Conclusion

As intuitively expected from the similarities in symptoms and clinical progress, quality of life issues are very similar in patients with chronic pancreatitis and pancreatic cancer. A quality of life assessment system designed for pancreatic cancer patients works effectively in patients with chronic pancreatitis, and can demonstrate significant differences between subgroups with chronic pancreatitis. Changes in quality of life with effective treatment have been observed and we are now able to measure quality of life objectively and quantifiably in prospective studies.

References

1. Streiner DL, Norman GR. Health measurement scales: a practical guide to their development and use. 2nd edn. Oxford: Oxford University Press, 1992.

2. Hayden KA, Moinpour CM, Metch B et al. Pitfalls in quality of life assessment. Lessons from a Southwest Oncology Group breast cancer clinical trial. Oncol Nurs Forum 1993; 20: 1415–9.
3. Donovan K, Sanson Fisher RW, Redman S. Measuring quality of life in cancer patients. J Clin Oncol 1989; 7: 959–68.
4. Gill TM. Quality of life assessment: values and pitfalls. J Royal Soc Med 1995; 88: 680–2.
5. Eypasch E, Williams JL, Wood-Dauphinee S et al. Gastrointestinal Quality of Life Index: development, validation and application of a new instrument. Br J Surg 1995; 82: 216–22.
6. Fitzsimmons D, Johnson CD, George S et al. Development of a disease-specific quality of life (QoL) questionnaire module to supplement the EORTC core cancer QoL questionnaire, the QLQ-C30 in patients with pancreatic cancer. EORTC Study Group on Quality of Life. Eur J Cancer 1999; 35: 939–41.
7. Johnson CD, Fitzsimmons D, Butturini G, Bornman P, Kahl S. Long-term outcome of Quality of Life in patients with chronic pancreatitis. Digestion 2000; 61: 298–9.
8. Sprangers M, Cull A, Groenvold M. EORTC Quality of Life Study Group. Guidelines for developing questionnaire modules. EORTC Brussels 1998.
9. Kahl S, Zimmermann S, Leodolter A et al. Quality of life in patients with chronic pancreatitis after medical treatment. Pancreatology 2001; 1: 149.
10. Tihanyi B, Csapó Zs, Farkas I et al. Quality of life and nutritional status after surgery for chronic pancreatitis: a longitudinal follow-up study. Pancreatology 2001; 1: 129.

Index

Page numbers in **bold type** refer to figures and/or tables.

E

F

G

T

U

V

W

Z